MEDICAL NEUROSCIENCE

Medical Neuroscience

Thomas C. Pritchard, Ph.D.

Department of Behavioral Science
Pennsylvania State University
College of Medicine
Hershey, Pennsylvania

Kevin D. Alloway, Ph.D.

Department of Neuroscience and Anatomy
Pennsylvania State University
College of Medicine
Hershey, Pennsylvania

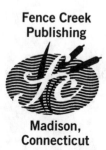

Fence Creek Publishing

Madison, Connecticut

Typesetter: Pagesetters, Brattleboro, VT
Printer: Port City Press, Baltimore, MD
Illustrations by Visible Productions, Fort Collins, CO
Distributors:

United States and Canada
Blackwell Science, Inc.
Commerce Place
350 Main Street
Malden, MA 02148
Telephone orders: 800-215-1000 or 781-388-8250
Fax orders: 781-388-8270

Australia
Blackwell Science, PTY LTD.
54 University Street
Carlton, Victoria 3053
Telephone orders: 61-39-347-0300
Fax orders: 61-39-347-5001

Outside North America and Australia
Blackwell Science, LTD.
c/o Marston Book Service, LTD.
P.O. Box 269
Abingdon Oxon, OX 14 4XN England
Telephone orders: 44-1-235-465500
Fax orders: 44-1-235-465555

1 2 3 4 5 6 7 8 9 10

TABLE OF CONTENTS

PREFACE

The tremendous growth in biomedical knowledge has caused significant changes in medical education during the last decade. These changes have been prompted by new research findings and by the realization that students cannot assimilate every factual detail in this expanding body of knowledge. This is especially true in medical neuroscience, which includes the subspecialties of anatomy, physiology, pharmacology, molecular biology, and genetics. To provide medical students with an adequate understanding of the nervous system, it is necessary to distill from neuroscience its essential elements that have significance for the practicing clinician. For these reasons, we have attempted to identify and explain those aspects of medical neuroscience that are essential for understanding the neurologic symptoms commonly encountered by physicians. In addition to describing the basic anatomic and physiologic principles of the nervous system, we have emphasized the clinical relevance of these concepts. As such, this book is not a comprehensive neuroscience textbook but rather a supplemental text that some students may wish to use to review for the board examinations. It has been written with the first- and second-year medical student in mind, but the presentation is within reach of students and professionals in allied health fields. Each chapter begins with a clinical case portraying a patient with neurologic symptoms and is followed by material necessary to achieve an accurate diagnosis. Questions and answers are provided at the end of each chapter to test the student's command of this information. Finally, a short list of recommended readings also is included for students who desire additional coverage of particular topics.

Thomas C. Pritchard and Kevin D. Alloway

ACKNOWLEDGMENTS

We would like to thank those who graciously provided photographic or artistic material. We are indebted to Mr. Roland Myers for the original electron micrographs appearing in Chapter 1 and to Dr. John Barr for the radiographs shown in Chapter 5. We also thank Dr. Linda Wilson-Pauwels for contributing several figures that appear in Chapter 4. We are especially grateful to Dr. Malcolm Carpenter for donating unpublished material for this book and for permitting us to use figures that appeared in his previous books.

We are thankful that we have numerous colleagues at Penn State who were willing to share their expertise by providing us with constructive criticisms of the preliminary drafts of this text. Thus, we extend our gratitude to Drs. Edward Bixler, Steven Dear, Thomas Gardner, Harold Harvey, John Hoover, Joan Lakoski, Linda Larson-Prior, Eric Lieth, Ralph Lydic, Robert Milner, and Ralph Norgren. Although our colleagues helped us immeasurably, we bear total responsibility for the selection of topics and for any inaccuracies that may appear in the final text (Dr. Pritchard took primary responsibility for writing Chapters 2, 5, 7, 8, 9, 11, and 12, while Dr. Alloway wrote the remaining chapters).

We would also like to thank Matt Harris for giving us the opportunity to add this book to the *Integrated Medical Sciences Series*. Matt's encouragement during the prolonged gestation of this book was much appreciated.

We are indebted to Jane Edwards and Michelle Arlotto for their meticulous editorial work. If it were not for Jane's exceptional organizational skills and good karma, this book would still be sloshing about in our word processors. We also thank the indexer, Larry Gilman, who saved us and the readers from some insidious errors. Finally, we thank Dave Carlson and the talented staff at Visible Productions whose artistic skills virtually bring the figures to life.

To my wife, Chris, for her love and support

To my colleagues, mentors, and friends,
Marshall Jones and Ralph Norgren

To Cathi, Christopher, and Lauren

INTRODUCTION

Medical Neuroscience is one of ten titles in the *Integrated Medical Sciences (IMS) Series* from Fence Creek Publishing. These books have been designed as course supplements and aids for board review for first- and second-year medical students. Rather than focusing on the individual basic science disciplines, the books in the *IMS Series* have been designed to highlight the points of integration between the sciences, including clinical correlations where appropriate. Each chapter begins with a clinical case, the resolution of which requires the application of basic science concepts to clinical problems. Extensive use of margin notes, figures, tables, and questions illuminates core biomedical concepts with which medical students often have difficulty.

Each book in the *IMS Series* shares common features and formats. Attempts have been made to present difficult concepts in a brief and focused format and to provide a pedagogical aid that facilitates both knowledge acquisition and also review.

Given the long gestation period necessary to publish a book, it is often impossible for publishers to keep pace with the changes and advances that occur so rapidly. However, the authors and the publisher recognize the need to have access to the most current information and are committed to keeping *Medical Neuroscience* as up to date as possible between editions. As the field of neuroscience evolves, updates to this text may be posted on our web site periodically at http://www.fencecreek.com.

We hope that the student finds the format and the text material relevant, interesting, and challenging. The authors, as well as the Fence Creek staff, welcome your comments and suggestions for use in future editions.

1

CELLULAR NEUROSCIENCE

INTRODUCTION OF CLINICAL CASE

A 34-year-old mother of three children was brought to the emergency room by her husband because she had difficulty breathing. She had recently been ill with the flu and had experienced varying degrees of weakness in swallowing during the past several days. Her face was expressionless, and she had trouble speaking because of weakness on both sides of her tongue and mouth. Both eyelids showed ptosis; the right eyelid was elevated 4 mm, and the left eyelid was elevated 6 mm. Her husband remarked that her eyelids had started drooping a few weeks earlier, but this problem seemed to disappear after a good night's sleep. The patient had normal pupillary light reflexes in both eyes but experienced double vision when gazing laterally. Her arms were weak and unable to maintain position when tested against resistance. Despite this weakness, deep tendon reflexes were present at the wrist and elbow of both arms. Both legs showed normal reflexes at the knee and ankles. Breathing was shallow but regular; inspiratory and expiratory pressure were both below normal. Blood pressure and heart rate were normal, but body temperature was elevated. The woman had been in excellent health all her life, exercised regularly, and did not suffer from fatigue. Her 60-year-old mother had rheumatoid arthritis, but all other members of her immediate family were in good health.

INTRODUCTION TO CELLULAR NEUROSCIENCE

Neurons process information and send it to other neurons. *Glia* support the metabolic functions of neurons.

The cells of the nervous system are broadly classified into two groups: neurons and glial cells. Neurons are highly specialized cells that use electrochemical signals to represent information that is communicated to specific regions of the brain. Groups of neurons are organized into circuits that process specific types of information and mediate a variety of integrative functions ranging from simple reflexes to more complex processes involving perception, cognition, and motor activity. By comparison, glial cells do not transmit signals but are needed to support the cellular and metabolic functions of neurons.

Neurons

Nerve cells are distinct from other cells in the body because of their unique ability to perform computations and transmit information rapidly over long distances. These properties are directly related to their geometric structure, the conductive properties of their membranes, and their functional interactions with other groups of neurons.

Most neurons have four distinct components: a soma, an axon, dendrites, and synaptic terminals. The dendrites receive information from other neurons and convey this information to the soma. The soma integrates information from multiple dendrites and determines whether to initiate an electrochemical impulse. These impulses are conducted along the length of the axon to synaptic terminals that contact other neurons or effectors such as muscles and glands.

SOMA

The terms *multipolar, bipolar,* or *unipolar* indicate the number of processes arising from the soma.

The cell body of a neuron is known as the soma or perikaryon. All dendritic and axonal processes originate from the soma; therefore, neurons are classified into multipolar, bipolar, or pseudounipolar groups according to the number of these processes (Figure 1-1).

FIGURE 1-1 ▶

Neuronal Classifications. Neurons are classified according to the number of dendritic and axonal processes that originate from the soma of the neuron.

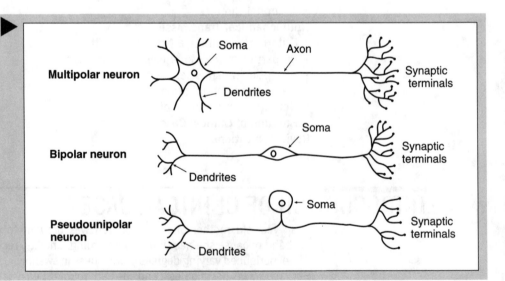

Multipolar neurons have multiple dendrites extending from a polygonal-shaped cell body. Although several primary dendrites may arise from its soma, a multipolar neuron only has a single axon. Most neurons in the central nervous system (CNS) are multipolar neurons and can be subdivided into additional categories, the most common being pyramidal cells, stellate cells, and basket cells.

Bipolar neurons have two processes that extend from opposite sides of a round or oval-shaped cell body. One process acts as a dendrite and receives synaptic contacts from other neurons; the other process acts as an axon and sends signals away from the cell body. Most bipolar neurons are in sensory structures such as the retina or the olfactory epithelium and transmit sensory signals from the periphery to the CNS.

A pseudounipolar neuron has a large, round cell body and gives rise to a single process that bifurcates shortly after leaving the soma. By dividing into two branches, the single process of a pseudounipolar neuron functions as both a dendrite and an axon. Most pseudounipolar neurons are located in the peripheral nervous system (PNS) where they send somatosensory signals from the skin, muscles, and joints to the CNS.

Subcellular Organelles. Neurons are among the most metabolically active cells in the body. This is due, in part, to their structural complexity and the need to manufacture components to maintain an extensive cytoskeleton and cellular membrane. In addition, neuronal function depends on concentrating several types of ions against a concentration gradient. The soma is the metabolic center of the neuron and contains most of the organelles involved in synthesizing the macromolecules used to mediate these functions. A large nucleus resides within the soma and usually contains at least one prominent nucleolus. The soma also contains an extensive endoplasmic reticulum (ER), Golgi apparatus, ribosomes, and many mitochondria to meet the metabolic demands of the neuron (Figure 1-2).

> The **soma** is the metabolic center of the neuron.

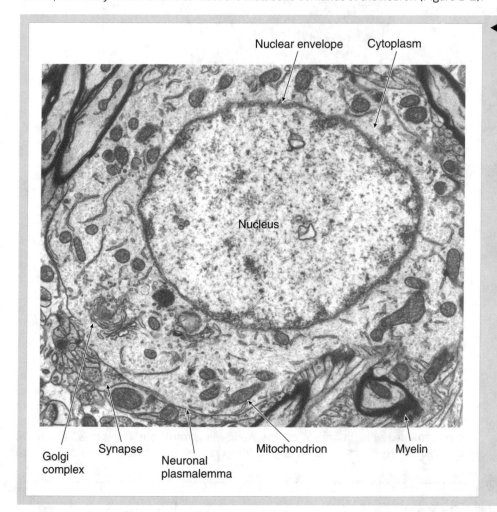

Nuclear envelope   Cytoplasm

Nucleus

Golgi complex   Synapse   Neuronal plasmalemma   Mitochondrion   Myelin

FIGURE 1-2
Neuronal Soma. *This electron micrograph illustrates the subcellular organelles in the soma of a neuron in the neostriatum. (Courtesy of Mr. Roland Myers, Pennsylvania State University College of Medicine, Hershey, Pennsylvania.)*

Most neurons have a high concentration of RNA in the nucleus and in the ribosomes associated with the rough endoplasmic reticulum (RER). The high concentration of nucleic acids in these structures makes the soma highly basophilic, and consequently, the soma is intensely stained by basic dyes. Neuroanatomists frequently use these dyes to stain the Nissl substance of the cell (i.e., organelles that contain nucleic acids) to differentiate brain regions according to the density and distribution of their neuronal soma.

DENDRITES

The cell bodies of most neurons give rise to a variable number of slender processes called dendrites. The term "dendrite" means tree-like, and most dendrites are highly branched processes that resemble the arborizations of a tree. Dendrites that extend directly from

Dendrites *are highly branched processes that receive inputs from other neurons and convey this information to the soma.*

the soma are called primary dendrites, and the typical neuron has only a small number of these. Primary dendrites subdivide into secondary dendrites, which then subdivide into smaller tertiary dendrites. For some neurons this process is repeated several times until a dense plexus of dendrites is formed (Figure 1-3).

FIGURE 1-3 ▶

Dendritic Arborizations. *A dense plexus of dendrites extends from the soma of a Purkinje neuron located in the cerebellum. (Courtesy of Dr. Linda Larson-Prior, Pennsylvania State University College of Medicine, Hershey, Pennsylvania.)*

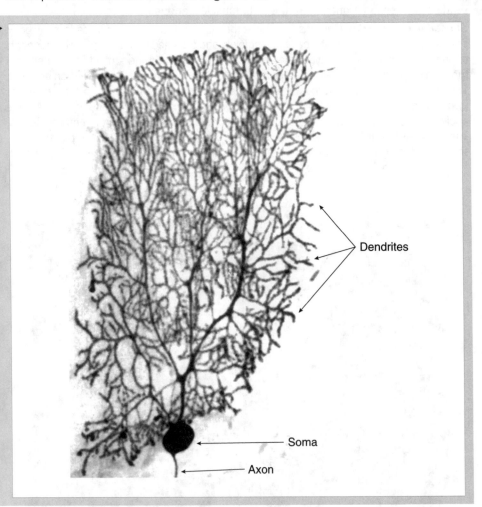

Dendrites provide a receptive area for integrating signals from other neurons. Communication between neurons occurs at specific sites on the dendritic arborization called synapses. The dendrite of a typical neuron may have hundreds or even thousands of synapses. Although some neurons have smooth dendrites, many neurons have dendrites that are studded with hundreds of small bud-like protrusions, or spines, which are specialized for receiving synaptic signals (Figure 1-4). Dendritic spines tend to be

FIGURE 1-4 ▶

Dendritic Spines. *(A) Drawing of a dendritic arborization at low magnification. (B) Drawing of spiny processes protruding from a dendrite viewed at high magnification. (C) Drawing of dendritic spines and their synaptic connections as seen through an electron microscope.*

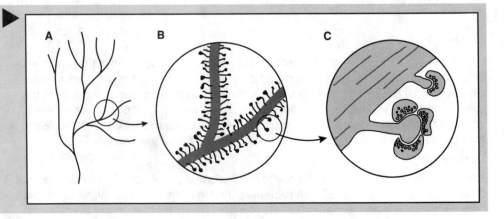

located on secondary, tertiary, or more distal dendritic branches. Although primary dendrites rarely contain spiny processes, they may receive many synapses. The soma may also have synapses, but these only comprise a small fraction of the total synaptic input.

Dendrites contain cytoplasm and an elaborate cytoskeletal system to maintain its complex structure. Neurofilaments and microtubules are present in small dendrites but are most numerous in the larger dendrites near the soma. Although few organelles are present in the distal dendrites, the primary dendrites contain mitochondria, ribosomes, and saccules of ER.

AXONS

The term "axon" was originally derived from the phrase "axial propagation." As that phrase implies, the axon is an elongated process that may extend for long distances before contacting other neurons. Each neuron has only one axon, and this process originates from the soma or from a small elevation of the soma called the axon hillock. Axons contain bundles of neurofilaments and microtubules, which provide structural support and play a critical role in transporting complex molecules and vesicular structures to the synaptic terminals. In contrast to dendrites, axons do not contain ribosomes and are not involved in protein synthesis (Figure 1-5).

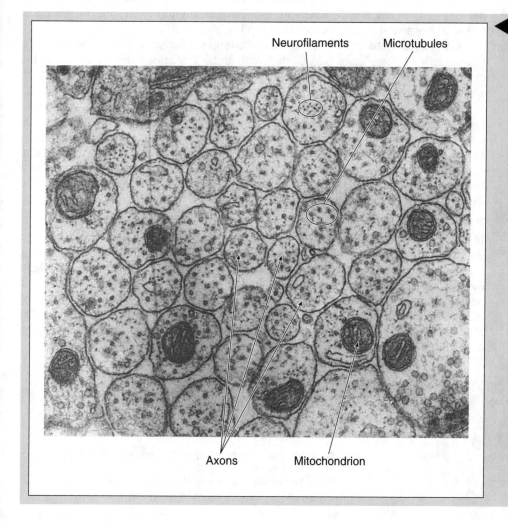

Neurofilaments   Microtubules

Axons   Mitochondrion

◀ **FIGURE 1-5**
Microtubules and Neurofilaments. *Several groups of microtubules and neurofilaments can be seen in this bundle of neuronal processes. (Courtesy of Mr. Roland Myers, Pennsylvania State University College of Medicine, Hershey, Pennsylvania.)*

An axon may split into collateral branches that terminate in different brain regions. Many axons bifurcate close to the axon hillock so that the local collateral branch may innervate adjacent neurons while the main branch projects to more distant targets. The main axonal branch may subdivide repeatedly to enable the neuron to communicate with more than one brain region. Upon entering the target region, an axon usually forms a plexus of endings that terminate on a population of postsynaptic neurons. The number of synaptic contacts that a neuron makes on a target neuron is highly variable, but it is not unusual for one neuron to form dozens of synaptic contacts on another neuron. A single synapse has very little effect on the activity of a neuron, and therefore, a neuron must form many synapses to exert significant influence on a target cell.

The main function of an axon is to conduct electrochemical impulses, known as action potentials, from the soma to the synaptic endings. Axons are electrically excitable because of the biophysical properties of their membranes and the differential concentration of specific ions in the intracellular and extracellular fluid. The conductive properties of the axon are discussed later in this chapter.

| *Axons* conduct electrochemical impulses to the synaptic terminals. |

SYNAPTIC TERMINALS

Synaptic terminals are specialized structures that allow one neuron to communicate with other neurons or effectors (i.e., muscles or glands). The terminal ending of an axon forms a distinct structure, the synaptic bouton, which lies in close apposition to the plasma membrane of its target cell. Synaptic boutons are slightly larger in diameter than an axon and are filled with mitochondria, synaptic vesicles, enzymes, and other neurochemicals. Synaptic vesicles contain neurotransmitter molecules that are released from the synaptic terminal in response to incoming electrochemical impulses. The release of neurotransmitter molecules enables a neuron to alter the electrochemical activity of other neurons that it contacts with its synaptic terminals. Neurotransmitters and the process of chemical transmission are discussed later in this chapter.

| *Synaptic terminals* release neurochemicals to communicate with other neurons. |

Synaptic boutons usually terminate on dendrites, their spines, or on the soma of a postsynaptic neuron (Figure 1-6). Such "axodendritic" or "axosomatic" synapses are the most common type of synapse in the CNS. Less frequent are "axoaxonic" synapses in which a synaptic bouton forms a synaptic contact on another terminal.

Although many synapses are formed by the terminal ending or synaptic bouton of an axon, other synapses are formed at multiple points along the course of an axonal arborization. These synaptic contacts are known as en passant ("in passing") synapses because they appear as a series of axonal enlargements or varicosities that contain vesicles filled with neurotransmitter molecules (Figure 1-7). En passant synapses allow a neuron to increase the number of its synaptic contacts on target cells without the biologic expense of maintaining additional axon collaterals.

AXOPLASMIC TRANSPORT

Most of the protein molecules and subcellular organelles needed to maintain the axon and its synaptic terminals are transported through the axon. This process, known as axoplasmic transport, is necessary because axons do not contain ribosomes or RER. Axoplasmic transport was demonstrated in 1948 when Paul Weiss observed the gradual accumulation of material in the axoplasm after ligating the sciatic nerve. Time-elapsed videomicroscopy and the analysis of transported radioactive amino acids have shown that a variety of particles are transported at different rates and in both directions through the axon (Table 1-1).

TABLE 1-1 ▶
Properties of Axoplasmic Transport

Direction	Rate (mm/d)	Transported Material
Anterograde		
Fast	200–400	Vesicles, neurotransmitters, membrane proteins, lipids
Medium	50–100	Mitochondria
Slow-a	0.2–1.0	Protein subunits for neurofilaments and microtubules
Slow-b	2–8	Clathrin, calmodulin, and metabolic enzymes
Retrograde		
Fast	150–300	Lysosomal packaged enzymes, and neurotrophic factors

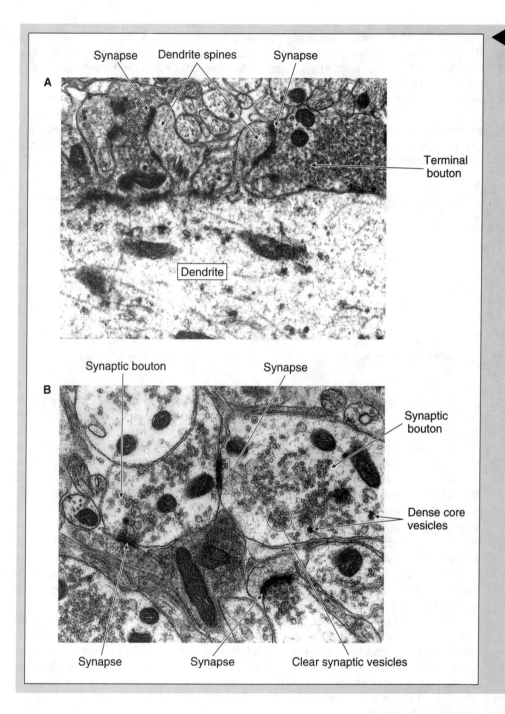

A

Synapse   Dendrite spines   Synapse

Terminal bouton

Dendrite

B

Synaptic bouton   Synapse

Synaptic bouton

Dense core vesicles

Synapse   Synapse   Clear synaptic vesicles

FIGURE 1-6
Axodendritic or Axoaxonic Synapses. *(A) Two dendritic spines receive contacts from axonal terminals packed with synaptic vesicles. (B) An axon terminal synapses with another axon terminal. Both terminals contain clear and dense-core vesicles. (Courtesy of Mr. Roland Myers, Pennsylvania State University College of Medicine, Hershey, Pennsylvania.)*

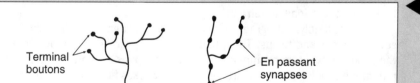

Terminal boutons

En passant synapses

FIGURE 1-7
Synaptic Terminals. *Axonal terminals may consist of clusters of single boutons or a series of synaptic contacts known as en passant synapses.*

Anterograde Movement. Anterograde transport involves the movement of material from the soma towards the synaptic terminals. Proteins and lipids synthesized by the RER and Golgi apparatus are assembled into organelles in the soma and enter the axon where they are moved by fast or medium anterograde transport (see Table 1-1). After entering the axon, these materials are rapidly shuttled through the axon by the microtubules. This process is mediated by a series of kinesin molecules, which alternately attach themselves to an organelle and move it a short distance before releasing it (Figure 1-8). Kinesin is a microtubule-associated adenosine triphosphatase (ATPase) molecule and requires oxidative metabolism for its function.

Microtubules provide a conduit for transporting vesicles and other macromolecules through the axon.

FIGURE 1-8 ▶

Kinesin. Axoplasmic transport in the anterograde direction is mediated by a series of kinesin molecules. Each kinesin molecule has a fan-tailed end that attaches to the organelle and a globular end that binds to the microtubule. Movement of the organelle occurs as one end of the kinesin molecule pivots around the center hinge.

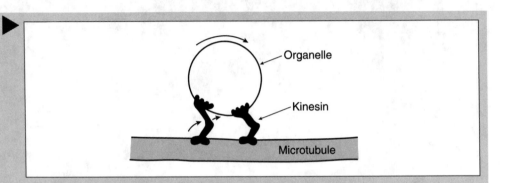

Other components of the neuron move in the anterograde direction but are transported relatively slowly. Cytoskeletal components and their associated proteins, for example, are slowly transported through the axon in their polymerized form. In fact, the neurofilaments and microtubules of an axon move continuously through the axon (0.2–1 mm/d) and are degraded by enzymatic depolymerization at the synaptic terminal. Other molecules such as clathrin, calmodulin, microfilaments, and several enzymes are also transported slowly through the axon (2–8 mm/d), but this mechanism of anterograde transport is poorly understood.

Retrograde Movement. Many subcellular organelles, enzymes, and membrane fragments are partially degraded and packaged into lysosomal vesicles to enable their retrograde transport to the soma. This process allows these materials to be recycled and used in the synthesis of new cellular components. Retrograde transport occurs rapidly and is mediated by dynein, another microtubule-associated ATPase that is similar to kinesin but operates in the reverse direction.

In addition to its scavenger function, retrograde transport has important developmental and regulatory functions. In the growing embryo, the terminals of developing axons find their appropriate cellular targets by taking up chemicals, such as nerve growth factor, which are released by the target cells. Nerve growth factor is retrogradely transported to the soma where it regulates the synthesis of material that is subsequently transported to the end of the growing axon. Similarly, in the fully developed adult, axons depend on the presence of neurotrophic factors released from the postsynaptic neuron. If the postsynaptic neuron degenerates, the loss of the neurotrophic factor often causes the presynaptic terminals to retract.

Unfortunately, retrograde transport also provides a mechanism for the spread of several viruses and toxins. Thus, herpes simplex, rabies, polio, and tetanus toxin enter the axons or synaptic terminals of peripheral nerves and are shuttled into the CNS by retrograde axoplasmic transport. Once these viruses find their way to the soma, they are able to exploit the metabolic functions of the nucleus and other organelles to replicate themselves.

Glial Cells

Glial cells do not transmit electrochemical signals but are essential for maintaining the biochemical environment in which neurons function. Thus, glial cells maintain the pH and osmolarity of the extracellular fluid within normal physiologic limits. In addition, glial cells enhance axonal conduction of electrochemical impulses, modulate neuro-transmission at synaptic junctions, and aid in nerve regeneration following peripheral nerve injury. The importance of glial cells in supporting neuronal functions is under-scored by the fact that they account for 70%–80% of all cells in the nervous system.

Based on their structural and functional features, neuroglial cells are classified into three major categories: astrocytes, oligodendrocytes, and microglia. Similar types of glial cells exist in the PNS and appear to serve equivalent functions. Schwann cells, the most common glial cells in the PNS, are similar to the oligodendrocytes of the CNS.

ASTROCYTES

Astrocytes have numerous branching processes that give them a stellate appearance. These processes terminate as "end feet" on the free surfaces of neuronal dendrites, cell bodies, and other structures. Astrocytic end feet frequently join together to form a secondary barrier that isolates the CNS from other tissues (Figure 1-9). For example, the outer surfaces of the brain and spinal cord are lined by astrocytic end feet that form the glial limitans membrane located below the pia mater (the inner layer of the meningeal membranes; see Chapter 2). Astrocytic end feet also cover the endothelial cells of all blood vessels in the CNS and provide an ancillary membrane in the blood–brain barrier.

Astrocytes
Isolate neurons from blood vessels
Metabolize the neurotransmitter gluta-mate
Provide structural support during develop-ment or injury

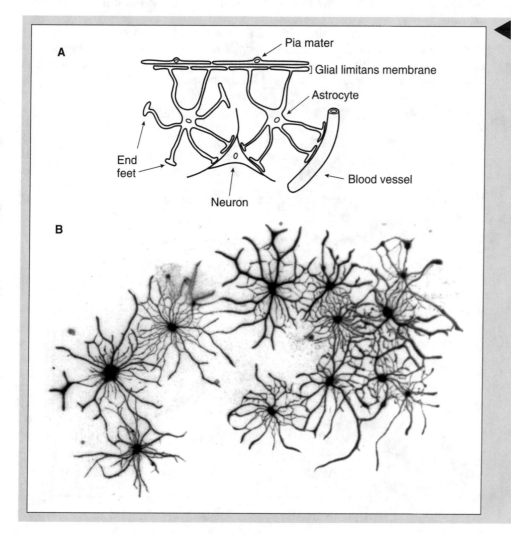

FIGURE 1-9
Astrocytes. (A) Astrocytes have processes that terminate as end feet on neurons, blood vessels, and the pia mater. (B) This photomicrograph shows the radiating processes of astrocytes growing in culture. (Courtesy of Dr. Robert Milner, Pennsylvania State University College of Medicine, Hershey, Pennsylvania.)

Astrocytes are important for controlling the molecular composition of the extracell-ular fluid in several ways. Astrocytic processes remove ions discharged into the extra-cellular fluid during the conduction of action potentials along the axon. Furthermore, astrocytes participate in the uptake and metabolism of certain neurotransmitters after they have been released from axonal terminals. When the neurotransmitter glutamate is released from synaptic terminals, for example, it is transported into neighboring astrocytes where it is converted into glutamine. Subsequently, the astrocytes release glutamine into the extracellular fluid where it is recovered by the nerve terminals and converted back to glutamate for neurotransmission.

Astrocytes also provide structural support during development and in response to injury. The developing neocortex contains a specific type of astrocyte, the radial glial cell, which provides a cellular substrate for migrating neurons. Furthermore, damage to the adult CNS often produces cell loss and leads to pockets of space that become filled by the proliferation of astrocytes. Because astrocytes are one of the few cell types that maintain their ability to proliferate in the mature brain, it is thought that astrocytes might be susceptible to chemical agents that alter cellular replication. This view may explain why most tumors in the CNS have an astrocytic origin.

OLIGODENDROCYTES

Oligodendrocytes form myelin insulation around axons in the CNS.

Oligodendrocytes are highly specialized glial cells that form the myelin insulation around the axons in the CNS. Myelination is the result of a cell–cell interaction in which surface proteins on the oligodendrocyte react to the presence of an axon by producing a sheet-like process that repeatedly wraps around the axon. The cytoplasm is squeezed from the glial process as it grows around the axon until, eventually, the axon is insulated from the extracellular fluid by multiple layers of myelin.

Oligodendrocytes are located within all of the major fiber tracts of the CNS. Each oligodendrocyte has multiple processes, each of which insulates a small segment of a single axon. Thus, multiple processes emerge from an oligodendrocyte like the tentacles of an octopus to wrap around the axons of several neurons (Figure 1-10).

FIGURE 1-10 ▶

Oligodendrocytes. *(A) Fiber tracts in the CNS contain axons wrapped by myelin sheaths extending from a single oligodendrocyte. Nodes of Ranvier represent sites between the myelin segments where ions can flow across the axonal membrane. (B) This photomicrograph illustrates a myelinating oligodendrocyte in the corpus callosum of an 8-month-old rat. The myelin segments of this oligodendrocyte envelop several axons having different orientations. (Courtesy of Dr. Steven Levison, Pennsylvania State University College of Medicine, Hershey, Pennsylvania.)*

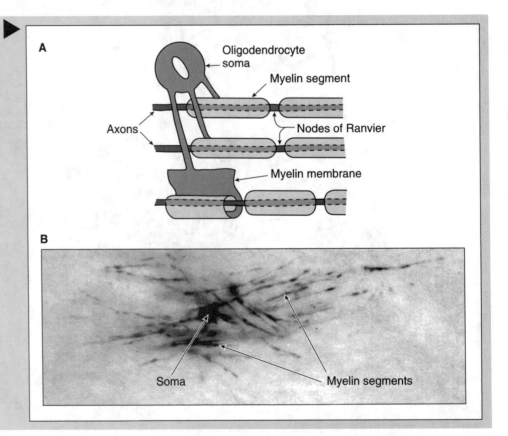

The myelin sheath surrounding a single axon is formed from many oligodendrocytes. Each myelinated axon is surrounded by a series of myelin segments, which are separated from each other by short intervals called nodes of Ranvier. The myelin segments insulate an axon from charged ions in the extracellular fluid; therefore, the nodes of Ranvier are the only part of the axonal membrane capable of conducting the ionic currents of an action potential. Because of this arrangement, myelination causes action potential impulses to "jump" from one node of Ranvier to the next. This process, known as saltatory conduction, results in axonal conduction velocities that are much faster than the conduction velocities of unmyelinated neurons.

Multiple Sclerosis (MS). Demyelinating diseases, such as MS, interfere with motor and sensory functions by disrupting the propagation of action potentials. Although the exact cause is unknown, the pathogenesis of MS is controlled by several factors, including genetic susceptibility, autoimmune mechanisms, and environmental conditions. MS causes degeneration of myelin sheaths in many of the major fiber systems of the CNS by destroying oligodendrocytes. The disease varies among individuals because several different fiber systems can be affected; the constellation of neurologic symptoms seen in patients with MS reflects the specific fiber tracts that are demyelinated.

MICROGLIA

Microglia comprise approximately 1% of the cells in the CNS. These cells originate from the mesoderm and migrate into the CNS during embryologic development. Microglial cells are small cells that function chiefly as scavengers. When CNS tissue is injured, microglial cells migrate to the injured region where they proliferate and devour the cellular debris. This mechanism of action and other evidence have prompted the view that microglia may also participate in certain autoimmune disorders.

SCHWANN CELLS

The Schwann cells of the PNS are structurally and functionally similar to the oligodendrocytes of the CNS. Schwann cells produce multiple layers of myelin sheaths that wrap around all but the smallest nerve fibers (Figure 1-11). Like the oligodendrocytes, the Schwann cell excludes the cytoplasm as it encircles the axon with its laminated wrapping. In contrast to an oligodendrocyte, however, a Schwann cell gives rise to only one process that produces a myelin sheath for a single axon.

> ***Schwann cells*** *form myelin insulation around axons in the PNS.*

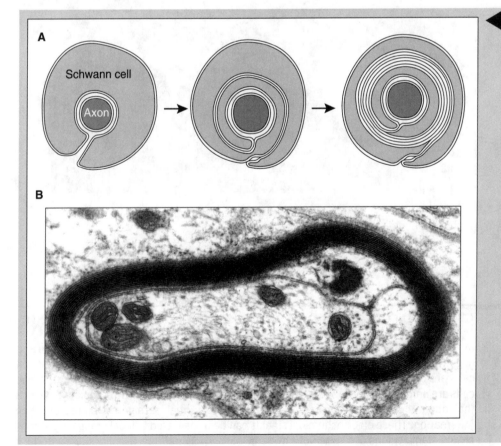

◄ ***FIGURE 1-11***

Myelination. *(A) Development of myelination around the axon of a peripheral neuron. The Schwann cell surrounds the axon and then spirals around the fiber repeatedly. The cell membranes fuse together as the cytoplasm is squeezed from each layer. (B) Electron micrograph illustrating multiple layers of myelin around a peripheral axon. The axon appears to be oval in shape because it was sectioned obliquely. (Courtesy of Mr. Roland Myers, Pennsylvania State University College of Medicine, Hershey, Pennsylvania.)*

The smallest axons in a peripheral nerve are not wrapped by layers of myelin but occupy invaginations in the plasmalemma of a Schwann cell (Figure 1-12). In these cases, a single Schwann cell supports multiple peripheral fibers, and as many as 20 unmyelinated axons can be ensheathed by a single Schwann cell.

FIGURE 1-12 ▶

Unmyelinated Axons. (A) Small diameter fibers occupy canal-like invaginations in the Schwann cell plasmalemma. (B) The electron micrograph shows two unmyelinated axons ensheathed by a nearby Schwann cell. (Courtesy of Mr. Roland Myers, Pennsylvania State University College of Medicine, Hershey, Pennsylvania.)

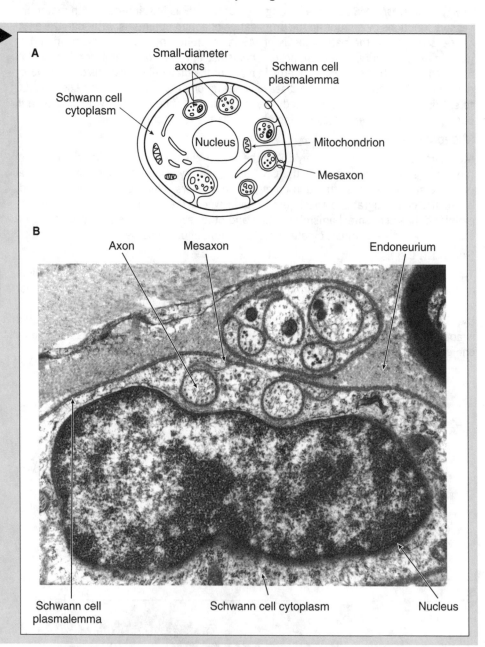

ELECTROCHEMICAL PROPERTIES OF NEURONS

In virtually all mammalian cells there is a slight imbalance in the number of positive and negative ions that are distributed across the cell's plasma membrane. Hence, nearly all cells are electrically charged with respect to the surrounding extracellular fluid. Nerve cells are unique, however, because their membranes are endowed with special properties that allow them to use changes in membrane potential as signals for representing information. These electrochemical signals can be transmitted to local groups of neurons or to distant regions of the nervous system.

Neuronal Membranes

The membrane of a neuron is a physical barrier that prevents molecules from diffusing freely into or out of the cell's cytoplasm. Constructed from a lipid bilayer that acts as an insulator, the neuronal membrane maintains the electrolytic concentration of several ions in the cytoplasm and extracellular fluid. Neurons maintain high concentrations of potassium (K^+) and negatively charged protein molecules in the cytoplasm (Table 1-2). Other ions, such as sodium (Na^+), chloride (Cl^-), and calcium (Ca^{2+}), are more highly concentrated in the extracellular fluid. Because of differences in the distribution of these electrically charged molecules, the cytoplasm usually has an excess of negative charges as compared to the extracellular fluid.

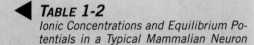

TABLE 1-2
Ionic Concentrations and Equilibrium Potentials in a Typical Mammalian Neuron

Ions	Intracellular (mM/L)	Extracellular (mM/L)	Nernst Potential (mV)
Potassium (K^+)	150	5.5	−86
Sodium (Na^+)	15	150	+60
Chloride (Cl^-)	10	125	−66
Calcium (Ca^{2+})	0.0001	2	+180
Organic anions[a]	130	1–2	. . .

[a] Intracellular anions do not cross the plasma membrane

The separation of positive and negative charges across a membrane results in a membrane potential or voltage. The membrane potential does not remain constant but fluctuates in response to synaptic inputs from other neurons. In the absence of synaptic input, the typical neuron has a resting membrane potential that ranges between −70 and −60 millivolts (mV) because the cytoplasm is slightly negative with respect to the surrounding extracellular fluid. The membrane potential of a neuron may change whenever charged ions (i.e., K^+, Na^+, Ca^{2+}, or Cl^-) flow through specialized pores or ion channels in the membrane. When the difference in charge across the membrane is reduced because positive ions enter the cytoplasm (or negative ions leave), the membrane potential moves closer to zero. This phenomenon is called depolarization. When the membrane potential becomes more negative because negative ions enter the cytoplasm (or positive ions leave), this phenomenon is called hyperpolarization.

GRADED POTENTIALS

Neurons release neurotransmitter molecules at their synaptic terminals to produce changes in the membrane potential of the postsynaptic neuron. Synaptic transmission may cause either depolarization or hyperpolarization depending on the type of neurotransmitter that is released and the ion channels that are activated. Local changes in the postsynaptic membrane potential of the dendrite or soma are called graded potentials because they vary in amplitude. Graded potentials are always monophasic and consist of either a depolarization or a hyperpolarization that spreads passively across the membrane. After rising rapidly to its peak amplitude, a graded potential gradually decays back to the neuron's resting membrane potential (Figure 1-13). Graded depolarizations are also known as excitatory postsynaptic potentials (EPSPs); graded hyperpolarizations are known as inhibitory postsynaptic potentials (IPSPs).

*A **graded potential** is a monophasic excitatory or inhibitory waveform of variable amplitude that spreads passively through the dendrite and soma.*

ACTION POTENTIALS

When a graded depolarization at the axon hillock exceeds a specific threshold level, the neuron produces a special electrochemical impulse known as an action potential (see Figure 1-13). Action potentials exhibit biphasic changes in membrane potential that are actively propagated through the axon until it reaches the synaptic endings. Unlike graded potentials, action potentials are all-or-none signals that remain constant in amplitude as they travel the length of the axon. On reaching the synaptic terminal, an action potential initiates a series of chemical events that culminates in the release of neurotransmitters from the presynaptic membrane. Neurons often produce a rapid series of action potentials, and changes in the timing of these impulses are important for coding specific types of information.

*An **action potential** is a biphasic waveform of constant amplitude that is actively conducted through the axon.*

FIGURE 1-13 ▶

Neuronal Membrane Potentials. *(A) An intracellular electrode records the membrane potential of a neuron that receives both inhibitory and excitatory inputs. (B) Release of inhibitory neurotransmitter causes a graded hyperpolarization; release of excitatory neurotransmitter causes a graded depolarization. Activation of several excitatory synapses in a brief time period depolarizes the membrane to threshold and produces an action potential.*

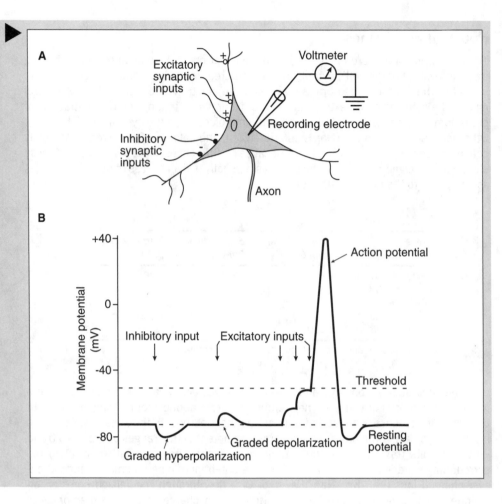

Pumps and Channels

Ion pumps transport ions against their concentration gradient. Ion channels transport ions down their concentration gradient.

The flow of charged ions across a neuronal membrane is controlled by two basic mechanisms. Ion pumps actively transport certain ions through the membrane against their concentration gradients. Ion channels, by contrast, allow passive diffusion of ions across the membrane according to their concentration gradients.

ION PUMPS

An ion pump is any protein molecule that has the ability to concentrate certain ions in the neuronal cytoplasm or the surrounding extracellular fluid. Several different types of ion pumps have been identified, and all of them require chemical energy to move ions against their concentration gradient. Many ion pumps, for example, depend on the hydrolysis of adenosine triphosphate (ATP) to transport ions across the membrane and thus are called ATPase pumps.

Na^+–K^+ Pump. The most important pump for understanding the membrane properties of a neuron is the Na^+–K^+-ATPase pump. Like many pumps, the Na^+–K^+ pump is an ion exchange pump that moves one ionic species in one direction while simultaneously moving a different ionic species in the opposite direction. The Na^+–K^+ pump relies on ion exchange to transport Na^+ from the cytoplasm to the extracellular fluid while simultaneously transporting K^+ into the cell (Figure 1-14). These processes are mutually dependent; removing K^+ from the extracellular fluid prevents Na^+ from being transported out of the cytoplasm.

The Na^+–K^+ pump is called an electrogenic pump because it produces an electric potential across the neuronal membrane. A small voltage potential develops across the membrane as the Na^+–K^+ pump removes three Na^+ ions from a neuron for every two K^+ ions that are transported into the cell. Although this process causes the cytoplasm to become more negative with respect to the extracellular fluid, the Na^+–K^+ pump has a

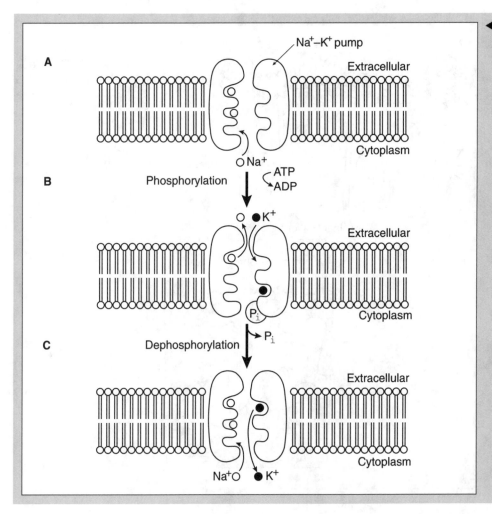

◀ FIGURE 1-14
Na⁺–K⁺ Pump. The Na⁺–K⁺ pump removes three Na⁺ ions from the cytoplasm for every two K⁺ ions transported into the cytoplasm. (A) Na⁺ ions leave the intracellular fluid and bind to specific sites on the Na⁺–K⁺ pump. (B) The Na⁺–K⁺ pump is phosphorylated by the conversion of ATP to ADP and releases three Na⁺ ions into the extracellular fluid as two 2 K⁺ bind to the Na⁺–K⁺ pump. (C) Dephosphorylation of the Na⁺–K⁺ pump causes the release of two K⁺ ions into the cytoplasm.

small influence on the resting membrane potential and absolutely no role in generating action potentials. Selective inhibition of the Na^+–K^+ pump with ouabain, a plant glycoside, does not prevent the generation of action potentials. After applying ouabain, the concentration gradients for Na^+ and K^+ eventually dissipate, but only after thousands of action potentials have occurred. The importance of the Na^+–K^+ pump lies in its ability to generate large concentration gradients that provide the driving force for the diffusion of Na^+ and K^+ when the membrane becomes selectively permeable to these ions.

ION CHANNELS

Many ion channels have been identified that provide stable openings in the plasma membrane for the diffusion of specific ions during certain conditions. Although most channels are selective for only one type of ion (e.g., K^+ channels), some channels permit diffusion of more than one ionic species.

Ion channels consist of several protein subunits that are bound to the lipid plasma membrane by uncharged lipophilic amino acid residues. Each subunit is a glycoprotein molecule that is composed of several transmembrane segments linked to each other by intracellular and extracellular loops of amino acids. When grouped together, the subunits form a cylindrical structure that encircles a water-filled channel through the plasma membrane (Figure 1-15).

The selectivity of an ion channel is determined by its geometric structure, the diameter of its pore, and the distribution of charged groups of amino acids within the pore. Ions can be blocked from passing through a channel by small loops of amino acid residues that project into the aqueous pore from the transmembrane subunits. These intrapore loops act as "gates" for controlling ionic currents through the channel. Electrostatic forces across the membrane may alter the conformational structure of the gate, thereby causing the channel to open or close.

FIGURE 1-15 ▶

Ion Channels. *(A) An example of an ion channel constructed from four protein sub-units, each of which has six membrane-spanning regions. The extracellular and intracellular loops act as gates that block ions from entering the pore. (B) The protein sub-units encircle a central water-filled pore.*

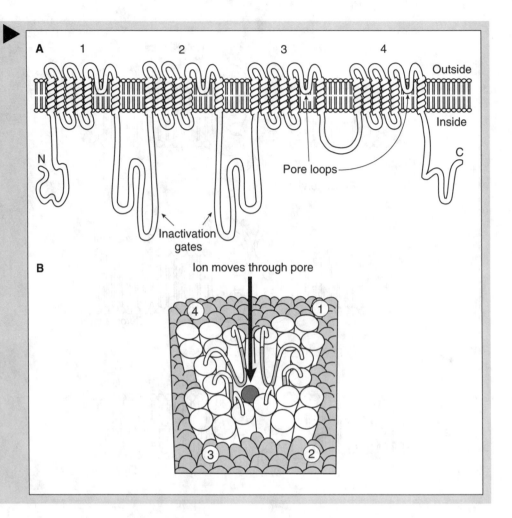

Voltage-gated Channels. Voltage-gated ion channels are located in all parts of a neuron's membrane, including the axon, and are essential for the propagation of action potentials to the axonal terminals. Voltage-gated ion channels are controlled by the magnitude and polarity of the potential difference across the plasma membrane. Voltage-gated ion channels are sensitive to shifts in membrane voltage because the pore loops or "gates" contain electrical charges that are either repelled by or attracted to the ionic charges lining the surfaces of the neuronal membrane. The electric polarity of the gate causes it to switch between the closed and open states as the membrane potential reverses its polarity.

Some ion channels, such as the voltage-gated K^+ channel, have only a single gate (Figure 1-16), while others, such as the voltage-gated Na^+ channel, have multiple gates (Figure 1-17). If all the gates are in the opened position, the channel permits the flow of hydrated ions. If one or more gates are closed, ions cannot pass through the channel. Ion channels that have more than one gate have special biophysical properties because different mechanisms may control each of the different gates.

Ligand-gated Channels. Ligand-gated ion channels are physically linked to receptors that are activated by specific neurotransmitters or other ligands having a similar molecular structure. When a neurotransmitter molecule binds to the receptor of a ligand-gated channel, the conformational structure of the ion channel changes to enable the gates to move from the closed to the open position. Ligand-gated channels are densest at sites that receive synaptic contacts and mediate the local EPSPs and IPSPs initiated by synaptic transmission. Thus, ligand-gated channels are embedded in the membrane of the soma, dendrites, or synaptic boutons but are not found in axons.

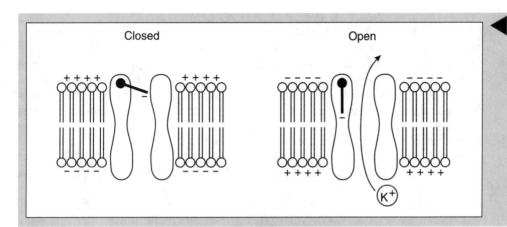

FIGURE 1-16
Voltage-gated K+ Channel. A single gate determines whether a voltage-gated K+ channel is in the open or closed state.

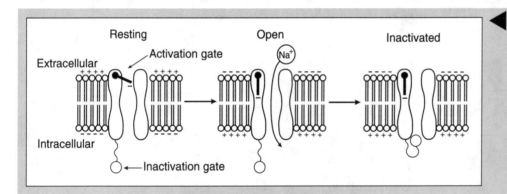

FIGURE 1-17
Voltage-gated Na+ Channel. Two gates control ion flow through a voltage-gated Na+ channel. The combination of opened and closed positions allows voltage-gated Na+ channels to exist in three different states. The activation gate is controlled exclusively by membrane voltage. The inactivation gate closes in a time-dependent manner soon after the membrane is depolarized.

Ionic Basis of Membrane Potentials

The membrane potential of a neuron is determined partly by the concentration of ions on each side of the neuronal membrane and partly by the permeability of the neuronal membrane. The intracellular and extracellular concentrations of K+, Na+, Ca2+, and Cl- usually stay in a fairly narrow range, but the permeability of the voltage-gated and ligand-gated ion channels may vary tremendously. Even if only a few ion channels are opened, an increase in the net flow of charges across the membrane can cause significant changes in the membrane potential. Shifts in membrane potential may occur in response to small ionic currents because most of the cytoplasm and extracellular fluid are electrically neutral. Only the ions lining the surfaces of the membrane actually determine the magnitude and polarity of the membrane potential (Figure 1-18).

Membrane potentials are determined by ion concentration gradients and by the ionic permeability of the membrane.

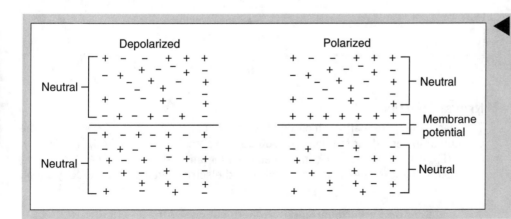

FIGURE 1-18
Membrane Potentials. Most of the extracellular fluid and neuronal cytoplasm is electrically neutral, and a small fraction of the ions moves across the membrane to produce a membrane potential. Charges contributing to the membrane potential line the surface of the membrane.

RESTING MEMBRANE POTENTIALS

Most neurons have resting membrane potentials that range between -60 and -70 mV. The negative polarity of the resting membrane potential is largely due to the increased permeability of voltage-gated K^+ channels in the resting membrane. To understand this phenomenon, consider what would happen if a neuron had a membrane potential that was neutral and the membrane was only permeable to K^+ (Figure 1-19). Under these conditions, K^+ would flow out of the neuron because K^+ is 30 times more concentrated in the cytoplasm than in the extracellular fluid (see Table 1-2). As K^+ leaves the cytoplasm, the membrane would begin to develop a potential difference due to the accumulation of negative charges inside the cell. In time, K^+ efflux would gradually slow down because of the increasing electrostatic attraction between the negatively charged cytoplasm and the positively charged K^+ ions. Eventually, K^+ influx and K^+ efflux would attain a state of equilibrium because the chemical force of the concentration gradient would be opposed by an electrical force of equal strength. Although some K^+ ions would still move across the neuronal membrane, flow would occur in both directions at equal rates to produce a net flow of K^+ that would be zero.

FIGURE 1-19 ▶

Ionic Basis for Resting Membrane Potentials. *A negative resting membrane potential develops if the membrane is selectively permeable to K^+. The membrane potential is initially zero but becomes negative as K^+ flows down its concentration gradient. Equilibrium is reached when the force of the chemical concentration gradient is counterbalanced by an electrical force acting in the opposite direction.*

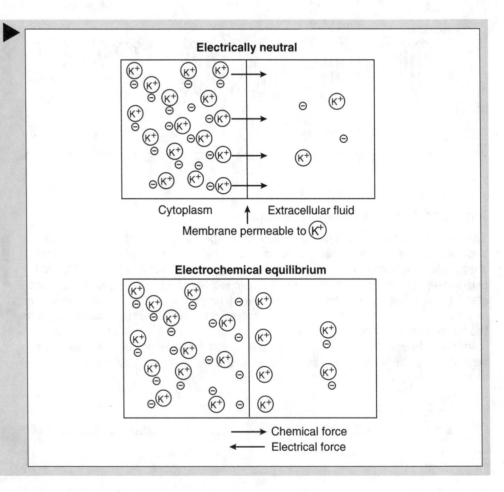

NERNST EQUATION

The membrane potential at which equilibrium occurs for a specific ion is called the equilibrium potential for that ion. The equilibrium potential for K^+ (E_{K^+}), Na^+ (E_{Na^+}), Ca^{2+} ($E_{Ca^{2+}}$), or Cl^- (E_{Cl^-}) can be calculated from a simple formula, the Nernst equation, which assumes that the chemical and electrical gradients are exactly equal:

Electric potential gradient = chemical concentration gradient   (1)

In the Nernst equation, the magnitude or driving force of the electric potential gradient is the product of the valence of the ion (z), Faraday's constant (F), and the membrane potential at that ion's equilibrium point (E):

$$\text{Electric potential gradient} = zFE \tag{2}$$

The driving force of the chemical concentration gradient is the product of the gas constant (R), the absolute temperature (T), and the natural logarithm of the ratio of the ionic concentrations in the extracellular and intracellular compartments:

$$\text{Chemical concentration gradient} = RT\ln[\text{ion}]_{out}/[\text{ion}]_{in} \tag{3}$$

By substituting expressions from equations 2 and 3 into equation 1 we get:

$$zFE = RT\ln[\text{ion}]_{out}/[\text{ion}]_{in} \tag{4}$$

The equilibrium potential (E) is the only unknown value and is expressed as the Nernst equation:

$$E = (RT/zF)\ln[\text{ion}]_{out}/[\text{ion}]_{in} \tag{5}$$

The Nernst equation can be simplified by substituting standard values for body temperature and the other physical constants and by converting to base 10. For ions with a valence of 1, the Nernst equation is expressed as:

$$E = 60 \, (\log_{10} [\text{ion}]_{out}/[\text{ion}]_{in}) \tag{6}$$

Using the concentration values in Table 1-2, the equilibrium potential for K^+ (E_{K^+}) is approximately −86 mV. By comparison, the equilibrium potential for Na^+ is +60 mV, while the equilibrium potential for Cl^- is −66 mV.

The equilibrium potential is an important concept because increases in the permeability of one type of ion channel shift the membrane potential towards the equilibrium potential for that ion. If a neurotransmitter causes an increase in the permeability of Na^+ channels, Na^+ flows down its concentration gradient into the cell until the membrane potential moves closer to the equilibrium potential of Na^+ (+60 mV). By contrast, an increase in the permeability of K^+ channels causes the membrane potential to shift towards the equilibrium potential for K^+ (−86 mV). An increase in the permeability of Cl^- channels usually has little effect on the membrane potential because the resting potential and the equilibrium potential for Cl^- are nearly identical (see Table 1-2).

Equilibrium potential is the membrane potential that results when a membrane is completely permeable to only one ionic species.

GOLDMAN EQUATION

The Nernst equation indicates the value that the membrane potential will attain if the membrane is permeable to only one ionic species, but this assumption is rarely true. In most neurons, some fraction of each type of ion channel is always open, and the membrane potential at any moment in time reflects the relative permeability of the membrane to ions that diffuse through different ligand-gated and voltage-gated channels. For this reason, the Goldman equation was developed to provide a general account of the relationship between membrane potential (V) and the relative permeability (P) of each population of ion channels:

$$V = 60 \, \log \frac{P_{K^+}[K^+]_{out} + P_{Na^+}[Na^+]_{out} + P_{Cl^-}[Cl^-]_{in}}{P_{K^+}[K^+]_{in} + P_{Na^+}[Na^+]_{in} + P_{Cl^-}[Cl^-]_{out}} \tag{7}$$

The Goldman equation is similar to the Nernst equation but applies whenever the membrane is permeable to more than one ion. In fact, if the permeability for two of the ions approaches zero, the Goldman equation becomes equivalent to the Nernst equation. The only difference between the Nernst and Goldman equations is that the latter does not contain a valence factor. This explains why the ratio of intracellular and extracellular concentrations is inverted for Cl^- ions.

The Goldman equation is important because it illustrates how the membrane potential is determined by both ionic concentration and the permeability of the membrane. If the membrane is permeable to only one ion, then the membrane potential shifts towards the equilibrium potential for that ion. If the membrane becomes permeable to more than one ion, the Goldman equation indicates that the resulting membrane potential is a function of the relative permeability of the membrane to the different ions. During a sudden increase in the permeability of one type of ion channel, the membrane potential rapidly shifts towards the equilibrium potential of the ion whose channels have suddenly opened.

Given the factors that influence the membrane potential, it is possible to understand why most neurons have a negative resting membrane potential between -60 and -70 mV. Because the resting membrane is highly permeable to K^+, an efflux of K^+ down its concentration gradient causes an accumulation of negative charges in the cytoplasm. Intracellular recordings have confirmed this explanation by showing how changes in the extracellular concentration of K^+, Na^+, and Cl^- have affected the resting membrane potential. When extracellular K^+ was increased, the resting membrane potential was significantly depolarized. When the extracellular and intracellular concentrations of K^+ were made equal, the resting membrane potential was 0 mV. By comparison, changing the extracellular concentrations of Na^+ or Cl^- only had a negligible effect on resting membrane potential. These findings indicate that the resting membrane potential is negative because the resting membrane is much more permeable to K^+ than to Na^+ or Cl^-. The resting membrane potential is not identical to E_{K^+}, however, because the resting membrane is slightly permeable to other ions.

> The **resting membrane potential** of most neurons is between -60 and -70 mV because the resting membrane is highly permeable to K^+.

Passive Membrane Properties of Neurons

Neurons are relatively poor conductors of passive ionic currents. To illustrate this principle, consider an experiment in which a micropipet is filled with a concentrated NaCl solution, and its tip is placed inside an axon. As the axon is depolarized by injecting Na^+ into the cytoplasm, the change in membrane potential is monitored by a set of electrodes placed at regular intervals along the axon (Figure 1-20). Assuming the depolarization is too weak to evoke an action potential, the change in membrane potential is greatest at the site of Na^+ injection and declines exponentially along the axon.

There are two reasons why the magnitude of depolarization is not equal at all points along the neuron's membrane. First, there is substantial resistance to the flow of ions

FIGURE 1-20 ▶

Passive Current Flow. *When small amounts of Na^+ are injected into a neuron, the level of depolarization is greatest at the site of injection. The level of depolarization declines with distance as Na^+ flows back across the membrane into the extracellular space.*

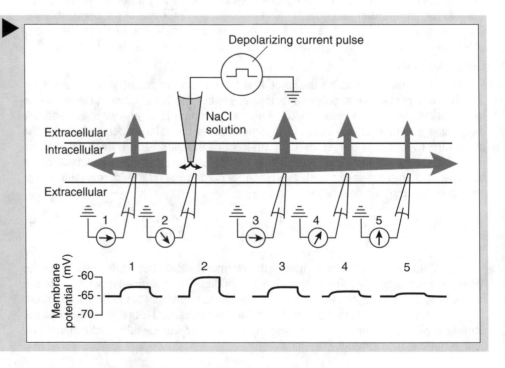

through the axon's cytoplasm because axons have a small diameter, and the resistance to flow varies inversely with the cross-sectional area of the conductor. Cytoplasmic resistance also increases with the length of the axon because ions are more likely to experience collisions as they travel a longer route through the cytoplasm. Secondly, the neuronal membrane is a leaky insulator. Many of the Na^+ ions injected into the cytoplasm will flow through the plasma membrane into the extracellular space. This efflux of Na^+ current allows the depolarization to dissipate with increasing distance from the injection site because fewer Na^+ ions are available to charge the inner surface of the membrane.

MEMBRANE TIME CONSTANTS

When Na^+ enters the cytoplasm, either experimentally or during neuronal activity, the change in membrane potential does not occur instantaneously. It takes time for membrane depolarization to develop because some of the Na^+ ions entering the cytoplasm return immediately to the extracellular fluid. Only Na^+ ions that remain in the cytoplasm contribute to the depolarization of the membrane potential. Eventually, as Na^+ continues to enter the cytoplasm, the membrane attains a steady state or peak amplitude of depolarization. The time it takes for the membrane to reach 63% of the peak depolarization is known as the membrane time constant τ_m (tau). The magnitude of the time constant depends on the resistance (R_m) and capacitance (C_m) of the membrane:

$$\tau_m = R_m \times C_m \qquad (8)$$

As equation 8 indicates, the time constant is proportional to the magnitude of the neuron's membrane resistance and to its membrane capacitance. Membrane resistance indicates how well the membrane prevents the passage of charged ions and is inversely proportional to the conductance of its ion channels. Hence, a membrane in which the ion channels are closed has a higher resistance than one in which the ion channels are open. The capacitance of a membrane indicates the capacity of the membrane to hold positive and negative charges. Relatively thin membranes can hold charges better than thicker membranes because electrostatic attraction decreases with increasing distance between the charged ions.

Neurons with long time-constants take longer to become depolarized in response to an excitatory input. The advantage of a long time-constant is that a given amount of Na^+ influx produces a larger depolarization because the incoming Na^+ does not return to the extracellular space as rapidly as in neurons with a short time-constant. Furthermore, when Na^+ influx ceases, membrane depolarization dissipates more slowly in neurons with long time-constants. Both of these characteristics contribute to a neuron's ability to integrate input from other neurons.

MEMBRANE LENGTH CONSTANTS

Sodium ions entering the cytoplasm at one region either pass immediately back to the extracellular space or travel through the axon a variable distance before exiting the neuron. The standard unit for measuring the passive spread of Na^+ current through the axon is the membrane length constant λ (lambda). The length constant represents the distance between the point of peak depolarization produced by Na^+ influx and the point where depolarization has declined to 37% of that peak value. Because Na^+ ions either flow through the cytoplasm or through the membrane, the length constant is related to the resistance offered by these two routes. Thus, λ is expressed as the square root of the ratio of the membrane resistance (R_m) to the internal resistance of the cytoplasm (R_i):

$$\lambda = (R_m/R_i)^{1/2} \qquad (9)$$

This equation for the length constant indicates that Na^+ current is more likely to spread farther along the axon if the membrane resistance is higher than the cytoplasmic resistance. The resistance offered by these routes is determined not only by their inherent conductivity but by the diameter of the axon. As the diameter of the axon increases, both R_m and R_i decrease. For a given length of axon, a thicker axon has a larger membrane area and more channels through which Na^+ may pass. Similarly, a thicker

*A **membrane time constant** indicates the length of time a charge is held by a membrane before dissipating.*

*A **membrane length constant** indicates the distance that a graded potential spreads passively before dissipating.*

axon allows Na$^+$ current to pass more easily through the cytoplasm in much the same way that water encounters less resistance when passing through a large hose than through a narrow hose. Because of differences in the relative growth of volume and surface area, R_i decreases more rapidly than R_m as axons become larger in diameter. Thus, when all other factors are equal, the length constant is longer for large-diameter axons than for small-diameter axons.

Length constants and time constants determine the effectiveness of a neuron in transmitting passive membrane potentials. In general, a subthreshold stimulus spreads further and persists longer in neurons having larger length and time constants. These are important properties because they increase the likelihood that multiple subthreshold depolarizations will sum together and reach the threshold for generating action potentials.

Ionic Basis of Action Potentials

When depolarization reaches a critical threshold level, the neuron responds by producing an action potential. In contrast to the passive current flow of a graded potential, an action potential is an all-or-none membrane potential that propagates the entire length of the axon without any decrement in its amplitude. Unlike graded potentials, which have monophasic shapes, action potentials have biphasic waveforms that reflect underlying changes in membrane permeability (or conductance) to Na$^+$ and K$^+$ (Figure 1-21).

FIGURE 1-21 ▶

Ionic Basis of Action Potentials. *Changes in the membrane conductance of Na$^+$ (g_{Na^+}) and K$^+$ (g_{K^+}) determine the action potential waveform (V_m).*

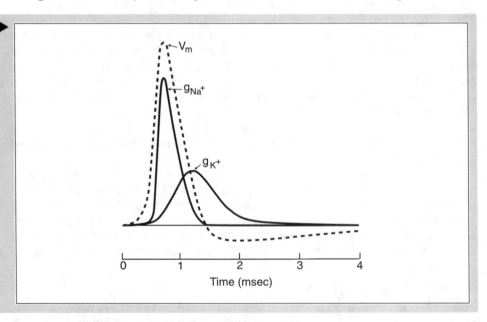

Action potentials are generated when the plasma membrane becomes permeable to Na$^+$ and the resulting influx of Na$^+$ is sufficient to depolarize the membrane to threshold. Once this critical value has been reached, the permeability of the membrane to Na$^+$ increases dramatically, and Na$^+$ rapidly enters the cell by flowing down its electrochemical gradients. This tremendous influx of Na$^+$ causes the membrane potential to become further depolarized and move toward the equilibrium potential for Na$^+$ (+60 mV). As the membrane potential approaches E_{Na^+}, however, the plasma membrane becomes more permeable to K$^+$, and K$^+$ flows out of the neuron. Eventually, Na$^+$ influx ceases because the voltage-gated Na$^+$ channels are unable to remain open for long periods and become inactivated during maintained depolarization (see Figure 1-17). The efflux of K$^+$ continues unopposed and causes the membrane potential to move back towards the equilibrium potential for K$^+$ until the resting membrane potential is re-established.

Action potentials are mediated by an influx of Na$^+$ and a delayed efflux of K$^+$.

VOLTAGE-DEPENDENT ION CURRENTS

Action potentials only occur when the membrane is depolarized to a critical level, and this suggests that changes in membrane permeability during an action potential are controlled by ionic charges on the membrane. In the 1940s, Alan Hodgkin and Andrew

Huxley tested this hypothesis by using the voltage-clamp technique to hold the membrane voltage of an axon at a constant level. By clamping the membrane potential at a constant level, they could study time-dependent changes in membrane permeability independent of the secondary shifts in membrane potential that must follow a change in membrane permeability. This was a significant advance because, if ion channel permeability is voltage-dependent, any change in permeability would allow a secondary shift in the membrane potential to produce additional changes in permeability.

The voltage-clamp experiments show that transmembrane ionic currents are voltage-dependent. Clamping the membrane at a constant level of depolarization causes an early inward current that is followed by a later outward current (Figure 1-22). The magnitude of the early inward current varies directly with the voltage and increases as the membrane potential is clamped at successively higher voltages ranging from -60 to 0 mV. Inward current reaches a peak amplitude at depolarizations maintained between 0 and +20 mV but becomes weaker when the membrane is clamped above +20 mV. If the membrane potential is clamped at the equilibrium potential for Na+ (+60 mV), the early inward current does not appear, and this indicates that Na+ influx mediates the early inward current. By comparison, the late outward current increases if the membrane is clamped at progressively higher levels of depolarization. When the membrane is clamped at the equilibrium potential for K+ (-86 mV), the late outward current is not present, suggesting that K+ efflux mediates the late outward current.

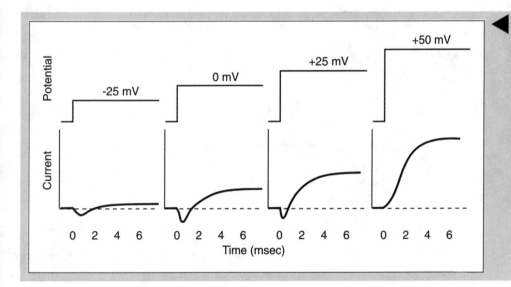

◀ **FIGURE 1-22**
Ionic Currents during Voltage Clamp.
These graphs show the results of clamping the membrane potential at successively higher levels of depolarization. At moderate levels of depolarization, current initially flows inward and then outward. When the membrane is depolarized to E_{Na^+} (+50 mV), all current flows outward.

Pharmacologic manipulations also indicate that the early inward and late outward currents of an action potential are mediated by Na+ and K+, respectively (Figure 1-23). Application of tetrodotoxin, a neurotoxic poison emitted by the puffer fish, selectively blocks Na+ channels and prevents the early inward current when the membrane is clamped at depolarized levels. Application of tetraethylammonium, which blocks K+ channels, prevents the late outward current without affecting the early inward current.

ION CHANNEL CONDUCTANCE

After establishing that action potentials were mediated by Na+ influx followed by K+ efflux, Hodgkin and Huxley used Ohm's law to calculate the changes in Na+ and K+ ion channel conductance as a function of membrane voltage. Ohm's law provides a mathematical expression of current (I) as it relates to voltage (V) and resistance (R):

$$I = V/R \qquad (10)$$

In terms of the flow of ionic current across a neuronal membrane, Ohm's law is expressed:

$$I_{ion} = (V_m - E_{ion})/R \qquad (11)$$

FIGURE 1-23 ▶

Ionic Basis of Early and Late Currents. (A) The neuron is clamped at a constant level of depolarization, and the change in membrane potential is recorded during different pharmacologic manipulations. (B) The membrane potential normally shows an early inward and a late outward current during depolarization. (C) When Na+ channels are blocked by tetrodotoxin, only the late outward current is present. (D) When K+ channels are blocked by tetraethylammonium, only the early inward current is present.

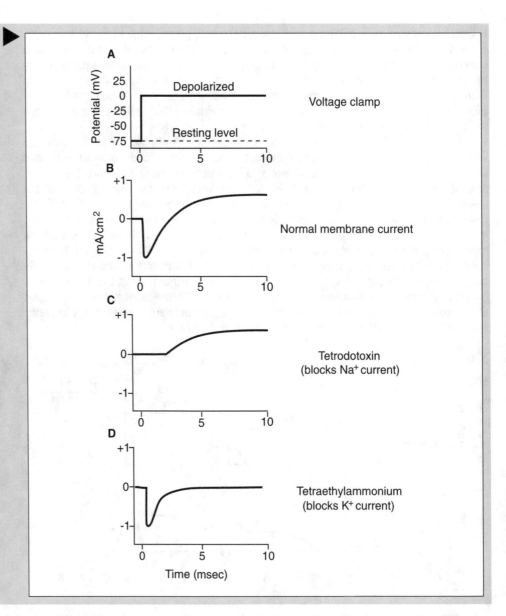

A

Voltage clamp

B

Normal membrane current

C

Tetrodotoxin
(blocks Na+ current)

D

Tetraethylammonium
(blocks K+ current)

Time (msec)

Ion channel conductance *indicates the relative ease with which an ion passes through a channel.*

where the difference between the resting membrane potential (V_m) and the equilibrium potential (E_{ion}) is the driving force that compels the ion across the membrane. Ion channel conductance (g_{ion}) indicates the permeability or relative ease of passing an ion through a channel. In mathematical terms conductance is the reciprocal of resistance and, after substitution, equation 11 becomes:

$$I_{ion} = g_{ion}(V_m - E_{ion}) \tag{12}$$

In the voltage-clamp experiments by Hodgkin and Huxley, a series of current measurements were taken in the presence and absence of extracellular Na+ to separately establish the flow of I_{Na^+} and I_{K^+} at different membrane potentials. When the membrane voltage (V_m) is experimentally controlled and the equilibrium potentials for Na+ and K+ are known, it is possible to calculate the conductances for these ions:

$$g_{Na^+} = I_{Na^+}/(V_m - E_{Na^+}) \tag{13}$$

$$g_{K^+} = I_{K^+}/(V_m - E_{K^+}) \tag{14}$$

Hodgkin's and Huxley's calculation of Na+ and K+ conductances at different levels of membrane depolarization indicated that these conductances are proportional to the level of depolarization. This relationship between ionic conductance and membrane potential indicates the presence of voltage-gated ion channels that are controlled by the polarity of ionic charges on the plasma membrane. Presumably, loops of amino acids in the channel's pore or groups of amino acids in the membrane-spanning domains have electrical charges that cause them to change their conformational position when the membrane polarity is altered. Such changes in the physical structure of a channel explain why shifts in membrane potential can selectively control the flow of ions through the channel (see Figures 1-16 and 1-17).

When a membrane is depolarized, the time course of the change in channel conductance is not identical for Na^+ and K^+ voltage-gated channels. Depolarization produces a rapid increase in Na^+ conductance and a delayed increase in K^+ conductance. This difference in timing allows Na^+ influx to precede K^+ efflux; otherwise, the membrane potential would never depolarize. If depolarization is prolonged over several milliseconds, however, Na^+ conductance quickly reaches a peak and then declines to reduce the flow of Na^+ into the cytoplasm. This suggests that voltage-gated Na^+ channels become inactivated even if the membrane remains in a constant state of depolarization. By comparison, depolarization causes a gradual increase in K^+ conductance that reaches an asymptotic level and persists for the duration of the depolarization (see Figure 1-23C). This indicates that K^+ channels remain open indefinitely when the membrane is depolarized.

Action potentials are mediated entirely by changes in the permeability of Na^+ and K^+ voltage-gated channels (see Figure 1-21). The rising phase of the action potential is due to the rapid influx of Na^+ produced by an increase in Na^+ conductance. The rate of Na^+ influx begins to slow as the membrane potential approaches E_{Na^+} so that the action potential reaches its peak amplitude when the Na^+ channels become inactivated. The falling phase of the action potential is mediated by the delayed activation of K^+ conductance. Potassium efflux is greatest just after the peak of the action potential and declines as the membrane potential approaches E_{K^+}. The membrane is briefly hyperpolarized as K^+ conductance does not return to resting levels until after the membrane voltage has declined below the normal resting potential.

THRESHOLD

The threshold for initiating action potentials may vary but is usually around -50 mV for most mammalian neurons. If a synaptic input does not activate enough voltage-gated Na^+ channels, a subthreshold EPSP is produced. When a neuron is at rest, K^+ conductance is higher than Na^+ conductance, and small depolarizations are countered by the efflux of K^+. As long as K^+ permeability is higher than Na^+ permeability, the efflux of K^+ slows depolarization and provides enough time to activate additional K^+ channels to restore the membrane potential to its resting level. As graded potentials become larger, Na^+ influx and K^+ efflux act as competing influences, and the membrane potential may briefly linger at a constant level of depolarization before returning to the resting level. If enough Na^+ enters the cell, however, Na^+ influx exceeds K^+ efflux and causes an exponential increase in Na^+ conductance, which cannot be offset by the delayed activation of additional K^+ channels. Hence, the threshold for an action potential is the membrane potential at which the rate of Na^+ influx surpasses the rate of K^+ efflux.

Threshold is the membrane potential at which Na^+ influx exceeds K^+ efflux.

AXONAL PROPAGATION OF IMPULSES

Once an action potential has been generated at the axon hillock, it propagates the entire length of the axon without stopping. This feature is related to the active and passive conduction properties of the membrane. When an action potential occurs, depolarizing current is passively conducted through neighboring parts of the axoplasm. Although the amount of current declines rapidly with distance (see Figure 1-20), it is strong enough to depolarize adjacent parts of the axon to threshold. On reaching threshold, the voltage-dependent Na^+ channels are activated, and consequently, more depolarizing current is available to spread passively to the next segment of the axon. Thus, the passive and active membrane properties cooperate with each other to generate an action potential in adjacent regions of the axon. This process is repeated continuously so that an action potential may propagate along the axon without any decrement in its amplitude (Figure 1-24).

FIGURE 1-24 ▶

Propagation of an Action Potential. An action potential requires active and passive flow of depolarizing current in the axoplasm. Na⁺ actively flows into the axon where the membrane is depolarized to threshold. The incoming current flows passively through the axon and causes neighboring regions of membrane to be depolarized. As the action potential propagates through the axon, the membrane potential returns to resting levels as K⁺ flows into the extracellular fluid.

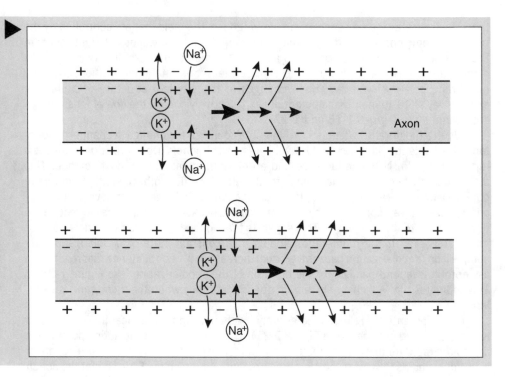

*The **refractory period** is the time interval during which Na⁺ channels are inactivated.*

REFRACTORY PERIODS

Immediately after an action potential has occurred, the neuron is unable to discharge again for a brief period of time. This interval, known as the refractory period, occurs because voltage-gated Na⁺ channels are inactivated during the falling edge of the action potential waveform (see Figure 1-17). The neuron is unable to discharge an action potential during this period regardless of the intensity of the depolarizing stimulus. As Na⁺ channels gradually recover from their state of inactivation, the neuron enters a relative refractory period and can discharge only in response to a large, suprathreshold depolarization. The duration of the refractory period varies across neurons as a function of the axonal density of certain types of ion channels.

The refractory period imposes an upper limit on the rate of activity that can be sustained by a neuron. This rate (in discharges/sec) is easily calculated by dividing one second of time (1000 msec) by the duration (in msec) of the refractory period. Another consequence of the absolute refractory period is that action potentials only travel in one direction after they are initiated at the axon hillock. Once an action potential propagates down the axon, inactivation of voltage-gated Na⁺ channels at the trailing edge of the waveform prevents any reversal in the direction of propagation.

CONDUCTION VELOCITY AND SALTATORY PROPAGATION

Each axon conducts action potentials at a constant velocity, but a wide range of conduction velocities have been recorded from different axons because the speed of propagation is proportional to axon diameter and the thickness of its myelination. Large-diameter axons are heavily myelinated and have fast conduction velocities; small-diameter axons are thinly myelinated and have moderate conduction velocities. The thinnest axons have no myelination and extremely slow conduction velocities.

Axon diameter and myelination control conduction velocity through their effects on the length constant of the membrane. As discussed earlier, the length constant varies as a function of the resistive properties of the membrane and cytoplasm. Large-diameter axons have lower cytoplasmic resistance, which allows for more rapid spread of passive depolarization. Thus, in response to an action potential at one point on the membrane, passive Na⁺ currents travel more efficiently through the cytoplasm of a large axon and enhance the velocity of impulse propagation.

Conduction velocity also increases as the resistance of the axon membrane increases. Myelination increases membrane resistance by adding another barrier to prevent the flow of ions from the axoplasm to the extracellular fluid. Because ionic current does not easily pass through the myelinated parts of the axon, incoming Na^+ current flows through the axoplasm until it reaches the next unmyelinated site at the next node of Ranvier. Nodes of Ranvier are spaced at regular intervals along the axon and are functionally different from myelinated parts of the membrane because they contain a much higher density of voltage-gated Na^+ channels. Consequently, an action potential evokes a depolarizing current that flows passively through the axoplasm to the next node of Ranvier and drives the membrane to threshold to produce another action potential. This process is repeated so that action potentials essentially jump from one node of Ranvier to the next. This rapid form of propagation is called saltatory conduction (Figure 1-25).

Myelination
Increases membrane resistance
Increases the membrane length constant
Increases axonal conduction velocity

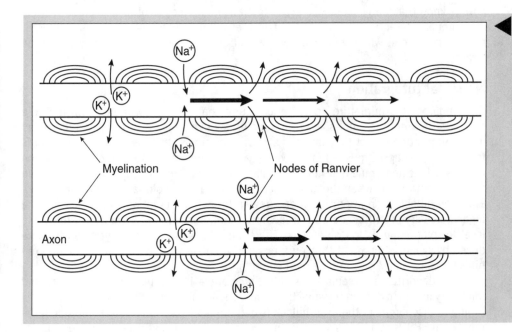

◀ **FIGURE 1-25**
Saltatory Conduction. *Myelination increases the resistance of the axonal membrane and prevents Na^+ from leaving the axon except at the nodes of Ranvier. Current flows passively through the axoplasm and depolarizes the axon to threshold at the next node of Ranvier. This process causes the action potential to propagate more quickly than in unmyelinated axons.*

NEURONAL INTERACTIONS

One of the major functions of the CNS is to integrate information from different sources. For this reason, the brain and spinal cord are organized into nuclei that process specific types of sensory, motor, autonomic, or cognitive information.

Definition of a Nucleus

A nucleus is a compact group of neurons whose connections are organized into functional circuits. The specific function of a nucleus depends on the type of information it receives, the pattern of its intrinsic neuronal circuits, and its projections to other nuclei. The main purpose of most nuclei is to perform some transformation on the input signals so that information useful to the organism can be extracted and sent to other brain regions for further processing.

All nuclei are composed of three basic components: (1) incoming axons and their synaptic terminals, (2) intrinsic neurons, and (3) principal neurons. Intrinsic neurons are called local circuit neurons or interneurons because all of their processes, including their axons, are located within a single nucleus. By comparison, the axon of a principal neuron is usually longer and always projects to other nuclei. Principal neurons are called projection neurons because their axons comprise all of the projection fibers found in the brain and spinal cord.

The specific interconnections between intrinsic and principal neurons determine how information is processed in a nucleus. These interconnections can be extremely

Intrinsic neurons *project locally.* **Principal neurons** *project to other nuclei.*

complex, and few rules govern the types of neuronal connections that may exist within a nucleus. For example, axonal projections may terminate on all neurons in a nucleus or only on certain classes of neurons in specific regions. Thus, incoming axons may have synaptic contacts on intrinsic neurons, principal neurons, or both sets of cells. Within a nucleus, intrinsic neurons may send local projections to other interneurons, to principal neurons, or to both sets of cells. Although principal neurons must project to other nuclei, it is not uncommon for principal neurons to have local collaterals that terminate on neighboring interneurons or on other principal neurons.

The physiologic interactions that occur between neurons within a nucleus or between nuclei are poorly understood and cannot be predicted from their neuronal connections. It was once thought that principal neurons always excite their target nuclei, but now we know that many nuclei can exert inhibitory influences on other nuclei. The variety of neuronal interactions is due to the fact that neurons use a wide range of different neurotransmitters, which produce diverse and complex effects on their postsynaptic targets.

Neuronal Integration

Every neuron is a miniature computational unit that integrates inputs from multiple sources. The dendrites and soma of a neuron usually receive excitatory and inhibitory inputs from hundreds or thousands of synaptic terminals. In general, excitatory inputs from several synapses must summate within a short interval of time to produce an action potential. The membrane potential of a neuron fluctuates continuously and results in an action potential only when the axon hillock reaches a threshold level of depolarization. The axon hillock is an important trigger region for action potentials because it has the highest density of voltage-gated Na^+ channels and, consequently, the lowest threshold level for producing action potentials. Therefore, changes in membrane potential produced by synaptic inputs at the dendrites and soma are usually conducted to the axon hillock before they result in an action potential.

The dendrites and soma constantly integrate a large number of excitatory and inhibitory inputs to determine when the neuron should discharge an action potential. The timing of discharges at the axon hillock is determined by several factors, including the number of EPSPs and IPSPs at a given moment, the spatial configuration of these inputs on the dendritic tree, and the passive membrane properties of the dendrites and soma. The passive membrane properties of a neuron are especially critical for determining how well a neuron can integrate synaptic inputs at separate dendritic sites or at separate points in time.

Excitatory inputs to a single synapse rarely produce action potentials. Instead, neuronal discharges are usually produced when multiple EPSPs are summed together from different synapses. Synaptic inputs to separate dendrites are unlikely to summate, however, unless the dendritic membrane has a long length-constant (Figure 1-26). Long length-constants allow EPSPs produced at one dendritic site to spread towards the soma where they may summate with EPSPs produced in other dendrites. This integrative process is known as spatial summation.

Consecutive inputs to the same synaptic site may also sum together in a process known as temporal summation. To integrate a sequence of inputs arriving at the same synapse, the postsynaptic membrane must have a long time-constant so that the first EPSP will persist long enough to summate with a subsequent EPSP (see Figure 1-26). Differences in the membrane time constant cause substantial differences in the postsynaptic effectiveness of a series of impulses arriving at the same synapse.

The time constant and length constant of a membrane are closely related to the membrane's resistive properties (see equations 8 and 9). Membrane resistance usually fluctuates, however, because ion channels constantly open and close in response to synaptic inputs. Therefore, time constants and length constants are not static qualities for a given neuron but vary continuously as the neuron receives different excitatory and inhibitory inputs. Hence, antecedent synaptic events may alter how a neuron responds to a particular set of inputs by changing the neuron's passive membrane properties.

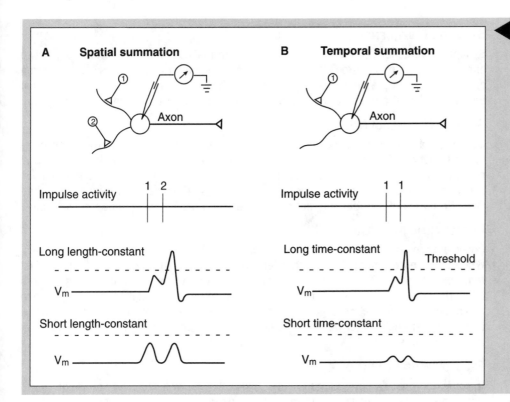

FIGURE 1-26
Spatial and Temporal Summation. (A) A pair of EPSPs produced by neurons 1 and 2 is likely to sum together if the postsynaptic neuron has a long length-constant. (B) A pair of EPSPs produced by consecutive impulses in neuron 1 is likely to sum together if the postsynaptic neuron has a long time-constant.

Synaptic Circuits

The spatial configuration of synaptic connections is extremely important for determining how neurons process information received from multiple sources. Certain synaptic arrangements occur frequently in the CNS and are identified by specific terms. Some of the more common synaptic circuits are illustrated in Figure 1-27.

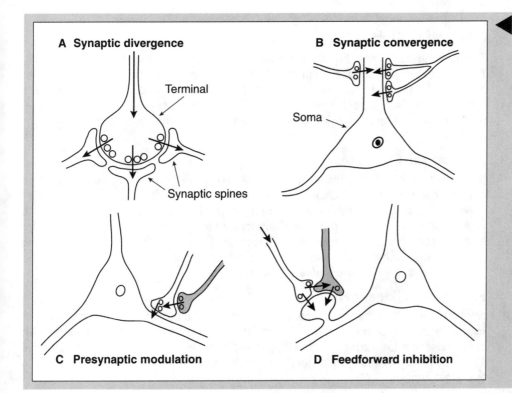

FIGURE 1-27
Synaptic Circuits. (A) Synaptic divergence allows an incoming signal to activate multiple postsynaptic neurons. (B) Synaptic convergence increases the likelihood that a postsynaptic neuron will discharge. (C) Presynaptic modulation is mediated by an axoaxonic synapse that modulates the efficacy of an axodendritic synapse. (D) Synaptic feedforward inhibition occurs when a synaptic terminal simultaneously activates a postsynaptic dendrite and a nearby inhibitory terminal (shaded). This synaptic arrangement produces an EPSP–IPSP sequence in the postsynaptic dendrite.

Synaptic Divergence

Synaptic divergence occurs when one synaptic terminal has functional synapses with two or more postsynaptic neurons. By contacting multiple dendrites, the presynaptic neuron can activate multiple neurons simultaneously. Thus, synaptic divergence is a physical arrangement that amplifies the physiologic influence of an incoming action potential.

Synaptic Convergence

Synaptic convergence occurs whenever multiple terminals synapse on the same postsynaptic neuron. The synaptic terminals may originate from one or many presynaptic neurons and can include inhibitory or excitatory influences. In either case, simultaneous activation of a group of convergent synapses increase the size or strength of the postsynaptic potential. Spatial summation requires the presence of synaptic convergence.

Presynaptic Modulation

Presynaptic modulation is mediated by neuronal circuits involving axoaxonic synapses. When one axon terminates on another terminal, neurotransmitter release from the first terminal alters the Ca^{2+} conductance of the second synaptic terminal. This process alters the amount of neurotransmitter that the second neuron can release in response to an action potential that propagates down its axon. Hence, presynaptic modulation may temporarily strengthen (or weaken) the efficacy of synaptic transmission between other pairs of neurons.

Feedforward Inhibition

In some neurons, synaptic excitation is quickly followed by a secondary phase of inhibition. This sequence of events is mediated by three synaptic processes in which an excitatory terminal forms synaptic contacts on a postsynaptic dendrite and on a neighboring inhibitory terminal (see Figure 1-27D). Neurotransmitter release from the excitatory terminal simultaneously depolarizes the postsynaptic dendrite and the neighboring inhibitory terminal. This causes the inhibitory terminal to release its neurotransmitter at a slight time delay, and the net effect in the postsynaptic dendrite is a rapid sequence of excitation followed by inhibition. Synaptic feedforward inhibition is used to restrict the duration of EPSPs because prolonged excitation can produce deleterious effects in many brain regions. Synaptic feedforward inhibition involves a combination of synaptic divergence, synaptic convergence, and presynaptic modulation.

Neuronal Circuits

There are basic patterns of neuronal connections that are repeated throughout the CNS. These basic patterns are often combined to form more sophisticated neural circuits that process information in specific ways. As shown in Figure 1-28, most neural circuits consist of combinations of the following types of connections: (1) feedforward excitation, (2) feedforward inhibition, (3) lateral inhibition, (4) recurrent inhibition, and (5) disinhibition.

Feedforward Excitation

Most principal neurons in the CNS are excitatory. These neurons frequently project to other excitatory neurons which, in turn, excite other neurons within the nucleus. In other cases, principal neurons may excite different groups of neurons that subsequently excite each other. Such disynaptic patterns of feedforward excitation provide an opportunity for neuronal convergence and divergence. Furthermore, the combination of monosynaptic and disynaptic excitatory connections can alter the timing of postsynaptic excitation and increase the probability of temporal summation.

Feedforward Inhibition

Afferent fibers often branch into collaterals that simultaneously activate populations of excitatory and inhibitory neurons. The inhibitory neurons are usually interneurons that are activated for the purpose of inhibiting the adjacent population of excitatory neurons. This mechanism of feedforward inhibition restricts the duration of neuronal EPSPs in the target nucleus.

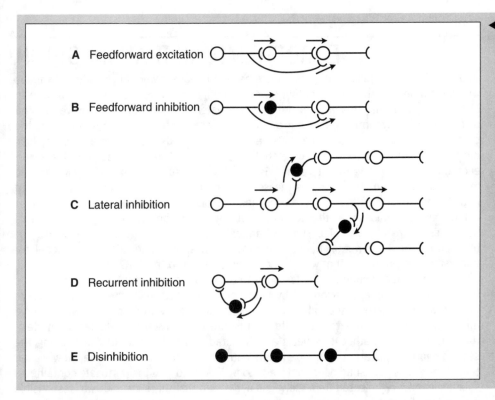

Neuronal Circuits. *Diagrams depict basic circuits found in many nuclei. Excitatory and inhibitory neurons are represented by unfilled and filled soma, respectively. Arrows illustrate the flow of excitatory activity. (A) Feedforward excitation alters the timing of excitatory transmission and provides an opportunity for synaptic divergence and convergence. (B) Feedforward inhibition limits the duration of excitatory activity in the third neuron. (C) Lateral inhibition restricts excitatory activity to a select population of neurons. (D) Recurrent inhibition limits the duration of activity in the first neuron. (E) Disinhibition involves serial connections between two inhibitory neurons. The third neuron is spontaneously active, and its output is regulated by the preceding inhibitory connections.*

Within the figure:
- A   Feedforward excitation
- B   Feedforward inhibition
- C   Lateral inhibition
- D   Recurrent inhibition
- E   Disinhibition

LATERAL INHIBITION

Lateral inhibition is a specific form of feedforward inhibition that restricts excitation to a small population of neurons. Lateral inhibitory connections are often, but not always, mediated by interneurons to enhance the disparity in activity between neighboring populations of neurons. Lateral inhibition is used in neuronal circuits of the visual, auditory, and somatosensory systems where the topographic extent of neuronal excitation is a neural code for representing stimuli in these systems.

RECURRENT INHIBITION

Recurrent inhibition is common throughout the CNS and is characterized by neurons that activate local inhibitory neurons that project back to the original neuron. Recurrent inhibition restricts the duration of repetitive discharges in the excitatory neuron and enhances the temporal resolution of its activity.

DISINHIBITION

Disinhibition occurs when at least two inhibitory neurons are connected in series with other neurons. Activation of the first inhibitory neuron inhibits the second neuron, which, consequently, removes inhibition from the third neuron in the series. Disinhibitory circuits provide more precise control of the discharge rate of the third neuron than direct excitation alone.

IMPORTANCE OF SYNAPTIC LOCATION

All synapses on a neuron are not equally important. Synaptic terminals on distal dendrites may exert less influence on a postsynaptic neuron than synapses on the soma or on the axon hillock. Inhibitory neurons often exploit this situation by forming the majority of synapses near trigger sites on the soma and axon hillock. Because the axon hillock has the lowest threshold for producing an action potential, inhibitory transmission at this site hyperpolarizes the membrane potential and prevents the neuron from discharging in response to excitatory inputs on the dendrites. For the same reason, inhibitory synapses on the dendritic tree are often located at branch points where inhibition would block excitation at either branch from reaching the soma and axon hillock.

Excitatory synapses form the majority of synapses on the dendrites. Inhibitory synapses form the majority of synapses on the soma and axon hillock.

NEUROCHEMICAL TRANSMISSION

In the early 1900s, most neuroanatomists believed neurons were physically continuous with each other and that neural activity spread through the nervous system as if it were an elaborate syncytium. This view of the nervous system was eventually disproved by the discovery of the synaptic cleft, a narrow space that separates axonal terminals from the postsynaptic membrane. But if neurons were not in physical contact with each other, how did they communicate? We now know that most neurons in the CNS communicate with each other by secreting minute quantities of chemical substances from their synaptic terminals. These chemicals act as messengers to produce electrochemical changes in neurons or muscles. Although synaptic transmission between neurons is more complicated than transmission at the neuromuscular junction, both types of neurochemical transmission are similar. In fact, neurochemical transmission was studied extensively at the neuromuscular junction because it provided a simple and accessible model for understanding processes that were later shown to occur in the CNS.

The presence of chemical transmitters in the nervous system was first demonstrated in a classic experiment performed by Otto Loewi in 1920. In this experiment, Loewi placed two frog hearts in separate chambers and electrically stimulated the vagus nerve innervating one of the hearts to slow its rate of contraction. He then collected a sample of the perfusate that bathed this heart and injected it into the chamber containing the second heart. Application of this perfusate caused the second heart to beat slower even though its vagus nerve had been removed. Loewi deduced that the perfusate contained a substance that was released from the vagus nerve, and that this substance was responsible for slowing the rate of contraction in both hearts. This substance was later identified as acetylcholine (ACh), the first chemical substance to be recognized as a neurotransmitter.

Criteria for Defining a Neurotransmitter

A neurotransmitter is any chemical released from neurons that changes the electrical activity of other neurons or of muscles. Although this definition is conceptually simple, it is not easy to identify which chemicals act as neurotransmitters, and formal criteria have been developed to determine whether a chemical compound should be classified as a neurotransmitter.

1. *The chemical must be present in the presynaptic neuron.* The chemical must be located presynaptically, preferably in the vesicles of the presynaptic bouton. As part of this criterion, the presynaptic neuron must contain the precursor molecules and synthetic enzymes for manufacturing the neurotransmitter.

2. *The chemical must be released from the presynaptic neuron during depolarization.* Although the chemical might be synthesized in the presynaptic neuron and reside in the presynaptic bouton, it must also be released from the presynaptic axon terminal when the axon conducts action potentials or is electrically stimulated. Furthermore, this process should occur in a Ca^{2+}-dependent manner.

3. *Application of the chemical to a postsynaptic neuron must mimic the physiological response produced by presynaptic stimulation.* The postsynaptic receptors should mediate identical responses when the chemical is released from the presynaptic terminal or applied exogenously. This criterion is also satisfied by showing that application of an antagonist blocks the synaptic response as well as the response to exogenous application of the neurotransmitter.

4. *There must be a mechanism for inactivating the chemical at the synapse.* Neurotransmitters usually have brief effects on the postsynaptic neuron because they are inactivated either by degradative enzymes, selective reuptake into the presynaptic nerve terminals, or uptake into adjacent glial cells. Diffusion of the neurotransmitter through the extracellular space may augment these inactivating mechanisms.

When all of these criteria are satisfied, the chemical's function as a neurotransmitter is firmly established. The identity of many neurotransmitters is still uncertain, however, because many experiments are required to satisfy these criteria. More than 100 chemicals in the nervous system meet some of these criteria, and these chemicals are called putative neurotransmitters.

Neurotransmitters are divided into two main groups: small-molecule neurotransmitters and neuropeptides. Small-molecule neurotransmitters include substances such as ACh, biogenic amines (e.g. dopamine), and small amino acids (e.g. glutamate). Neuropeptides, on the other hand, are composed of 3–35 amino acids and include the opioid peptides, pituitary peptides, and peptides that have additional functions in the gastrointestinal tract. A partial list of compounds that are considered neurotransmitters are listed in Table 1-3.

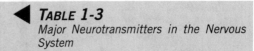

TABLE 1-3
Major Neurotransmitters in the Nervous System

Small Molecules	Neuropeptides
Biogenic amines	**Opioid peptides**
Acetylcholine	Leucine enkephalin
Dopamine	Methionine enkephalin
Norepinephrine	β-Endorphin
Epinephrine	Dynorphins
Serotonin	
Histamine	**Pituitary peptides**
	Oxytocin
Amino acids	Vasopressin
Aspartate	Adrenocorticotropic hormone
γ-Aminobutyric acid	Thyroid-stimulating hormone
Glutamate	
Glycine	**Gastrointestinal peptides**
Homocysteine	Cholecystokinin
Taurine	Substance P
	Neurotensin
Nucleotides	Gastrin
Adenosine	Insulin
Adenosine triphosphate	Glucagon
	Somatostatin
Retrograde	
Nitric oxide	**Others**
	Angiotensin
	Bradykinin
	Neuropeptide Y

SMALL-MOLECULE NEUROTRANSMITTERS

Small-molecule neurotransmitters are produced by short biosynthetic pathways involving substrates derived from carbohydrate metabolism. The enzymes for synthesizing these neurotransmitters are produced by free polysomes in the soma's cytoplasm. These enzymes and the neurotransmitter precursor are then moved to the synaptic endings by slow axoplasmic transport. The enzyme converts the small precursor molecule into a neurotransmitter, and this reaction usually occurs in the synaptic cytosol. After synthesis, small-molecule neurotransmitters are transported from the cytosol into synaptic vesicles by an ATP-dependent pump (or transporter) located in the vesicular membrane. Neurotransmitters are sequestered in vesicles to protect them from enzymatic degradation and to provide a mechanism for releasing precise quantities of neurotransmitter into the synaptic cleft during neurotransmission. Some of the small-molecule neurotransmitters are contained in small (40–60 nm), translucent vesicles whereas other neurotransmitters, especially the biogenic amines, are packaged in small (40–60 nm) or medium-sized (90–120 nm) dense-core vesicles.

Small-molecule neurotransmitters are synthesized in the synaptic terminal cytosol.

NEUROPEPTIDES

Neuropeptide synthesis occurs within the soma and involves genetic transcription. Large polypeptide molecules are synthesized by a series of reactions that take place in the RER. Newly synthesized polypeptides are transported to the Golgi apparatus, which packages the polypeptide into a vesicle. Subsequently, the polypeptide is broken into several smaller molecules by a series of steps involving proteolytic cleavage, glycosylation,

Neuropeptides are synthesized in the soma for vesicular transport through the axon.

phosphorylation, and other chemical reactions. Vesicles containing neuropeptides are rapidly transported through the axon by microtubules until they reach the synaptic terminal. Synaptic terminals with neuropeptides usually contain medium-sized (90–120 nm) or large (200–250) vesicles with a granular or electron-dense core.

NEUROPEPTIDES AND SMALL-MOLECULE NEUROTRANSMITTERS ARE CO-LOCALIZED

Neurons may synthesize more than one neurotransmitter, and it is not unusual to observe different types of synaptic vesicles in the same synaptic terminal (Figure 1-29). Although some neurons contain more than one neuropeptide, it is extremely rare for a neuron to synthesize more than one of the small-molecule neurotransmitters. Many neurons, however, contain one type of small-molecule neurotransmitter and at least one type of neuropeptide. In neurons that contain both types of neurotransmitters, the small-molecule neurotransmitters are located in the smaller vesicles, whereas the neuropeptides are located in large, dense-core vesicles. The small vesicles are generally docked closest to the active sites on the presynaptic membrane, while the dense-core vesicles tend to be located further away from the active sites. Because of this differential location, small vesicles release their contents sooner than the dense-core vesicles. Furthermore, the small vesicles fuse with the presynaptic membrane in response to low rates of neuronal discharges, whereas the dense-core vesicles require higher rates of neuronal activity before they release their neuropeptides into the synaptic cleft. Thus, the presence of two types of neurotransmitter in a synapse provides many neurons with two modes of neurochemical transmission.

Small-molecule neurotransmitters are in small (40–60 nm), clear vesicles. *Biogenic amines* are in small (40–60 nm) or medium (90–120) vesicles with a dense core. *Neuropeptides* are in medium (90–120 nm) or large (200–250 nm) vesicles with a dense core.

FIGURE 1-29 ▶
Co-localization of Translucent and Dense-Core Vesicles. Synaptic terminals in the hypothalamus contain small translucent vesicles and large vesicles with a dense granular core. The former contain small molecule transmitters, the latter contain neuropeptides. Unlike most synapses, many hypothalamic terminals release neurotransmitters into the extracellular space for diffusion into nearby blood vessels. (Courtesy of Ms. Tina Rutherford and Dr. Robert Page, Pennsylvania State University College of Medicine, Hershey, Pennsylvania.)

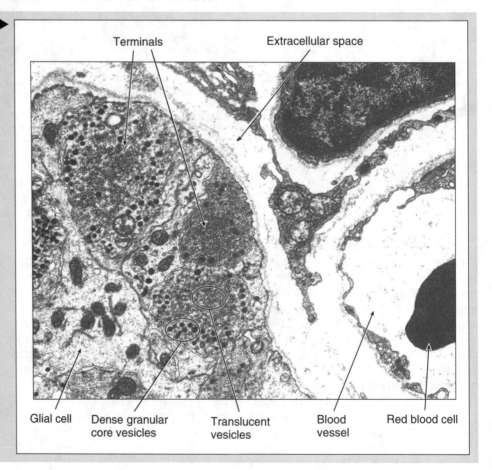

Properties of the Major Neurotransmitters

Although many different neurotransmitters are used by the nervous system, some are more prevalent and have been studied more intensively. This section briefly describes the major neurotransmitters, their distribution, functional importance, and biosynthetic and inactivation pathways.

ACETYLCHOLINE

ACh is the major neurotransmitter of the PNS. It is present at all neuromuscular junctions, in preganglionic neurons of the sympathetic system, and in the preganglionic and postganglionic neurons of the parasympathetic system. ACh is also present in the CNS, especially in the brainstem tegmentum and in the ventral forebrain. ACh acts as an excitatory neurotransmitter at the neuromuscular junction and at most synapses in the CNS and PNS.

ACh is synthesized from acetyl coenzyme A (acetyl CoA) and choline in a reaction catalyzed by the enzyme choline acetyltransferase (Figure 1-30). Acetyl CoA is derived from pyruvate generated during glycolysis; the choline precursor is transported across the presynaptic membrane by a transporter molecule. After ACh is released into the synaptic cleft, its effect on the postsynaptic receptors is terminated by a hydrolytic enzyme, acetylcholinesterase (AChE). The synaptic cleft contains high concentrations of AChE, which catalyzes ACh into acetate and choline. Choline in the synapse and extracellular fluid is transported into the synaptic ending where it is recycled into another ACh molecule.

> **Acetylcholine** is located in the following:
> Neuromuscular junctions
> Sympathetic and parasympathetic ganglia
> Brainstem tegmentum
> Ventral forebrain and cerebral cortex

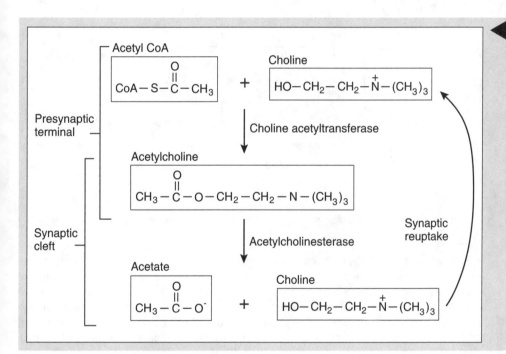

FIGURE 1-30

Acetylcholine Metabolism. *Acetylcholine (ACh) is synthesized from acetyl CoA and choline in the presynaptic terminal. After its release into the synaptic cleft, ACh is metabolized into acetate and choline, and the latter is transported into the synaptic terminal and recycled into ACh.*

Numerous compounds have been developed that interact at peripheral cholinergic synapses. Organophosphates, such as mustard gas and a variety of insecticides, derive their lethal properties by irreversibly binding to AChE and preventing the hydrolysis of ACh. These anticholinesterases allow ACh to accumulate at the neuromuscular junction, thereby causing extended depolarization of the muscle, which renders it insensitive to subsequent ACh release. Consequently, exposure to these chemicals leads to death because of respiratory paralysis.

In the cerebral cortex, ACh modulates synaptic interactions and is necessary for normal cognitive functions. ACh enhances neuronal responses to other noncholinergic inputs, and its loss has been implicated in Alzheimer's disease, a form of dementia that is associated with profound memory loss. Pharmacologic intervention with anticholinesterases has shown some therapeutic effects in ameliorating some of these cognitive symptoms and is currently used to treat Alzheimer's disease.

GLUTAMATE

Glutamate is an excitatory neurotransmitter that has been found in virtually every brain region. It is likely that glutamate is released from at least half of the brain's synapses.

Glutamate is a fast-acting excitatory neurotransmitter that is found in virtually every region of the brain.

Glutamate is the neurotransmitter that is used by most principal neurons for relaying excitatory signals from one nucleus to another in the CNS.

Glutamate is an amino acid that is synthesized in synaptic terminals from glutamine (Figure 1-31). The conversion to glutamate is catalyzed by the mitochondrial enzyme glutaminase. Once glutamate is released at a synapse, it is quickly removed by high-affinity glutamate transporters located on glial cells and on presynaptic terminals. Glial cells contain an enzyme, glutamine synthetase, which converts glutamate to glutamine. The glutamine is then released from the glial cells and transported into glutamatergic terminals where it is recycled into another glutamate molecule.

FIGURE 1-31

Glutamate Metabolism. Glutamate is synthesized from glutamine in the presynaptic terminal. Following synaptic release, glutamate is transported into surrounding glial cells where it is converted into glutamine.

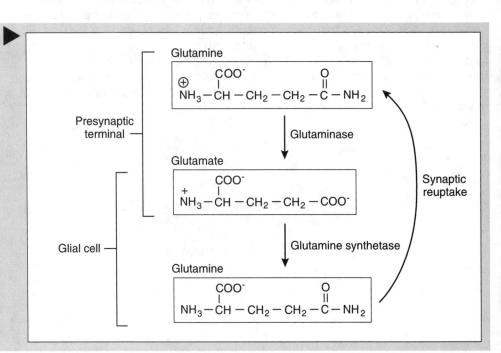

High concentrations of glutamate have toxic effects on neurons.

Glutamate Excitotoxicity, Ischemia, and Epilepsy. Excessive levels of extracellular glutamate can overstimulate neurons and cause them to die. In animals, a diet high in glutamate is correlated with neuronal degeneration in the retina and in other brain regions. Glutamate toxicity results from the excessive activation of postsynaptic receptors that open Ca^{2+} channels. The increase in Ca^{2+} influx activates Ca^{2+}-dependent proteases in postsynaptic cells, and these proteases can produce free radicals, which damage the neuron's plasma membrane and its cytoplasmic organelles.

Glutamate-induced neurotoxicity may explain the relationship between ischemia (a reduction in blood flow) and subsequent brain damage. When a cerebral blood vessel is occluded, even for a short period of time, the extracellular glutamate concentration increases significantly. Extracellular glutamate rises to toxic levels because glutamate reuptake into synaptic terminals is an energy-dependent process, which slows down when oxygen is unavailable. Recent studies have shown that glutamate antagonists, which block the receptors mediating Ca^{2+} influx, can reduce the amount of neuronal damage that occurs during ischemia.

Glutamate excitotoxicity may also be responsible for the repetitive nature of epileptic seizures. Epilepsy is a neurologic disease that is mediated by excessive neuronal activity in the hippocampal formation or cerebral cortex. Excessive neural activity in these regions increases the extracellular concentration of glutamate, and this may have toxic effects on other neurons, especially inhibitory interneurons. Samples of the cerebral cortex from animals or individuals suffering from epileptic seizures show a significant loss of neurons that use γ-aminobutyric acid (GABA) as an inhibitory neurotransmitter. Synaptic release of GABA suppresses neuronal activity, and loss of GABAergic neurons during an epileptic episode is thought to increase the probability and severity of subsequent seizures. In fact, most anticonvulsant drugs act by enhancing GABAergic inhibition. Thus, epileptic seizures are treated mainly by suppressing the activity of neurons that release glutamate.

GABA AND GLYCINE

GABA and glycine are the main inhibitory neurotransmitters used by neurons in the CNS. Most brain areas contain GABAergic neurons, but glycine is distributed mainly in the spinal cord. Neurons that use GABA or glycine play an important role in preventing prolonged neuronal excitation. GABAergic terminals often form "baskets" or "pericellular nests" of inhibitory synapses around the soma of certain types of neurons. By opening Cl^- channels in the postsynaptic membrane, GABAergic transmission holds the membrane potential of the soma and axon hillock at subthreshold levels. Hence, inhibitory synapses located near the axon hillock can effectively prevent EPSPs in the distal dendrites from initiating action potentials.

GABA is synthesized from glutamate by glutamate decarboxylase (GAD), an enzyme found only in neurons using GABA as a neurotransmitter (Figure 1-32). Pyridoxal phosphate, a vitamin B_6 derivative, is an essential cofactor for GAD activity. Insufficient amounts of vitamin B_6 in the diet cause a decrease in GABA synthesis and can lead to seizures. Many types of neurons and glial cells contain specific transporter molecules that remove GABA from the synaptic cleft. Extracellular GABA that is transported into

GABA is a fast-acting inhibitory neurotransmitter that is found in many local circuit neurons in most areas of the brain.

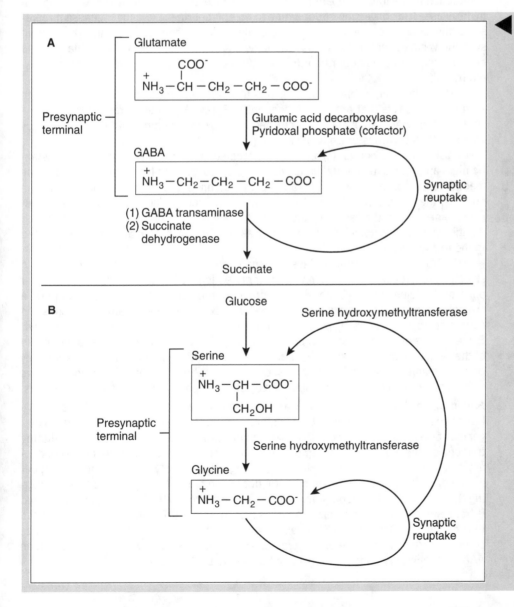

FIGURE 1-32
GABA and Glycine Metabolism. *(A) γ-Aminobutyric acid (GABA) is synthesized from glutamate in the presynaptic terminal. After synaptic release, GABA is either transported back into the terminal or metabolized into succinate via the tricarboxylic acid cycle. (B) Glycine is synthesized from serine by mitochondrial enzymes. After synaptic release, glycine is transported into the synaptic terminal for recycling.*

GABAergic terminals is recycled for subsequent synaptic transmission, whereas GABA taken into other types of neurons or glial cells is converted into succinate as part of the tricarboxylic acid cycle, which produces ATP. In this latter pathway, GABA is degraded by GABA transaminase to form succinic semialdehyde, which is then metabolized by succinic semialdehyde dehydrogenase. Both of the enzymes in this metabolic pathway are in mitochondria, which are located in synaptic terminals. Inhibiting these enzymes causes an increase in extracellular GABA, and inhibitors of GABA transaminase are widely used as anticonvulsants.

Glycine is synthesized from serine by a mitochondrial enzyme, serine hydroxymethyltransferase. After its synaptic release, glycine is removed from the synaptic cleft by transporters on the synaptic terminals and is recycled into synaptic vesicles.

CATECHOLAMINES

Dopamine, norepinephrine, and epinephrine are called catecholamines because they contain an amine group attached to a catechol (6 carbon ring with two hydroxyl groups). These neurotransmitters are similar in their molecular structure, and all are derived from the same dietary amino acid, tyrosine (Figure 1-33). Tyrosine is converted by tyrosine hydroxylase to dihydroxyphenylalanine (L-dopa). Tyrosine hydroxylase is the rate-limiting enzyme in catecholamine production and is present in all catecholaminergic neurons. Next, L-dopa is converted to dopamine by aromatic amino acid decarboxylase (AAAD). In noradrenergic neurons, dopamine is converted to norepinephrine by dopamine-β-hydroxylase. The conversion of dopamine to norepinephrine is unusual because it represents the only case where a small molecule neurotransmitter is synthesized within synaptic vesicles, not in the cytosol. Finally, a small percentage of catecholaminergic neurons convert norepinephrine into epinephrine by means of phenylethanolamine-*N*-methyltransferase.

Catecholaminergic transmission is inactivated by synaptic reuptake involving high affinity transporters that are Na^+-dependent ATPases. After being transported into the synaptic terminal, catecholamines are degraded by monoamine oxidase (MAO) or by catechol *O*-methyltransferase (COMT).

Most dopamine-containing neurons are located in two midbrain nuclei, the substantia nigra and ventral tegmental area, which project rostrally to the basal ganglia and the medial frontal cortex. Almost all noradrenergic neurons are located in a single brainstem nucleus, the locus ceruleus. The locus ceruleus projects diffusely throughout the neuraxis, especially to the telencephalon and the brainstem. Compared to dopamine and norepinephrine, few nuclei use epinephrine as a neurotransmitter, and these are located in the rostral part of the medulla.

Catecholamines are localized in a few discrete brain regions and regulate the forebrain circuits mediating mood and arousal.

One function of catecholamines is to modulate the overall tone of neural activity in selected brain regions. Consistent with their projections to the limbic forebrain and other parts of the telencephalon, the level of activity in the catecholamine pathways plays a critical role in regulating psychological mood. A decrease in catecholamine transmission causes depression, a serious psychiatric disorder that may lead to suicide if not treated. Some classes of antidepressants act by inhibiting MAO or by blocking synaptic reuptake of the catecholamines. On the other hand, excessive catecholaminergic stimulation may produce mania or psychotic illnesses such as schizophrenia. Most antipsychotic drugs interfere with catecholamine transmission by blocking postsynaptic dopamine receptors.

Parkinsonism. Parkinson's disease is a neurodegenerative disorder produced by selective loss of dopaminergic neurons in the substantia nigra. Parkinsonism is characterized by a general poverty of locomotor activity, an increase in muscular rigidity, and oscillating tremors of the head and forelimbs. Although the exact relationship between dopaminergic transmission and its role in regulating motor activity is poorly understood, our knowledge of the biosynthetic pathway for dopamine presents an opportunity for managing this disease. Unlike dopamine, L-dopa can pass through the blood–brain barrier and is transported into the terminals of neurons that contain AAAD where L-dopa is converted into dopamine. Because AAAD is also located in the periphery and may metabolize L-dopa before it crosses the blood–brain barrier, L-dopa is usually administered with an AAAD inhibitor, carbidopa, that does not cross the blood–brain barrier.

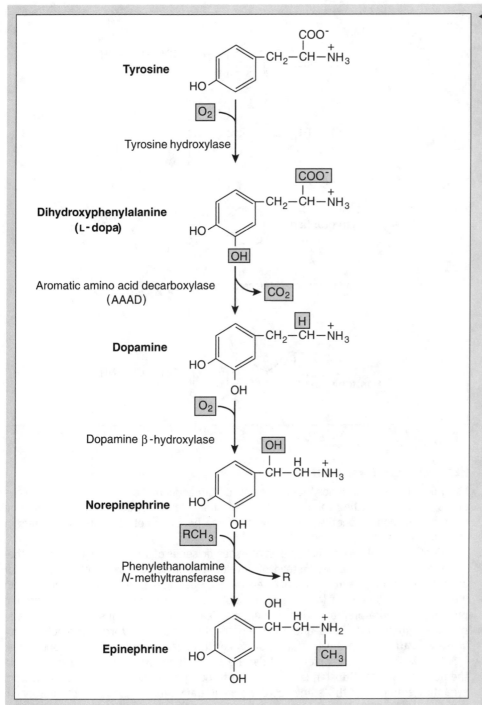

FIGURE 1-33

Catecholamine Metabolism. Tyrosine is a necessary amino acid precursor for the biosynthesis of dopamine, norepinephrine, and epinephrine. Tyrosine hydroxylase is the rate-limiting enzyme for synthesizing these catecholamines. AAAD = aromatic amino acid decarboxylase.

SEROTONIN

Serotonin (5-hydroxytryptamine, 5-HT) is synthesized from tryptophan, a common amino acid, which is obtained in the diet. Tryptophan is selectively transported into serotonergic neurons where it is converted into serotonin by the rate-limiting enzyme, tryptophan hydroxylase (Figure 1-34). Serotonin is found in the raphe nuclei located along the midline of the brainstem. The raphe nuclei have diffuse ascending and descending pathways that innervate widespread regions of the telencephalon, diencephalon, and spinal cord. Serotonergic transmission has been implicated in the regulation of mood and plays a critical role in controlling different states of arousal (i.e., sleep, wakefulness).

FIGURE 1-34 ▶

Serotonin Metabolism. The amino acid tryptophan is converted into serotonin by tryptophan hydroxylase and aromatic amino acid decarboxylase (AAAD). 5-HT = hydroxytryptamine.

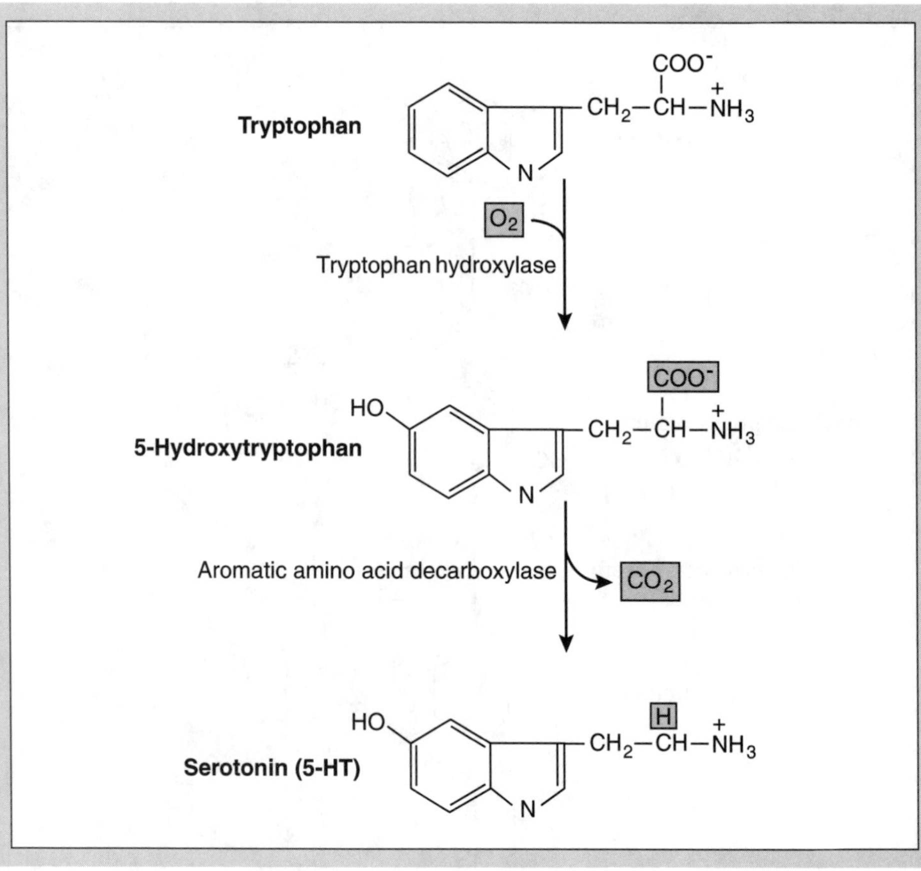

PEPTIDE NEUROTRANSMITTERS

Many peptides are hormones that are released from endocrine cells or endocrine regions of the brain such as the hypothalamus and pituitary gland. In addition to their hormone functions at their respective target organs, some peptides act as neurotransmitters in specific regions of the PNS and CNS.

Peptide neurotransmitters consist of a specific series of amino acids that are synthesized in the neuronal soma. Instead of developing a specific biosynthetic pathway for each neuropeptide, neurons produce several neuropeptides from a much larger protein molecule that contains a long series of peptides (Figure 1-35). The original protein precursor, called a prepropeptide, undergoes cleavage of its initial signal sequence to produce a propeptide. Subsequently, the propeptide undergoes further proteolytic processing that results in the formation of its constituent molecules, the neuropeptides.

Substance P and the opioid peptides are among the most studied neuropeptides in the nervous system. Substance P is located in peripheral nerves and is released from synaptic terminals in the spinal cord where it transmits nociceptive information in response to peripheral tissue damage. Opioid peptides in the spinal cord antagonize substance P neurotransmission and suppress the perception of pain. There are at least two dozen opioid peptides, and they are grouped into three major classes: endorphins, enkephalins, and dynorphins. All of the opioid peptides have central effects that, to a greater or lesser degree, are mimicked by morphine or other narcotic drugs. The opioid peptides are distributed throughout the brain and play a major role in the behavioral response to pain and other forms of stress.

One prepropeptide molecule may serve as a precursor for many neuropeptide molecules.

Synaptic Transmission

Synaptic transmission is a complex process initiated by the arrival of action potentials at the synaptic terminal. The terminal responds by releasing one or more neurotransmitters into the synaptic cleft. After diffusing across the synapse, the neurotransmitter causes an excitatory or inhibitory response in the postsynaptic element. Although some details in

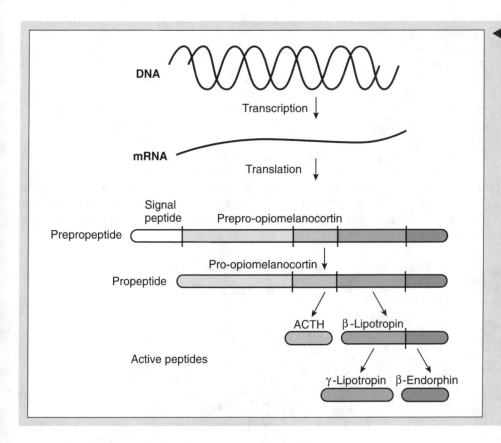

DNA

Transcription ↓

mRNA

Translation ↓

Signal peptide   Prepro-opiomelanocortin

Prepropeptide

Pro-opiomelanocortin ↓

Propeptide

ACTH   β-Lipotropin

Active peptides

γ-Lipotropin   β-Endorphin

FIGURE 1-35
Neuropeptide Synthesis. *The opioid peptides are synthesized in the soma and involve genetic transcription and translation to produce large polypeptides that act as precursor molecules. Subsequent cleavage of the prepropeptide leads to the production of several smaller neuropeptides. ACTH = adrenocorticotropic hormone.*

this process are not completely understood, the basic mechanisms of synaptic transmission have been elucidated.

SYNAPTIC MORPHOLOGY

Most neurochemical synapses in the CNS are formed by synaptic terminals on the dendrites of postsynaptic neurons (see Figure 1-6). A number of metabolic processes occur within synaptic terminals, and many mitochondria are needed to provide energy for these processes. Synaptic boutons also contain many synaptic vesicles to maintain a reservoir of releasable neurotransmitter molecules. These vesicles tend to aggregate near active sites in the presynaptic membrane so that they can release their contents into the synaptic cleft immediately following the arrival of an action potential. Synaptic clefts are narrow, no more than 20–50 nm wide, and neurotransmitter molecules can diffuse across this space in a fraction of a millisecond. The postsynaptic membrane contains specific receptors that bind neurotransmitter molecules released from the presynaptic neuron.

Synapses are often classified according to their ultrastructural appearance. Asymmetric synapses have clear round vesicles and a prominent postsynaptic density, which is noticeably thicker than the presynaptic membrane. By comparison, the presynaptic and postsynaptic membranes of symmetric synapses are the same thickness, and the synaptic vesicles tend to be oval or flattened. Originally it was thought that asymmetric synapses were excitatory and symmetric synapses were inhibitory, but physiologic studies have shown that the excitatory or inhibitory effects of a neurotransmitter are determined by the type of neurotransmitter receptors in the postsynaptic membrane. Furthermore, there is no correlation between the presence of dense-core vesicles or small translucent vesicles and the physiologic response produced in the postsynaptic neuron. Thus, the structure of a synaptic vesicle is not a reliable indicator of its synaptic function.

The physiologic effects of a neurotransmitter are determined by the postsynaptic receptors.

MECHANISM OF NEUROTRANSMITTER RELEASE

The general sequence of events occurring during synaptic transmission are shown schematically in Figure 1-36. When an action potential reaches the synaptic terminal, the

Depolarization of the synaptic terminal allows Ca^{2+} influx to mediate neurotransmitter release.

incoming depolarization activates voltage-gated Ca^{2+} channels located throughout the presynaptic membrane. Opening these channels allows Ca^{2+} to enter the terminals by flowing down its concentration gradient. The influx of Ca^{2+} activates several Ca^{2+}-sensitive proteins in the synaptic terminal, many of which cause the vesicular membrane to fuse with "active sites" in the presynaptic membrane. Neither the proteins involved in this process nor the mechanism by which Ca^{2+} mediates vesicular fusion with the presynaptic membrane are precisely known. Vesicular fusion causes the vesicle to release its neurotransmitter into the synaptic cleft, and the neurotransmitter molecules diffuse across the synaptic cleft where they bind to specific receptors in the postsynaptic membrane. Neurotransmitter molecules interact with different types of postsynaptic receptors and cause an increase (or sometimes a decrease) in the permeability of specific ion channels. The resulting change in ionic current alters the membrane potential of the postsynaptic neuron, and this increases or decreases the probability that an action potential will be initiated.

FIGURE 1-36

Neurochemical Transmission. *Depolarization causes synaptic vesicles to fuse with the presynaptic membrane and release their neurotransmitters. Although vesicles are originally produced in the soma and transported to the terminal by microtubules, segments of the presynaptic membrane are retrieved and recycled into synaptic vesicles by an endosome.*

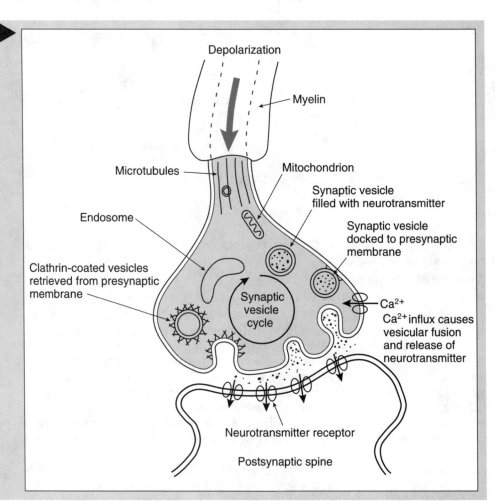

Depolarization

Myelin

Microtubules

Mitochondrion

Synaptic vesicle filled with neurotransmitter

Synaptic vesicle docked to presynaptic membrane

Endosome

Clathrin-coated vesicles retrieved from presynaptic membrane

Synaptic vesicle cycle

Ca^{2+}

Ca^{2+} influx causes vesicular fusion and release of neurotransmitter

Neurotransmitter receptor

Postsynaptic spine

RECYCLING OF SYNAPTIC VESICLES

When synaptic vesicles fuse with the presynaptic membrane, there is a temporary increase in the amount of membrane in the synaptic terminal. The surface area of a synaptic terminal fluctuates within certain limits but is prevented from unlimited expansion because the presynaptic membrane is used to form new synaptic vesicles (see Figure 1-36). On the lateral edge of the synaptic terminal, away from the active sites, small segments of the plasma membrane invaginate and are pinched off from the presynaptic membrane to form clathrin-coated vesicles. Subsequently, these coated vesicles merge into an intracellular organelle, the endosome, which recycles the segments of presynaptic membrane into new vesicles. When a newly formed vesicle emerges from the endosome, neurotransmitter molecules are pumped into the vesicle from the cytosol. Once loaded with neurotransmitter, the vesicle migrates to active sites in the synapse and docks with the presynaptic membrane until fusion occurs. This sequence of events occurs repeatedly and is called the synaptic vesicle cycle.

Neuromuscular Junctions

A neuromuscular junction is a special type of synapse formed by the terminal of a peripheral motor neuron and a skeletal muscle fiber (Figure 1-37). Motor nerves have beaded synaptic terminals called motor end-plates because they resemble a collection of saucers. Unlike central synapses, which may employ a variety of different neurotransmitters, all motor neurons release ACh from their terminal end-plates to cause contraction of skeletal muscle fibers. ACh is the only neurotransmitter that is released at the neuromuscular junction; thus, there is no mechanism by which peripheral nerves may directly inhibit muscle fibers from contracting.

Motor end-plates are motor neuron terminals at the neuromuscular junction.

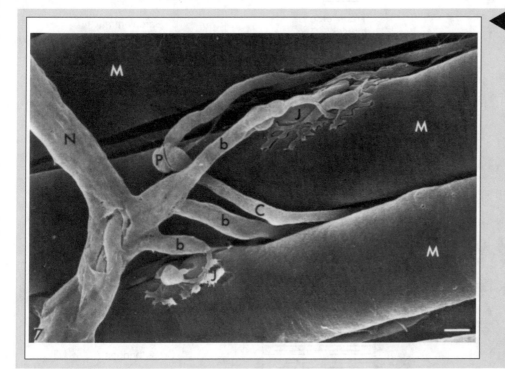

FIGURE 1-37
Neuromuscular Junctions. This scanning electron micrograph depicts neuromuscular junctions in the sternothyroid muscle of a hamster. The peripheral nerve fiber (N) has collateral branches (b) which form junctions (J) with individual motor nerve fibers (M). A capillary (C) and pericyte (P) are also present. (Source: Reprinted with permission from Desaki J, Uehara Y: The overall morphology of neuromuscular junctions as revealed by scanning EM. Neurocytol J 10:107, 1981.

ACh release at the neuromuscular junction resembles the process of chemical transmission at synapses in the CNS. An invading action potential depolarizes the motor end-plate, and this opens the voltage-gated Ca^{2+} channels. The immediate influx of Ca^{2+} causes the synaptic vesicles to fuse with the presynaptic membrane and release ACh into the cleft separating the motor end-plate from the muscle fiber.

Cholinergic transmission at the neuromuscular junction causes a rapid sequence of events that leads to muscular contraction (Figure 1-38). First, ACh molecules diffuse across the neuromuscular junction to activate cholinergic receptors lining a delicate membrane, the sarcolemma, which surrounds all striated muscle and lies on the postsynaptic side of the neuromuscular junction. Activation of cholinergic receptors causes an influx of Na^+ that produces a localized depolarization known as an end-plate potential. The end-plate potential opens voltage-gated Na^+ channels and produces an action potential similar to action potentials in a neuronal axon. Once initiated, the action potential travels across the surface of the muscle cell and into transverse tubules, which perforate the muscle at regular intervals. Propagation of the action potential through the transverse tubules stimulates Ca^{2+} release from the lateral sacs of the sarcoplasmic reticulum, a cylindrical network of membranous tubules that envelop each myofibril.

FIGURE 1-38 ▶

Muscle Fibers. Muscles are composed of actin and myosin filaments. Cross-bridges between the actin and myosin fibers are activated by Ca²⁺ released from the lateral sacs of the sarcoplasmic reticulum (shown in the upper myofibril). Muscle contraction is driven by small movements of the cross-bridges, which force the actin and myosin filaments to move in opposite directions.

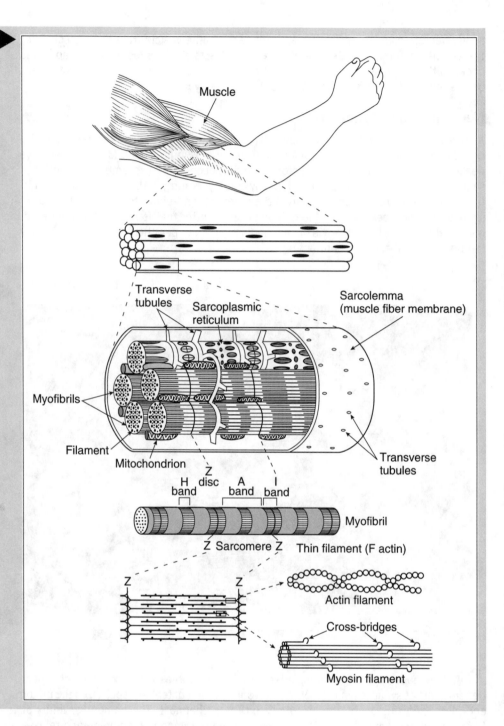

The sudden release of Ca^{2+} into myofibrils initiates contraction of the muscle by activating movements of the cross-bridges that link the myosin and actin filaments.

QUANTAL RELEASE OF ACETYLCHOLINE

Microelectrode recordings have shown that individual muscle fibers develop extremely small end-plate potentials in the absence of impulses in the motor nerve fiber. These potentials, called miniature end-plate potentials, occur spontaneously but are too weak to generate action potentials in the sarcolemma of the muscle fiber. Miniature end-plate potentials have an extremely small amplitude, which is remarkably constant across different muscles. Careful measurements of the larger end-plate potentials indicate that their amplitudes are integer multiples of the amplitude of a miniature end-plate potential. This suggests that a miniature end-plate potential represents the effect of a single synaptic vesicle releasing its reservoir of ACh. Each synaptic vesicle is thought to hold an incremental volume or "quantum" of neurotransmitter. Synaptic vesicles in the motor

Each synaptic vesicle releases a discrete quantity or "quantum" of neurotransmitter.

end-plates appear identical in size, and each one is estimated to contain about 10,000 molecules of ACh.

Neurotransmitter Receptors

Postsynaptic receptors respond to specific neurotransmitter molecules in the synaptic cleft by altering the flow of ionic currents through specific channels in the plasma membrane. One major difference between chemical transmission at neuromuscular junctions and neuronal synapses is the diversity of postsynaptic responses that can be mediated by neurotransmitters in the CNS. Whereas neuromuscular junctions use ACh to produce rapid depolarization and contraction of muscle fibers, CNS synapses release neurotransmitters that produce a variety of postsynaptic effects. When a neurotransmitter binds to a postsynaptic receptor in the CNS, the membrane potential may move closer to or away from the threshold level for initiating an action potential. Many postsynaptic receptors have been identified for most putative neurotransmitters, and the variety of receptor subtypes is reflected by the diversity of postsynaptic responses evoked by a given neurotransmitter. This is an important functional property of the CNS because a neuron must release the same neurotransmitter from all of its axonal collaterals. The different types of postsynaptic receptors enable collateral branches of a neuron to produce divergent responses in different regions of the brain.

Many clinical drugs used to treat psychiatric illnesses achieve their therapeutic effects by blocking neurotransmitter receptors. As more is learned about the pharmacokinetics of different receptor subtypes, it is hoped that this information can be used to design drugs that act with greater receptor specificity. Thus, it may be possible to develop drugs that ameliorate certain symptoms yet produce fewer unwanted side effects.

Two major classes of neurotransmitter receptor are recognized based on their mechanisms for changing the postsynaptic membrane potential. One group of neurotransmitter receptors are called ionotropic or ligand-gated ion channels because the neurotransmitter receptor and the ion channel are a single entity. In contrast, metabotropic or G-protein–coupled receptors are physically separated from the ion channel, but are able to control its conductance indirectly through a series of metabolic steps.

IONOTROPIC RECEPTORS

Ionotropic receptors are usually composed of five protein subunits that span the plasma membrane to form a pentameric structure that encircles a central water-filled pore or channel (Figure 1-39). The protein subunits extend into the synaptic cleft where their extracellular domain contains a site for binding a neurotransmitter molecule or other ligands having a structure similar to the endogenous transmitter. Neurotransmitter binding produces a conformational change in the protein subunit that enables an increase (or decrease) in the conductance of the ion channel. This change in ionic conductance is usually independent of membrane potential. Once the ion channel is open, however, the driving force of ionic current through the channel is proportional to the difference between the membrane potential and the equilibrium potential for the flowing ions.

> **Ionotropic Receptors**
> Neurotransmitter receptor and ion channel are linked.
> Receptor activation alters channel conductance rapidly.

Ionotropic receptors are located at synapses where a rapid response to presynaptic activity is required. Ionotropic receptors produce rapid changes in membrane potentials because neurotransmitter binding directly alters the conductance of the ion channel with no intermediate steps. Ionotropic receptors usually mediate postsynaptic changes within a few milliseconds of neurotransmitter binding, and their postsynaptic responses are very brief, perhaps a tenth of a second. Some ionotropic receptors have been carefully characterized and are prevalent throughout the nervous system. Among these are the cholinergic receptors at the neuromuscular junction, the glutaminergic receptors that mediate fast EPSPs, and the GABAergic receptors that mediate fast IPSPs.

Nicotinic Acetylcholine Receptors. Cholinergic receptors at the neuromuscular junction are called nicotinic receptors because nicotine also activates these ACh receptors. The isolation and purification of nicotinic receptors has revealed that each receptor consists of five protein subunits that unite to form a pentamer around a central pore. Each subunit contains four transmembrane amino acid sequences that are coiled into a helical structure. The nicotinic ACh receptors at the neuromuscular junction contain two α-subunits,

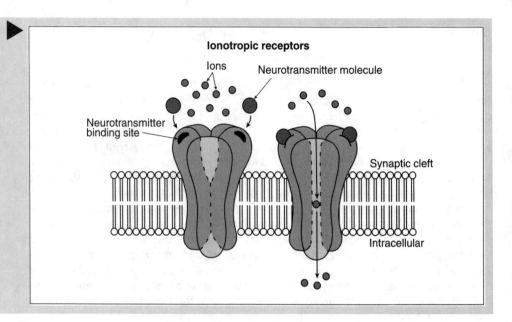

FIGURE 1-39

Ionotropic Receptors. A typical ligand-gated ionotropic receptor consists of five protein subunits that surround a central pore. In this case, binding of two neurotransmitter molecules to the binding site causes the ion channel to open.

Different protein subunits may combine to form specific receptor subtypes that possess unique physiologic characteristics.

a β-subunit, a γ-subunit and a δ-subunit. Each α-subunit has a binding site for ACh that can bind nicotine or other cholinergic ligands such as α-bungarotoxin, a snake venom.

The five subunits form a funnel-shaped pore that has a large entrance and a small diameter near the cytoplasmic side of the channel. When two ACh molecules bind to the extracellular domains of the α-subunits, the interior of the channel undergoes a conformational change that allows both Na+ and K+ ions to flow through the channel. If the muscle fiber is hyperpolarized, the influx of Na+ into the sarcolemma of the muscle fiber is much greater than the efflux of K+ into the synaptic cleft.

Nicotinic ACh receptors in the CNS differ from those at the neuromuscular junction. In the CNS, a nicotinic ACh receptor contains three α-subunits and two β-subunits. This small change renders these nicotinic receptors insensitive to α-bungarotoxin.

Glutamate Receptors. Although several families of glutamate receptors have been identified in the past two decades, additional research will be needed before the functional properties of the glutamate receptor subtypes are completely understood. In general, glutamate receptors can be broadly classified into one family of metabotropic receptors (mGluR), which are activated by quisqualate and related compounds, and a larger family of ionotropic receptors, which are activated either by α-amino-3-hydroxyl-5-methyl-4-isoxazole-propionate (AMPA), kainic acid (kainate), or *N*-methyl-D-aspartate (NMDA). The postsynaptic effects of glutaminergic transmission vary widely throughout the brain because some glutamate synapses have one glutamate receptor subtype, whereas other synapses contain many glutamate receptor subtypes.

The AMPA and kainate receptor subtypes are formed by five subunits that are assembled around a central pore. Six different protein subunits can be used to form the pentameric stucture of a specific AMPA or kainate receptor. Hence, there are dozens of glutamate receptors that can be constructed from different combinations of these subunits, and these receptor subtypes may differ in their functional properties. Glutamate-induced activation of an AMPA or kainate receptor usually causes a rapid increase in channel conductance to Na+ and K+. If the postsynaptic membrane is hyperpolarized, a rapid influx of Na+ will evoke an EPSP.

The NMDA receptor is formed by a family of five subunits that can combine in different permutations to form dozens of NMDA receptor subtypes. These receptors differ from the AMPA and kainate receptors, however, in that glutamate activation of the NMDA receptors causes an increase in the conductance of Ca2+ as well as Na+ and K+. As a result, NMDA receptor activation increases the intracellular concentration of Ca2+. In addition, NMDA receptors are unique because Mg2+ ions are strongly attracted to the Ca2+ channel when the membrane is hyperpolarized and will block Ca2+ from passing through the channel. Therefore, NMDA receptors are activated by glutamate only if the

Mg^{2+} block has been removed by previous depolarization of the membrane. Thus, NMDA receptors are one of the few ligand-gated receptors that are also voltage-dependent. Current flow through an NMDA-controlled ion channel is more likely to occur when the postsynaptic neuron is depolarized by convergent excitatory synapses from a large number of presynaptic neurons. These properties suggest that NMDA receptor activation might signal when the postsynaptic neuron has received excitatory inputs from two or more afferent pathways. Such a mechanism appears to play a role in strengthening synaptic efficacy during learning and memory.

GABA Receptors. There are two GABA receptor subtypes: $GABA_A$ and $GABA_B$. The $GABA_A$ receptors are ionotropic while the $GABA_B$ receptors are metabotropic receptors. $GABA_A$ receptors have a pentameric structure similar to the ligand-gated ion channels described for glutamate and ACh. There are five different protein subunits (α, β, γ, δ, ρ) that can combine to produce several $GABA_A$ receptor subtypes. Activation of any of these $GABA_A$ receptors causes a rapid increase in the conductance of Cl^- across the plasma membrane. The equilibrium potential for Cl^- is close to the resting membrane potential of most neurons so Cl^- influx through a $GABA_A$ channel may produce little, if any, change in the neuron's membrane potential. Nonetheless, when Cl^- conductance is increased, the membrane potential becomes less responsive to EPSPs arriving from other synapses, and the probability of a neuronal discharge is significantly reduced.

There are numerous drugs that act at GABAergic synapses by binding with different subunits of the $GABA_A$ receptor. Tranquilizers such as diazepam bind to the α- and β-subunits while barbiturates such as phenobarbital bind to the γ-subunits. These drugs act as modulators that enhance the binding of GABA and, thus, promote the inhibitory effects of GABAergic transmission. Hence, the clinical effectiveness of these drugs is based on their ability to increase suppression of neuronal activity in certain brain regions. Alcohol also acts at GABA receptors, and this explains why combining alcohol with tranquilizers or barbiturates has a powerful synergistic effect on behavior.

METABOTROPIC RECEPTORS

Metabotropic receptors are physically separated from their ion channels and, therefore, must activate intermediate proteins to regulate channel conductance (Figure 1-40). These metabolic steps take time, and this means that synaptic transmission involving metabotropic receptors is relatively slow. Postsynaptic responses mediated by metabotropic receptors may last for hundreds of milliseconds or much longer.

Unlike ionotropic receptors, metabotropic receptors consist of a single protein entity that has seven membrane spanning regions. Metabotropic receptors are also called G-protein receptors because they activate proteins associated with guanosine triphos-

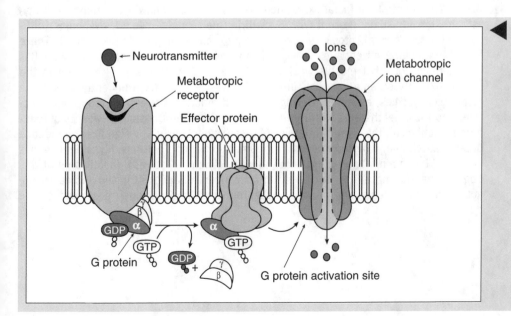

FIGURE 1-40
Metabotropic Receptors. Metabotropic receptors control ion channels through a series of intermediate steps involving activation of G proteins. In some metabotropic receptors, the G proteins activate a cascade of intracellular enzymes or cause long-lasting changes in genetic expression. GTP = guanosine triphosphate; GDP = guanosine diphosphate.

Metabotropic Receptors
Neurotransmitter receptor and ion channel are separate.
Receptor activation alters intermediate proteins.
Change in ionic conductance occurs slowly.

phate (GTP) or guanosine diphosphate (GDP). The extracellular domain of a metabotropic receptor has a neurotransmitter binding site, whereas the intracellular domain has a site for binding G-protein molecules.

When the receptor is inactive, the G proteins contain three subunits (α, β, γ) of which the α-subunit is linked to GDP. When a neurotransmitter molecule binds to the receptor, the GDP is exchanged for GTP, and the α-GTP subunit dissociates from the $\beta\gamma$-subunits. Both the α-GTP and the $\beta\gamma$-subunits are capable of activating other effector proteins that control ion channel conductance.

Activated G proteins may act directly at certain ion channels to produce a postsynaptic response. Direct interaction with the ion channel allows G proteins to mediate postsynaptic responses in a few milliseconds, but these responses do not occur as quickly as responses mediated by ionotropic receptors. In other cases, the G proteins must activate a complex cascade of biochemical signals, and this process requires even more time. Metabotropic receptors may also alter gene expression to regulate the synthesis of enzymes or other proteins involved in synaptic transmission. Protein synthesis requires more time and is probably involved in mediating some of the long-lasting changes in synaptic efficacy that are needed for memory.

Muscarinic Acetylcholine Receptors. Perhaps the best-characterized example of a metabotropic receptor is the muscarinic ACh receptor found in the heart and CNS. Muscarine is a cholinergic agonist that slows cardiac contraction and reduces the frequency of action potentials in many neurons in the CNS. These responses occur because muscarinic receptors activate G proteins that open K^+ channels; the resulting efflux of K^+ causes rapid hyperpolarization. This effect can be mimicked by injecting the $\beta\gamma$-subunits into the cell. Furthermore, muscarinic activation of the α-subunit causes rapid closing of both Ca^{2+} and Na^+ channels, and this complements the inhibitory effects produced by the $\beta\gamma$-subunits.

RESOLUTION OF CLINICAL CASE

Most neurology problems involve a constellation of clinical symptoms. It is the responsibility of the physician to recognize the profile of clinical signs associated with common neurologic disorders. The case in this chapter describes the classic symptoms of myasthenia gravis, an autoimmune disorder caused by the formation of antibodies directed against nicotinic ACh receptors in skeletal muscle. The loss of cholinergic receptors impairs the response of muscles to ACh released from peripheral motor neurons. Most patients with this disease initially experience weakness in the extraocular muscles and the muscles controlling facial expression, swallowing, and chewing. Patients with myasthenia gravis usually present with dysarthria (inarticulate speech), dysphagia (difficulty with swallowing), ptosis (drooping eyelids), and diplopia (double vision). These symptoms are intermittent and may even disappear for weeks before occurring again. It is important to note that muscle weakness, not fatigue, is an essential element in the diagnosis of myasthenia gravis. If untreated, myasthenia gravis frequently affects the respiratory muscles, especially during periods of emotional stress or respiratory infection, and most deaths are attributed to respiratory failure. Consistent with its autoimmune mechanism, the primary relatives of these patients exhibit a significant incidence of other autoimmune disorders such as rheumatoid arthritis or lupus. Myasthenia gravis is treated by administering drugs that inhibit acetylcholinesterase; inactivation of this degradative enzyme enhances the synaptic concentration of ACh and increases the activation of the remaining nicotinic receptors that have not been destroyed by the disease.

REVIEW QUESTIONS

Directions: For each of the following questions, choose the **one best** answer.

1. Which of the following events would hyperpolarize a typical neuron?
    (A) A decrease in Cl⁻ conductance
    (B) An increase in K⁺ conductance
    (C) An increase in Na⁺ conductance
    (D) An increase in Ca²⁺ conductance
    (E) Toxin-induced poisoning of the Na⁺–K⁺ pump

2. Myelination causes an increase in the conduction velocity of action potentials because
    (A) it decreases the length of the refractory period
    (B) it decreases the capacitance of the axonal membrane
    (C) it decreases the axon's membrane resistance
    (D) it lowers the equilibrium potential for Na⁺
    (E) it increases the length constant of the axon

3. Which pair of items is unlikely to be located in the same synaptic terminal?
    (A) Dense-core vesicles and clear synaptic vesicles
    (B) Substance P and glutamate
    (C) Acetylcholine (ACh) and glutamate
    (D) Tyrosine hydroxylase and dopamine
    (E) Mitochondria and clear synaptic vesicles

4. The repetitive seizures that characterize epilepsy are caused by excessive release of
    (A) glutamate
    (B) γ-aminobutyric acid (GABA)
    (C) acetylcholine (ACh)
    (D) norepinephrine
    (E) substance P

5. L-Dopa ameliorates the symptoms of Parkinson's disease because
    (A) tyrosine hydroxylase is missing in patients with Parkinson's disease and L-dopa must be administered as a dietary supplement
    (B) it crosses the blood–brain barrier and activates postsynaptic dopamine receptors
    (C) it crosses the blood–brain barrier and is converted to dopamine by neurons that contain aromatic amino acid decarboxylase (AAAD)
    (D) it crosses the blood–brain barrier and is converted to dopamine by dopaminergic terminals
    (E) Parkinson's disease is caused by a defective gene that interferes with the synthesis of L-dopa

ANSWERS AND EXPLANATIONS

1. The answer is B. A typical neuron has a resting membrane potential of −65 mV. The equilibrium potential for K+ is nearly −90 mV, and an increase in K+ conductance would shift the neuron's membrane potential towards −90 mV. Any change in Cl− conductance would have little effect on the resting potential because the equilibrium potential for Cl− is close to the resting potential. Increases in the conductance of either Na+ or Ca2+ would depolarize the membrane potential. Poisoning the Na+−K+ pump would not cause an immediate change in membrane potential but would allow the membrane potential to gradually dissipate during the production of action potentials.

2. The answer is E. Myelination causes an increase in membrane resistance but does not alter the internal resistance of the axoplasm. The length constant is the ratio of these terms, and by increasing the membrane resistance, myelination enables ionic current to flow further through the axoplasm. Refractory periods are determined by voltage-gated ion channels, not by myelination. Myelination causes a decrease in membrane capacitance, but this does not affect the velocity of action potentials. The equilibrium potential for Na+ is not affected by myelination.

3. The answer is C. Mitochondria, dense-core vesicles, and small clear vesicles are frequently seen in the same synaptic terminal. All small molecule neurotransmitters are synthesized in the synaptic terminal, and both dopamine and its rate-limiting enzyme, tyrosine hydroxylase, are co-localized in dopaminergic terminals. Neuropeptides and small-molecule neurotransmitters (e.g., substance P and glutamate) are frequently located in the same synaptic terminal. It is rare, however, for two small-molecule neurotransmitters (e.g., glutamate and ACh) to be synthesized in the same neuron.

4. The answer is A. Excessive release of glutamate causes an excessive influx of Ca2+ and activates Ca2+-dependent proteases, which leads to the formation of free radicals. Destruction of GABAergic neurons by free radicals releases glutaminergic neurons from the inhibitory effects of GABA and increases the probability that glutamate will cause further damage. ACh, norepinephrine, and substance P are not strongly implicated in epilepsy.

5. The answer is C. Dopaminergic neurons degenerate in patients with Parkinson's disease, but dopamine cannot be used to treat this disease because it does not cross the blood−brain barrier. The precursor to dopamine, L-dopa, enters the brain after systemic administration and can be converted into dopamine by nondopaminergic neurons that contain the enzyme AAAD. There is no evidence that Parkinson's disease is caused by a lack of tyrosine hydroxylase or by a defective gene that interferes with tyrosine hydroxylase.

ADDITIONAL READING

Cooper JR, Bloom FE, Roth RH: *The Biochemical Basis of Neuropharmacology*. New York, NY: W. H. Freeman, 1991.

Hall Z: *An Introduction to Molecular Neurobiology*. Sunderland, MA: Sinauer Associates, 1992.

Hodgkin AL: *The Conduction of the Nervous Impulse*. Springfield, IL: Charles C Thomas, 1967.

Katz B: *Nerve, Muscle, and Synapse*. New York, NY: McGraw-Hill, 1966.

Nicholls DG: *Proteins, Transmitters, and Synapses*. Boston, MA: Blackwell Scientific, 1994.

Rothman JE: Mechanisms of intracellular protein transport. *Nature* 372:55–63, 1994.

Shepard GM: *The Synaptic Organization of the Brain*, 3rd ed. New York, NY: Oxford University Press, 1990.

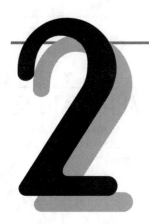

GENERAL ORGANIZATION OF THE NERVOUS SYSTEM

CHAPTER OUTLINE

INTRODUCTION OF CLINICAL CASE

When T. R., a 67-year-old retired plumber, was brought to the emergency room by his wife, he was experiencing shortness of breath and nausea and had a flushed complexion. T. R. reported having a severe headache, which in his own words was "the worst of his life." Onset of the headache several hours earlier was sudden and poorly localized. The patient reported having a few headaches over the last year but several over the past 2 weeks; none responded to self-medication with aspirin. This headache, unlike the others, was accompanied by a stiff neck. The patient's blood pressure was 170/100 mm Hg, his pulse was 90 beats/min, and his respiration rate was 20 breaths/min, but labored. As the physical examination continued, the patient became disoriented, incoherent, stuporous, and finally lost consciousness. The physician ordered a full series of computed tomography (CT) scans of the head and, pending the outcome of the scans, a lumbar puncture.

TERMINOLOGY AND NOMENCLATURE

This chapter, after introducing basic terminology that will be used in this book, will preview the organization of the nervous system. The remaining sections of this chapter include more detailed descriptions of the embryologic development of the nervous system as well as its vasculature, ventricular system, and meningeal covers.

Neuroscientists use a specialized lexicon to describe accurately the complex three-dimensional organization of the nervous system. To students beginning their study of neuroanatomy, this terminology may seem imposing, but given time, it will prove its worth.

Orientation

The longitudinal orientation of the mammalian nervous system is best appreciated in a quadruped species such as the rat. As Figure 2-1 illustrates, the nervous system of the rat has clear rostral and caudal ends that correspond to its nose and tail. The rat's ventral (or anterior) surface presses against the substrate, while its dorsal (or posterior) surface forms the back. In humans, the brain has a pronounced flexure that orients the forebrain almost perpendicular to that of the spinal cord (see Figure 2-1). At spinal and lower brainstem levels, the terms *dorsal* and *ventral* have the same meaning in bipeds and quadrupeds. Further rostrally, however, this flexure affects the meaning of some terms. For example, the terms dorsal and ventral continue to describe structures that lie above or below the long axis of the brain, but the terms *anterior* and *posterior* relate to the rostrocaudal axis, that is, toward or away from the front of the head.

Three other terms use the midline as their reference point. *Median* means on the midline, while *medial* means toward the midline. Note that a structure may be medial to another yet may not lie on the midline. *Lateral* means away from the midline. Use of the words "lateral" and "medial" typically requires that some referent be used as well; for example, "nucleus A lies lateral to nucleus B."

FIGURE 2-1 ▶

Axes of the Central Nervous System. The directions of orientation used to describe the brain of the rat (panel A), whose brain is linear, and the human (panel B), whose brain has a pronounced flexure. (Source: Reprinted with permission from Martin JH: Neuroanatomy Text and Atlas, Stamford, CT: Appleton & Lange, 1996, p 22.)

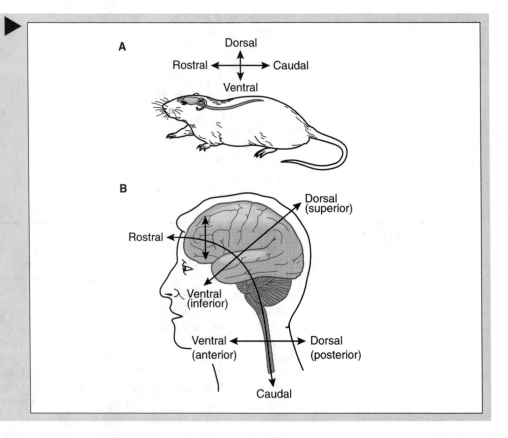

Planes of Section

Sections of the nervous systems are typically shown in one of the three major planes: *sagittal*, *coronal* (transverse), or *horizontal* (Figure 2-2). A sagittal section divides the specimen into left and right portions. When this specimen is cut on the midline, it is referred to as a *midsagittal* section; other sections offset from the midline are in parasagittal planes. A section of the brainstem or spinal cord perpendicular to its long axis would be in the *transverse* plane. A similar section in the forebrain, that is, rostral to the flexure of the neuraxis, would be in the coronal plane. Sections made in the horizontal plane divide the specimen into dorsal and ventral segments. It is common for neuroradiographic studies of the forebrain to be done in the horizontal plane; in the brainstem, it is rare. Oblique sections do not conform to any of these planes.

Three Major Planes of Section
Sagittal
Coronal
Horizontal

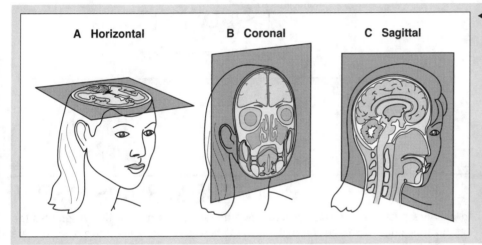

A Horizontal   B Coronal   C Sagittal

FIGURE 2-2
Planes of Section. *Panels A, B, and C illustrate the horizontal, coronal, and sagittal planes of section that are used to describe the human brain.*

Pathways

Mastery of the organization of the central nervous system (CNS) requires a detailed understanding of its circuitry. A variety of terms are used to distinguish the many types of CNS pathways (Figure 2-3). A collection of axons is called a *tract, fasciculus*, or *lemniscus*. The term *funiculus* refers to a longitudinal bulge in the spinal cord formed by one or more underlying tracts. Pathways whose origin, course, and destination remain on the same side of the nervous system project *ipsilaterally*; those that cross the midline project *contralaterally*. Crossing or *decussating* pathways are common in the nervous system and account for a number of observations including control of the body's musculature by the contralateral side of the brain. Another type of crossing pathway is a *commissure*, which interconnects corresponding regions on each side of the brain or spinal cord.

Afferent pathways, which carry information to a nucleus, are often distinguished from *efferent pathways*, which carry information from a nucleus. These terms also may be used without reference to a particular nucleus. For example, an afferent projection carries sensory information (e.g., a sour taste) while an efferent projection has a motor function (e.g., innervation of the biceps muscle). Another way to distinguish afferent and efferent pathways is to add the suffix "*-fugal*" or "*-petal*" to the nuclear root. For example, efferent projections of the cerebral cortex are corticofugal projections while its afferent projections are corticopetal. In both instances there may be multiple cortical connections, but none are identified with this nomenclature. Another way to specify a pathway is to combine the source and destination nuclei into a new word. For example, a cerebellothalamic projection goes from the cerebellum to the thalamus. This nomenclature designates both the source and destination of the pathway without designating either as sensory or motor in function.

FIGURE 2-3 ▶
Pathways. *Diagram showing the assembly of axons into progressively larger fiber bundles and the names used to distinguish between those bundles that cross the midline and those that do not.*

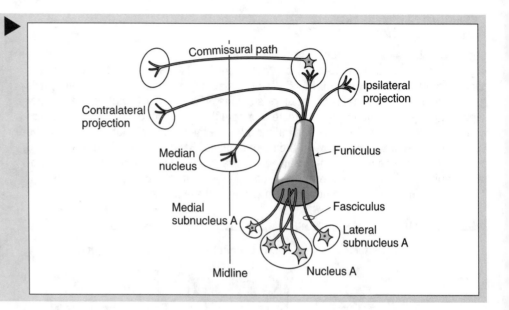

THE NERVOUS SYSTEM

In many respects, the nervous system has a hierarchical structure that resembles the organization chart of a large corporation. In the nervous system, executive decisions are made at the highest level, the cerebral cortex. Information gathered by receptors located in various sense organs is analyzed by subcortical nuclei, the neural equivalent of corporate departments. When this information reaches the cerebral cortex, it is analyzed further, and a plan of action is determined. Specific regions in the cerebral cortex communicate these decisions to subordinate systems in the brainstem and spinal cord, which implement the orders.

This neural hierarchy, like its corporate counterpart, enables routine tasks such as reflexes and autonomic regulation to proceed with limited supervision by the cerebral cortex. More complex tasks or those that involve cognition require participation of the cerebral cortex.

Central Nervous System

The nervous system consists of two anatomic divisions: the CNS, which consists of the brain and spinal cord, and the *peripheral nervous system*. The brain can be further subdivided into five parts: (1) *telencephalon*, (2) *diencephalon*, (3) *mesencephalon*, (4) *metencephalon*, and (5) *myelencephalon*. The peripheral nervous system is composed of the 12 cranial nerves and 31 pairs of spinal nerves.

The telencephalon forms the most rostral part of the brain and is represented by the cerebral cortex and several buried nuclei, the basal ganglia. The diencephalon lies beneath the telencephalon and, consequently, cannot be seen except for the small portion at the base of the brain that is encircled by the optic tracts and the temporal lobe. The diencephalon is composed of four parts: thalamus, hypothalamus, subthalamus, and epithalamus. The mesencephalon, metencephalon, and myelencephalon constitute the brainstem, which lies exposed along the ventral surface of the brain. The spinal cord, the most caudal part of the CNS, is continuous with the myelencephalon and extends to the base of the vertebral column.

TELENCEPHALON

The telencephalon consists of the cerebral cortex and the subcortical nuclei of the basal ganglia.

The **telencephalon** consists of the cerebral cortex and the basal ganglia.

The **diencephalon** is composed of the thalamus, hypothalamus, subthalamus, and epithalamus.

The **brainstem** consists of the mesencephalon, metencephalon, and myelencephalon.

Cerebral Cortex. The cerebral cortex is a highly convoluted, laminated structure whose appearance is consistent but not identical among individuals. Each convolution, or *gyrus*, is separated from neighboring gyri by a deep incisure called a *sulcus* (pl. sulci). The largest sulcus, the longitudinal fissure, divides the brain into left and right hemispheres. Each hemisphere consists of six lobes whose boundaries are determined by other prominent gyri and sulci. Four of these six lobes are named after the overlying bones of the skull: the frontal, parietal, temporal, and occipital. The two remaining lobes, which are not visible externally, are the insular and the limbic lobes.

> The groove between two gyri is a **sulcus**.

> The **longitudinal** or **midsagittal sulcus** divides the brain into left and right halves.

The two most prominent landmarks on the lateral cortical surface are the central sulcus or fissure of Rolando and the lateral sulcus or Sylvian fissure (Figure 2-4). The central sulcus separates the frontal and parietal lobes. The lateral sulcus runs along the lateral margin of the frontal and parietal lobes and serves as the dorsal boundary for the temporal lobe.

> The **central sulcus** separates the frontal and parietal lobes.

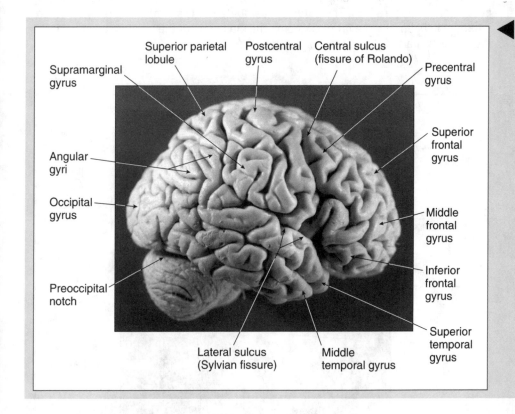

FIGURE 2-4
Lateral Surface of the Brain. *Anterior is to the right.*

Labels on figure: Supramarginal gyrus; Superior parietal lobule; Postcentral gyrus; Central sulcus (fissure of Rolando); Precentral gyrus; Superior frontal gyrus; Angular gyri; Middle frontal gyrus; Occipital gyrus; Inferior frontal gyrus; Preoccipital notch; Superior temporal gyrus; Lateral sulcus (Sylvian fissure); Middle temporal gyrus

The *frontal lobe*, the largest of the six lobes, includes all of the cortex rostral to the central sulcus and dorsal to the cingulate sulcus. The precentral gyrus, which forms the anterior bank of the *central sulcus*, includes the primary motor cortex. The premotor cortex, which has important connections with the primary motor area, is located immediately rostral to the precentral gyrus. Further rostrally, the frontal lobe consists of the superior, middle, and inferior frontal gyri, which are arranged as horizontal tiers. The inferior frontal gyrus consists of three parts: the pars orbitalis, the pars triangularis, and the pars opercularis. In the dominant hemisphere, the pars triangularis and opercularis constitute Broca's area, an important region for motor control of language.

> The **lateral sulcus** separates the temporal lobe from the frontal and parietal lobes.

> The **motor cortex** is located on the precentral gyrus.

The *parietal lobe* includes all cortex dorsal to the cingulate gyrus between the central sulcus and the anterior border of the occipital lobe. The parieto-occipital border is an imaginary line projecting from the parieto-occipital sulcus on the medial surface of the hemisphere to the pre-occipital notch on the lateral aspect of the hemisphere. The lateral sulcus separates the parietal and temporal lobes. The postcentral gyrus, which forms the posterior bank of the central sulcus, contains the primary somatosensory cortex and has a topographical representation of the contralateral body surface. The intraparietal sulcus divides the remainder of the parietal lobe into the superior and inferior parietal

> **Broca's area** is located on the inferior frontal gyrus.

> The **somatosensory cortex** is located on the postcentral gyrus.

lobules. A lobule is a small lobe or one of the primary divisions of a lobe. The superior parietal lobule organizes one's immediate extrapersonal space. The inferior parietal lobule contains the supramarginal and angular gyri, two regions that integrate information from adjacent somatosensory, auditory, and visual areas.

The *temporal lobe* occupies the ventral bank of the lateral sulcus and fills the entire middle cranial fossa. The temporal lobe and the parietal lobe share the same posterior border. The external surface of the temporal lobe is divided into superior, middle, and inferior gyri, all of which lie parallel to the Sylvian fissure. The superior temporal gyrus, which forms the ventral bank of the Sylvian fissure, contains the transversely oriented gyri of Heschl. This region serves as primary auditory cortex and has important connections with other auditory processing and language comprehension areas in the parietal and frontal lobes. More lateral parts of the temporal lobe, such as the inferior temporal gyrus, mediate pattern recognition and higher-order processing of visual information. The ventral surface of the temporal lobe is formed by the occipitotemporal and parahippocampal gyri (Figure 2-5). The *parahippocampal gyrus* is an important relay for sensory information bound for the limbic system. The medial tip of the parahippocampal gyrus, the *uncus*, is part of the primary olfactory cortex.

The **primary auditory cortex** *resides within the gyri of Heschl.*

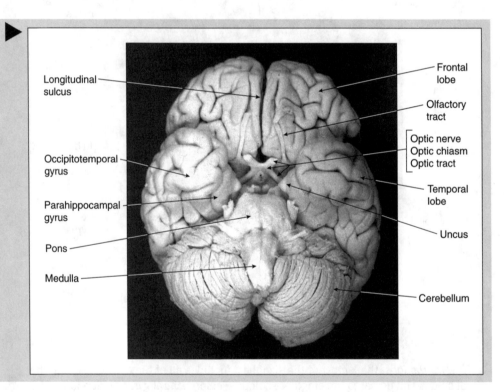

FIGURE 2-5
Inferior Surface of the Brain. Anterior is to the top.

Longitudinal sulcus

Occipitotemporal gyrus

Parahippocampal gyrus

Pons

Medulla

Frontal lobe

Olfactory tract

Optic nerve
Optic chiasm
Optic tract

Temporal lobe

Uncus

Cerebellum

The **primary olfactory cortex** *is located along the medial aspect of the temporal lobe.*

The **primary visual cortex** *is located in the occipital lobe.*

Operculum *means "cover" in Latin.*

The *occipital lobe*, lying caudal to the parietal and temporal lobes, comprises the posterior pole of the cerebral cortex. It is the smallest of the four true lobes and is devoted exclusively to vision. The primary visual cortex lies along the banks of the calcarine sulcus, which is located on the medial surface of the occipital lobe (Figure 2-6). Higher-order visual areas, which begin as a series of bands around the primary visual area, extend rostrally into the caudal parietal and temporal lobes.

The *insula* and the *limbic lobe* are considered synthetic lobes because their boundaries with adjacent areas of the brain are less clear. The insula, located deep within the lateral sulcus, can be visualized only after separating the temporal lobe from the frontal and parietal lobes (Figure 2-7). The parts of the frontal, parietal, and temporal lobes that cover the insula are called the opercular cortex. The rostral insula, in addition to serving as the primary gustatory cortex, has been implicated in cardiovascular, pulmonary, and gastric function.

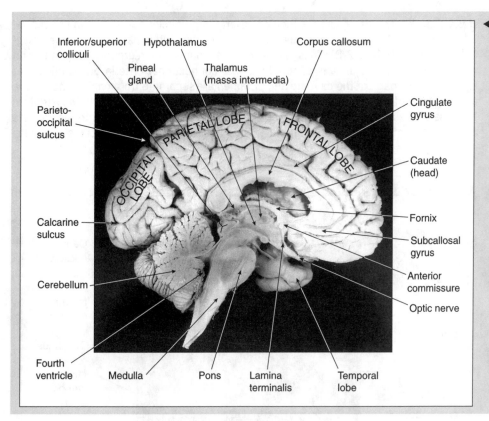

FIGURE 2-6
Medial Surface of an Unstained Brain in the Midsagittal Plane. *Anterior is to the right.*

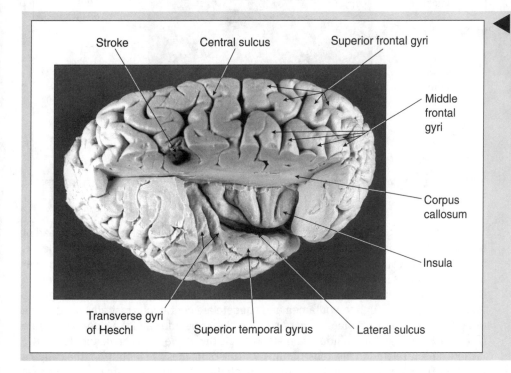

FIGURE 2-7
Dorsolateral Aspect of the Brain. *(Anterior is to the right). A wedge has been removed from the frontoparietal cortex to reveal the underlying insula. The primary auditory cortex is located on the transverse gyri of Heschl along the superior aspect of the temporal lobe. The dark stain along the superior surface of the parietal lobe is a small hemorrhagic stroke, which was large enough to be symptomatic, but not fatal.*

The limbic lobe, located on the medial surface the frontal, parietal, and temporal lobes, includes the subcallosal, cingulate, and parahippocampal gyri as well as the hippocampal formation. Collectively, these regions form a broad arc that surrounds the diencephalon. The hippocampal formation and other parts of the limbic cortex play a critical role in memory formation. The functions of the subcallosal and cingulate gyri are not well understood but appear to involve visceral aspects of emotional expression.

The **primary gustatory cortex** is located in the rostral insula.

Basal Ganglia. The basal ganglia include several large nuclei buried within the ventral telencephalon: the caudate nucleus, the putamen, the globus pallidus, and the amygdaloid complex (Figure 2-8). These nuclei may be grouped and regrouped, depending on whether embryologic, anatomic, functional, or connectional criteria are applied. For example, most parts of the caudate and putamen are separated from one another by the anterior limb of the internal capsule, but they often are referred to as the neostriatum because of their functional similarity. The term "corpus striatum" refers to the caudate nucleus, putamen, and globus pallidus, while the term "lenticular nucleus" includes only the globus pallidus and putamen.

> The **basal ganglia** include the caudate nucleus, the putamen, the globus pallidus, and the amygdala.

FIGURE 2-8 ▶
Unstained Coronal Section of the Brain Showing the Basal Ganglia.

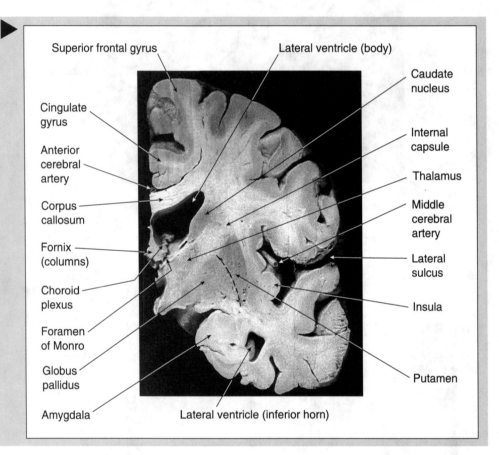

The caudate nucleus consists of three parts: a head, a body, and a tail. The head of the caudate is a massive structure that forms the lateral wall of the lateral ventricle. As the body of the caudate nucleus stretches posteriorly, it becomes progressively smaller until it terminates like a tail within the inferior horn of the lateral ventricle. The putamen is the largest nucleus of the basal ganglia, but it can be seen only in sections through the telencephalon. Although the putamen and caudate are continuous rostrally, most of the putamen lies between the lateral margin of the globus pallidus and the external capsule (Figure 2-9). The globus pallidus is an embryologic derivative of the diencephalon, but it is more closely related to the neostriatum by virtue of its massive input from the caudate nucleus. The corpus striatum has been implicated in sensorimotor integration because damage to these structures often accompanies movement disorders such as Parkinson's disease, Huntington's chorea, and Tourette's syndrome.

The amygdala is an almond-shaped cluster of small nuclei located within the rostral pole of the temporal lobe beneath the uncus (see Figure 2-8). Although embryologically and anatomically the amygdaloid complex is considered to be a part of the basal ganglia, its connections with the hypothalamus and its involvement in emotional behavior suggest that it is more closely aligned with the limbic system.

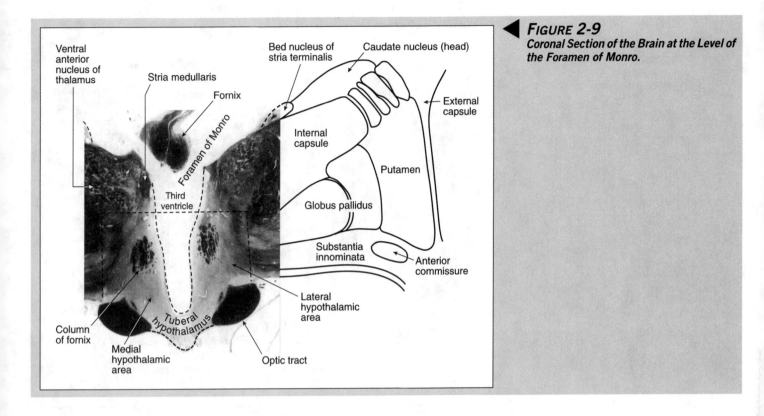

DIENCEPHALON

The diencephalon consists of four parts: the thalamus, the hypothalamus, the sub-thalamus, and the epithalamus. The ventral surface of the diencephalon lies exposed at the base of the brain, but its dorsal surface, which serves as the floor of the lateral ventricle, is hidden by the overlying corpus callosum and cerebral cortex (Figure 2-10; see Figure 2-9). From the lamina terminalis to the posterior commissure, the internal capsule serves as the lateral boundary of the diencephalon. The slit-like third ventricle located on the midline divides the diencephalon into symmetrical halves. The junction between the thalamus and the hypothalamus is demarcated by the hypothalamic sulcus, a modest indentation in the wall of the third ventricle. The optic nerve is the only cranial nerve that enters the brain through the diencephalon (see Figures 2-5 and 2-10).

Thalamus. The thalamus is the largest division of the diencephalon, and both anatomically and physiologically it represents an important nexus for many systems of the brain (see Figure 2-10). Several dozen thalamic subnuclei traverse the full length of the diencephalon from the interventricular foramen to the posterior commissure. The structural diversity of the thalamus reflects it functional breadth. Every sensory system uses the thalamus as an obligate relay during its ascent to neocortex. Several nuclei in the thalamus serve as relays in the feedback loop between the cerebellum and the primary motor cortex. The remaining thalamic nuclei play vital roles in consciousness, arousal, and sleep.

Hypothalamus. The hypothalamus forms the ventral walls and floor of the third ventricle from the lamina terminalis to the caudal border of the mamillary bodies (see Figures 2-9 and 2-10). Laterally, the hypothalamus abuts the medial margin of the internal capsule, the subthalamic nucleus, and the lenticular fasciculus. The hypothalamus, along with the hypophysis, plays a critical role in vegetative, regulatory, and cognitive functions related to maintenance of core temperature, regulation of food and fluid consumption, initiation of sleep, reproduction, maternal behavior, and endocrine function. The intimate relationship between the hypothalamus and the autonomic nervous system has earned it the nickname, "head autonomic ganglion."

Epithalamus. The epithalamus includes the pineal gland and the habenular nuclei, which are located in proximity to the posterior commissure. The pineal gland, known in

The **hypothalamus** works in concert with the **hypophysis**.

FIGURE 2-10 ▶
Unstained Brainstem and Cerebellum Shown in Figure 2-6. Anterior is to the right.

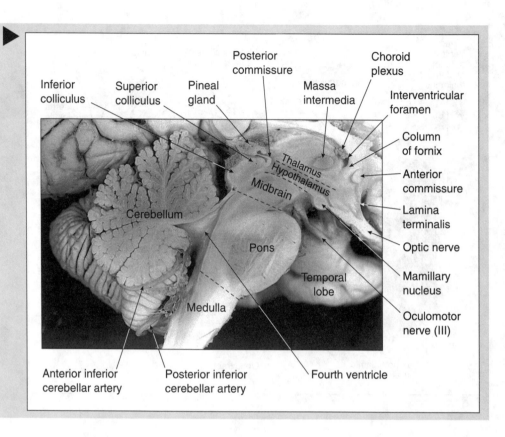

Tectum means "roof" in Latin.

antiquity as the "seat of the soul," is partially responsible for regulating the body's diurnal rhythm.

Subthalamus. The subthalamus is a lens-shaped nucleus located beneath the internal capsule and lateral to the hypothalamus. Although derived from the diencephalon, it is more closely related to the globus pallidus and usually is discussed along with the basal ganglia.

BRAINSTEM

The brainstem includes, from rostral to caudal, the midbrain (mesencephalon), the pons (metencephalon), and the medulla (myelencephalon) [see Figures 2-6 and 2-10]. Each division contains intrinsic nuclei as well as ascending and descending pathways that play key roles in the sensory, motor, and vegetative functions of the nervous system. Sensory nuclei in the brainstem process somatosensory, auditory, vestibular, or gustatory information received from the cranial nerves. Motor nuclei located throughout the brainstem control the muscles of the head, face, eyes, and intraoral cavity. These motor nuclei participate in normal reflexes as well as volitional movements initiated by the cerebral cortex. Other brainstem nuclei receive afferent information from the thoracic and abdominal viscera.

The brainstem is divided into dorsal and ventral regions by the cerebral aqueduct in the midbrain and the fourth ventricle in the pons. The ventral region, called the *tegmentum*, contains cranial nerve nuclei, the reticular formation, and a variety of ascending and descending fiber tracts. The dorsal surface of the midbrain and pons is called the *tectum* because it serves as the roof plate for these regions of the brainstem. The medulla has no tectum; its dorsal surface is formed by the floor of the fourth ventricle. The fourth ventricle is enclosed by the overlying cerebellum and its three massive cerebellar peduncles.

Midbrain (Mesencephalon). The junction between the diencephalon and mesencephalon is marked by the pineal gland, the habenula, the posterior commissure, and the crus cerebri. The rostral border of the midbrain coincides with the transition between the third ventricle and the cerebral aqueduct. The midbrain is the smallest division of the brainstem.

The tectal region of the midbrain contains two pairs of swellings, the *superior* and *inferior colliculi*, also known as the corpora quadrigemina (Figure 2-11; see Figure 2-10). The trochlear nerve (IV), which emerges immediately posterior to the inferior colliculus, is the only cranial nerve that exits the dorsal surface of the brainstem. The midbrain tegmentum is dominated by the red nucleus, parts of the reticular formation, and several other sensory and motor nuclei. The ventral part of the midbrain contains a darkly pigmented nucleus, the substantia nigra, and the crus cerebri. The oculomotor nerve emerges from the interpeduncular fossa, the prominent midline cistern formed by the massive pillars of the crus cerebri (Figure 2-12).

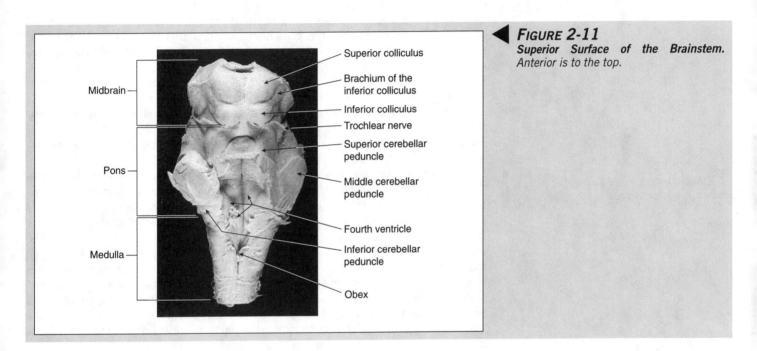

FIGURE 2-11
Superior Surface of the Brainstem. *Anterior is to the top.*

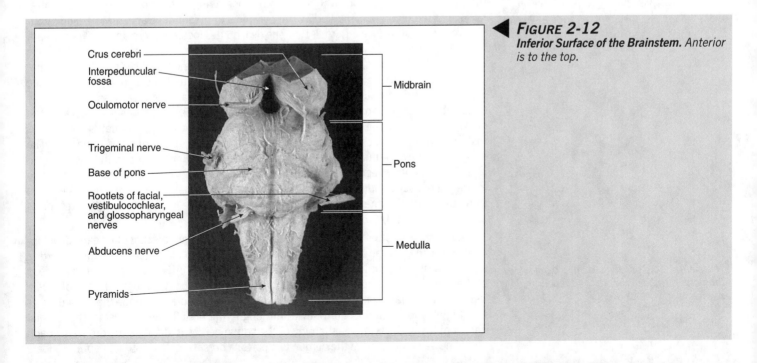

FIGURE 2-12
Inferior Surface of the Brainstem. *Anterior is to the top.*

Pons (Metencephalon). The ventral surface of the pons has a distinctive bulge formed by the pontine nuclei and several prominent myelinated pathways (see Figure 2-12). The pontine nuclei act as a functional bridge between the cerebral cortex and the cerebellum. The efferent projections from the pontine nuclei form the broad band of transversely oriented fibers that cross the midline, wrap around the lateral aspect of the pons, and form the middle cerebellar peduncle. The middle cerebellar peduncle is the largest afferent pathway of the cerebellum.

The dorsal surface of the pons forms the rostral half of the floor of the fourth ventricle. The floor of the fourth ventricle is marked by the facial colliculi, a pair of bumps produced by fibers of the facial nerve wrapping around the abducens nucleus. Four cranial nerves emerge from the pons or the cerebellopontine angle: the motor and sensory roots of the trigeminal nerve (V), the abducens nerve (VI), the facial motor and intermediate nerves (VII), and the vestibulocochlear nerve (VIII).

The cerebellum, a derivative of the rhombic lip of the metencephalon, forms the roof of the fourth ventricle above the pons and medulla and is the largest tenant of the posterior fossa (see Figures 2-5, 2-6, and 2-10). Projections from almost every sensory system enable the cerebellum to modulate balance, muscle tone, and fine motor control. Although the cerebellum is divided into cortical and subcortical parts, its internal and external architecture differ significantly from that of neocortex.

The dorsal surface of the cerebellum is separated from the occipital lobe by a dural sheath, the tentorium, while its ventral surface forms a canopy above the fourth ventricle. The cerebellum is anchored to the brainstem by three stout pillars, the superior, middle, and inferior cerebellar peduncles.

> *The myelinated core of the cerebellum is called the* **arbor vitae**.

The cerebellar cortex is divided into two hemispheres by the narrow vermal region on the midline. Each hemisphere contains hundreds of gyri called folia whose small size and tight packing obscure the cerebellum's few named sulci. As in the cerebellum, these sulci divide the cerebellar cortex into lobes. The three lobes of the cerebellum, from rostral to caudal, are the paleocerebellum, the neocerebellum, and the archicerebellum. The primary fissure, the deepest of all cerebellar sulci, separates the paleocerebellum from the neocerebellum. The posterolateral fissure marks the boundary between the neocerebellum and the archicerebellum. The heavily myelinated afferent and efferent axons of the cerebellar cortex form the core of the cerebellum, the arbor vitae. Buried within the arbor vitae are four paired nuclei that channel almost all cerebellar output to the rest of the brain. All afferent and efferent connections of the cerebellum traverse one of the three peduncles that connect the cerebellum to the brainstem.

Medulla (Myelencephalon). The medulla extends from the caudal border of the pons to the pyramidal decussation, which marks the beginning of the spinal cord. The ventral surface of the medulla is marked by the pyramids or pyramidal tracts that lie along both sides of the midline (see Figure 2-12). The oval bulges located lateral to the pyramids are formed by the underlying inferior olivary nuclei. In cross-section, the inferior olive resembles a crumpled paper bag and extends almost the entire length of the medulla.

> *The* **cerebellopontine angle** *is located at the junction of the cerebellum, pons, and medulla.*

The dorsal surface of the medulla cradles the caudal half of the fourth ventricle (see Figure 2-11). The caudal medulla is marked by several protuberances or tubercles caused by underlying nuclei. The bulging tubercle gracilis, which lies just lateral to the obex, is caused by the underlying nucleus gracilis. The tubercle cuneatus, which lies rostrolateral to the tubercle gracilis, marks the location of the nucleus cuneatus. The lump formed by the nucleus of the trigeminal tract is called the tuberculum cinereum.

The medullary tegmentum, like that of the pons and midbrain, contains a dense reticular core surrounded by other sensory and motor nuclei. Four cranial nerves emerge from the medulla: the glossopharyngeal nerve (IX), the vagus nerve (X), the spinal accessory nerve (XI), and the hypoglossal nerve (XII).

Spinal Cord. The spinal cord retains the elongated shape reminiscent of its early development from the neural tube. Though continuous with the brainstem, the spinal cord is noticeably smaller, and its internal and external features differ substantially from those of the brainstem. The spinal cord communicates with the body through 31 pairs of *spinal nerves*. The spinal nerves give the spinal cord a segmented appearance that obscures its functional and anatomic continuity. Although functionally analogous to the cranial nerves of the brainstem, the anatomy of the spinal nerves is significantly different. Each spinal nerve emerges from the cord in two parts: a *dorsal root* consisting of afferent fibers

> *The spinal cord is divided into* **cervical, thoracic, lumbar, sacral,** *and* **coccygeal** *segments.*

and a *ventral root* consisting of efferent fibers (see Chapter 4, Figure 4-6). To identify specific levels of the spinal cord, the spinal nerves and their corresponding vertebral segments (i.e., cervical, thoracic, lumbar, sacral, coccygeal) are numbered consecutively from rostral to caudal (e.g., fifth cervical vertebra or C5).

The spinal cord in transverse section reveals a butterfly-shaped neuronal core surrounded by an annulus of ascending and descending myelinated tracts (see Chapter 4, Figure 4-6). This concentric organization resembles the brainstem, where the core tegmental region is surrounded by long ascending and descending tracts. The central gray consists of three parts, the dorsal, ventral, and lateral horns, which, generally speaking, are involved with sensory, motor, and autonomic activity, respectively.

Peripheral Nervous System

The peripheral nervous system is composed of all nerve fibers located outside the brain and spinal cord. These components include the cranial nerves originating from the brainstem and the paired spinal nerves emerging from the cord. The cranial nerves are listed in Table 2-1 and will be described in more detail elsewhere in the text. Functionally, the peripheral nervous system is frequently divided into somatic and autonomic divisions.

The **dorsal root**: *afferent fibers.*

The **ventral root**: *efferent axons.*

The **peripheral nervous system**: *12 cranial nerves and 31 spinal nerves.*

◄ **TABLE 2-1**
Cranial Nerves

Number	Name	Components	Function	CNS Insertion
I	Olfactory	Sensory	Olfaction	Telencephalon
II	Optic	Sensory	Vision	Diencephalon
III	Oculomotor	Mixed	Eye movement	Mesencephalon
IV	Trochlear	Motor	Eye movement	Mesencephalon
V	Trigeminal	Mixed	Sensation from face and mouth Mastication	Metencephalon
VI	Abducens	Motor	Eye movement	Metencephalon
VII	Facial	Mixed	Facial expression Taste	Metencephalon
VIII	Vestibulocochlear	Sensory	Hearing and balance	Metencephalon
IX	Glossopharyngeal	Mixed	Sensation from pharynx, taste buds, and vascular system Gag reflex	Myelencephalon
X	Vagus	Mixed	Autonomic control and sensation	Myelencephalon
XI	Spinal accessory	Motor	Shoulder and neck movement	Myelencephalon
XII	Hypoglossal	Motor	Tongue movement	Myelencephalon

SOMATIC DIVISION

The somatic division of the peripheral nervous system includes both sensory and motor components. The sensory elements include the neurons and axons associated with the dorsal root and cranial nerve ganglia. The area of the body innervated by a single dorsal root is known as its dermatome (see Chapter 4, Figure 4-14).

The motor component of the somatic division consists of the ventral root and cranial nerve axons. Most motor axons within the ventral roots derive from motor neurons located in the ventral horn of the spinal cord. The musculature innervated by a single ventral root is referred to as a myotome. The ventral roots also contain visceral efferent fibers that originate in the lateral horn.

AUTONOMIC DIVISION

The autonomic division of the peripheral nervous system has components of central and peripheral origin and consists of three separate but intertwined parts: the *sympathetic*, the *parasympathetic*, and the *enteric nervous systems*. In emergency situations, the sympathetic system readies the body for "fight or flight." The parasympathetic system predominates during quiescent periods when it is safe to "rest and digest." The coopera-

Autonomic Nervous System
Sympathetic division
Parasympathetic division
Enteric division

Sympathetic functions: *fight or flight.*

Parasympathetic function: rest and digest.

tive action of the sympathetic and parasympathetic systems enables the body to meet varying environmental challenges. Both sympathetic and parasympathetic divisions originate in the CNS and project to peripherally located ganglia prior to reaching their target organs. The enteric nervous system controls the smooth muscles of the gastrointestinal tract, usually independently of the sympathetic and parasympathetic systems.

EMBRYOLOGIC DEVELOPMENT OF THE NERVOUS SYSTEM

The complexity of the adult nervous system belies its simple embryonic form. The adult nervous system retains the tubular form of the embryo, but certain areas, most notably the cerebral cortex, have undergone tremendous growth and elaboration.

Neural Tube and Spinal Cord

The neural tube is the predecessor of the ventricular system.

Approximately 18 days after fertilization, the ectodermal lining destined to become skin thickens and differentiates into the *neural plate*, the earliest vestige of the nervous system. As the neural plate begins to elongate, its lateral edges arch medially and fold around the *neural groove*, the hallmark of the keyhole stage of development (Figure 2-13). With further elaboration these folds approach one another at the midline and fuse. Fusion spreads both rostrally and caudally until the entire neural plate has been converted into a tube, usually by day 28. A thin membrane called the *lamina terminalis* closes the rostral end of the *neural tube* at the *anterior neuropore*, while distal closure takes place at the *posterior neuropore*. The lumen of the neural tube is the predecessor of the adult ventricular system. Formation of the neural tube pinches off a small cluster of cells called the *neural crest* that develops into Schwann cells, the meninges, and the neurons of the cranial, dorsal root, and autonomic ganglia (see Figure 2-13).

Closure of the neural tube is complete by embryologic day 28.

By the fourth postnatal week a longitudinal groove called the *sulcus limitans* develops in the wall of the neural tube (Figure 2-14). The sulcus limitans divides the neural

FIGURE 2-13 ▶

Development of the Neural Tube. *(A) The keyhole stage is marked by the development of the neural groove, the precursor of the neural tube. Formation of the neural groove is induced by the underlying notochord along the midline of the embryo. As cross sections 1 and 2 show, the neural groove first develops in the center of the embryo. (B) Closing of the neural groove forms the neural tube (cross section 3). Closure of the neural tube begins in the center of the embryo and spreads to both ends. Cross section 3 shows the closed neural tube with neural crest located dorsally.*

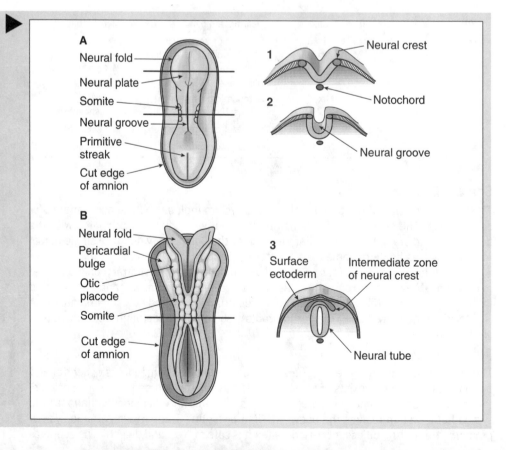

tube into a dorsal *alar plate* and a ventral *basal plate*. With further differentiation, sensory neurons will develop from the alar plate while the basal plate will serve motor functions. This functional partition is best illustrated by the spinal cord where sensory and motor functions are mediated by the dorsal and ventral horns, respectively. Vestiges of the sulcus limitans can be traced within the neural tube as far rostrally as the midbrain. In the brainstem, just as in the spinal cord, the sulcus limitans serves as the boundary between alar (sensory) and basal (motor) regions of the hindbrain. The sulcus limitans is an important landmark for organizing the cranial nerve sensory and motor nuclei into longitudinal columns that stretch from the medulla to the midbrain (see Chapter 4).

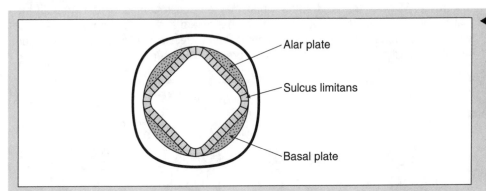

FIGURE 2-14
Cross Section of the Neural Tube. The alar (dorsal) and basal (ventral) plates are separated from one another by the sulcus limitans.

During early prenatal development the spinal cord extends to the caudal tip of the vertebral column (Figure 2-15). As growth of the spinal cord slows, however, its caudal tip recedes from the end of the spinal canal. At birth, the spinal cord ends at the L3 vertebra but by adulthood, the caudal tip of the spinal cord extends only as far as the L1–L2 level. This mismatch forces the nerve roots from the lumbar, sacral, and coccygeal segments to descend within the lumbar cistern before exiting the spinal canal below the vertebra for which each is named. Use of the lumbar cistern for spinal taps is discussed later in this chapter and again in Chapter 3.

The spinal cord, which ends at the L3 vertebra at birth, extends only as far as the L1–L2 level in adults.

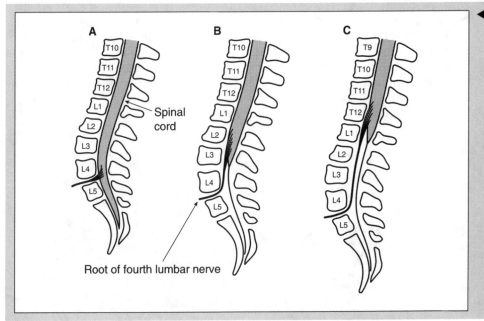

FIGURE 2-15
Relationship between the Spinal Cord and the Vertebral Column during Early Embryologic Development (A), at Birth (B), and in the Adult (C).

Clinical Aspects of Embryologic Development

Closure of the anterior and posterior neuropores is essential for normal development of the nervous system. Incomplete closure of either neuropore produces severe neurologic deficits, which are readily apparent at birth. Failure of the anterior neuropore to close

Faulty closure of the anterior neuropore causes anencephaly.

prevents formation of the telencephalon, a condition known as *anencephaly*. Most anencephalic infants are either dead at birth or die shortly thereafter.

Faulty closure of the posterior neuropore results in *spina bifida*, a malformation of the vertebral column in which one or more vertebral arches remain open (Figure 2-16A). The neurologic importance of spina bifida varies widely. Spina bifida occulta occurs in 15%–25% of the population, but it has no clinical significance because the defect is not accompanied by meningeal or neural herniation (Figure 2-16B). Herniation of the dura through the vertebral defect is called a *meningocele* (Figure 2-16C). The most serious form of spina bifida, a *meningomyelocele*, includes meningeal and spinal cord herniation (Figure 2-16D). All forms of spina bifida may be accompanied by the Arnold-Chiari malformation, a caudal displacement of the brainstem and cerebellum. Although most symptoms of spina bifida are caused by mechanical stress placed on the nervous system, seemingly unrelated abnormalities may be present elsewhere in the body.

> *Faulty closure of the posterior neuropore causes **spina bifida**.*

FIGURE 2-16 ▶

Formation of the Vertebral Arch. (A) Normal. (B) Spina bifida occulta. Although the vertebral arch is missing, neither the arachnoid nor spinal cord have herniated through the defect. One marker for spina bifida occulta is a patch of hair on the overlying skin. (C) Meningocele. Herniation of the arachnoid through the vertebral defect. (D) Meningomyelocele. Herniation of the spinal cord and arachnoid through the vertebral defect makes this the most serious form of spina bifida.

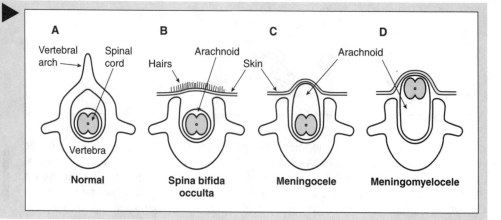

Primary Brain Vesicles and the Ventricular System

Following closure of the anterior neuropore during embryonic week 4, the rostral half of the central canal dilates into three chambers or primary brain vesicles: the *prosencephalon* (forebrain), the *mesencephalon* (midbrain), and the *rhombencephalon* (hindbrain; Figure 2-17A). By week 5, the prosencephalon has differentiated into the telencephalon and the diencephalon while the rhombencephalon has divided into the metencephalon and the myelencephalon (Figure 2-18; see Figure 2-17B). The only primary vesicle that does not subdivide during development is the mesencephalon, which forms the midbrain (Figure 2-19).

> *The three-vesicle embryonic brain is comprised of the **prosencephalon**, **mesencephalon**, and **rhombencephalon**.*

FIGURE 2-17 ▶

Three-Vesicle (A) and Five-Vesicle Stages (B) of Embryonic Development.

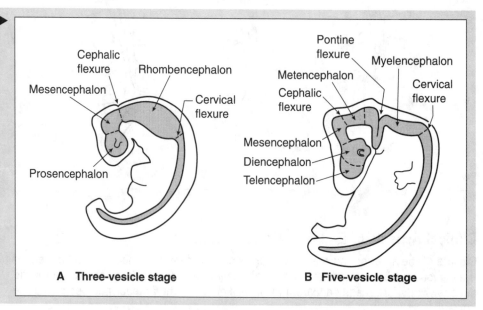

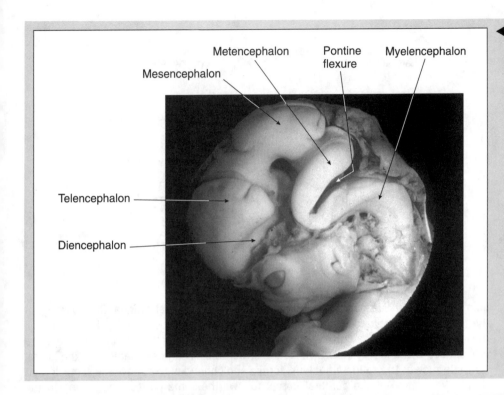

Metencephalon Pontine Myelencephalon
flexure
Mesencephalon

Telencephalon

Diencephalon

FIGURE 2-18
The Brain in Situ of an 8-Week-Old Embryo. (Source: *Courtesy of Dr. Malcolm B. Carpenter, Professor and Chairman Emeritus, Uniformed Armed Services University of the Health Sciences, Bethesda, Maryland.*)

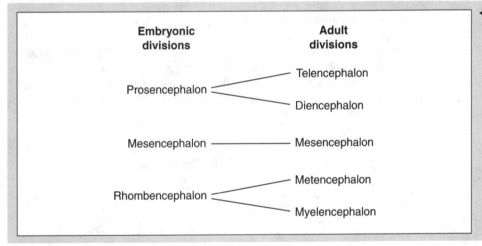

Embryonic divisions	Adult divisions
Prosencephalon	Telencephalon
	Diencephalon
Mesencephalon	Mesencephalon
Rhombencephalon	Metencephalon
	Myelencephalon

FIGURE 2-19
Divisions of the Embryonic and Adult Nervous System.

Growth and elaboration of the tissue surrounding the primary brain vesicles determine the size and shape of the brain's ventricles (Figure 2-20). For example, as the cerebellum develops from the alar plate, the central canal widens into the fourth ventricle. The small, roundish cerebral aqueduct, by comparison, reflects the modest development of the mesencephalon. In the diencephalon, the third ventricle is compressed into a vertically oriented slit during proliferation of the thalamus and hypothalamus. The most profound changes to the ventricular system reflect the explosive growth of the telencephalon. Each telencephalic hemisphere contains a lateral ventricle, which assumes the shape of a ram's horn as the telencephalon gradually envelopes the underlying diencephalon. Despite these changes in the shape and size of the ventricular system, it remains a continuous system where cerebrospinal fluid (CSF) produced in the lateral ventricles is able to flow into the third and fourth ventricles and finally into the subarachnoid space where it is resorbed into the venous system.

Forebrain

The telencephalon develops from the two telencephalic vesicles that form at the rostral end of the prosencephalon (see Figure 2-20). Each outpocket develops into a cerebral

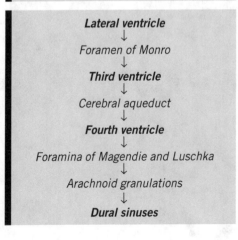

The cerebral aqueduct also is known as the ***aqueduct of Sylvius***.

Lateral ventricle
↓
Foramen of Monro
↓
Third ventricle
↓
Cerebral aqueduct
↓
Fourth ventricle
↓
Foramina of Magendie and Luschka
↓
Arachnoid granulations
↓
Dural sinuses

FIGURE 2-20 ▶
Ventricular System as Seen from Above during Late Embryonic Development.

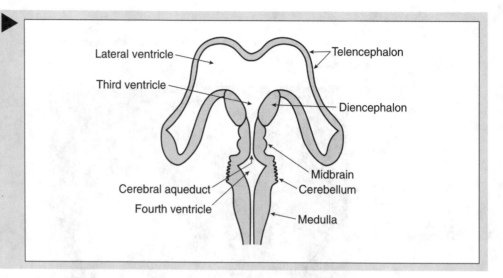

hemisphere while cells near the midline form the massive basal ganglia. Development of the telencephalon spreads from the lamina terminalis first rostrally and then caudally, the latter being more pronounced. The caudal expansion pulls the lateral ventricle into a pronounced C-shape (Figure 2-21). Neural structures closely associated with the lateral ventricle such as the caudate nucleus, fornix, and choroid plexus, have the same arched shape. Maturation of the cerebral cortex follows the same pattern, beginning in the frontal lobe and then spreading caudally through the parietal and occipital lobes. The rapid development of the frontal lobe traps and begins burying the more slowly growing insular cortex within the depths of the lateral sulcus. Final interment of the insula commences around the time of birth as the temporal lobe increases its size. Development of the telencephalon also covers the dorsal aspects of the diencephalon, mesencephalon, and cerebellum. As the cerebral hemispheres fill the limited confines of the cranium, its smooth (lissencephalic) surface folds into gyri. Although the major sulci are present at birth, others form during the next several years.

FIGURE 2-21 ▶
Sagittal View of the Internal Structure of the Cerebrum. (A) The ventricular system. (B) Caudate nucleus. (C) Hippocampus, fimbria, and fornix. (D) Amygdala and stria terminalis. (Source: Adapted with permission from Haines DE: Fundamental Neuroscience New York, NY: Churchill Livingstone, 1997, p 214.)

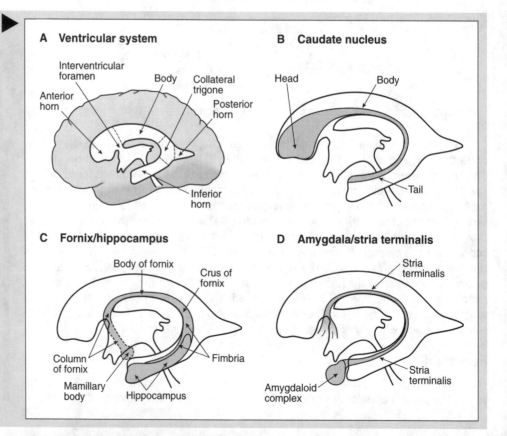

MENINGES AND THE VENTRICULAR SYSTEM

The human brain, whose consistency resembles that of meringue, requires an extraordinary degree of protection to survive the rigors of everyday life, not to mention rugby, soccer, and skateboarding. The skull provides the first level of protection, but other mechanisms must prevent the brain from pressing against the inner surface of the skull. This protection is afforded by the *meninges*, a membranous canopy that suspends the brain within its bony vault. Additional cushioning is provided by the CSF. The brain's need for chemical stability, though perhaps not as obvious, is just as important. Two complex systems, the *blood–brain barrier* and the *blood–CSF barrier*, enable the brain to draw nutrients from the vasculature system while insulating it from the chemical flux in the rest of the body.

Meninges

The *dura mater*, the *arachnoid*, and the *pia mater* form a laminated structure that, collectively, is referred to as the meninges.

Dura Mater. The dura mater, the outermost layer of the meninges, is a thick, parchment-like membrane that serves two functions. First, by stabilizing the CNS within the skull and vertebral column, the dura protects these delicate structures from trauma. Second, the dura contains specialized cavities called sinuses, which link the venous system of the brain with the systemic circulation.

The dura consists of collagen and flattened fibroblasts arranged into an outer periosteal layer that adheres tightly to the skull and an inner meningeal layer that is attached to the underlying arachnoid. The *periosteal layer* is confined to the cranium; the *meningeal layer*, however, exits the skull through the foramen magnum and lines the entire inner surface of the vertebral column. The caudal end of the spinal dura is woven into a tight cord, the coccygeal ligament, that anchors the spinal cord to the sacrum of the vertebral column (Figure 2-22). The dura protects the brain and the spinal cord from trauma by suspending them within their bony casings. The brain is provided additional stability by the *falx cerebri*, a sickle-shaped dural reflection located within the midsagittal sulcus (Figure 2-23). The falx cerebri extends from the crista galli of the ethmoid bone to the internal occipital protuberance where it joins the *tentorium cerebelli*. The tentorium is a broad dural reflection interposed between the dorsal surface of the cerebellum and the overlying occipital cortex. The tentorium effectively partitions the brain into a supratentorial compartment that contains the forebrain and the upper brainstem and an infratentorial compartment that contains the cerebellum and the lower brainstem. The midbrain passes through the lone opening in the tentorium, the tentorial notch. Gross inspection of the brain reveals two other dural reflections, the falx cerebelli and the diaphragma sellae. The falx cerebelli is the cerebellar analog of the falx cerebri. The *diaphragma sellae* forms a partition between the base of the brain and the pituitary fossa, the bony receptacle of the hypophysis.

Layers from the Skull to the Brain
Skull
Epidural space
Dura
Subdural space
Arachnoid
Pia
Brain

Dura mater means "tough mother" in Latin.

The ***falx cerebri*** lies within the midsagittal sulcus.

The ***tentorium*** separates the cerebellum from the overlying occipital cortex.

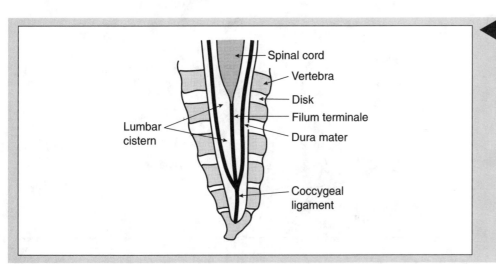

◀ **FIGURE 2-22**
The Caudal End of the Dural Sac. *The filum terminale secures the spinal cord to the dural sac. The coccygeal ligament anchors the dural sac to the base of the vertebral column. The cauda equina, which fills the lumbar cistern, is not shown.*

FIGURE 2-23 ▶
The Dura Mater and the Falx Cerebri Dissected Free from the Skull and Brain. *This section of the dura mater was removed from the frontoparietal region and is shown from the front. Occult blood in the midsagittal sinus gives this normally hollow structure its darkened appearance.*

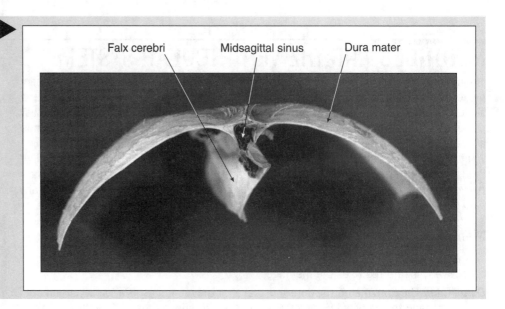

Falx cerebri   Midsagittal sinus   Dura mater

Dural sinuses, naturally occurring cavities between the periosteal and meningeal layers of the dura, link the venous circulation of the brain with the systemic circulation (Figure 2-24; see Figure 2-23). The most common site for a sinus is along the edges of the dural folds. All sinuses eventually drain into the internal jugular vein after first converging at the *confluens of the sinuses*. The confluens of the sinuses is located at the internal occipital protuberance and is formed by the anastomosis of three major sinuses:

Sinuses *are cavities between the meningeal and periosteal layers of the dura.*

1. **Superior sagittal sinus.** Located on the midline above the falx cerebri, the superior sagittal sinus drains both cerebral hemispheres posteriorly toward the confluens.

2. **Straight sinus.** Located on the dorsal ridge of the cerebellum, the straight sinus collects venous blood from deep structures of the brain via the vein of Galen and empties into the confluens.

3. **Inferior sagittal sinus.** The inferior sagittal sinus runs posteriorly along the ventral edge of the falx cerebri and reaches the confluens via the straight sinus.

Venous blood, after passing through the confluens, drains into the left and right *transverse sinuses* located along the posterolateral margin of the tentorium. The transverse sinus also receives venous output from the cavernous and petrosal sinuses (see Figure 2-24).

FIGURE 2-24 ▶
Lateral View of the Head Showing Major Dural Sinuses. *(Source: Reprinted with permission from Browder I, Kaplan MA: Cerebral Dural Sinuses and Their Tributaries. Springfield, IL: Charles C Thomas, 1976, p 11.)*

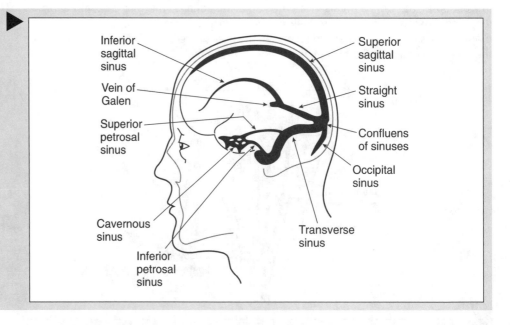

Inferior sagittal sinus
Vein of Galen
Superior petrosal sinus
Cavernous sinus
Inferior petrosal sinus
Superior sagittal sinus
Straight sinus
Confluens of sinuses
Occipital sinus
Transverse sinus

1. **Cavernous sinuses.** The cavernous sinuses are located along the lateral margin of the sella turcica, the bony saddle that partially encapsulates the hypophysis. The proximity of the cavernous sinus to the hypothalamus, the hypophysis, the internal carotid artery, and numerous cranial nerves (III, IV, VI, and the ophthalmic and maxillary branches of V) makes this a clinically important structure. The cavernous sinus drains into the superior and inferior petrosal sinuses.

2. **Superior and inferior petrosal sinuses.** The superior and inferior petrosal sinuses drain the cavernous sinus into the transverse sinus and the internal jugular vein, respectively.

3. **Anterior and posterior intercavernous sinuses.** This anastomotic venous grid surrounds the stalk of the pituitary gland at the base of the diencephalon and thus connects the left and right cavernous sinuses.

Venous blood carried by the transverse sinuses returns to the heart and the systemic circulation via the internal jugular artery.

Arachnoid Mater. The arachnoid mater consists of fibroblasts arranged into an outer sheet and an underlying web or trabeculae (Figure 2-25). The framework formed by the trabeculae not only secures the meningeal dura to the underlying pia mater, but also creates the *subarachnoid space*, which contains CSF, arteries, veins, and cranial nerve roots. CSF formed within the ventricular system uses the subarachnoid space as a conduit to return to the venous circulation. Passage from the subarachnoid space to the venous circulation takes place through specialized structures called arachnoid villi located in the walls of the superior sagittal sinus. Each villus is formed by an evagination of the outer arachnoid membrane into the lumen of the dural sinus. Flow of CSF through the villus occurs when fluid pressure in the subarachnoid space exceeds that of the dural sinus. Because reversal of the pressure gradient stops the discharge of CSF from the subarachnoid space, from a functional standpoint, each villus resembles a one-way valve.

Arachnoid villi act as one-way valves between the subarachnoid space and the venous system.

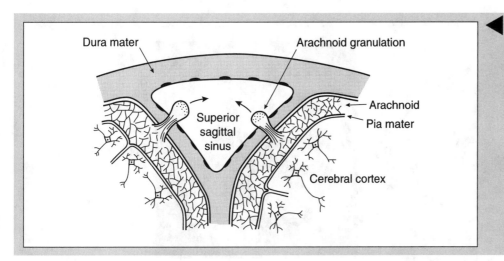

Dura mater

Arachnoid granulation

Arachnoid

Pia mater

Superior sagittal sinus

Cerebral cortex

◀ ***FIGURE 2-25***
Cross Section of the Midsagittal Sinus Showing Two Arachnoid Granulations.

Because the arachnoid follows the contours of the skull more closely than the brain, the width of the subarachnoid space increases in those areas where the brain's surface does not lie close to the skull. These enlargements of the subarachnoid space are called *cisterns*. The largest cistern, the *cisterna magna*, is located between the base of the cerebellum and the dorsal surface of the medulla. One of the most clinically relevant is the *lumbar cistern*, which is located in the spinal canal beyond the caudal end of the spinal cord. The lumbar cistern contains CSF as well as the nerve roots that form the cauda equina (see Chapter 3). Percutaneous punctures of the lumbar cistern are used routinely to obtain samples of CSF and to deliver therapeutic agents to the CNS (see Chapter 4, Figure 4-2). Two additional cisterns are the interpeduncular and cerebellopontine.

Cisterns are CSF-filled cavities formed between the arachnoid and the pia mater.

Pia Mater. The innermost meningeal layer is the pia mater, a delicate membrane that clings to the contours of the brain. The pia lacks the strength of the dura and arachnoid, but its tight adhesion to the entire cortical surface distributes the suspensory forces that secure the brain within the cranium. The pial lining of the spinal cord has two elaborations that secure the cord within the spinal canal. A series of pial bands called denticulate ligaments anchor the lateral aspect of the spinal cord to the arachnoid and dural membranes. The denticulate ligaments run the full length of the spinal cord. The caudal end of the spinal cord is secured to the end of the dura sac by a tough pial filament called the filum terminale.

Clinical Aspects Related to the Meninges

Hematomas. Hematomas are pools of occult blood formed by either arterial or venous hemorrhage. When intracranial hematomas displace and compress the brain, there may be irreversible brain damage. It is not uncommon for the point of maximum compression to be distant to the site of hematoma formation as in uncal herniations (see Chapter 4). During acute hematoma formation patients exhibit headaches, lethargy, and mental confusion that may progress to coma.

Hematomas may form within the parenchyma, but the most common sites are juxtaposed to the dura. Normally, the dura is securely attached to the inner tablet of the skull and the underlying arachnoid, but trauma may cause separation of these layers and hemorrhagic bleeding. Epidural bleeding into the space between the periosteal dura and the skull is usually of arterial origin. Subdural hematomas are usually caused by rupture of bridging veins, the short segment of the superficial cerebral veins that cross the arachnoid space (Figure 2-26). Subdural hematomas form along the border between the meningeal dura and the underlying arachnoid layer. Epidural and subdural hematomas represent life-threatening medical emergencies that require immediate care.

Hematomas are pools of occult blood of either arterial or venous origin.

Subdural hematomas are usually caused by rupture of bridging veins that cross the arachnoid space.

FIGURE 2-26
Computerized Axial Tomography Scan of Trauma-induced Subdural Hematoma over the Left Frontoparietal Area. Note the shift of the midline to the patient's right. (Source: Courtesy of Dr. John Barr, Pennsylvania State University College of Medicine, Hershey, Pennsylvania.)

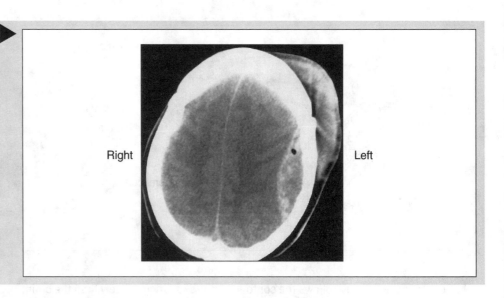

Right   Left

Meningiomas are tumors of the meninges, which displace rather than invade the parenchyma of the brain.

Meningiomas. Meningiomas are a class of slow-growing tumors that originate in the meninges, usually where the arachnoid villa, cranial nerves, or blood vessels pierce the dura. The most common site of meningioma formation is along the falx cerebri. Meningiomas rarely invade the parenchyma, so their damage is caused primarily through compression and displacement of the brain. These tumors are accompanied by headaches and seizures; more specific symptoms related to brain compression are seen in advanced cases. The slow but inexorable growth of meningiomas requires surgical intervention, but regrowth, usually within 5 years, is common.

Ventricular System

The ventricular system, the adult derivative of the embryonic neural tube, helps protect, stabilize, and nourish the CNS. Many parts of the ventricular system contain choroid plexus and its plasma-like secretion, CSF. The ventricular system consists of four chambers: the paired lateral ventricles, the third ventricle, and the fourth ventricle.

Lateral Ventricles. The lateral ventricles are paired, C-shaped cavities within the telencephalon. The lateral ventricle consists of four parts, the anterior horn, the body, and the posterior and inferior horns (Figure 2-27). The *anterior horn* ends abruptly within the white matter of the frontal lobe, its medial wall formed by the septum pellucidum and the fornix. The head of the caudate nucleus lines its lateral wall while the corpus callosum forms the roof. The *body of the lateral ventricle* is located further caudally, its floor formed by the thalamus and the caudate nucleus. As the body of the lateral ventricle sweeps further posteriorly, it joins the inferior and posterior horns at the *collateral trigone*. The *posterior horn* terminates within the white matter of the occipital lobe, partially surrounded by fibers of the corpus callosum. The *inferior horn* descends and enters the temporal lobe and proceeds rostrally until terminating immediately caudal to the amygdala. The inferior horn is bounded dorsomedially by the tail of the caudate nucleus and ventrally by the hippocampus.

> **Four Parts of the Lateral Ventricle**
> *Anterior horn*
> *Body*
> *Posterior horn*
> *Inferior horn*

> The **collateral trigone** also is known as the **atrium.**

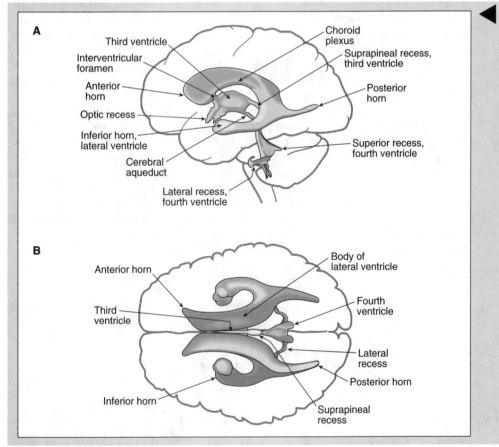

FIGURE 2-27
(A) Lateral view of the ventricular system.
(B) Dorsal view of the ventricular system.
Anterior is to the left.

Third Ventricle. The third ventricle is a vertically oriented, slit-like cavity in the diencephalon, bounded anteriorly by the lamina terminalis and laterally by the thalamus and hypothalamus. At its rostral end, the third ventricle communicates with the paired lateral ventricles through the interventricular foramen (foramen of Monro). Caudally, the third ventricle tapers to a narrow channel, the aqueduct of Sylvius, that burrows through the mesencephalon before opening into the fourth ventricle.

> The **foramen of Monro** connects the lateral and third ventricles.

> The **cerebral aqueduct** connects the third and fourth ventricles.

*Foramen of **M**agendie: **M**edial
Foramen of **L**uschka: **L**ateral*

Fourth Ventricle. The fourth ventricle forms a diamond-shaped depression on the roof of the pons and medulla. The walls of the fourth ventricle are formed by the cerebellum and the superior cerebellar peduncle. Two membranes, the anterior and posterior medullary vela (sing., velum), separate the fourth ventricle from the overlying cerebellum. Posteriorly, the fourth ventricle tapers to a point, the obex, and joins the central canal of the spinal cord. Because the central canal is only open at its rostral end, little CSF enters. Almost all CSF flows from the fourth ventricle into the subarachnoid space through three perforations in the vela: the *foramen of Magendie* and the paired *foramina of Luschka*. The foramen of Magendie is a jagged opening near the midline of the posterior medullary velum while the paired foramina of Luschka are located in the lateral recess of the fourth ventricle at the pontomedullary junction.

Choroid Plexus

***CSF** is produced by the choroid plexus.*

CSF that supports and protects the CNS is produced primarily by the choroid plexus. The choroid plexus is a band of highly vascularized, microvillous tissue within the lateral, third, and fourth ventricles. In the lateral ventricle, the choroid plexus forms a loose trail from the foramen of Monro to the tip of the inferior horn. A dense accumulation of choroid plexus within the collateral trigone called the glomus calcifies with age and may appear on radiographic films. Some of the choroid plexus in the body of the lateral ventricle enters the third ventricle through the *foramen of Monro*. The choroid plexus is not found in the anterior or posterior horn of the lateral ventricle or the cerebral aqueduct. The choroid plexus in the fourth ventricle hangs like moss from the posterior medullary velum and spills through the foramina of Luschka into the subarachnoid space of the cerebellopontine cistern.

The histologic structure of the choroid plexus can be best understood in the context of its embryologic development. Initially, the nutritional requirements of the neural tube are met by diffusion of solutes from the intrauterine fluid of the womb. As the neural tube grows and its demand for nutrients exceeds what diffusion can provide, most of the nourishment is derived from the fledgling vasculature system. Blood vessels, after their appearance on the surface of the neural tube, penetrate the pia and the underlying parenchyma. When this process occurs along the roof plates of the third and fourth ventricle, the invading arterioles, venules, and pia fuse with the underlying ependymal lining of the ventricles to form the choroid plexus (Figure 2-28). The vascular elements lie at the core of the choroid plexus while the ependymal cells form its lining. The surface of the ependymal cells consists of numerous large folds or villi covered with microvilli. These cells, now specialized for the secretion of CSF, are the choroidal epithelium.

FIGURE 2-28 ▶
Development of the Choroid Plexus. *(A) Blood vessels initially develop on the outer surface of the pia. (B) As the blood vessels invade the parenchyma, they take the pia with them. (C) Blood vessels that penetrate the ventricle form the choroid plexus by fusing with the trapped pia and ependymal lining of the ventricle. (Source: Adapted with permission from Martin JM: Neuroanatomy Text and Atlas, Stamford, CT: Appleton & Lange, 1996, p 39.)*

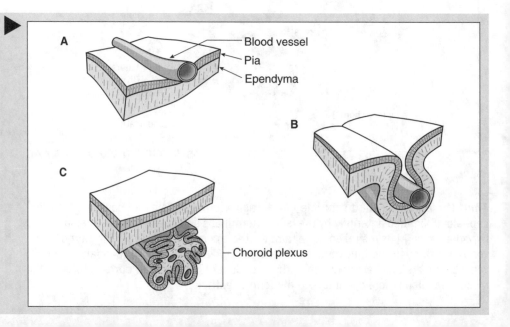

Cerebrospinal Fluid

CSF is a clear, plasma-like liquid that bathes the ventricular and pial surfaces of the ventricles and the subarachnoid space surrounding the brain and spinal cord. The CSF, which is known as the third circulation, flows from the lateral ventricles through the foramina of Monro into the third ventricle before squeezing through the cerebral aqueduct into the fourth ventricle. Once in the fourth ventricle, the CSF empties into the subarachnoid space through the foramina of Magendie and Luschka. The impetus for CSF flow is provided by pulsation of the choroidal arteries within the ventricles and the coordinated beating of the cilia of the choroidal epithelium. When the hydrostatic force of the CSF exceeds the venous pressure, CSF moves from the subarachnoid space through the arachnoid granulations into the superior sagittal sinus. CSF in the subarachnoid space surrounding the spinal cord is resorbed into the lymphatic system through the perilymphatic spaces along the spinal veins.

The primary function of the CSF is to prevent the brain from striking the inner surface of the skull during quick or violent head movements. The protection afforded by the CSF derives from the brain's natural buoyancy, which evenly distributes the weight of the brain to all of the meningeal surfaces.

The buoyancy provided by the CSF reduces the effective weight of the brain by 97%.

Almost 70% of the CSF is derived from the choroid plexus through secretion and filtration of blood plasma. The remaining 30% of the CSF represents water-soluble metabolic waste discharged by the neuropil surrounding the ventricles. Compared to blood plasma, CSF has lower concentrations of glucose, calcium (Ca^{2+}), protein, and potassium (K^+) and higher concentrations of sodium (Na^+), magnesium (Mg^{2+}), and chloride (Cl^-). The concentrations of B and T lymphocytes, monocytes, and neutrophils normally are low. Changes in the chemical composition of the CSF can be an important diagnostic tool for a variety of disorders. For example, bacterial meningitis and brain abscesses cause the CSF glucose concentration to plummet and the neutrophil count to increase. Viral meningitis, on the other hand, has little effect on the glucose concentration. Multiple sclerosis causes an increase in the lymphocyte count as well as the concentration and makeup of immunoglobulin. Increased protein levels may signal a subarachnoid hemorrhage or a CNS tumor. A cautionary note should be added here: obtaining a CSF sample via a lumbar puncture in patients suspected of having elevated intracranial pressure risks herniation of the cerebellar tonsils through the cisterna magnum. Tonsillar herniation compresses the lower brainstem causing apnea, circulatory collapse, and coma; prompt treatment is required to avoid death.

Changes in the chemical composition of CSF can be an important diagnostic tool.

Daily secretion of CSF, approximately 450–500 mL, far exceeds the 120 mL capacity of the average adult brain. Normally, excess CSF is resorbed and intracranial pressure is maintained within normal limits. Certain pathologic conditions such as congenital malformations and developmental or mass lesions may interfere with normal CSF equilibrium and cause *hydrocephalus*, an excess accumulation of CSF in the cranium. The presenting symptoms of hydrocephalus may include dizziness, headaches, nausea, and vomiting. If intracranial pressure has increased, papilledema may be present (see Chapter 10). Radiographs of the skull may show enlarged ventricular spaces proximal to the occlusion and thinning of the cerebral cortex (Figure 2-29). Hydrocephalus in infants causes skull enlargement with widened fontanelles and, left untreated, will cause severe physical and mental retardation and, ultimately, death.

Hydrocephalus is caused by excess CSF.

Hydrocephalus is often but not always associated with an increase in intracranial pressure. Hydrocephalus accompanied by an increase in intracranial pressure is classified as either noncommunicating or communicating, depending on whether an obstruction to CSF flow is present. Obstructions within the ventricular system or the subarachnoid space that prevent the normal flow of CSF toward the arachnoid villi cause *noncommunicating hydrocephalus*. Every part of the ventricular system except the lateral ventricle is vulnerable to obstruction, but the most common site is the cerebral aqueduct because of its small diameter. Extraventricular obstructions are less common but may occur almost anywhere in the subarachnoid space. Common causes of noncommunicating hydrocephalus include congenital stenosis of the cerebral aqueduct, posthemorrhagic blood clots, intracranial neoplasms, tuberculosis, and meningitis.

FIGURE 2-29
Ventricular Enlargement and Thinning of the Cerebral Cortex Due to Noncommunicating Hydrocephalus. Anterior is to the top. (Source: *Courtesy of Dr. John Barr, Pennsylvania State University College of Medicine, Hershey, Pennsylvania.*)

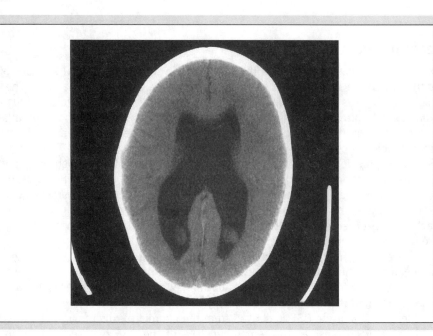

In the absence of an intra- or extraventricular occlusion, the diagnosis of a *communicating hydrocephalus* is made. Common causes of communicating hydrocephalus include oversecretion of CSF, impaired CSF absorption, and venous insufficiency. Impairment of CSF absorption may be caused by clogging of the arachnoid villi with either red blood cells, following a subarachnoid hemorrhage, or with protein in cases of CNS tumors. The preferred method of treatment for all forms of hydrocephalus is surgical implantation of a shunt that either bypasses the obstruction or drains excess CSF from the head into the heart or the peritoneal cavity.

Chemical Isolation of the Brain

The brain's reliance on the vascular system for its nourishment exposes it to the chemical flux in the rest of the body. The chemical integrity of the CNS is protected by the blood–brain barrier and the blood–CSF barrier. Both barriers are the structural partitions between the blood and the CSF, and interstitial fluid compartments of the CNS.

*The **blood–brain barrier** and **blood–CSF barrier** are formed by tight junctions in the walls of arterial capillaries.*

The blood–brain and blood–CSF barriers are formed by the walls of arterial capillaries within the CNS. All capillaries consist of an endothelial wall, a basal lamina, and an outer sheath of astrocytic foot processes (Figure 2-30). In the body, solutes pass freely from capillaries to the interstitial space through the fenestrated endothelial cell walls. In the brain, solute flow is obstructed by tight junctions between adjacent endothelial cells. Additional barriers are formed by the basal lamina and astrocytes whose foot processes form a continuous sheath around each capillary. These barriers allow water, small lipid-soluble solutes, and gases such as oxygen and carbon dioxide to enter either the CSF or the brain. Capillary cell walls are slightly permeable to Na^+, K^+, and Cl^- but are impermeable to large plasma proteins and large organic molecules. This selective permeability complicates treatment of intracranial disorders because antibiotics, antineoplastic agents, and many other therapeutic agents are unable to enter the brain. It is possible to bypass the blood–brain barrier by injecting drugs into the ventricular system, usually at the lumbar cistern. Drugs administered intraventricularly enter the brain by diffusing through the pia mater and the ependymal lining of the ventricles.

The circumventricular organs lack a blood–brain barrier.

Despite the widespread distribution of these barriers along the capillaries within the brain and choroid plexus, several brain areas have no barrier system. These areas have fenestrated capillaries that allow solutes to pass freely into and out of the brain. For example, various hormones secreted by the adenohypophysis and neurohypophysis pass directly into the systemic circulation. The pineal gland, which also lacks a blood–brain

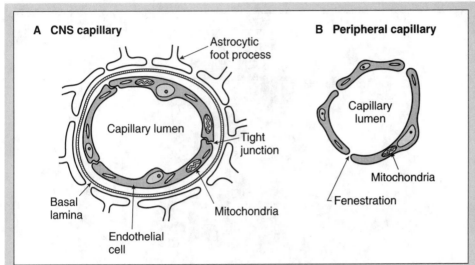

FIGURE 2-30
Central and Peripheral Capillaries. (A) The relative impermeability of capillaries in the CNS derives from the tight junctions between the endothelial cells and the continuous lining of astrocytic foot processes. (B) Capillaries in the systemic circulation have a fenestrated lining of epithelial cells that permits most solutes to pass freely between the blood and the interstitial spaces in the tissue. CNS = central nervous system.

barrier, secretes melatonin directly into the systemic circulation. Other circumventricular areas such as the area postrema, the subfornical organ, the organum vasculosum of the lamina terminalis, and the median eminence are chemoreceptor zones that monitor changes in body fluids such as plasma osmolarity and blood glucose levels. Because many brain tumors lack a barrier system, they readily absorb contrast agents that are detectable by magnetic resonance imaging (MRI) and CT scans.

BLOOD SUPPLY OF THE BRAIN AND SPINAL CORD

Humans can survive for several weeks without food and for several days without water. When the brain's supply of oxygen is interrupted for as little as 30 seconds, however, brain metabolism is affected. Following 1 minute of anoxia, neural activity begins to falter; by 5 minutes, irreversible cell death begins, followed minutes later by certain death. The brain's vulnerability derives from its high metabolic requirements and severely limited stores of oxygen and glucose. The responsibility for delivering continuous supplies of oxygen and glucose to the brain lies with the elaborate vascular matrix that derives from the carotid and vertebral arteries.

Arterial Supply

Carotid Artery Circulation. The common carotid artery ascends the neck, bifurcates, and forms the external and internal carotid arteries. The external branch supplies the face while the internal branch enters the skull and supplies the brain. The *internal carotid artery* has four segments: the *cervical*, the *intrapetrosal*, the *cavernous*, and the *cerebral* (Figure 2-31). The cervical branch of the internal carotid artery is located in the neck between the carotid bifurcation and the petrous bone of the skull. The intrapetrosal segment lies within the carotid canal of the petrous bone. As the internal carotid artery enters the cranium, it passes through the cavernous sinus close to the oculomotor, trochlear, trigeminal, and abducens nerves. The cerebral segment begins as the internal carotid artery emerges from the cavernous sinus. The intracavernous and cerebral segments of the internal carotid artery form an S-shaped region called the *carotid siphon*. The cerebral segment gives rise to three major arteries: the ophthalmic, the posterior communicating, and the anterior choroidal. The *ophthalmic artery* supplies the optic nerve and retina, as well as the paranasal sinuses and parts of the nose. The anterior choroidal artery passes posterolaterally, enters the inferior horn of the lateral ventricle through the choroidal fissure, and supplies blood to the choroid plexus, the globus pallidus, the hippocampal formation and parts of the internal capsule, the amygdala, and the tail of the caudate (Figure 2-32). The *posterior communicating artery* is the link in the

Four Segments of the Internal Carotid Artery
Cervical
Intrapetrosal
Intracavernous
Cerebral

FIGURE 2-31 ▶

Angiogram in the anterior–posterior plane showing the distributions of the internal carotid artery (ICA), anterior cerebral artery (ACA), and the middle cerebral artery (MCA). (Source: Courtesy of Dr. John Barr, Pennsylvania State University College of Medicine, Hershey, Pennsylvania.)

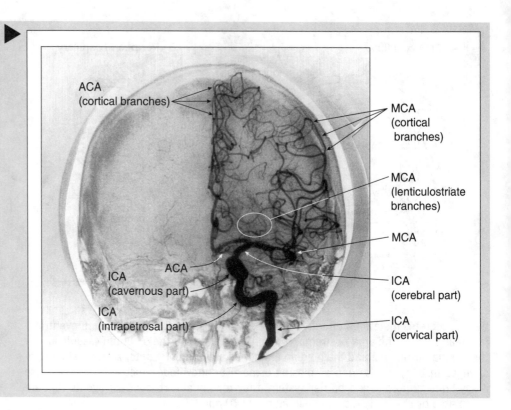

FIGURE 2-32 ▶

Circle of Willis. *ACA = anterior cerebral artery; AICA = anterior inferior cerebellar artery; ICA = internal carotid artery; MCA = middle cerebral artery; PCA = posterior cerebral artery; PICA = posterior inferior cerebellar artery; SCA = superior cerebellar artery.*

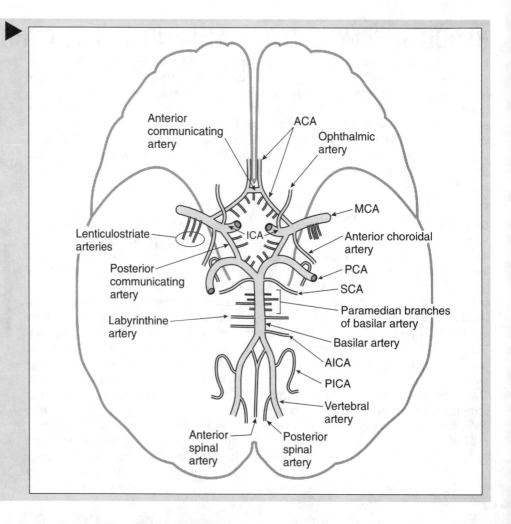

circle of Willis that connects the internal carotid artery with the posterior circulation arising from the *vertebral artery* (see Figure 2-32). The internal carotid artery ends at the bifurcation of the anterior and middle cerebral arteries.

From its origin at the internal carotid artery, the *anterior cerebral artery (ACA)* courses rostromedially, crosses the optic nerve, and enters the interhemispheric fissure (Figure 2-33). Two branches of the ACA, the frontopolar and orbital arteries, supply the frontal pole and the orbital and medial surfaces of the frontal cortex. Two larger branches, the callosomarginal and the pericallosal arteries, arch posteriorly around the genu of the corpus callosum and supply blood to the entire medial surface of the frontal and parietal lobes and part of the adjacent lateral convexity. Occlusion of the callosomarginal branch may produce anesthesia, paralysis, or both of the contralateral lower limbs.

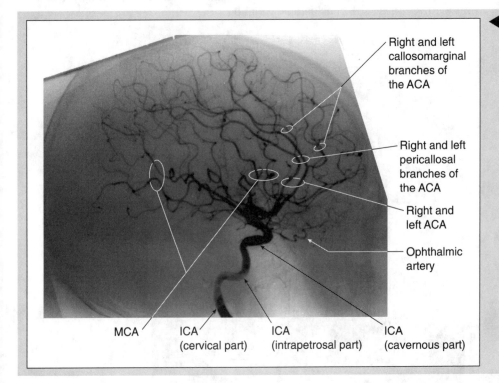

Right and left callosomarginal branches of the ACA

Right and left pericallosal branches of the ACA

Right and left ACA

Ophthalmic artery

MCA   ICA (cervical part)   ICA (intrapetrosal part)   ICA (cavernous part)

FIGURE 2-33
Lateral Angiogram Following Injection of the Internal Carotid Artery. *Anterior is to the right. ACA = anterior cerebral artery; ICA = internal carotid artery; MCA = middle cerebral artery.*

The *middle cerebral artery (MCA)*, which represents the continuation of the internal carotid artery, has the largest and most complex distribution of the major cerebral arteries. From its origin near the circle of Willis, the MCA passes laterally between the insula and the rostral pole of the temporal lobe. During its course, small penetrating branches of the lenticulostriate arteries enter the brain through the anterior perforated substance and supply blood to most of the anterior and posterior limbs of the internal capsule as well as parts of the globus pallidus and the putamen. The first major branches of the MCA are the anterior temporal artery and the orbitofrontal artery. The anterior temporal artery and the orbitofrontal artery emerge from the lateral sulcus and blanket the superior and middle temporal gyri and the lateral gyri located in the orbitofrontal cortex, respectively. Occlusion of the anterior temporal artery affects the primary auditory cortex and the adjacent auditory association cortices. In the dominant hemisphere severe language deficits result if this damage includes Wernicke's area, which is located at the terminus of the lateral sulcus.

The main trunk of the MCA remains within the lateral sulcus and spreads across the insula. Some small penetrating arteries supply the insula itself, but most ascend and make a hairpin turn at the circular sulcus, descend along the inner surface of the operculum, emerge from the lateral sulcus, and fan out across the frontoparietal cortex. The Rolandic and pre- and post-Rolandic arteries supply the primary motor and somatosensory cortices located along the banks of the central sulcus (fissure of Rolando).

The middle cerebral artery is the continuation of the internal carotid artery.

The lenticulostriate arteries perfuse the lentiform nucleus, which is part of the striatum.

Obstruction of the Rolandic branches produces motor and somatosensory deficits of the contralateral torso, upper limbs, or head. Such an infarct usually spares the lower limbs, whose cortical representations are buried within the longitudinal fissure and are perfused by the ACA.

Vertebral Artery Circulation. The vertebral arteries derive from the subclavian artery and ascend to the brain by passing through the foramina of the upper six cervical vertebrae. After entering the cranial vault through the foramen magnum, the paired vertebral arteries run along the ventrolateral margin of the medulla until they join as the basilar artery at the pontomedullary junction (Figure 2-34; see Figure 2-32). Four major arteries emerge from the vertebral artery: the *posterior meningeal artery*, the *posterior inferior cerebellar artery (PICA)*, and the *anterior* and *posterior spinal arteries*. The paired vertebral arteries perfuse the brainstem and cerebellum as well as part of the spinal cord, but their territories show considerable variation.

Four Major Arteries Emerge from the Vertebral Artery
Posterior meningeal artery
Posterior inferior cerebellar artery
Anterior spinal artery
Posterior spinal artery

FIGURE 2-34
Angiogram in the Anterior–Posterior Plane Following Injection of the Vertebral Artery. AICA = anterior inferior cerebellar artery; PICA = posterior inferior cerebellar artery; PCA = posterior cerebral artery; SCA = superior cerebellar artery. (Source: Courtesy of Dr. John Barr, Pennsylvania State University College of Medicine, Hershey, Pennsylvania.)

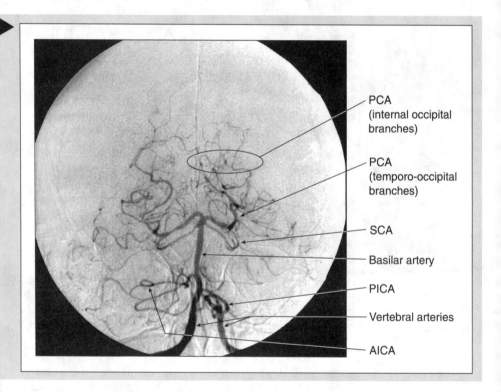

PCA (internal occipital branches)

PCA (temporo-occipital branches)

SCA

Basilar artery

PICA

Vertebral arteries

AICA

The posterior meningeal artery is one of three arteries that supply the dura of the posterior fossa, the other two being the occipital and pharyngeal arteries.

The PICA, the largest branch of the vertebral artery, supplies parts of the rostral medulla and cerebellum (Figure 2-35; see Figures 2-32 and 2-34). Proximal branches perfuse the dorsolateral quadrant of the medulla, which contains nuclei of cranial nerves V, VII, IX, and X. More distal branches perfuse the cerebellum. Occlusion of the vertebral or the PICA produces a constellation of deficits known as the lateral medullary syndrome (Wallenberg's syndrome) and Horner's syndrome (see Chapter 4).

Further caudally, the medulla is supplied by the vertebral arteries and the proximal parts of the anterior and posterior spinal arteries (see Figures 2-32 and 2-35). The anterior spinal artery is formed by the fusion of two small branches that emerge from the vertebral arteries (see Figure 2-32). The anterior spinal artery perfuses a U-shaped area along the midline. Medullary structures located further laterally are supplied by the vertebral artery. Sudden occlusion of the anterior spinal artery within the medulla produces an inferior alternating hemiplegia (see Chapter 4). Proximal branches of the posterior spinal artery perfuse the dorsolateral quadrant of the medulla while its more distal branches descend to the conus medullaris of the spinal cord.

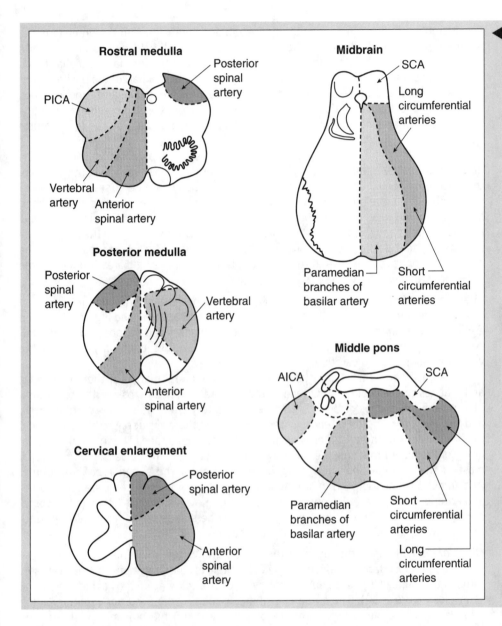

Rostral medulla

PICA

Posterior spinal artery

Vertebral artery

Anterior spinal artery

Posterior medulla

Posterior spinal artery

Vertebral artery

Anterior spinal artery

Cervical enlargement

Posterior spinal artery

Anterior spinal artery

Midbrain

SCA

Long circumferential arteries

Paramedian branches of basilar artery

Short circumferential arteries

Middle pons

AICA

SCA

Paramedian branches of basilar artery

Short circumferential arteries

Long circumferential arteries

FIGURE 2-35
Arterial Supply of the Brainstem and Spinal Cord. AICA = anterior inferior cerebellar artery; PICA = posterior inferior cerebellar artery; SCA = superior cerebellar artery.

The anterior and posterior spinal arteries provide the primary vascular supply for the upper cervical segments (see Figure 2-35). Caudal to the cervical level, the continuity of the spinal arteries is maintained by anastomotic connections with radicular arteries, which are of segmental origin. Unfortunately, the radicular arteries are not distributed evenly along the length of the spinal cord. Infarcts are more common at those levels of the spinal cord where the radicular supply is sparse (i.e., T1–T4, L1). From its position within the anterior median fissure, the anterior spinal artery supplies the anterior two-thirds of the spinal cord. The posterior spinal artery supplies a wedge-shaped area of the posterior spinal cord. Interestingly, the paired posterior spinal arteries supply about one-third as much blood as the single anterior spinal artery does to the spinal cord. The perimeter of the lateral funiculus is supplied by the halo of superficial arteries of the arterial vasocorona.

The spinal cord is perfused by the anterior spinal artery, the paired posterior spinal arteries, and radicular arteries.

Basilar Artery Circulation. At the pontomedullary junction, the vertebral arteries anastomose to form the *basilar artery*, which ascends the pons within the basilar sulcus (see Figure 2-32). The basilar artery has three major branches: the *labyrinthine artery*, the *anterior inferior cerebellar artery (AICA)*, and the *superior cerebellar artery* as well as many smaller, unnamed branches. The labyrinthine artery travels with the eighth cranial nerve through the internal auditory meatus to the inner ear where it supplies the auditory and vestibular apparatus. The distribution of the AICA, like its posterior namesake, varies

Three Major Branches of the Basilar Artery
Labyrinthine artery
Anterior inferior cerebellar artery
Superior cerebellar artery

considerably but usually includes the brainstem and cerebellum. In the brainstem, the AICA supplies the middle cerebellar peduncle and the choroid plexus of the fourth ventricle. In the cerebellum, its territory includes most of the inferior cerebellar hemisphere. The superior cerebellar artery originates from the rostral part of the basilar artery, passes immediately caudal to the root fibers of the oculomotor nerve, and supplies blood to most of the rostral cerebellum. Proximal branches perfuse the crus cerebri, parts of the superior and middle cerebellar peduncles, and part of the choroid plexus of the fourth ventricle.

The unnamed branches of the basilar artery include the *paramedian* and the *short and long circumferential arteries*. The paramedian branches perfuse the pontine nuclei, the middle cerebellar peduncle, and descending corticofugal fibers (see Figures 2-32 and 2-35). Structures located further laterally in the pons are supplied by the short circumferential branches of the basilar artery. The long circumferential branches curve around the pons and supply blood to most of the nuclei and tracts within the dorsolateral pontine tegmentum. In the caudal pons, the long circumferential arteries overlap the proximal branches of the AICA; further rostrally they overlap the field area supplied by the superior cerebellar artery.

Posterior Cerebral Artery. As the basilar artery reaches the interpeduncular fossa, it bifurcates and forms the right and left posterior cerebral arteries (see Figures 2-32 and 2-34). An anastomosis between the posterior cerebral artery and the posterior communicating artery, one segment in the circle of Willis, provides continuity between the vertebrobasilar and the carotid circulations (see below).

The posterior cerebral artery passes around the lateral margin of the crus cerebri and reaches the ventrolateral surface of the cerebral cortex by crossing the tentorium. The two main branches of the posterior cerebral artery are the temporo-occipital artery and the internal occipital artery. The temporo-occipital artery supplies the inferior and medial surfaces of the posterior two-thirds of the temporal lobe. The internal occipital artery or its major branches, the parieto-occipital artery and the calcarine artery, supply most of the occipital lobe and a significant portion of the superior parietal lobule. Anastomotic connections often are found where the territories of the posterior, middle, and anterior cerebral arteries oppose one another. The anastomoses between the posterior and middle cerebral arteries along the calcarine sulcus may preserve visual function following infarcts of the occipital lobe (see Chapter 10).

Circle of Willis. Despite the fact that the carotid and vertebral arteries supply different and largely nonoverlapping regions of the CNS, there is continuity between these vessels through the circle of Willis, an anastomotic ring of arteries lying on the floor of the cranial vault (see Figure 2-32). The circle of Willis is formed by the posterior communicating arteries, which connect the internal carotid arteries with the proximal portion of the posterior cerebral artery, as well as by the anterior communicating artery, which connects the left and right anterior cerebral arteries. In the event of a stroke, the circle of Willis should allow one side of the brain to be fed by the arteries from the opposite side. In reality, there is little collateral circulation in most individuals because the anterior and posterior communicating arteries are either too small or missing. The circle of Willis is, however, a common site for cerebral aneurysms which, if left untreated, may bleed into the subarachnoid space and cause serious neurologic deficits.

Venous Drainage

The venous organization of the spinal cord resembles its arterial supply in that the longitudinal vessels lying on the anterior and posterior surfaces of the cord are supplemented by a series of radicular veins. While some venous blood ascends and enters the jugular veins, most of it leaves the spinal canal through epidural plexuses that drain into nearby segmental veins.

Venous drainage of the brain does not run in parallel to its arterial supply. Instead, venous drainage of the brain is accomplished through an elaborate system of veins that shunts blood into the sinuses that eventually drain into the internal jugular vein for return to the systemic circulation. Depending on their location, cerebral veins are classified as superficial or deep. Superficial veins lie on the surface of the cerebral cortex and drain

The paired posterior cerebral arteries are the continuation of the basilar artery.

*In some individuals, the **circle of Willis** is capable of providing collateral circulation following a stroke.*

into the large sinuses between the meningeal and periosteal layers of the dura. Deep veins, which serve the internal structures of the brain, empty into the great cerebral vein which, in turn, drains into the straight sinus.

Superficial Veins. The superficial venous circulation differs from the arterial system in two ways: (1) the venous system is more variable, and (2) anastomoses are the rule rather than the exception in the venous system.

The superficial veins most consistently observed are the superior and inferior cerebral veins, the superficial middle cerebral vein, and two large anastomotic veins, the superior anastomotic vein of Trolard and the inferior anastomotic vein of Labbé (Figure 2-36). The superior cerebral veins drain the medial parts of the frontal and parietal lobes into the superior sagittal sinus. The inferior cerebral veins drain the ventral surface of the cerebrum into the sinuses that line the base of the calvarium. The superficial middle cerebral vein, which runs within the lateral sulcus, drains the adjacent temporal, frontal, and parietal lobes into the transverse sinus. Some of the flow of the superficial middle cerebral vein is diverted to the superior sagittal sinus by the superior anastomotic vein of Trolard; additional flow is siphoned off by the inferior anastomotic vein of Labbé to the transverse sinus.

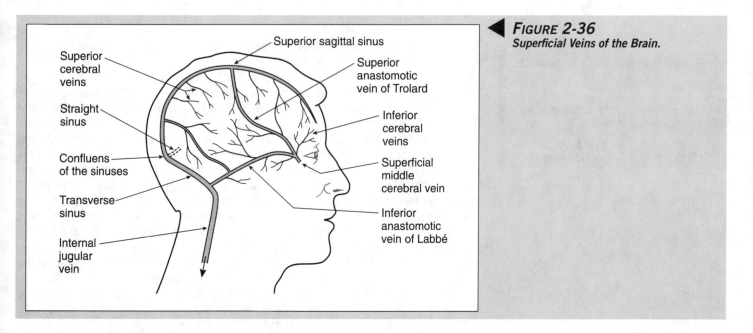

FIGURE 2-36
Superficial Veins of the Brain.

Deep Cerebral Veins. The two most important deep cerebral veins are the *internal cerebral vein* and the *basal vein of Rosenthal*; both empty into the *great vein of Galen* (Figure 2-37). The internal cerebral veins, after collecting venous blood from the striatum, the thalamus, the hippocampus, and the choroid plexus of the lateral ventricle, run posteriorly along the dorsomedial edge of the thalamus. At the posterior border of the thalamus, the left and right cerebral veins fuse on the midline and form the great vein of Galen. The basal vein of Rosenthal collects venous blood from the medial surface of the temporal pole, the orbital gyri of the frontal lobe, and the insular-opercular cortices before emptying into the great vein of Galen. The great vein of Galen, after receiving the bilateral discharge from the basal and internal cerebral veins, courses under the splenium of the corpus callosum and enters the straight sinus, which runs along the midline ridge of the tentorium before joining the confluens of the sinuses.

Clinical Aspects

Cerebrovascular accidents are one of the leading causes of mortality and morbidity in the world. The arterial and venous blood supply of the CNS is vulnerable to trauma, disease (e.g., heart disease, diabetes), and the normal aging process. Other factors such as heredity and life style (e.g., cigarette smoking, diet, level of exercise) play important roles as well.

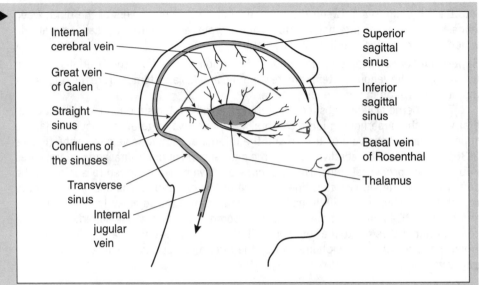

FIGURE 2-37 ▶

Deep Veins of the Brain.

Internal cerebral vein

Great vein of Galen

Straight sinus

Confluens of the sinuses

Transverse sinus

Internal jugular vein

Superior sagittal sinus

Inferior sagittal sinus

Basal vein of Rosenthal

Thalamus

---

*Strokes are either **hemorrhagic** or **ischemic**.*

*The area of cell death associated with stroke is called an **infarct**.*

*Debris lodged in an artery is an **embolism**.*

Strokes. Strokes are caused by a sudden interruption of the arterial blood supply causing vascular insufficiency (ischemic or embolic stroke) or arterial, venous, or capillary bleeding into the neuropil (hemorrhagic stroke). Effective medical care requires the differential diagnosis of ischemic versus hemorrhagic stroke. Anticoagulant therapy, a prudent course of treatment for an embolic stroke, would be catastrophic for a patient in the midst of a hemorrhagic stroke. The area of cell death caused by a stroke is called an infarct.

Ischemic or embolic strokes are caused by circulating debris called emboli that occlude the vasculature of the brain or the arteries leading to the brain. Stroke onset is usually abrupt and the clinical signs are usually focal and static. The clinical presentation reflects the location of the ischemic tissue, which may not necessarily be the site of the occlusion. For example, contralateral paresis and sensory loss in the arm and face might be caused by occlusion of the middle cerebral artery or the internal cerebral artery.

In some cases, an embolic stroke is preceded by a *transient ischemic attack (TIA)*, an episode lasting less than 24 hours during which the patient shows all of the neurological signs of a stroke. A TIA is believed to be caused by small emboli that dissolve over the course of the episode. A TIA is time-limited and self-resolving.

Hemorrhagic strokes are caused by intracranial bleeding into the parenchyma, usually by an artery (see Figure 2-7). While some damage is caused by inadequate perfusion, most is caused by physical disruption of the tissue itself. If the hemorrhage is not contained quickly, additional damage may be caused by increased intracranial pressure. The majority of hemorrhagic strokes are of supratentorial origin, with the basal ganglia and thalamus being the most common loci. Clinical signs associated with hemorrhagic strokes depend on the size and location of the infarct, but headache, vomiting, and focal sensorimotor deficits are the most common. Symptoms typically progress, and the patient's condition worsens until the bleeding is controlled. Intracranial hemorrhages are common in hypertensive patients because their arterial walls are stiff and brittle. Other causes of hemorrhagic stroke include aneurysms, arteriovenous malformations, trauma, and tumors.

An aneurysm is a dilation of an artery caused by a congenital weakness in the arterial wall.

Aneurysms. An aneurysm is a congenital dilatation of an artery caused by weakness in the arterial wall (Figure 2-38). Saccular or berry aneurysms, the most common type of intracranial aneurysm, are rounded dilatations attached to the main artery by a narrow pedestal. Approximately 95% of all saccular aneurysms are located on branch points associated with the anterior circulation, (i.e., anterior and middle cerebral arteries, carotid artery, anterior rim of the circle of Willis). The first sign of an aneurysm is usually a severe headache caused by bleeding into the subarachnoid space. Left untreated, an aneurysm may burst or become a source of emboli. The most effective treatment is isolation of the aneurysm body from the general circulation by placing a small clip on its pedestal.

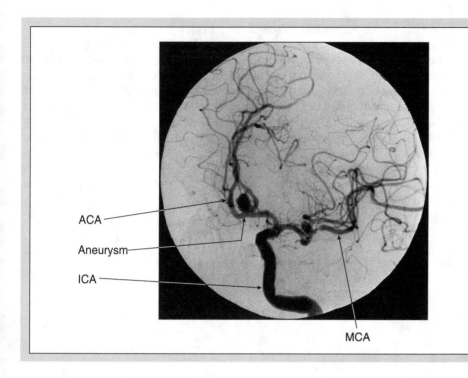

ACA

Aneurysm

ICA

MCA

FIGURE 2-38
Angiogram Showing a Saccular Aneurysm on the Anterior Communicating Artery. *ACA = anterior cerebral artery; ICA = internal carotid artery; MCA = middle cerebral artery. (Source: Courtesy of Dr. John Barr, Pennsylvania State University College of Medicine, Hershey, Pennsylvania.)*

Arteriovenous Malformations. Arteriovenous malformations (AVMs) are congenital, arteriovenous shunts (Figure 2-39A). Although focal in nature, AVMs may enlarge with age and become symptomatic. Because these arteriovenous anastomoses bypass the normal capillary bed, the adjacent neuropil may linger in a chronic ischemic state. Patients also may present with seizures or neurologic deficits caused by hemorrhage through the abnormally thin walls of these blood vessels. Large or troublesome AVMs require surgical removal, which is best done after the most tortuous vasculature has been embolized (Figure 2-39B).

Arteriovenous malformations are congenital shunts between the arterial and venous systems.

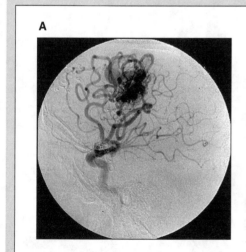

A

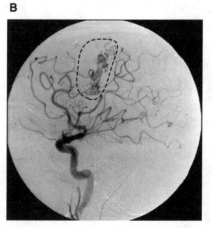

B

FIGURE 2-39
Arteriovenous Malformation of the Anterior Cerebral Artery before (A) and after (B) Embolization. *The dotted lines in B show the former distribution of the arteriovenous malformation. Some of the opacities in the postembolization radiograph are matrix inserted by the surgeon to facilitate embolization. (Source: Courtesy of Dr. John Barr, Pennsylvania State University College of Medicine, Hershey, Pennsylvania.)*

RESOLUTION OF CLINICAL CASE

T. R. was in the acute phase of a subarachnoid hemorrhage when he arrived at the emergency room. The headache was caused by bleeding into the subarachnoid space, probably by a saccular aneurysm. Saccular aneurysms may leak sporadically before more serious bleeding forces the patient to seek emergency care. In this case, T. R. experienced intermittent headaches during the preceding few weeks when there may have been seepage from the aneurysm. Aspirin did little to relieve the pain and, indeed, may have exacerbated the bleeding. During the current episode, the bleeding was worse, and the symptoms more serious. The progression of the patient's symptoms to the point of unconsciousness makes this a life-threatening situation. The physician, suspecting a subarachnoid hemorrhage, has ordered a CT scan, the technique of choice for visualizing occult blood. If bleeding is confirmed, pharmacologic intervention would be instituted to prevent vasospasm. Bleeding, which may increase intracranial pressure, would dictate that the order for the lumbar puncture be canceled. Once the location of the aneurysm has been determined with a series of angiograms, the decision will be made as to whether this aneurysm can be clipped.

REVIEW QUESTIONS

Directions: For each of the following questions, choose the **one best** answer.

1. Which of the following neurologic defects is caused by failure of the anterior neuropore to close?
    (A) Spina bifida
    (B) Anencephaly
    (C) Syringomyelia
    (D) Meningomyelocele
    (E) Hydrocephalus

2. Which of the following conditions is most likely to involve venous blood?
    (A) Hemorrhage
    (B) Stroke
    (C) Epidural hematoma
    (D) Subdural hematoma
    (E) Aneurysm

3. Which of the following sites is most commonly used to obtain a sample of the cerebrospinal fluid (CSF)?
    (A) Lateral ventricle
    (B) Lumbar cistern
    (C) Subarachnoid space
    (D) Cerebellopontine cistern
    (E) Superior sagittal sinus

4. Which of the following correctly describes the sequence of cerebrospinal flow within the ventricular system?
    (A) Lateral ventricle → foramen of Magendie → third ventricle → fourth ventricle → midsagittal sinus → arachnoid villi
    (B) Third ventricle → lateral ventricle → cerebral aqueduct → fourth ventricle → foramen of Magendie → arachnoid villi → midsagittal sinus
    (C) Lateral ventricle → foramen of Monro → third ventricle → fourth ventricle → midsagittal sinus → arachnoid villi
    (D) Third ventricle → lateral ventricle → foramen of Magendie → fourth ventricle → arachnoid villi → midsagittal sinus
    (E) Lateral ventricle → third ventricle → cerebral aqueduct → fourth ventricle → foramen of Magendie → arachnoid villi → midsagittal sinus

5. Which of the following blood vessels forms part of the circle of Willis?
    (A) Internal carotid artery
    (B) Middle cerebral artery
    (C) Superior cerebellar artery
    (D) Ophthalmic artery
    (E) Cavernous sinus

6. If blue dye were injected into the femoral artery, which area would remain its normal color?

    (A) Choroid plexus

    (B) Pineal gland

    (C) Thalamus

    (D) Area postrema

    (E) Liver

ANSWERS AND EXPLANATIONS

1. The answer is B. Failure of the anterior neuropore to close prevents development of the forebrain. Spina bifida is an incomplete closure of the vertebral arch of the spinal vertebrae caused by faulty closure of the posterior neuropore. Syringomyelia is an enlargement of the central canal that is not a developmental defect but rather one caused by trauma such as whiplash. Hydrocephalus is an enlargement of the cerebral ventricles caused by excessive production or incomplete resorption of CSF.

2. The answer is D. Subdural hematomas are usually caused by leakage from veins that bridge the arachnoid space. Epidural hematomas are caused by rupture of arteries that lie between the periosteal dura and the skull. Strokes, which may be hemorrhagic or embolic, most often interrupt arterial blood flow to part of the nervous system. Aneurysms are defects in the arterial wall that may leak or rupture into the parenchyma or subarachnoid space.

3. The answer is B. The lumbar cistern is used to sample CSF because, done properly, there is little danger of damaging the spinal cord or spinal nerves. The lateral ventricle, subarachnoid space, and cerebellopontine cistern contain CSF, but drawing samples from these areas would be difficult for the physician and dangerous to the patient. The superior sagittal sinus contains venous blood.

4. The answer is E. The correct sequence of cerebrospinal flow is lateral ventricle → third ventricle → cerebral aqueduct → fourth ventricle → foramen of Magendie → arachnoid villi → midsagittal sinus.

5. The answer is A. The proximal part of the internal carotid artery joins the circle of Willis before continuing as the middle cerebral artery. The superior cerebellar artery branches from the basilar artery and does not form part of the circle of Willis. The ophthalmic artery is a branch of the middle cerebral artery. The cavernous sinus is a venous reservoir located underneath the circle of Willis.

6. The answer is C. The blood–brain barrier would prevent the blue dye from entering the brain. The choroid plexus would turn blue because it is on the vascular side of the barrier. There is no blood–brain barrier at the area postrema or the pinal gland, both of which would turn blue. The liver, part of the systemic circulation that has fenestrated capillaries, also would be blue.

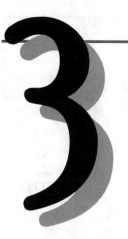

3

SPINAL CORD AND PERIPHERAL NERVES

INTRODUCTION OF CLINICAL CASE

A 30-year-old man was attacked by gang members and brought to the emergency room of a local hospital. Examination revealed multiple bruises and lacerations on the head and arms; the patient also suffered a piercing knife wound in the back, just to the right of midline at the first thoracic vertebra (T1). During the examination, the man was conscious and described the incident with the gang. He showed no signs of confusion, and all mental functions appeared normal. Pupillary, gag, and corneal reflexes were normal; a full range of eye movements was present; the tongue protruded on midline, and facial expression was normal. The man moved both arms and his left leg, but voluntary movements were completely absent in the right leg. Deep tendon reflexes were absent in the right leg, which exhibited flaccid paralysis. There was no response to pinprick on the left side of the body below T3. The right side was responsive to pinprick, but sensation for light touch and vibration was lost on the right side below T1. Another examination 2 months later revealed similar findings except the right leg showed hyperactive deep tendon reflexes, and Babinski's sign was present upon stroking the plantar surface of the right foot.

INTRODUCTION TO THE SPINAL CORD

The spinal cord represents the caudal end of the central nervous system (CNS). In conjunction with the peripheral nerves, the spinal cord forms a functional system that is essential for the sensory and motor activities of the body. The peripheral nervous system contains thousands of nerve fibers that transmit sensory activity to the spinal cord and motor commands to skeletal muscles. As part of the CNS, the spinal cord contains a network of circuits that perform many tasks related to sensory integration and muscular coordination. The functional integrity of these circuits is evaluated by examining limb reflexes, muscular strength, and cutaneous sensitivity. Impairment of spinal cord or peripheral nerve function can be recognized by many symptoms and is likely if the patient exhibits weakness, paralysis, or insensitivity to sensory stimulation.

GROSS ANATOMY OF THE SPINAL CORD

The spinal cord is a cylindrical structure that extends through the neural canal of the vertebral column. The rostral end of the spinal cord continues into the medulla through the foramen magnum, and its caudal end terminates in the conus medullaris as shown in Figure 3-1. The spinal cord develops from the caudal two-thirds of the neural tube, and in the earliest stage of embryologic development, it occupies the entire length of the vertebral column. However, as the embryo develops, the caudal end of the spinal cord ascends with respect to the spine so that, at birth, the conus medullaris lies at the third lumbar vertebra (L3). The differential growth of the spinal cord and vertebral column continues for some time until, by adulthood, the conus medullaris has risen to the first lumbar vertebra (L1). As the conus medullaris rises, an elongated space emerges in the caudal end of the spinal canal and forms the lumbar cistern. Nerve roots emerging from lumbosacral segments descend through the lumbar cistern and are called the "cauda equina" because they resemble a horse's tail. Hypodermic needles can be inserted into the lumbar cistern without damaging the spinal cord (Figure 3-2). This technique is used frequently to withdraw cerebrospinal fluid for its diagnostic value or to inject drugs to anesthetize the spinal cord during labor and delivery.

Cauda equina resembles a horse's tail.

Lumbar cistern is used for spinal taps.

The 31 pairs of spinal nerves that emerge from the spinal cord impose a segmental organization that is used for identifying different levels of the spinal axis. Each segment is numbered according to the vertebra associated with the departing spinal nerve: 8 cervical (C1–C8), 12 thoracic (T1–T12), 5 lumbar (L1–L5), 5 sacral (S1–S5), and 1 coccygeal. In the cervical segments, nerves C1–C7 emerge rostral to the vertebra with the same number; nerve C8 emerges rostral to the first thoracic vertebra. The remaining spinal nerves emerge caudal to the corresponding vertebra (Figure 3-3).

Vertebral Column

The bony vertebrae and spinal nerves are arranged in a spatial configuration that permits flexible support of the vertebral column during normal motor activities. As shown in Figure 3-4, the spinal cord is protected by virtue of its position within the neural canal of the bony vertebrae. Generally, an intervertebral disk is located between each vertebral body; exceptions are the sacrum and coccyx, which are fused vertebrae. The disks act as shock absorbers and are composed of the nucleus pulposus, a soft, pulpy material surrounded by denser connective tissue called the annulus fibrosus. Longitudinal ligaments attached to the vertebral bodies hold the disks in place when the vertebral column bends during movement. Each spinal nerve passes through the intervertebral foramen

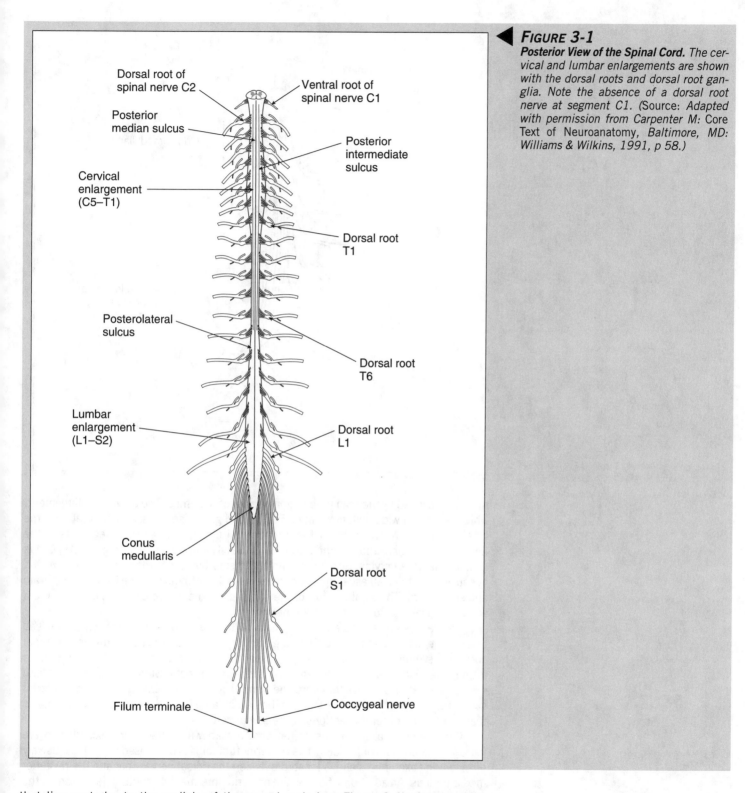

FIGURE 3-1
Posterior View of the Spinal Cord. *The cervical and lumbar enlargements are shown with the dorsal roots and dorsal root ganglia. Note the absence of a dorsal root nerve at segment C1. (Source: Adapted with permission from Carpenter M: Core Text of Neuroanatomy, Baltimore, MD: Williams & Wilkins, 1991, p 58.)*

that lies posterior to the pedicle of the neural arch (see Figure 3-4). Among older individuals, the disks may rupture and herniate into the neural canal (Figure 3-5). If the herniated disk impinges upon the spinal cord or nerve root, it causes severe pain, paralysis, or loss of sensation.

Longitudinal Organization of the Spinal Cord

The spinal cord varies in diameter throughout its length because of differences in the number of neurons and axons that innervate different parts of the body. The cord has two enlargements, one at the cervical level and another at the lumbar level; these enlarge-

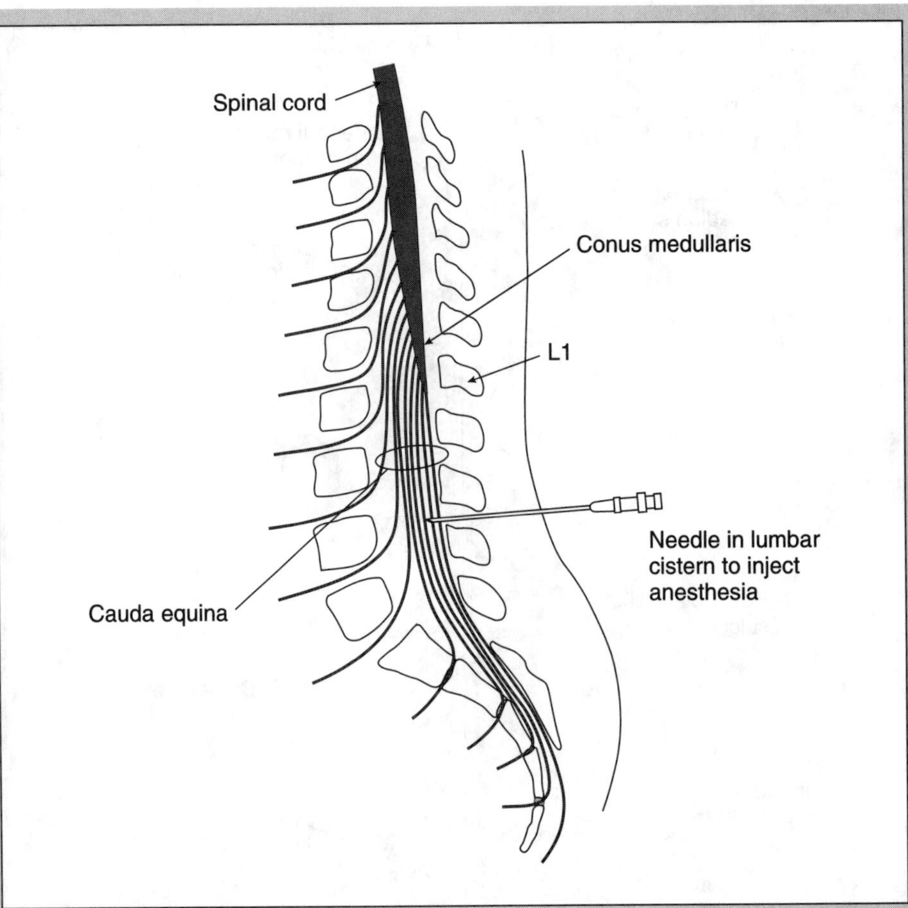

Spinal cord
Conus medullaris
L1
Needle in lumbar cistern to inject anesthesia
Cauda equina

FIGURE 3-2
Injection into the Lumbar Cistern. *This lateral view shows a lumbar puncture to inject narcotics into the lumbar cistern.*

ments are caused by the high innervation density of the limbs. The cervical enlargement, which is 1.5 cm wide, extends from C5 to T1 and gives rise to nerve roots that form the brachial plexus. Nerve roots for the lumbosacral plexus emerge from segments in the lumbar enlargement that extends from L1 to S2. The upper cervical region (C1–C4) is smaller than the cervical and lumbar enlargements but larger than the thoracic region because it contains all ascending and descending fiber tracts passing between the brain and spinal cord. The smallest part of the spinal cord, the thoracic region, is only 1.0 cm wide and gives rise to the intercostal nerves.

Several fissures extend along the length of the spinal cord. On the midline, the deep anterior median fissure and the shallow posterior median septum nearly divide the spinal cord into symmetrical halves along the sagittal plane (Figure 3-6). On each side, a posterolateral sulcus marks the entry of dorsal nerve roots. Similarly, an anterolateral sulcus is located at the site where the ventral nerve roots emerge from the anterior surface of the cord. The nerve roots and their associated fissures provide gross landmarks that distinguish different sections of the spinal cord.

Collections of axons in the spinal cord are known as tracts or fasciculi and are located in three pairs of funiculi. The posterior funiculus is composed almost exclusively of ascending axon fibers and is located between the dorsal nerve roots and the posterior median sulcus. An additional fissure, the posterior intermediate septum, is present in the cervical and upper thoracic segments (C1–T6) and subdivides the posterior funiculus into the posterior columns. The lateral funiculus contains a mixture of ascending and descending tracts and is located between the dorsal and ventral nerve roots. The anterior funiculus also contains a mixture of ascending and descending tracts and is located between the ventral nerve roots and the anterior median fissure.

Transverse Organization of the Spinal Cord

A transverse section through an unstained spinal cord reveals a central gray region surrounded by three pairs of white funiculi (see Figure 3-6). The central gray region is

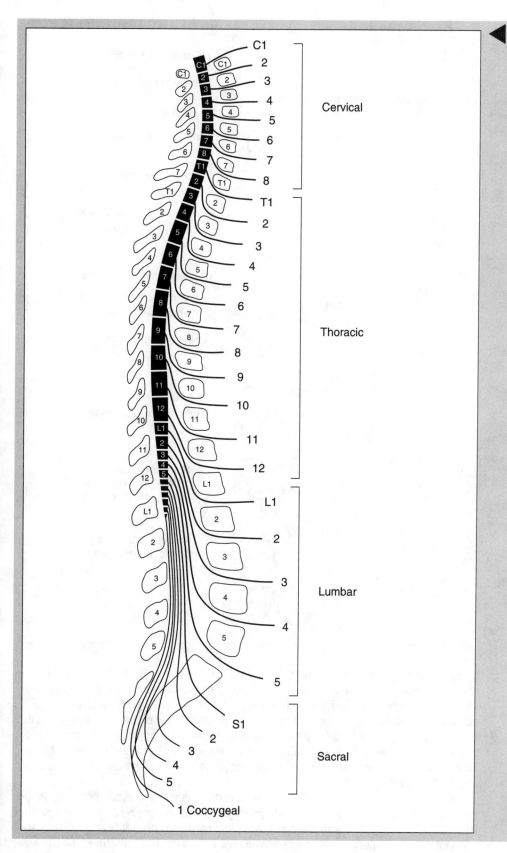

Cervical

Thoracic

Lumbar

Sacral

FIGURE 3-3
Spinal Cord and Vertebral Segments. This drawing shows the relationship between the bony vertebral bodies and the spinal nerves emerging from different segments of the spinal cord.

FIGURE 3-4 ▶

Bony Vertebrae. *(A) Superior view of a typical vertebra. (B) Lateral view. (C) Lateral view showing spinal nerves emerging from the intervertebral foramina of successive vertebrae. (Source: Reprinted with permission from DeMyer W: Neuroanatomy, Baltimore, MD: Williams & Wilkins, 1988, p 66.)*

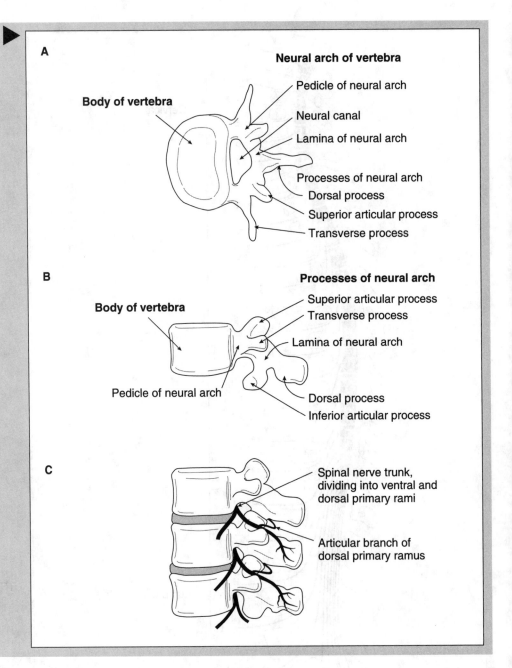

characterized by symmetrical pairs of posterior and anterior horns that resemble the wings of a butterfly. Because transverse sections of the human spinal cord are usually shown with the posterior horns on top, many find it acceptable to refer to the dorsal (i.e., posterior) or ventral (i.e., anterior) horns. The gray appearance of the central region is due to a high density of neuronal cell bodies and their dendritic processes. By comparison, the surrounding funiculi have a pale appearance because they are composed of myelinated fiber tracts. The gray and white matter regions are infiltrated by small blood vessels and glial supporting cells.

Different levels of the spinal cord can be distinguished on the basis of size, shape, and the relative proportions of white and gray matter. In addition, certain nuclei and fiber tracts are found only at specific levels of the spinal cord and contribute to the differential appearance of segments examined transversely. A flow chart illustrating how the size, shape, and topography of white and gray matter can be used to determine the level of the spinal cord is presented in Figure 3-7.

Cervical Levels. Transverse sections in the cervical cord have an oval shape dominated by large funiculi. Cervical segments have large funiculi because: (1) ascending fiber systems are augmented as they proceed rostrally toward the brainstem, and (2) descending

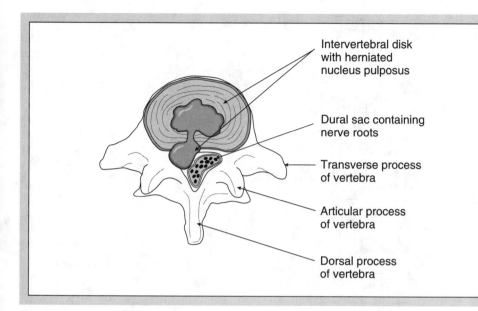

FIGURE 3-5
Herniated Disk. Transverse view of a herniated disk at the level of the lumbar cistern. The herniation compresses nerve roots that innervate the lower back and legs. (Source: Reprinted with permission from DeMyer W: Neuroanatomy, Baltimore, MD: Williams & Wilkins, 1988, p 67.)

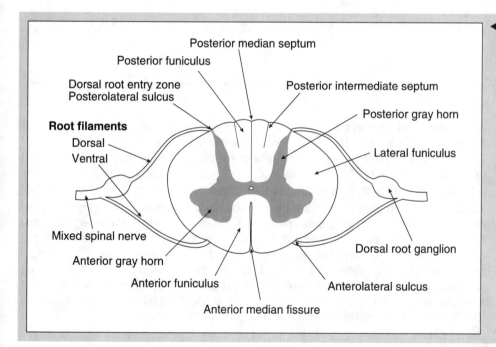

FIGURE 3-6
Spinal Cord Landmarks. This drawing identifies the major landmarks of the spinal cord. The central gray region is surrounded by three pairs of funiculi consisting of myelinated fiber tracts. The dorsal and ventral roots enter the spinal cord and are closely associated with the posterior and anterior gray horns, respectively.

tracts are maximal in size in the rostral cord and gradually taper in diameter as specific fibers terminate in successive caudal levels. In the posterior funiculus, the posterior intermediate sulcus and underlying septum form the boundary between the fasciculus gracilis and the more lateral fasciculus cuneatus. In all cervical segments, the lateral edge of the dorsal horn is marked by the reticular process, which is composed of groups of corticospinal fibers moving laterally from the pyramidal decussation into the lateral funiculus. Lower cervical segments, C5–C8, have enlarged posterior and anterior horns, the latter being especially prominent because it contains the large number of motor neurons required to innervate the muscles of the arm and hand. Figure 3-8 compares transverse views of cervical segments with other levels of the spinal cord.

Thoracic Levels. With the exception of thoracic segment T1, transverse sections through the thoracic cord are smaller because the central gray region requires only a small number of neurons to innervate the intercostal muscles of the trunk. Thoracic segments have a small lateral horn that protrudes into the lateral funiculus, halfway between the slender posterior and anterior horns. The lateral horn contains the inter-

FIGURE 3-7 ▶

Determination of Spinal Level. *This flow chart can be used to determine the approximate level of a transverse section of spinal cord.*

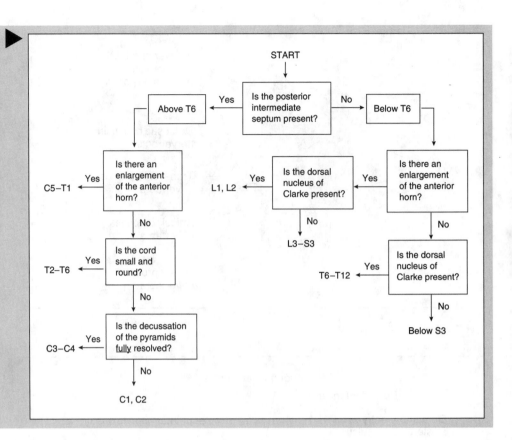

mediolateral cell column that gives rise to efferent preganglionic sympathetic fibers of the autonomic nervous system. All thoracic segments contain the dorsal nucleus of Clarke, a group of large neurons at the base of the posterior horn that is especially well developed in segments T10–T12 (see Figure 3-8). Upper thoracic segments T1–T6 are distinguished from lower thoracic segments by the presence of the fasciculus cuneatus.

Lumbar Levels. Transverse sections through the lumbar cord have large posterior and anterior horns with a relatively small proportion of white matter. In lumbar segments, the fasciculus gracilis has a boomerang shape and is relatively narrow compared to sections of the thoracic spinal cord. Upper lumbar segments L1–L2 have a lateral horn and a prominent dorsal nucleus of Clarke, but both of these landmarks are absent in lower lumbar segments L3–L5 where the anterior horn extends much further into the lateral funiculus. The increased size of the anterior horn is due to the addition of motor neurons that innervate the muscles of the lower limb (see Figure 3-8).

Sacral Levels. Sections through the sacral cord are characterized by small amounts of white matter, a relatively large proportion of gray matter, and a thick gray commissure in the center of the cord. With successively more caudal sections, sacral segments diminish in size, and the three funiculi become progressively thinner. Coccygeal segments resemble sacral segments in appearance but have a smaller diameter (see Figure 3-8).

CYTOARCHITECTURE OF THE CENTRAL GRAY REGION

The central gray region of the spinal cord is composed of a network of neurons with different sizes and shapes that vary in the pattern of their afferent and efferent connections. Neurons in the central gray region receive afferent projections from dorsal root ganglia, from neurons in other parts of the central gray region (intersegmental connections), and from neurons located in many parts of the brainstem or cerebral cortex (suprasegmental connections). Neurons in the central gray region innervate peripheral targets, such as muscles and autonomic ganglia, or they project to other parts of the CNS. Spinal cord neurons whose processes remain entirely in the CNS can project locally (interneurons), to neighboring segments of the central gray region (intersegmental connections), or to nuclei in the brainstem or thalamus (suprasegmental connections).

Rexed Laminae

The earliest studies of spinal cord cytoarchitecture led to several anatomic descriptions of the central gray matter, but the terminology was inconsistent, and only a few nuclear groups were widely recognized. In 1952, Rexed made thick transverse sections of the spinal cord and discovered a distinct laminar pattern composed of columns of neurons extending through the longitudinal axis of the cord. The classification system of Rexed uses Roman numerals to identify nine laminae progressing ventrally from the superficial aspect of the dorsal horn (lamina I) to the motor neurons of the ventral horn (lamina IX). The region surrounding the central canal is classified as lamina X.

The laminar classification system of Rexed is used by most anatomists, but it is difficult to detect transitions in cytology unless the histologic sections are at least 100 μm thick. Some nuclei are confined to a single Rexed lamina; in such cases, the name of the nucleus may be used interchangeably with the laminar designation. In other cases, spinal cord nuclei extend across Rexed laminae or are located in one part of a specific lamina. Table 3-1 indicates the anatomic relationships and identified functions of several nuclei located at different levels of the spinal cord.

◀ **TABLE 3-1**
Subdivisions of the Central Gray Region

Spinal Nucleus	Rexed Lamina	Spinal Levels	Functions
Dorsomarginal nucleus	I	All	Anterolateral system
Substantia gelatinosa	II	All	Modulates pain and temperature
Nucleus proprius	III, IV, V	All	Sensory processing, anterolateral system
Not named	VI	Enlargements	Proprioceptive processing
Dorsal nucleus of Clarke	VII	C8–L2	Posterior spinocerebellar tract
Intermediomedial nucleus	VII	All	Receives visceral afferents
Intermediolateral nucleus	VII	T1–L3	Preganglionic sympathetic cells
Sacral parasympathetic nucleus	VII	S2–S4	Preganglionic parasympathetic cells
Not named	VIII	All	Receives descending supraspinal inputs
Medial motor neurons	IX	All	Innervates axial musculature
Lateral motor neurons	IX	Enlargements	Innervates limb muscles
Phrenic nucleus	IX	C3–C5	Innervates diaphragm
Spinal accessory nucleus	IX	Medulla-C5	Innervates sternocleidomastoid and trapezius

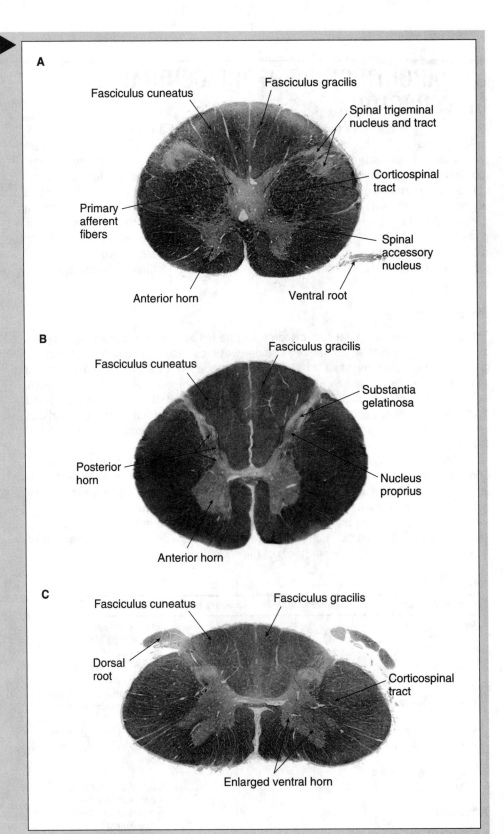

FIGURE 3-8

Transverse Sections of the Spinal Cord. *Selected levels of the spinal cord reveal characteristic differences in the size, shape, and topography of the central gray and surrounding white matter regions. (A) Section through C1, just caudal to the pyramidal decussation. (B) Section through C4, just rostral to the cervical enlargement. (C) Section of the cervical enlargement at C7. (D) Section through the thoracic level of the spinal cord at T10. (E) Section through the lumbar enlargement at L3. (F) Section through the sacral level of the spinal cord.*

◀ *FIGURE 3-8*

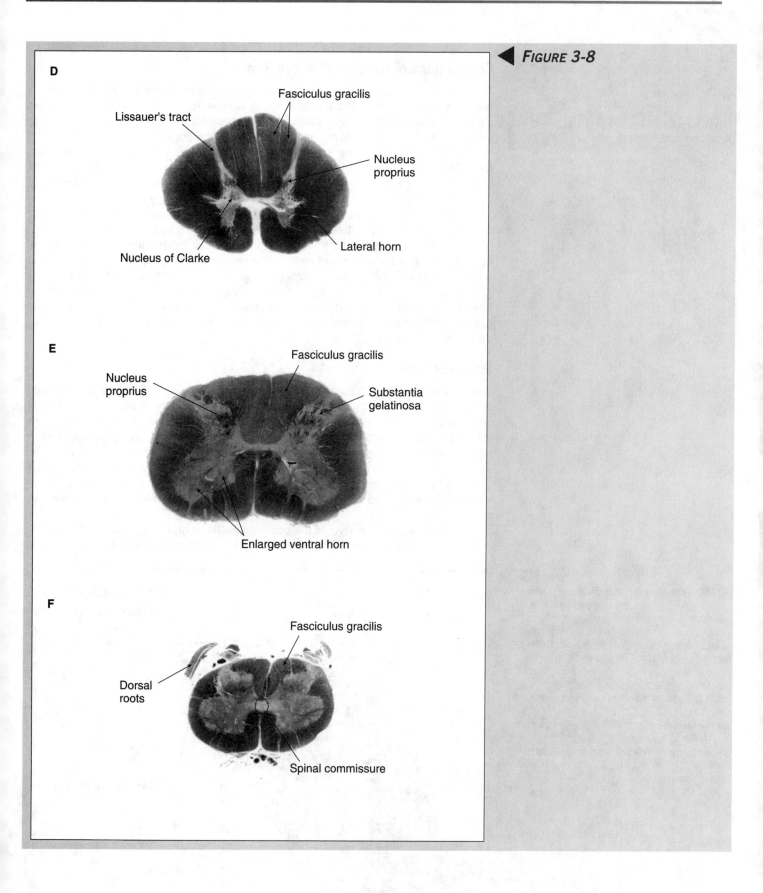

D

Lissauer's tract

Fasciculus gracilis

Nucleus proprius

Lateral horn

Nucleus of Clarke

E

Nucleus proprius

Fasciculus gracilis

Substantia gelatinosa

Enlarged ventral horn

F

Dorsal roots

Fasciculus gracilis

Spinal commissure

Connections of the Spinal Nerve Roots

The functional anatomy of the central gray region can be understood by considering the functional connections of the dorsal and ventral nerve roots. All dorsal nerve root fibers convey sensory impulses, and virtually all of these fibers have collateral axons that terminate in the posterior horn. Hence, neurons in the posterior horn receive synaptic inputs from fibers conveying sensory information from the skin, joints, and muscles. Nerve fibers entering the posterior horn are classified as general somatic afferents (GSA) or general visceral afferents (GVA), and their cell bodies are located in the dorsal root ganglia.

By comparison, at least 80% of the ventral nerve root fibers have efferent functions. These efferent fibers originate from cell bodies located in the anterior or lateral horns. Ventral root fibers originating from the lateral horn are preganglionic general visceral efferent (GVE) fibers of the autonomic nervous system. Ventral nerve root fibers that originate from cell bodies in the anterior horn are classified as general somatic efferents (GSE) and are responsible for innervating skeletal muscles. A small portion (~ 15%) of fibers in the ventral nerve root do not follow this functional convention, and these appear to be nociceptive afferents that enter the cord through the ventral rather than through the dorsal root entry zone.

Posterior Horn

The posterior horn is primarily sensory in nature and lies between the lateral and posterior funiculi. Lissauer's tract lies dorsolateral to the posterior horn at the dorsal root entry zone. Many afferent fibers send bifurcating axons rostrally and caudally in Lissauer's tract for a few segments before entering the posterior horn. After leaving Lissauer's tract, small-diameter nociceptive fibers enter the lateral aspect of the posterior horn, while the wider cutaneous fibers proceed more medially as shown in Figure 3-9. Both sets of fibers use excitatory neurotransmitters; glutamate is found in the terminals of cutaneous fibers, whereas glutamate and substance P are co-localized in the terminals of the nociceptive fibers.

Depending upon the level of the cord, the posterior horn is composed of five or six cell layers (Rexed laminae) that vary according to thickness, neuronal composition, and

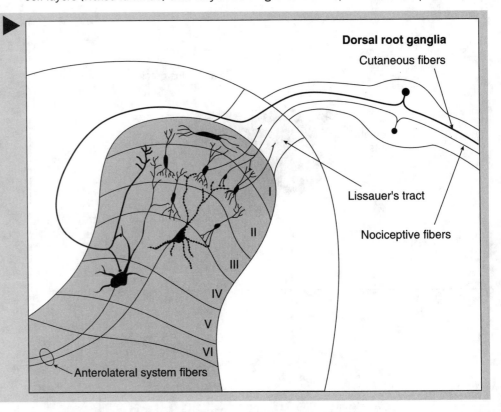

FIGURE 3-9
Cytoarchitecture of the Posterior Horn.
The posterior horn is composed of Rexed laminae I–VI in which each layer is characterized by different types of neurons. Large- and small-diameter afferent fibers enter the cord through Lissauer's tract before diverging into medial and lateral groups. The larger fibers enter the medial side of the posterior horn and terminate in laminae II, IV, and V, whereas the thin fibers enter laterally to terminate in laminae I, II, IV, and V. Laminae I, IV, and V contain projection neurons whose axons cross the midline before ascending into the lateral funiculus.

Dorsal root ganglia
Cutaneous fibers
Lissauer's tract
Nociceptive fibers
Anterolateral system fibers

anatomic connections. The superficial rim of the posterior horn contains a thin layer of neurons known as Rexed lamina I or the posteromarginal nucleus (see Figure 3-9). The posteromarginal nucleus receives inputs primarily from thin fibers conveying nociceptive information. Lamina II, located below the posteromarginal nucleus, has a pale appearance resembling gelatin and is known as the substantia gelatinosa. The substantia gelatinosa has small neurons with high concentrations of enkephalin and receives synaptic terminals from both cutaneous and nociceptive nerve fibers. Neurons in Rexed laminae III and IV form the nucleus proprius (proper sensory nucleus) and receive inputs mainly from myelinated cutaneous fibers and, to a lesser extent, from nociceptive nerve fibers. Rexed lamina IV is the thickest layer of the dorsal horn and contains many large multipolar neurons. Neurons in Rexed lamina V extend across the neck of the dorsal horn and receive inputs from both cutaneous and nociceptive afferents. Neurons forming Rexed lamina VI are located along the base of the dorsal horn but are present only at the cervical and lumbar enlargements. The medial part of lamina VI receives input from Golgi tendon organs, muscle spindles, and nociceptive free nerve endings. The lateral part of lamina VI receives inputs from the cerebral cortex that are concerned with motor function.

Local Pain Circuits. The posterior horn plays a significant role in coding the intensity and quality of somatosensory sensations, especially those related to pain. Most neurons located in laminae I, IV, and V, and some in laminae VI and VII, respond to intense thermal or tissue-damaging stimulation and send long ascending projections to parts of the brainstem and thalamus involved in nociception. Posterior horn neurons that convey pain information to supraspinal levels are identified as the anterolateral system because their axons are located in the anterior part of the lateral funiculus. Although these neurons respond maximally to inputs from nociceptive nerve fibers, they also receive inputs from cutaneous nerve fibers. Due to the convergence of these submodalities, neurons in the anterolateral system discharge at low frequencies during cutaneous (nonnoxious) stimulation and at high frequencies during more intense or painful stimulation as illustrated by Figure 3-10. Given these response properties, neurons in the anterolateral system are said to respond over a wide dynamic range. This indicates that pain intensity is coded, in part, by the rate of activity among fibers in the anterolateral system.

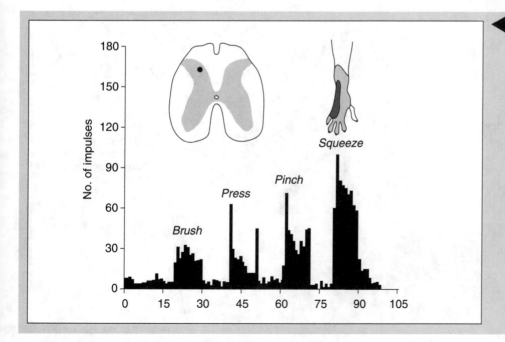

◄ **FIGURE 3-10**
Convergent Responses in the Posterior Horn. *Many neurons in the posterior horn respond with increasingly greater rates of activity as the stimulation progresses in intensity. This response was recorded from a neuron located in lamina I in the lumbar enlargement of a monkey. The neuron's receptive field was located on the foot as shown.* (Source: *Adapted with permission from Willcockson WS, et al: Effects of iontophoretically released peptides on primate spinothalamic tract cells.* J Neurosci 4:743, 1984.)

Physiologic studies have shown that enkephalin is a powerful neurotransmitter that inhibits the responsiveness of neurons contributing to the anterolateral system (see Figure 3-9). The enkephalinergic neurons of the substantia gelatinosa send their axons dorsally into lamina I and into the overlying Lissauer's tract where they ascend or descend for three to four segments before reentering laminae I and II. Although the substantia gelatinosa does not send axons ventrally into laminae III, IV, and V, neurons in those underlying layers send dendrites up into the substantia gelatinosa where they receive enkephalinergic innervation. In addition, the substantia gelatinosa receives serotonergic and noradrenergic projections from the brainstem. Serotonergic fibers from the raphe magnus (in the pons) and noradrenergic fibers from the nucleus paragigantocellularis (in the medulla) activate the substantia gelatinosa, causing it to release enkephalin and inhibit the anterolateral system. Hence, the substantia gelatinosa controls or "gates" the efficacy of transmission between peripheral pain fibers and the projection neurons of the anterolateral system. This view, known as the gate-control theory of pain transmission, was first proposed by Melzack and Wall in 1967 and is illustrated in Figure 3-11. The gate-control theory explains why descending projections from the brain may decrease the intensity of pain sensations and, under extreme circumstances, may prevent pain from reaching consciousness. In addition, because the substantia gelatinosa receives cutaneous inputs, it is possible to activate this system by gently stimulating the skin; this explains why we derive some pain relief by rubbing a skin injury. Opiates and other narcotic drugs relieve pain because their molecular structure allows them to act as agonists at enkephalin-binding sites (pre- and postsynaptic receptors) in the posterior horn.

> **Substantia gelatinosa** is a neural gate for blocking pain.

Lateral Horn and Intermediate Region

The region between the posterior and anterior horns contains several nuclei that lie in different parts of Rexed lamina VII. These nuclei receive a variety of afferent connections, including inputs from primary sensory afferents, intersegmental connections from other parts of the spinal cord, and descending inputs from the cerebral cortex and other parts of the brain (suprasegmental connections). The nuclei in lamina VII differ widely in

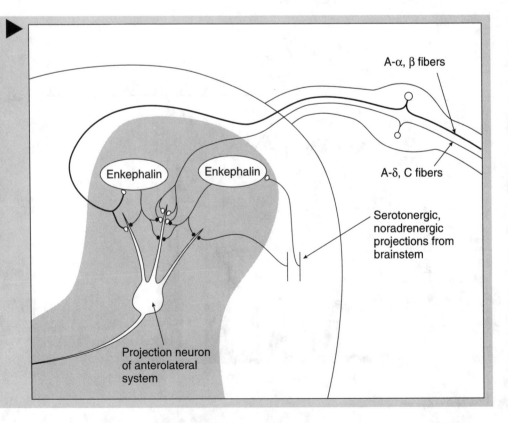

FIGURE 3-11 ▶

Pain Control Circuits in the Posterior Horn.
A schematic illustration of the gate-control mechanism for modulating nociception in the posterior horn. Inhibitory synapses are indicated by filled terminals; excitatory synapses are indicated by open terminals. Enkephalinergic neurons in the substantia gelatinosa inhibit projection neurons directly and also inhibit the release of excitatory transmitters from the C fibers. Enkephalinergic neurons can be activated either by cutaneous stimulation (A-α fibers) or by serotonergic and noradrenergic fibers descending from the brainstem. Projection neurons in the anterolateral system exhibit wide dynamic responses because they receive inputs from both cutaneous and nociceptive afferents.

A-α, β fibers

Enkephalin   Enkephalin

A-δ, C fibers

Serotonergic, noradrenergic projections from brainstem

Projection neuron of anterolateral system

their functions according to differences in their afferent and efferent connections (see Table 3-1).

The dorsal nucleus of Clarke lies in the medial part of lamina VII from C8 to L2 and contains large neurons that receive inputs from several muscle receptors, including annulospiral endings, flower spray endings, and Golgi tendon organs. When viewing transverse sections of the spinal cord, the dorsal nucleus of Clarke is most prominent in the lower segments of the thoracic cord. Axonal projections from the dorsal nucleus of Clarke form the posterior spinocerebellar tract, which ascends to the cerebellum through the lateral funiculus. This is one of the pathways that conveys sensory information about the position and dynamic activities of the muscles to the cerebellum.

The intermediolateral nucleus is a cholinergic cell column located in the lateral horn from T1 to L2. It contains large preganglionic sympathetic neurons whose axons emerge from the ventral root. Although the lateral horn does not extend into sacral levels, a group of cholinergic neurons occupies a similar position in the lateral part of lamina VII from S2 to S4 and gives rise to the preganglionic parasympathetic fibers of the pelvic nerves.

An intermediomedial nucleus lies ventral to the dorsal nucleus of Clarke and receives afferent projections from peripheral fibers innervating the thoracic and abdominal viscera. The intermediomedial nucleus extends the entire length of the cord and sends local projections to the intermediolateral nucleus of the lateral horn. Additional neurons in the vicinity of the intermediolateral nucleus, but closer to the posterior horn, receive convergent inputs from visceral and somatic afferent neurons and send ascending projections into the anterolateral system. These projections may be responsible for the phenomenon of "referred pain" in which the pain associated with myocardial infarction, kidney infection, or visceral muscle sensations are perceived as radiating into the arm, upper chest, lower back, or other areas of the body.

Anterior Horn

The anterior horn lies between the lateral and anterior funiculi and contains large and small neurons concerned with voluntary movements as well as movements associated with a variety of reflexes. Consistent with this role, the ventral horn receives descending inputs from brain regions concerned with motor functions, including the cerebral cortex, the red nucleus, and the reticular formation. To execute reflexes, neurons in the anterior horn receive sensory information from peripheral receptors either directly from dorsal nerve roots or indirectly from intersegmental pathways originating from neurons in the posterior horn (Figure 3-12).

The anterior horn contains laminae VIII, IX, and the ventral parts of lamina VII (see Figure 3-12). Lamina VIII varies in size and is located mainly in the medial part of the ventral horn, especially at levels associated with the spinal enlargements. Lamina VIII receives descending inputs from the brainstem that are important for modulating motor tone. The motor neurons that innervate peripheral skeletal muscles reside in clusters that form lamina IX.

Alpha-Motor Neurons. The functional significance of the anterior horn lies in the presence of alpha- (α-) motor neurons and their emerging axons that form the ventral root. Alpha-motor neurons are large, multipolar neurons in lamina IX that innervate the extrafusal fibers of striated muscle that are responsible for executing skeletal movements. All α-motor neurons release acetylcholine (ACh) at the neuromuscular junction. All descending motor commands converge onto α-motor neurons, which prompted Sherrington to refer to the axons of the α-motor neurons as the "final common pathway."

Alpha-motor neurons are referred to as the final common pathway.

Gamma-Motor Neurons. Lamina IX also contains smaller neurons, known as gamma- (γ-) motor neurons, that innervate the short intrafusal fibers of striated muscle. Gamma-motor neurons also release ACh at their synapses with the intrafusal fibers, which form a major component of muscle spindles and play a key role in the regulation of muscle tone. The γ-motor system is explained in further detail later in this chapter.

Motor Neuron Nuclei. Small collections of α- and γ-motor neurons are topographically organized to innervate specific groups of muscles. Medial groups of motor neurons

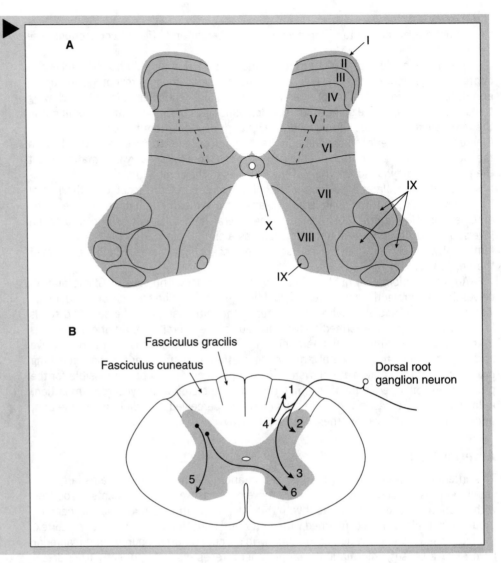

FIGURE 3-12 ▶

Afferent Connections in the Central Gray Region. *(A) Relative location of Rexed laminae in the central gray region. (B) Major routes for transmission of afferent information in the spinal cord. Primary afferent fibers project to several areas including: (1) the fasciculus gracilis or fasciculus cuneatus, (2) the posterior horn, and (3) the anterior horn. Some collateral fibers descend several segments before terminating in the central gray region (route 4). Many posterior horn neurons transmit afferent information ipsilaterally (route 5) or contralaterally (route 6) to the anterior horn of neighboring levels of the spinal cord. Routes 2, 3, 4, 5, and 6 are important for mediating spinal reflexes.*

Fasciculus gracilis

Fasciculus cuneatus

Dorsal root ganglion neuron

Phrenic Nucleus
Cut C4, breathe no more.

innervate the axial musculature (e.g., the intercostal muscles). The lateral groups are relatively small in thoracic levels but are substantially larger in the cervical and lumbar enlargements because they innervate muscles in the upper and lower limbs. For example, in the cervical enlargement, the motor neurons located most laterally innervate the most distal muscles of the hand, while neurons located more medially innervate the muscles controlling the shoulder and upper arm (Figure 3-13). A second functional organization is superimposed on the anterior horn so that motor neurons innervating the extensors are located more ventrally than those innervating the flexors.

One of the most important motor nuclei in the spinal cord is the phrenic nucleus, a small cell column located in lamina IX from C3 to C5 that innervates the diaphragm. Together with motor neurons controlling the intercostal muscles, the phrenic nucleus controls inspiration and receives descending projections from the motor cortex (voluntary control) and regions of the caudal brainstem (involuntary autonomic control) that determine the rhythm, rate, and depth of respiratory movements during the different stages of sleep. Damage to the phrenic nucleus or nerve results in respiratory paralysis and leads to death unless there is immediate intervention.

Poliomyelitis. Poliomyelitis is an acute viral disease that destroys the anterior horns and causes degeneration of α-motor neurons. Although the severity and spatial extent of the infected sites can vary, the disease invariably produces muscular paralysis and atrophy. In addition to attacking the spinal cord, poliomyelitis may destroy motor nuclei in the brainstem, thereby impairing swallowing and respiration. At present, the spread of polio is almost entirely prevented by childhood vaccination.

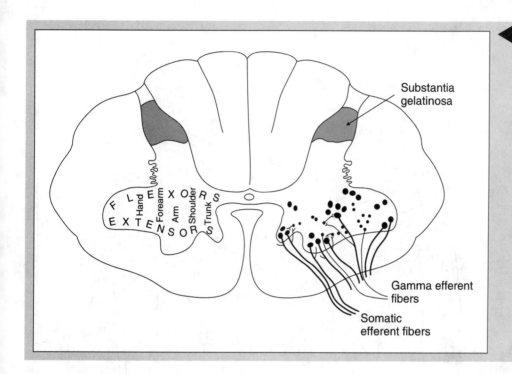

FIGURE 3-13
Topography of the Motor Neurons. The left side *of the diagram indicates the general position of motor neurons innervating the flexors or extensors of the upper limb. The* right side *indicates the presence of segregated populations or clusters of motor neurons supplying specific muscle groups. Each cluster contains α- and γ-motor neurons as well as local inhibitory neurons known as Renshaw cells. Axon collaterals from the motor neurons activate the Renshaw cells to provide feedback inhibition.* (Source: *Reprinted with permission from Carpenter M:* Core Text of Neuroanatomy, *Baltimore, MD: Williams & Wilkins, 1991, p 73.)*

SPINAL NERVES

Peripheral nerves are responsible for afferent and efferent communication between the body and the CNS. The cell bodies of afferent nerve fibers are located in the dorsal root ganglia, near the dorsal root entry site. Peripheral afferent neurons are classified as pseudounipolar neurons because only a single axonal process emanates from the soma before bifurcating into a distal branch that innervates the periphery and a proximal branch that enters the spinal cord. The peripheral area innervated by a single dorsal nerve root is called a dermatome. The collection of dermatomes innervated by all of the dorsal nerve roots forms a standard dermatomal map that is used clinically to determine the spinal segments associated with impaired sensitivity (Figure 3-14).

The efferent fibers of the ventral nerve root originate from cell bodies located in the lateral or ventral horns of the spinal cord. After departing from the spinal cord, these efferent fibers merge with the distal processes of the afferent fibers to form a mixed spinal nerve. Efferent fibers originating from motor neurons in lamina IX proceed to the skeletal muscles and terminate in neuromuscular junctions. The topographic sequence of muscles innervated by neighboring ventral nerve roots is not arranged in a clear linear sequence like the dermatomal map; consequently, the dermatomal map is also used to state clinical findings relating to level of muscle impairment.

Spinal nerves contain fibers of varying diameters, Schwann cells, connective tissue coverings, and blood vessels (Figure 3-15). The entire nerve is wrapped by an outer layer of epineurium that forms a loose connective sheath. Composed of collagen and fibroblasts, the highly elastic epineurium is continuous with the dura and usually ends near the distal termination of small nerve branches. Another connective covering, the perineurium, wraps around bundles of myelinated and unmyelinated nerve fibers. The perineurial cells continue to the distal ends of some nerves to form encapsulated endings such as pacinian corpuscles and muscle spindles. The innermost layer of connective tissue, the endoneurium, ensheathes individual nerve fibers and provides an important substrate for the regrowth of peripheral nerve fibers after injury.

Compound Action Potentials

A cross section of peripheral nerve shows that the diameter of individual fibers may vary substantially (Figure 3-16). The largest nerve fibers are approximately 20 μm in diameter and are heavily myelinated, whereas the smallest nerve fibers are less than 1 μm in

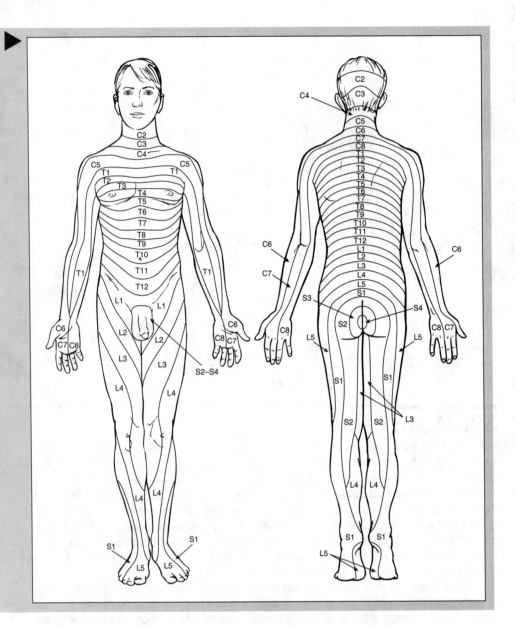

Figure 3-14

Figure 3-14

Dermatome Map. *Each dermatome represents the body region that receives afferent innervation from a specific dorsal nerve root. The dermatome map shows the pattern of innervation for all segments of the spinal cord and is divided into cervical, thoracic, lumbar, and sacral regions.*

diameter and are unmyelinated. In the 1930s, a series of electrophysiology experiments by Erlanger and Gasser demonstrated the functional importance of the variance in fiber diameter. As shown in Figure 3-16, when the distal part of a peripheral nerve is electrically stimulated, a compound action potential is recorded by an electrode located more proximally. A compound action potential contains several peaks or waves of activity that represent the summated response of multiple fibers having similar conduction velocities. By comparing the peaks in a compound action potential to the distribution of fiber diameters in a peripheral nerve, it was possible to deduce that conduction velocity was directly related to fiber diameter. Indeed, the conduction velocity (in m/sec) of a large-diameter fiber can be estimated by multiplying the diameter (in µm) by a factor of 5 or 6. For smaller fibers, multiplying the diameter by a factor of 4 provides an accurate estimate of conduction velocity.

The waves in a compound action potential represent different types of nerve fibers that neurophysiologists have classified into corresponding functional categories (Table 3-2). The first wave of activity, the "A" wave, corresponds to fast-conducting impulses transmitted along large-diameter, heavily myelinated fibers. The first wave contains several smaller peaks identified by the Greek letters α, β, γ, and δ. A Roman numeral system was developed to categorize nerve fibers according to their diameter, and the two systems are used interchangeably, although some fiber groups are classified in one system but not in the other. The fastest axons, A-α fibers, conduct action potentials at

TABLE 3-2
Peripheral Nerve Fiber Classifications

Location	Classification	Function	Axon Diameter (μm)	Conduction Velocity (m/sec)
Dorsal Roots				
	Ia (A-α)-GSA	Muscle spindles	12–20	70–120
	Ib (A-α)-GSA	Golgi tendon organs	10–18	60–100
	II (A-β)-GSA	Flower spray endings	6–12	35–70
	II (A-β)-GSA	Tactile receptors	6–12	35–70
	III (A-δ)-GSA	Pain, temperature	1–6	10–40
	IV (C)-GSA	Pain, temperature	< 1	0.5–2
Ventral Roots				
	α-GSE	Extrafusal muscle fibers	12–20	70–120
	γ-GSE	Intrafusal muscle fibers	3–6	15–40

Note. GSA = general somatic afferents; GSE = general somatic efferents.

60–120 m/sec. A-α axons include all nerve fibers important for muscle performance, such as α-motor neurons and afferent fibers innervating muscle spindles and Golgi tendon organs. The next fastest (35–70 m/sec) group are the A-β fibers that innervate a variety of mechanoreceptors responsible for cutaneous sensations. The γ-motor neurons have conduction velocities (15–40 m/sec) that are substantially slower, although not as slow as the thinly myelinated A-δ fibers that mediate sensations of sharp pain, cold, or heat. The second wave, composed of "B" fibers, reflects activity in preganglionic sympathetic fibers that originate from cell bodies in the lateral horn. These nerve fibers are lightly myelinated but only conduct at 3–15 m/sec. Preganglionic sympathetic fibers leave the ventral root soon after emerging from the anterior horn and proceed toward the

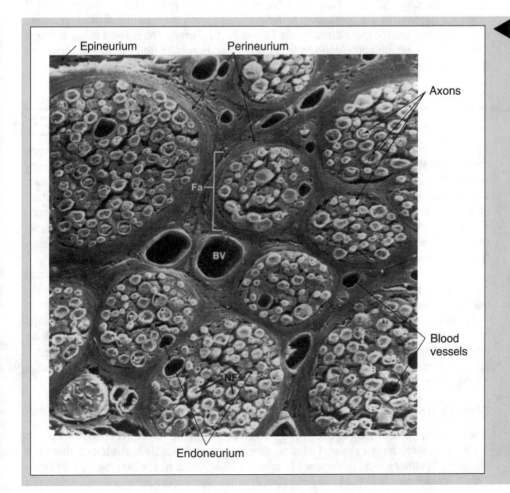

FIGURE 3-15
Transverse View of a Peripheral Nerve. *This scanning electron micrograph shows a freeze-fractured preparation of peripheral nerve. A band of loose connective tissue, the epineurium, encircles groups of fibers called fascicles (Fa). Each fascicle is covered by perineurium, and individual nerve fibers (NF) within the fascicle are wrapped by a thin layer of endoneurium. Blood vessels (BV) are located within the endoneurium or perineurium to supply nutrients to the nerve. (Source: Reprinted with permission from Kessel R, Kardon R: Tissues and Organs. San Francisco, CA: W. H. Freeman, 1979, p 79.)*

FIGURE 3-16 ▶

Compound Action Potentials. (A) The distal portion of a peripheral nerve is electrically stimulated while a pair of recording electrodes monitor changes in membrane potentials at a more proximal site. (B) Compound action potentials are recorded as a series of waves that correspond to activity transmitted along populations of fibers with different diameters and conduction velocities.

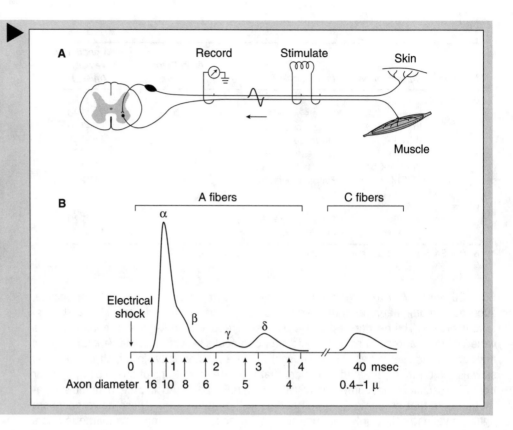

sympathetic chain ganglia. Consequently, the summated potentials for the group of B fibers are not seen in the compound action potential when the stimulating and recording electrodes are located more distally (see Figure 3-16). Finally, the slowest group of fibers are "C" fibers, which correspond to small-diameter, unmyelinated axons that innervate free nerve endings and convey sensations of dull, aching pain.

SPINAL REFLEXES

The peripheral nerves and spinal cord work together to mediate a variety of sensory, motor, and visceral activities of the body. Among these activities, spinal reflexes may occur independently of descending inputs from the brain, although, in most instances, supraspinal influences modulate muscle tone and may inhibit or enhance the execution of a spinal reflex. It is important to recognize that spinal nerves and their central connections in the spinal cord form a functional unit because spinal reflexes are frequently tested in the clinic to assess the functional integrity of the spinal cord and its connections with the peripheral nerves.

Reflexes are involuntary, stereotypical movements that are mediated by a small number of neural elements. All reflexes involve sequential activation of the following components: (1) peripheral sensory receptors, (2) afferent nerve fibers, (3) efferent nerve fibers, and (4) effectors such as smooth or skeletal muscles. In addition, many spinal reflexes involve one or more central gray interneurons that receive sensory information from the afferent nerve fibers and transmit impulses intersegmentally to different populations of motor neurons. Hence, reflexes vary in complexity according to the neuronal connections needed to coordinate the constituent muscles performing the reflex.

Stretch Reflexes

The simplest spinal reflex is called the stretch or myotactic reflex because it occurs in response to stretching a skeletal muscle. When a skeletal muscle is stretched, there is a tendency for the muscle to contract to prevent its intrinsic fibers from being damaged. This is seen clinically in the knee jerk reflex in which tapping the patellar tendon causes a slight stretch of the quadriceps muscle, which responds by contracting and moving the lower leg in a quick jerk. To understand myotactic reflexes and their clinical importance, it is necessary to understand the structure of muscle spindles and the function of the γ-motor system.

Muscle Spindles. Striated muscles are composed primarily of elongated extrafusal fibers that decrease their length when stimulated by ACh. Muscle spindles, by comparison, are specialized sensory receptors distributed throughout striated muscles that respond to muscle stretch and, thus, provide information about changes in muscle length to the CNS. Muscle spindles contain a small number of intrafusal fibers whose ends are attached to the longer extrafusal fibers. Two types of intrafusal fibers have been characterized, and both of these have a multinucleated, central region that extends into a pair of elongated, contractile regions as shown in Figure 3-17. One type, the nuclear bag fiber, has a broad nuclear area in which the nuclei are clustered together in a central "bag" region. Nuclear chain fibers, on the other hand, are slender in shape because the nuclei are aligned in single file. Muscle spindles contain a variable number of these fibers but usually have 2–3 nuclear bag fibers and 4–8 nuclear chain fibers. The sensory fibers that detect changes in muscle length innervate an encapsulated region located in the central part of the intrafusal fibers.

Muscle spindles detect muscle stretch.

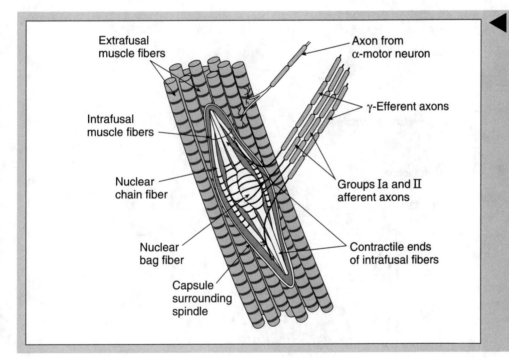

FIGURE 3-17
Anatomy of a Muscle Spindle. *Nuclear bag and nuclear chain fibers are innervated by a single group Ia annulospiral ending that wraps around the central portion of both sets of intrafusal fibers. Smaller afferents, group II flower spray endings, also innervate the nuclear chain fibers. The contractile ends of both types of intrafusal fibers receive efferent inputs from γ-motor neurons.*

Extrafusal muscle fibers

Axon from α-motor neuron

γ-Efferent axons

Intrafusal muscle fibers

Nuclear chain fiber

Groups Ia and II afferent axons

Nuclear bag fiber

Contractile ends of intrafusal fibers

Capsule surrounding spindle

Muscle spindles contain two types of neural innervation. Primary endings (group Ia) consist of a single, large-diameter axon that enters the encapsulated receptor and branches into collaterals that wrap around the central nuclear region of each intrafusal fiber present in the muscle spindle. These primary afferents are called annulospiral endings because they make a spiral as they encircle the intrafusal fiber. Secondary endings (group II) are formed by thinner axons that only innervate the nuclear chain fibers on each side of the annulospiral ending. Secondary endings are also called flower spray endings because they form a "spray" of contacts that resemble a flower. Functionally, primary and secondary endings are inactive in the absence of tension along the middle region of the intrafusal fiber and discharge when this region is stretched. Because intrafusal fibers are connected in parallel to the extrafusal fibers, they are stretched whenever the extrafusal muscle is stretched.

The myotactic reflex is the simplest of all reflexes because it is mediated by a neural loop containing only two neurons and a single synapse (Figure 3-18). Afferent fibers from muscle spindles (Ia, II) enter the posterior horn and proceed to lamina IX, where they synapse with α-motor neurons. Consequently, stretching a muscle and its muscle spindles causes a series of impulses to be sent directly to those motor neurons responsible for contracting the stretched muscle. Thus, the myotactic reflex is an extremely quick and reliable response to muscle stretch because it is mediated by monosynaptic connections between fast-conducting nerve fibers.

FIGURE 3-18 ▶

Myotactic Reflex Circuit. *Tapping the patellar tendon causes the quadriceps muscle to be stretched. The primary afferents to the muscle spindles are activated, and the incoming impulses cause monosynaptic excitation of α-motor neurons that project to the extrafusal fibers of the quadriceps. This causes a quick extension known as the knee jerk response.*

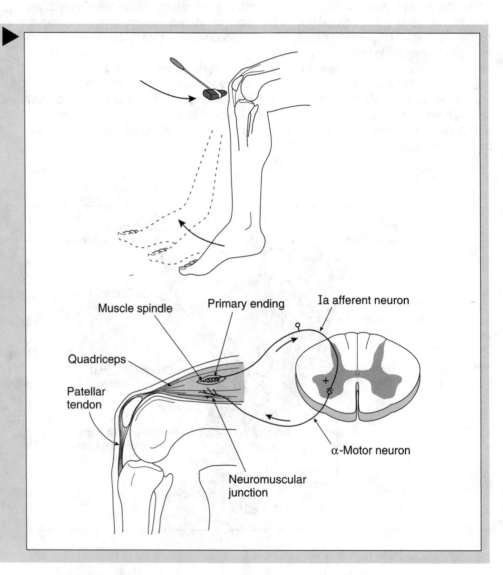

Muscle spindle   Primary ending   Ia afferent neuron

Quadriceps

Patellar tendon

α-Motor neuron

Neuromuscular junction

Gamma-Motor System. Intrafusal muscle fibers receive efferent innervation to maintain the sensitivity of muscle spindles over a wide range of muscle lengths. The contractile ends of the nuclear bag and chain fibers are innervated by γ-motor neurons originating in the anterior horn. Contraction of the intrafusal fibers does not contribute to the overall strength of the muscle because the intrafusal fibers are smaller and less numerous than extrafusal fibers. Rather, the intrafusal fibers contract to maintain tension in the central region of the muscle spindle when the muscle shortens during muscle contraction (Figure 3-19). This process enables muscle spindles to remain in a state of readiness regardless of muscle length. Intrafusal and extrafusal muscle fibers contract simultaneously during movements; this process is called alpha–gamma coactivation.

Gamma-motor neurons regulate muscle spindles.

Two types of γ-motor neurons are activated during different phases of muscular activity. One type innervates nuclear bag fibers and appears to regulate stretch sensitivity during the dynamic phase of muscle stretch. The other type innervates nuclear

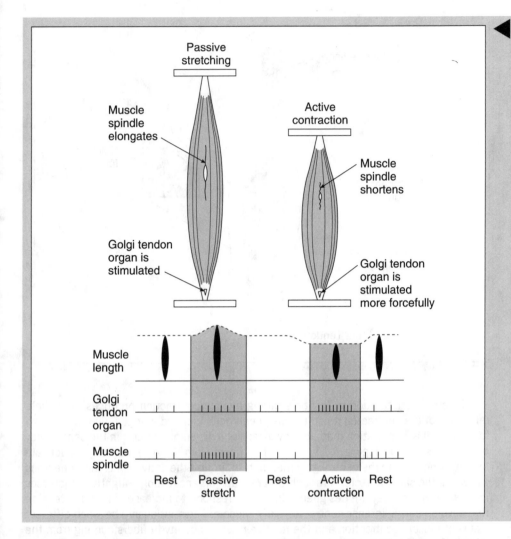

FIGURE 3-19
Muscle Receptor Mechanisms. This drawing compares the activity of afferent fibers from the Golgi tendon organs and muscle spindles during different states of muscle contraction. Muscle spindles are parallel to the extrafusal fibers of a muscle and become more active when the muscle is passively stretched. If the muscle contracts because of incoming impulses along the motor neurons, there is no tension along the muscle spindle, and the muscle spindle is silenced. Because of their location, Golgi tendon organs are in series with the muscles and are moderately active when the muscle is passively stretched; however, they become more active when the muscle actively contracts.

chain fibers, apparently to regulate spindle sensitivity during the static phase of muscle stretch. In general, the γ-motor system acts as a feedback loop that enables the nervous system to acquire information continuously about the status of the muscles even as the tension and length of a muscle change in the course of a movement.

The pathways mediating myotactic reflexes are also involved in maintaining muscle tone. Muscle tone is not an inherent property of muscle tissue but involves a minimal degree of contraction that is imposed by the nervous system without conscious effort. Descending supraspinal tracts regulate muscle tone by engaging the γ-motor system to increase the tension on the nuclear bag region and activate the annulospiral receptors. Increased activity in Ia fibers activates α-motor neurons to maintain a minimum degree of contraction. Muscles normally show muscle tone, and the lack of muscle tone is considered a pathologic sign of ventral root damage.

Tendon Reflexes

Golgi tendon organs reside in the myotendinous junction and signal the degree of tension that develops along a tendon during muscle contraction. Each Golgi tendon organ consists of a network of collagenous fibers surrounded by a membranous capsule (Figure 3-20). A large sensory fiber (group Ib) enters the receptor and splits into several processes that infiltrate the collagen bundles. The Ib fibers of the Golgi tendon organs increase their activity as tension increases during active muscle contraction. In contrast to muscle spindles, Golgi tendon organs are less responsive when pulling directly on the tendon because most of the tension develops along the passively stretched muscle fibers. Because Golgi tendon organs are connected "in series" with the extrafusal muscle fibers, slight contractions of a few extrafusal fibers produces a noticeable increase in tendon tension that, in turn, increases activity in Ib fibers.

Golgi tendon organs detect tendon tension.

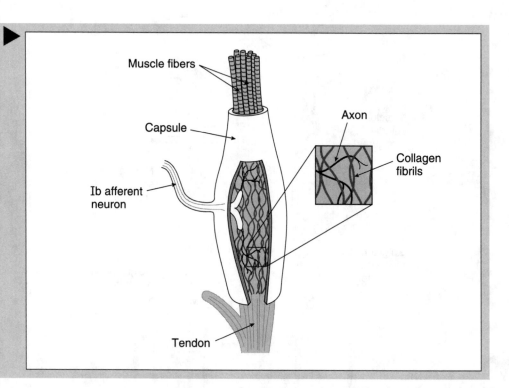

FIGURE 3-20
Anatomy of a Golgi Tendon Organ. Encapsulated receptors located in the myotendinous junctions are innervated by a large Ib fiber that arborizes into a plexus of endings scattered throughout a mass of collagen fibers.

Electrical stimulation of Ib fibers during muscle contraction produces immediate relaxation of the contracted muscle. This phenomenon, called autogenic inhibition, is a form of feedback inhibition mediated by means of a disynaptic circuit in the central gray region. As shown in Figure 3-21, afferent Ib fibers from Golgi tendon organs activate inhibitory neurons in the central gray that, in turn, inhibit the activity of α-motor neurons supplying the same muscle. Although Golgi tendon organs respond slightly to increases in muscle length, they are designed primarily to respond to increases in tendon tension that develop during intense contractions of a muscle. The relationship between different states of muscle contraction and the relative rates of activity in fibers coming from the muscle spindles and Golgi tendon organs is illustrated in Figure 3-19.

FIGURE 3-21
Autogenic Inhibition. When a muscle is in a state of contraction, incoming impulses from the Golgi tendon organs excite spinal interneurons that, in turn, cause inhibition of the α-motor neurons supplying the contracted muscle. This circuit is responsible for mediating the clasp-knife reflex.

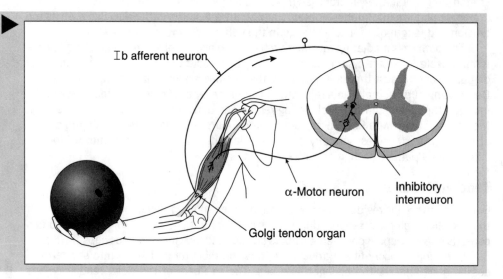

Clasp-Knife Reflex

Although the exact role of the Golgi tendon organs during normal motor activity is not clear, the influence of autogenic inhibition can be observed in patients sustaining certain spinal cord injuries. In cases where the corticospinal tract has been severed, patients are unable to control their limbs voluntarily because the descending projections from the motor cortex to the anterior horn have been damaged. If the dorsal and ventral roots remain intact, spinal cord reflexes are still present but are greatly modified by the loss of the supraspinal inputs. In such cases, the limbs show spasticity as indicated by an increase in muscle tone and resistance to passive movements. If sufficient force is applied to a limb, it will gradually flex until a point is reached where all resistance disappears and the limb folds suddenly like the blade of a pocket knife. This "clasp-knife" response is due to autogenic inhibition that develops when tendon tension surpasses the threshold level of responsiveness for the Golgi tendon organs.

Spasticity is characterized by stiff, hypertonic muscles.

Flexor and Crossed Extension Reflexes

The central gray region of the spinal cord contains an integrated network of neuronal connections that coordinate the output of the motor neurons that innervate antagonistic muscle groups on both sides of the body. These spinal circuits were first inferred in the late 1800s by Sherrington and others who investigated spinal reflexes in animals after transecting the upper cervical regions of the spinal cord. Intersegmental circuits not only mediate spinal reflexes but provide an anatomic system that is engaged by suprasegmental connections to help coordinate both sides of the body during walking and other complex movements that involve bilateral coordination.

The function of intersegmental connections is easily demonstrated by the simultaneous movements that form the flexor and crossed extension reflexes. A flexor reflex is a rapid withdrawal of a limb that is triggered by a noxious stimulus such as stepping on a tack. Such stimulation causes free nerve endings in the foot to transmit pain signals to different groups of spinal cord neurons (Figure 3-22). In response to this nociceptive input, intersegmental circuits are activated that lift the ipsilateral foot (flexor or withdrawal reflex) and extend the contralateral leg (crossed extension reflex).

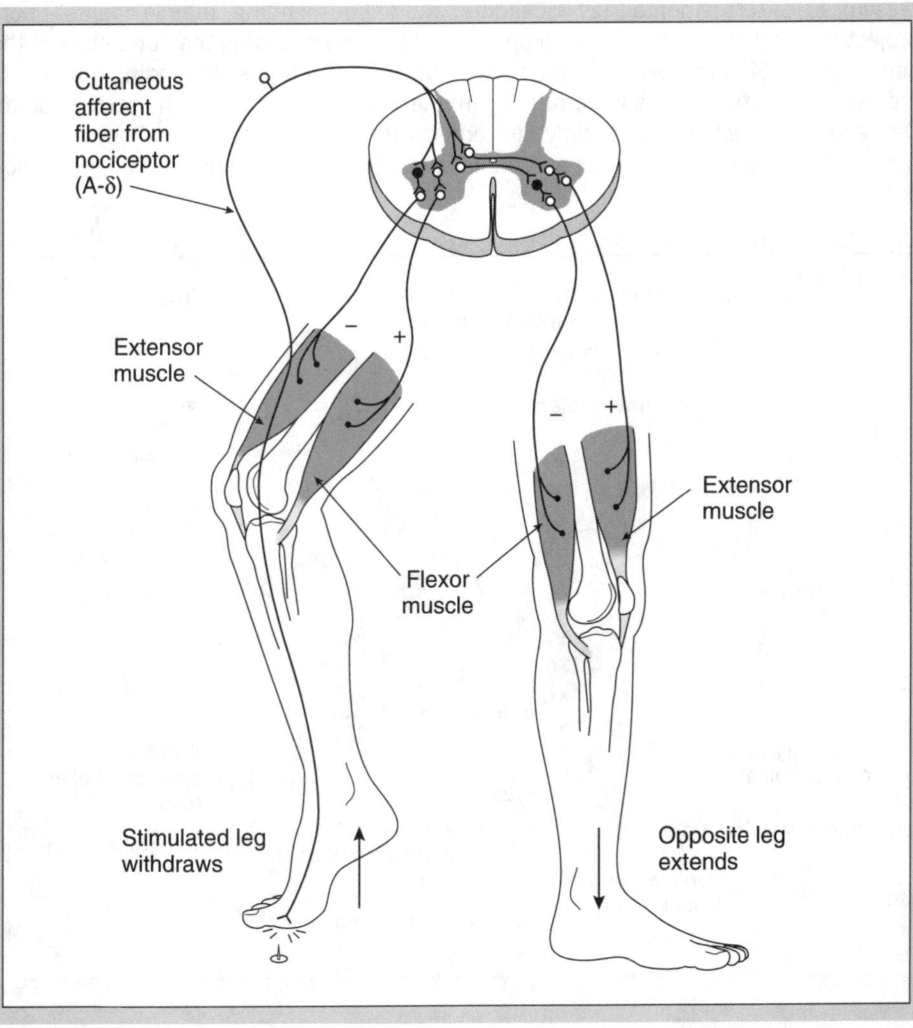

◀ *FIGURE 3-22*
Flexor and Crossed Extension Reflexes. *In response to noxious inputs, intersegmental circuits in the spinal cord mediate limb withdrawal while simultaneously causing extension of the opposite limb. Flexor and extensor movements of each limb are mediated by parallel sets of neural connections that activate one set of muscles while inhibiting the antagonist muscles. These hard-wired connections illustrate the principle of reciprocal innervation.*

Principle of Reciprocal Innervation. The withdrawal and crossed extension reflexes involve activation of several multisynaptic circuits connecting neighboring segments of the spinal cord. An essential feature of these intersegmental circuits is the reciprocal innervation of agonist and antagonist muscle groups (see Figure 3-22). Once inside the central gray region, primary afferent fibers diverge to control different muscle groups in each limb. Thus, the flexor response is controlled by neurons projecting to two populations of interneurons in the ipsilateral anterior horn: (1) one set that excites α-motor neurons innervating the flexors and (2) another set that inhibits α-motor neurons innervating the extensors. Without reciprocal innervation, antagonistic muscles would not be coordinated, and a limb would not move smoothly.

Intersegmental projections connecting the two sides of the spinal cord are an elaboration of the principle of reciprocal innervation. Extension of the contralateral leg depends on posterior horn neurons that project across the midline to the contralateral anterior horn. Similar to the circuits mediating ipsilateral flexion, these fibers also activate two populations of interneurons: (1) one set that excites the extensor α-motor neurons and (2) another set that inhibits the flexor α-motor neurons.

> **Reciprocal innervation** is activation of one muscle with inhibition of its antagonist.

SPINAL CORD TRACTS

Three pairs of funiculi surround the central gray region and contain myelinated fibers that communicate information to and from the spinal cord. Bundles of fibers having the same origin, course, and terminations are organized into tracts or fasciculi in specific regions of the spinal cord (Figure 3-23). Essentially, three types of fiber tracts are present: (1) intersegmental, (2) ascending, and (3) descending. Intersegmental fibers project rostrally or caudally in the propriospinal tract surrounding the outer edge of the central gray region and are involved in mediating spinal reflexes. Ascending fiber tracts are sensory in function and terminate in the thalamus, cerebellum, or brainstem. Descending projections are mainly concerned with motor functions and serve to connect parts of the cerebral cortex and brainstem with neurons in the central gray region of the spinal cord.

FIGURE 3-23 ▶
Ascending and Descending Spinal Tracts. This diagram indicates the size and position of the spinal tracts in the paired funiculi. Ascending tracts are shown on the right side, while descending tracts are shown on the left side.

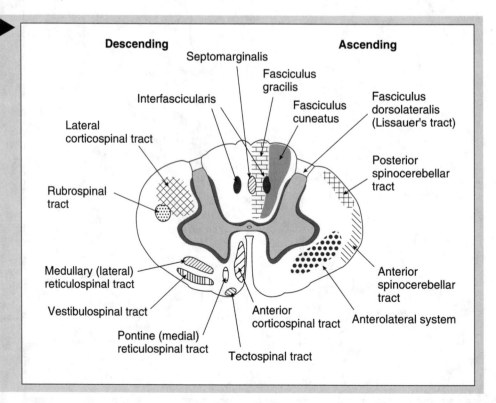

Ascending Tracts

A variety of encapsulated mechanoreceptors and free nerve endings are distributed throughout the skin, joints, and muscles. These receptors transduce cutaneous stimuli or other somatic sensations related to pain, temperature, or kinesthesia. These sensory modalities reach conscious awareness because the sensory signals they convey are ultimately transmitted to the cerebral cortex. All somatosensory sensations that reach consciousness ascend the spinal cord through either the posterior column–medial lemniscal system or through the anterolateral system. A third ascending system, the spinocerebellar pathway, is responsible for conveying information from muscle spindles and Golgi tendon organs to the cerebellum, which plays a major role in muscular coordination. Information ascending the spinocerebellar pathways is not consciously perceived.

Ascending spinal tracts have traditionally been described as having specific sensory functions. This view has arisen largely because many afferent fibers represent specific submodalities and project primarily into one of the ascending spinal tracts. It would be more accurate, however, to recognize that most afferent fibers entering the spinal cord have collaterals that allow sensory information of a given modality to be distributed to several spinal tracts. Indeed, most of the ascending tracts convey sensory information from more than one modality, and most modalities ascend through multiple routes. Consistent with this view, patients that sustain damage in one of the ascending pathways may have some remaining sensitivity to the modality that was conveyed by the damaged tract; however, these individuals usually exhibit some behavioral impairment, especially in tasks that require integration of multiple sensory channels. In other instances, the loss of a sensory tract may produce temporary effects, and an individual may report recovery of the affected sensations as other pathways compensate for the damaged tract. Although these mechanisms are poorly understood, this type of recovery indicates that there is some functional redundancy across the ascending spinal tract systems.

POSTERIOR COLUMNS

The posterior columns are located in the posterior funiculus and contain a pair of myelinated fiber tracts, the fasciculus gracilis and fasciculus cuneatus, that lie on both sides of the midline. The fasciculus gracilis lies adjacent to the midline and ascends the entire length of the spinal cord until it terminates in the nucleus gracilis at the caudal end of the medulla. The fasciculus cuneatus is present only at segments rostral to T6 and lies lateral to the fasciculus gracilis. The fasciculus cuneatus also extends to the rostral end of the spinal cord but terminates in the nucleus cuneatus just lateral to the nucleus gracilis. All fibers in the posterior columns remain ipsilateral to their site of origin (Figure 3-24).

Most fibers comprising the posterior columns are derived from primary afferent neurons whose cell bodies are located in the dorsal root ganglia. These fibers are mainly large-diameter axons (A-β) that innervate a variety of encapsulated receptors. The posterior columns transmit cutaneous information from the skin, kinesthetic information from encapsulated joint endings, and some proprioceptive information from deep receptors located in the muscles. These fibers enter the medial part of the dorsal root entry zone and bifurcate into two main branches that extend rostrally and caudally along the lateral edge of the posterior column for a few segments. Collateral axons emerge from these branches at regular intervals and project to the posterior horn where they mediate spinal reflexes and process nociceptive inputs. Many of these fibers terminate exclusively in the spinal cord, but others ascend the spinal cord and terminate in the caudal medulla.

The posterior columns are somatotopically organized so that the lower part of the body is represented medially and the upper body laterally. Fibers coming from each dorsal root form a laminated pattern that extends parasagittally through the posterior columns. This arrangement occurs because, at successive segments of the spinal cord, primary afferent fibers are added laterally to those fibers ascending from lower levels. Thus, fibers coming in from the foot, leg, and lower trunk lie closest to the midline in the fasciculus gracilis. Rostral to T6, fibers innervating the upper trunk, arm, shoulder, neck, and posterior head lie progressively more lateral in the fasciculus cuneatus.

The increased number of fibers coming from the legs and arms causes considerable

FIGURE 3-24 ▶

Posterior Column–Medial Lemniscal System. Primary afferents conveying tactile and kinesthetic information bifurcate at the dorsal root entry zone. The main axon collateral ascends ipsilaterally in the posterior column and terminates in the caudal medulla. Fibers representing the lower trunk or leg ascend in the fasciculus gracilis and terminate in the nucleus gracilis. Fibers representing the upper trunk or arm ascend in the fasciculus cuneatus and terminate in the nucleus cuneatus. Second-order neurons in the nuclei gracilis and cuneatus cross the midline and ascend in the medial lemniscus to the ventroposterolateral (VPL) nucleus of the thalamus. Third-order neurons in the VPL nucleus project to the primary somatosensory cortex in the postcentral gyrus. The posterior columns and medial lemniscal pathways maintain a somatotopic organization throughout their course of projection.

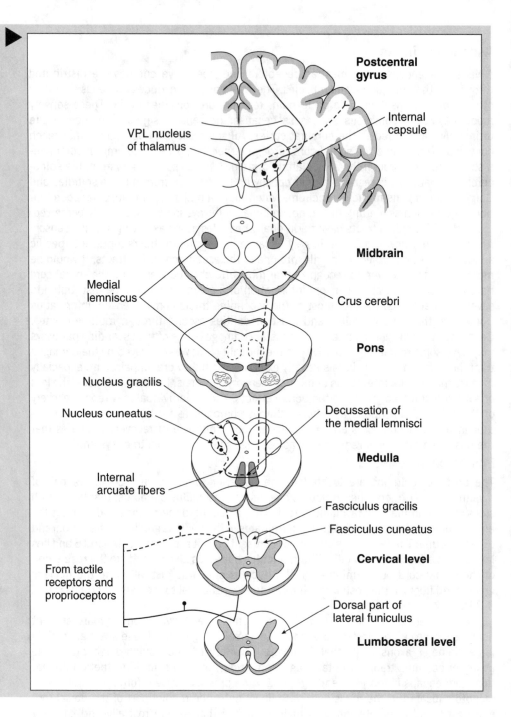

widening of the fasciculus gracilis and fasciculus cuneatus at the lumbar and cervical enlargements, respectively. In addition, the posterior columns contain two smaller tracts, which enable sensory information to descend short distances within the cord. The fasciculus interfascicularis and the septomarginal fasciculus perform these tasks for the cervical and lumbar regions of the cord, respectively (see Figure 3-23).

According to classical teaching, the posterior columns were composed exclusively of first-order neurons (i.e., primary afferent neurons). More recent studies indicate that 20%–25% of the fibers in the posterior columns originate from second-order neurons whose cell bodies are located in the posterior horn. The posterior horn receives inputs from several different submodalities, and neurons in this region exhibit multimodal response properties. Furthermore, a given segment of the posterior horn receives inputs from primary afferent neurons that innervate neighboring dermatomes. The convergence of information across adjacent dermatomes suggests that neurons in the posterior horn are important for integrating information across a wide region of skin. This view is

Posterior Columns
Cutaneous, kinesthetic sensations
Spatial integration
Complex tactile discriminations

consistent with evidence showing that transections of the posterior columns do not interfere with the ability to detect a tactile stimulus, although they significantly impair the ability to perform more complex discriminations. For example, patients with damage to the posterior columns are seriously impaired on a two-point discrimination task: they can neither determine the direction of stimulus movement on the skin nor identify letters traced on the skin. In addition, the fasciculus cuneatus contains fibers from encapsulated joint endings, and damage to this fasciculus interferes with the ability to judge the shape or size of an object placed in the palm.

Medial Lemniscal System. Neurons contributing to the posterior columns comprise the first part of a multisynaptic route for transmitting somatosensory information to the cerebral cortex. The posterior columns are composed largely of first-order neurons, although some second-order neurons are present. Because neurons in the nucleus gracilis and nucleus cuneatus comprise the second link of this multisynaptic route to the cortex, they are called second-order neurons. These neurons project across the midline and ascend contralaterally through a narrow tract called the medial lemniscus. The medial lemniscus terminates on third-order neurons located in the ventroposterolateral (VPL) nucleus of the thalamus. Neurons in the thalamic VPL nucleus project ipsilaterally to the postcentral gyrus of the cerebral cortex, which is also known as the primary somatosensory area. The posterior column–medial lemniscal system is composed exclusively of neurons with wide, heavily myelinated axons that transmit cutaneous information from the periphery to consciousness with minimal delay.

> **Lemniscus** is a ribbon-like tract.

Tabes Dorsalis. Tabes dorsalis is a manifestation of tertiary neurosyphilis that results in the destruction of the dorsal root ganglia and their central processes, especially the myelinated fibers in the fasciculus gracilis. Initially, this disease is characterized by intermittent pain and paresthesia (i.e., an abnormal burning or prickly sensation) caused by irritation of the dorsal roots. In time, the principal symptoms produced by degeneration of the posterior columns include loss of cutaneous sensations, diminished tendon reflexes, loss of muscle tone, and marked impairment of the sense of limb position. To compensate for the loss of position and kinesthetic sense, the patient walks with a broad-based, ataxic gait with eyes directed to the floor.

> **Tabes Dorsalis**
> Posterior columns are destroyed.
> Impairment of kinesthesia
> Broad-based, ataxic gait

ANTEROLATERAL SYSTEM

The anterolateral system consists of a collection of fibers ascending through the anterior part of the lateral funiculus. It is a crossed, multisynaptic pathway whose fibers originate mainly from neurons in Rexed laminae I, IV, and V. Neurons in the anterolateral system project across the midline through the anterior white commissure of the spinal cord and proceed towards the lateral funiculus where they asend the spinal cord and terminate in a variety of brainstem targets (Figure 3-25). Four groups of fibers have been distinguished in the anterolateral system on the basis of their anatomic projections: (1) spinothalamic, (2) spinoreticular, (3) spinomesencephalic, and (4) spinotectal tracts.

The spinothalamic tract is the most well-known tract in the anterolateral system because of its clinical importance for conscious awareness of pain and temperature information. Neurons contributing to the spinothalamic tract, however, do not respond exclusively to noxious stimulation. Because spinothalamic neurons have extensive dendritic arborizations throughout the posterior horn, they receive convergent inputs from different types of primary afferent neurons. Consequently, spinothalamic neurons may exhibit moderate discharge rates during cutaneous stimulation and higher rates of activity during more intense, noxious stimulation. As indicated by Figure 3-10, spinothalamic neurons have a wide dynamic range of responsiveness that enables them to signal stimulus intensity. Other neurons in the spinothalamic tract respond primarily to cutaneous inputs and show little if any response to noxious stimulation. Thus, fibers responding to cutaneous and nociceptive inputs are intermingled in the anterolateral system; this may explain why loss of the posterior columns does not completely destroy the ability to detect cutaneous stimulation.

> **Anterolateral System:** Conveys pain to the brain

Pain Perception. Some evidence suggests that different perceptual qualities of pain are mediated by different groups of fibers in the anterolateral system. One group of fibers, called the neospinothalamic tract, originates mainly from laminae I and V and terminates in the VPL nucleus of the thalamus. These neurons receive inputs primarily from A-δ

> **Neospinothalamic Tract**
> Conveys sharp, well-localized pain
> Receives input from A-δ fibers

FIGURE 3-25 ▶

Anterolateral System. *Primary nociceptive afferents enter the spinal cord and terminate on neurons in the posterior horn. Second-order neurons, originating in laminae I, IV, and V, cross the midline to ascend the spinal cord through the anterior part of the lateral funiculus. While traversing the brainstem, different fibers terminate in the reticular formation (spinoreticular), the periaqueductal gray region (spinomesencephalic), the superior colliculus (spinotectal), or the thalamus (spinothalamic). Spinothalamic fibers terminate in the ventroposterolateral (VPL) nucleus or in the intralaminar nuclei. The intralaminar nuclei also receive multisynaptic projections from the reticular formation; this is an additional route by which nociceptive information reaches the thalamus. The thalamic nuclei project to cerebral cortex, where the conscious perception of pain takes place.*

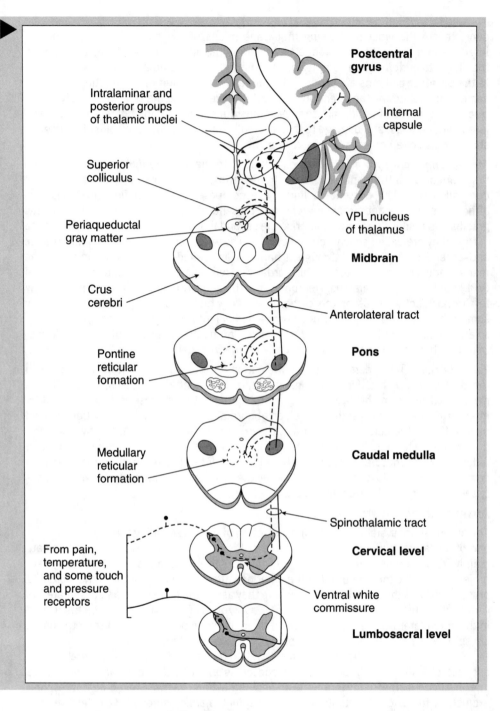

fibers and appear to be responsible for fast conduction of well-localized sensations of sharp, prickly pain. The paleospinothalamic tract, on the other hand, originates from neurons located more deeply in the posterior horn and projects to the central lateral and other intralaminar thalamic nuclei. Additional neurons in the anterolateral system terminate in the reticular formation, which transmits pain information multisynaptically to the intralaminar nuclei of the thalamus. In contrast to the VPL nucleus, the intralaminar thalamus is not somatotopically organized. Consistent with this evidence, paleospinothalamic and spinoreticular fibers probably mediate sensations of dull, aching pain that are conveyed more slowly by unmyelinated C fibers and subsequent multisynaptic pathways.

Chronic Pain. In the past, neurosurgeons transected the anterolateral pathways to relieve suffering in patients with intractable pain. These surgeries, called cordotomies, usually produced immediate analgesia if the transection occurred two segments above the highest dermatome exhibiting pain. Cuts at a higher level are necessary because nocicep-

Paleospinothalamic and Spinoreticular Tracts
Convey dull, aching, slow pain
Receive inputs from C fibers

tive fibers ascend in Lissauer's tract before entering the posterior horn, and fibers contributing to the anterolateral system also ascend one or two segments as they decussate through the spinal commissure. Furthermore, surgical transection must affect the deepest fibers lying adjacent to the ventral horn because superficial cuts would only interfere with spinothalamic and spinoreticular fibers representing the most caudal dermatomes of the body. At each level of the spinal cord, spinothalamic fibers are added medially to those fibers ascending from more caudal segments. Hence, the anterolateral system has a mediolateral somatotopic organization that is opposite to the posterior columns.

Anterolateral cordotomies produce immediate contralateral analgesia, but the effect usually lasts only a few months. The reason the patient's pain returns is not entirely understood, but it is thought to involve a few spinothalamic fibers that either ascend the spinal cord ipsilaterally or else were located just beyond the scalpel cut. Presumably, the terminal synapses of these remaining fibers become more efficacious in transmitting pain information to the thalamus following degeneration of the lesioned fibers. Whatever the explanation, this phenomenon illustrates the functional plasticity of the spinal cord pathways.

Syringomyelia. In contrast to the recovery of pain sensations following a lateral cordotomy, there is no functional recovery of pain sensibility if the loss is produced by syringomyelia. As the name implies, syringomyelia involves the formation of an elongated cavity or syrinx around the region of the central canal. This is a chronic disease that occurs either because of congenital defects in the neural tube or because the central part of the cord is destroyed by gliosis following certain types of trauma. In either case, syringomyelia is distinguished by a dissociated sensory loss in which pain and thermal sensitivity are impaired while the sense of touch is preserved because the decussating spinothalamic fibers are destroyed by the central location of the cavity. Syrinx formation is most common in consecutive segments in the cervicothoracic region and produces bilateral loss of pain sensitivity in the shoulders and arms. As the syrinx enlarges laterally and affects the ventral horns, the patient experiences weakness and atrophy of the upper limbs.

Syringomyelia
Bilateral sensory loss of pain and temperature
Produced by cavities in central gray region

SPINOMESENCEPHALIC AND SPINOTECTAL TRACTS

Additional fibers in the anterolateral system proceed to rostral levels of the brainstem, where they terminate either in the periaqueductal gray (spinomesencephalic) or in deep layers of the superior colliculus (spinotectal). The spinomesencephalic tract projects to parts of the periaqueductal gray that contain high concentrations of endorphin, a type of neuropeptide important for controlling pain. The periaqueductal gray sends descending projections to serotonergic neurons located in the raphe magnus of the pons and to noradrenergic neurons located in the nucleus paragigantocellularis of the medulla. Both of these regions, in turn, send projections to the posterior horn and inhibit postsynaptic responses to nociceptive inputs either directly or indirectly by activating enkephalinergic neurons in the substantia gelatinosa (see Figure 3-11). Thus, the spinomesencephalic tract is the afferent limb of a feedback loop that is critical for supraspinal regulation of pain sensitivity. The superior colliculus is involved in controlling eye and head movements during changes in visual attention. Hence, the spinotectal tract directs visual attention to body regions experiencing intense somatosensory stimulation.

SPINOCEREBELLAR TRACTS

The spinocerebellar pathways transmit proprioceptive information from the limb muscles and their joints to the cerebellum. Proprioception is the sensory modality concerned with limb position and includes the sense of stationary position and the sense of limb movement known as kinesthesia. Thus, the spinocerebellar tracts convey information about the length, tension, and position of the limb muscles; this information is used for controlling posture and coordinating fine movements. The posterior and anterior spinocerebellar tracts convey proprioceptive information from the muscles and joints of the lower body; the cuneocerebellar tract conveys proprioceptive information from the upper body. These tracts originate from second-order neurons that receive primary inputs from deep receptors located in the muscles and joints (Figure 3-26). Although some proprioceptive and kinesthetic information is transmitted by the posterior column–medial lemniscal system to the cerebral cortex and enters the sphere of consciousness, we are not consciously aware of information sent to the cerebellum.

FIGURE 3-26 ▶

Spinocerebellar Pathways. Primary afferents from muscle spindles and Golgi tendon organs in the leg muscles enter the spinal cord and terminate in the dorsal nucleus of Clarke or in other regions of the posterior horn. The posterior spinocerebellar tract is an uncrossed tract that originates from the dorsal nucleus of Clarke. The anterior spinocerebellar tract is a crossed tract that originates from second-order neurons in laminae V, VI, and VIII. Primary afferents from receptors in the hand and arm muscles ascend through the ipsilateral fasciculus cuneatus before terminating in the external cuneate nucleus. The cuneocerebellar tract originates from the external cuneate nucleus. The posterior spinocerebellar and cuneocerebellar tracts enter the inferior cerebellar peduncle and terminate in the ipsilateral cerebellar cortex. The anterior spinocerebellar tract enters the superior cerebellar peduncle and crosses the midline a second time before terminating in cerebellar cortex.

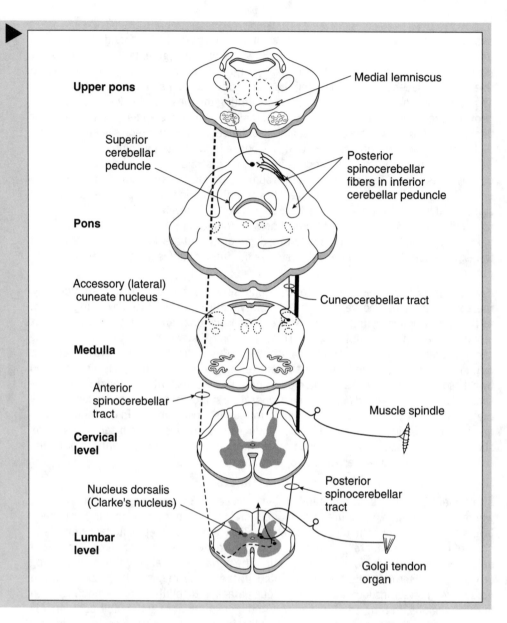

Upper pons — Medial lemniscus

Superior cerebellar peduncle

Posterior spinocerebellar fibers in inferior cerebellar peduncle

Pons

Accessory (lateral) cuneate nucleus

Cuneocerebellar tract

Medulla

Anterior spinocerebellar tract

Muscle spindle

Cervical level

Nucleus dorsalis (Clarke's nucleus)

Posterior spinocerebellar tract

Lumbar level

Golgi tendon organ

Posterior Spinocerebellar Tract. The posterior spinocerebellar tract originates from neurons in the dorsal nucleus of Clarke located in Rexed lamina VII. Clarke's nucleus extends from segments C8 to L2, and it receives inputs from muscle spindles, Golgi tendon organs, encapsulated joint endings, and, to a lesser extent, from touch and pressure endings of the leg and lower trunk. Since the dorsal nucleus of Clarke does not extend below L3, afferent fibers entering more caudal levels of the cord ascend through the fasciculus gracilis before terminating in the dorsal nucleus of Clarke. This explains why Clarke's nucleus is so large and appears more prominent in segments T10–T12 than in more rostral sections of the thoracic cord. Axons emerging from the dorsal nucleus of Clarke enter the lateral funiculus and ascend ipsilaterally in a superficial layer of fibers lying ventrolateral to the dorsal root entry zone. In the brainstem, the posterior spinocerebellar tract merges with other fibers entering the inferior cerebellar peduncle and terminates in the ipsilateral vermis of the cerebellum.

Anterior Spinocerebellar Tract. The anterior spinocerebellar tract differs from the posterior spinocerebellar tract in several ways. First, it originates from cells scattered throughout Rexed laminae V, VI, and VII in spinal segments caudal to L1. Second, the neurons of the anterior spinocerebellar tract receive inputs from a more diverse group of afferent sources including Golgi tendon organ fibers, several mechanoreceptor fibers, and descending spinal tracts. Finally, the anterior spinocerebellar tract is a crossed pathway. Second-order neurons contributing to this tract project across the midline and ascend as a superficial layer of fibers just lateral to the anterolateral system. However, instead of entering the cerebellum through the inferior cerebellar peduncle, these fibers continue further rostrally and enter the cerebellum through the superior cerebellar peduncle and recross the midline to innervate the ipsilateral vermis of the cerebellum.

Cuneocerebellar Tract. Proprioceptive information coming from the arm does not ascend the spinal cord in segregated fiber bundles like the posterior or anterior spinocerebellar tracts representing the leg. Instead, type Ia and Ib fibers from the arm enter the ipsilateral fasciculus cuneatus and ascend into the medulla, where they terminate on second-order neurons in the lateral cuneate nucleus (also called the accessory or external cuneate nucleus). The lateral cuneate nucleus lies lateral to the nucleus cuneatus and is functionally considered to be the upper limb equivalent of the dorsal nucleus of Clarke. Efferent fibers from the lateral cuneate nucleus form the cuneocerebellar tract and merge with other fibers of the inferior cerebellar peduncle before terminating in the ipsilateral vermis of the cerebellum. Some anatomists contend that another pathway, the rostral spinocerebellar tract, is the upper limb equivalent of the anterior spinocerebellar tract, but there is little information regarding this tract in humans.

Descending Tracts

Many regions of the brain send descending projections to the spinal cord to execute skeletal movements or to modulate the transmission of incoming sensory inputs. All of these descending systems terminate on neurons located in the central gray of the spinal cord. The corticospinal tract is the major pathway for controlling voluntary movements, and it is the only tract that transmits impulses from the cerebral cortex down to the spinal cord. The actions of the corticospinal system are supplemented by other descending fiber systems that originate in the brainstem and play a role in modulating muscle tone and spinal reflexes. These descending pathways include the rubrospinal, reticulospinal, vestibulospinal, and tectospinal tracts.

CORTICOSPINAL TRACTS

Voluntary, highly skilled movements are dependent on neural impulses transmitted through the corticospinal tract. Corticospinal fibers originate from neurons in the cerebral cortex and descend ipsilaterally through the internal capsule and crus cerebri before passing through the pyramidal tract on the anterior surface of the medulla (Figure 3-27). At the spinomedullary junction, approximately 90% of the corticospinal fibers cross the midline through the pyramidal decussation and continue their descent as the lateral corticospinal tract (Figure 3-28). The lateral corticospinal tract resides in the posterior part of the lateral funiculus, just medial to the posterior spinocerebellar tract. Lateral corticospinal fibers are somatotopically organized so that fibers destined to reach the most caudal levels of the cord are located most laterally while those terminating in the cervical cord are located most medially. Approximately 8% of the corticospinal fibers remain uncrossed on the anterior surface of the spinal cord to form the anterior corticospinal tract. Fibers of the anterior corticospinal tract eventually cross the midline at the spinal cord segment in which they terminate. Only about 2% of the corticospinal fibers descend uncrossed within the lateral funiculus.

Consistent with its role in motor control, most fibers in the corticospinal tract originate from motor regions in the cerebral cortex. Slightly more than 30% of the fibers originate from the primary motor cortex (Brodmann area 4), and another 30% come from the premotor cortex (Brodmann area 6). Surprisingly, nearly 40% of corticospinal fibers originate from somatosensory cortical areas, and these fibers terminate in the posterior horn to modulate the transmission of afferent inputs. The lateral corticospinal tract descends the entire length of the spinal cord, but more than half ($\sim$ 55%) of its axons terminate in cervical regions representing the neck and upper limbs. Approximately 25% of corticospinal fibers terminate in the lumbosacral enlargement to control the lower limbs while the remaining fibers terminate throughout the thoracic segments. Although some ($\sim$ 10%) corticospinal fibers terminate directly on the α-motor neurons, most fibers terminate on nearby interneurons that, in turn, control the output of the α-motor neurons. The corticospinal tract is concerned primarily with controlling flexor muscles because the

FIGURE 3-27 ▶

Upper and Lower Motor Neurons. *The cor-ticospinal tract originates in cerebral cor-tex and descends through the internal capsule and brainstem before entering the spinal cord and descending to different levels of the spinal cord. Corticospinal neurons are upper motor neurons that ter-minate in the anterior horn to innervate lower motor neurons. The lower motor neu-rons comprise the final common pathway to the peripheral muscles.*

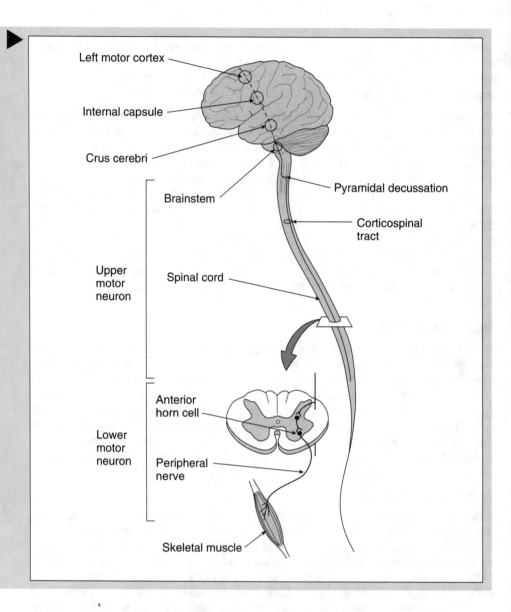

flexors are responsible for the fine, dextrous movements used by the arm and hand to manipulate objects.

Upper and Lower Motor Neurons. Motor neurons giving rise to the ventral spinal roots or to the motor fibers of the cranial nerves are referred to as "lower motor neurons." These neurons constitute the final common pathway because they provide the final link be-tween the nervous system and the muscles of the head and body (see Figure 3-27). Neurons that project to the final common pathway are called "upper motor neurons." The corticospinal tract is composed of upper motor neurons, and this phrase is often used to refer to the lateral corticospinal tract.

When lower motor neurons lose their innervation due to disease or trauma, the muscles atrophy and exhibit flaccid paralysis. Neurologic signs of a lower motor neuron lesion include: (1) loss of muscle tone (hypotonia), (2) absence of spinal reflexes (areflexia), (3) muscular atrophy, and (4) muscular fasciculations. It is thought that fasciculations occur because the synaptic terminals release ACh at the neuromuscular junction while the motor neuron degenerates.

Symptoms of an upper motor lesion are produced by damaging the corticospinal tract at any level of the neuraxis. Lesions of the corticospinal tract result in distinct neurologic symptoms that differ from symptoms produced by lower motor neuron pathol-ogy. A lesion of the corticospinal tract is usually indicated if muscles participate in spinal reflexes but are not under voluntary control. Transection of the lateral corticospinal tract

Lower Motor Neuron Lesions
Hypotonia
Areflexia
Muscle atrophy
Fasciculations

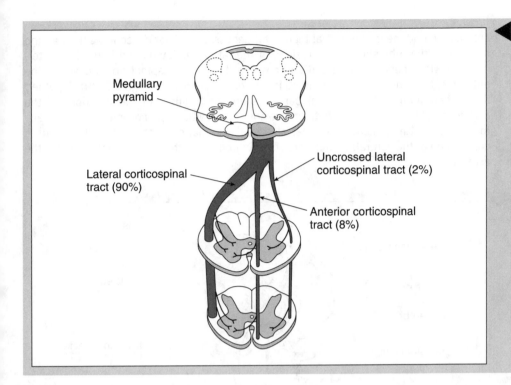

Medullary pyramid

Lateral corticospinal tract (90%)

Uncrossed lateral corticospinal tract (2%)

Anterior corticospinal tract (8%)

FIGURE 3-28
Pyramidal Decussation. *The pyramidal tract lies along the anterior surface of the medulla and contains corticospinal fibers exclusively. At the spinomedullary junction, approximately 90% of the corticospinal fibers cross the midline through the pyramidal decussation and descend through the lateral funiculus as the lateral corticospinal tract. Most of the remaining fibers descend ipsilaterally as the anterior corticospinal tract, and these fibers eventually cross the midline at the level of termination. (Source: Reprinted with permission from Carpenter M: Core Text of Neuroanatomy. Baltimore, MD: Williams & Wilkins, 1991, p 97.)*

causes spasticity, which is a state of heightened muscular tone (hypertonia) and rigidity. Spastic paralysis is characterized by hyperactive deep tendon (myotatic) reflexes and increased resistance to passive movement of the limb. Corticospinal lesions cause spinal reflexes to exhibit rapid reverberations or clonus because the reflexive movements are no longer modulated by descending inputs. Pathologic reflexes such as the clasp-knife phenomenon and Babinski's sign are also observed with upper motor neuron lesions. Babinski's sign is a dorsiflexion of the toes in response to lightly stroking the sole of the foot; although it generally indicates loss of corticospinal function, it is also seen in intoxicated adults and in infants before the corticospinal tract has fully developed.

Upper Motor Neuron Lesions
Spasticity
Clonus
Hyperactive tendon reflexes
Clasp-knife phenomenon
Babinski's sign

Amyotrophic Lateral Sclerosis. Amyotrophic lateral sclerosis is a progressive disease of unknown etiology that affects upper and lower motor neurons without altering the sensory systems. This disease causes degeneration of the corticospinal tracts and anterior horn neurons; consequently, signs of both upper and lower motor neuron paralysis are present. The muscles of the arm and hand gradually show signs of lower motor neuron lesions, including weakness, atrophy, and fasciculations. Until the anterior horn cells are affected, the patient exhibits upper motor neuron signs, including hyperreflexia, clonus, and Babinski's sign. Motor neurons in the brainstem are also affected, and much later, the disease impairs bladder and bowel function as the descending autonomic fibers degenerate.

Amyotrophic Lateral Sclerosis
Progressive, diffuse degeneration
Destroys lower and upper motor neurons
Leads to muscular paralysis

Spinal Shock. When the descending tracts of the spinal cord are severely injured, a period of spinal shock ensues that is characterized by flaccid paralysis and areflexia. Spinal shock occurs even if the ventral roots are intact, and it usually lasts for several weeks or months. Eventually, the limbs become spastic and exhibit hyperactive deep tendon reflexes. The reason for the temporary loss of reflex activity is not understood, but it appears to involve the loss of facilitating influences exerted by descending fiber systems on the reflex circuits of the spinal cord. As the descending fibers degenerate, connections in the reflex circuits become stronger, and their functions are reestablished to a greater degree than seen prior to the injury. Patients with spinal shock lose bladder function temporarily and must be catheterized to reduce distention of the bladder until reflex voiding develops.

Spinal Shock
Temporary loss of reflexes, muscle tone
Produced by spinal cord trauma

RUBROSPINAL TRACT

The red nucleus is a large nuclear structure in the midbrain that receives direct ipsilateral projections from motor and premotor cortical regions (Brodmann areas 4 and 6) via corticorubral pathways. The rubrospinal tract originates from magnocellular neurons and crosses the midline in the ventral tegmental decussation. After descending through the brainstem, the rubrospinal tract resides in the lateral funiculus and is partially intermingled with fibers of the lateral corticospinal tract. Rubrospinal fibers descend the entire length of the cord and terminate in laminae V, VI, and VII (Figure 3-29). Together, the corticorubral and rubrospinal pathways appear to augment the functions of the corticospinal tract because both tracts are concerned with flexor movements. In animals, for example, it has been shown that electrical stimulation of the red nucleus causes contraction of the contralateral flexors while inhibiting motor neurons that innervate the extensors.

FIGURE 3-29 ▶

Tectospinal and Rubrospinal Pathways. *The rubrospinal tract originates in the red nucleus and crosses through the ventral tegmental decussation before descending through the brainstem and spinal cord. Rubrospinal fibers terminate in laminae V, VI, and VII and are involved in controlling flexor movements. The tectospinal tract originates in the deep layers of the superior colliculus and crosses the midline through the dorsal tegmental decussation. The tectospinal tract descends through the anterior funiculus and terminates on neurons in laminae VI, VII, and VIII of the upper cervical segments.*

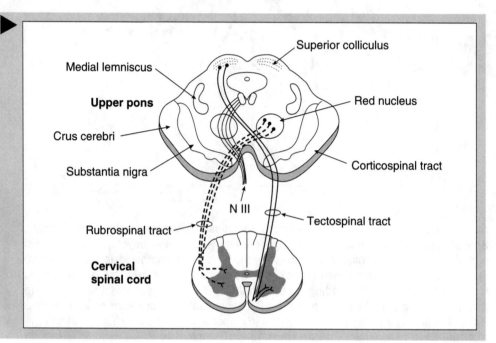

TECTOSPINAL TRACT

The tectospinal tract originates from the deep layers of the superior colliculus and crosses the midline in the dorsal tegmental decussation (see Figure 3-29). Tectospinal fibers descend in the anterior funiculus and project to neurons located in laminae VI, VII, and VIII of spinal segments C1 to C4. The superior colliculus receives projections from the visual, auditory, and somatosensory systems and integrates these sensory modalities to construct a representation of extrapersonal space. The superior colliculus is responsible for directing changes in visual attention and has connections with several motor nuclei that orient the head and eyes to novel stimuli in the visual field or to different parts of the body. By projecting to neurons in the upper four segments of the spinal cord, the tectospinal tract provides a route by which the superior colliculus controls the position of the head and neck.

RETICULOSPINAL TRACTS

The reticular formation exerts widespread influences throughout the neuraxis, including the modulation of activity in the α-motor and γ-motor systems. Many of the actions of the reticular formation are undoubtedly directed by corticoreticular fibers that originate from premotor cortical area 6 and terminate bilaterally in the pontine and medullary reticular nuclei. These nuclei, in turn, send descending projections to the ipsilateral spinal cord. The lateral reticulospinal tract originates from large neurons in the medullary reticular formation (nucleus gigantocellularis), whereas the medial reticulospinal tract originates from the pontine reticular formation (nucleus oralis and caudalis). Although these tracts are segregated, both sets of fibers terminate mainly in the medial and ventral regions of laminae VII, VIII, and IX through all levels of the spinal cord (Figure 3-30). The reticulospinal tracts can facilitate or inhibit spinal circuits involved in reflexive or voluntary movements. Because of widespread influences from motor and somatosensory cortices,

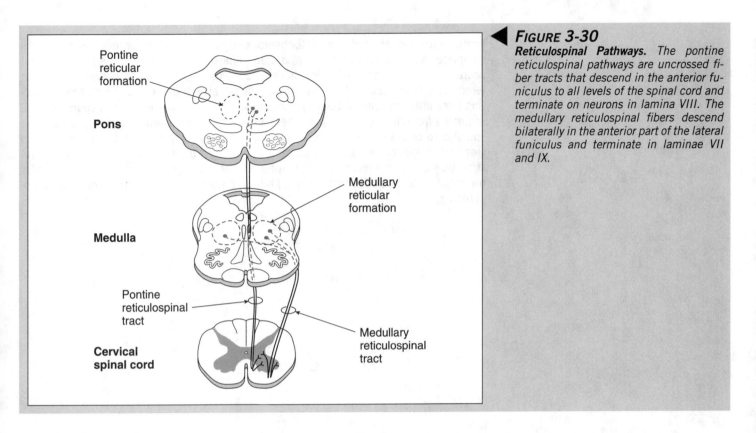

Reticulospinal Pathways. *The pontine reticulospinal pathways are uncrossed fiber tracts that descend in the anterior funiculus to all levels of the spinal cord and terminate on neurons in lamina VIII. The medullary reticulospinal fibers descend bilaterally in the anterior part of the lateral funiculus and terminate in laminae VII and IX.*

the corticoreticulospinal pathways are a major alternative to the corticospinal tract in controlling spinal motor neurons.

The reticular formation is essential for controlling the autonomic activities of the spinal cord. Visceral regions of the reticular formation contain neurons that receive inputs from the hypothalamus and from parasympathetic nuclei associated with the cranial nerves and their related nuclei (see Chapter 4). Descending fibers in the lateral reticulospinal tract project to sympathetic and parasympathetic centers of the spinal cord that are concerned with cardiovascular and respiratory function. These fibers modulate heart rate, respiratory rate, blood pressure, perspiration, and pupillary dilation, and they control some processes in the gastrointestinal and urinary systems.

VESTIBULOSPINAL TRACTS

The lateral and medial vestibular nuclei send separate descending projections to the spinal cord through the lateral and anterior funiculi, respectively. These are mainly uncrossed fiber projections that terminate in laminae VII and VIII, which, in turn, interact with the α-motor and γ-motor neurons of lamina IX. Both the medial and lateral vestibulospinal tracts facilitate muscle stretch reflexes and enhance contraction of extensor muscles, especially during reflexive movements that occur in response to falling. The vestibulospinal pathways coordinate the movements of the eyes, head, and limbs in response to angular or linear acceleration. The functions of these pathways are discussed later in this book (see Chapter 8).

RESOLUTION OF CLINICAL CASE

The clinical case at the beginning of this chapter presents symptoms that characterize the Brown-Séquard syndrome. Although rare, this syndrome is a classic demonstration of symptoms that illustrate the differential course of the ascending and descending spinal tracts. After recovery from spinal shock, limbs lying caudal to the hemisection develop spastic paralysis on the ipsilateral side. Voluntary movements of the limb are absent because the lateral corticospinal tract has been transected ipsilaterally. Deep tendon reflexes are hyperactive, and resting muscle tone is elevated because the muscles continue to be innervated by α-motor neurons originating from the anterior horn. There is complete loss of touch, proprioception, and kinesthetic sense because the ipsilateral posterior columns and spinocerebellar tracts are damaged. The perception of pain and temperature is lost contralaterally two segments below the wound because the transection interrupts the anterolateral system whose fibers decussate over the course of 1–2 segments from their site of origin. There are many instances where a focal lesion in the spinal cord or brainstem may produce a constellation of symptoms affecting opposite sides of the body because the decussating fibers of one tract are usually near other neural structures that present ipsilateral symptoms when damaged. Hence, it is important for the clinician to recognize that crossed findings provide a clear indication of focal neuropathology.

REVIEW QUESTIONS

Directions: For each of the following questions, choose the **one best** answer.

1. During a traffic accident, an individual suffered a complete dislocation of the spinal cord at C4–C5. Following surgical stabilization of the spine and a long-term course of rehabilitation, which of the following findings would you expect to see 1 year after the accident?

   (A) Preservation of cutaneous and pinprick sensations below the lesion

   (B) Hypotonia of the limb muscles

   (C) Hyperactive deep tendon reflexes

   (D) Areflexia

   (E) Normal volitional bladder emptying

2. Both arms of a patient exhibit impairment of pain and temperature sensation, but tactile sense is preserved. These symptoms indicate the patient is suffering from which of the following conditions?

   (A) Syringomyelia

   (B) Tabes dorsalis

   (C) Amyotrophic lateral sclerosis

   (D) Brown-Séquard syndrome

   (E) Complete transection of the cord at C4

3. Weakness, fasciculations, and atrophy of the muscles of the hands and arms without sensory loss suggest a pathologic process involving which of the following structures?

   (A) Lateral horn

   (B) Anterior horn

   (C) Lateral corticospinal tract

   (D) Posterior horn

   (E) Dorsal root ganglia

4. Narcotics injected into the lumbar cistern exert their analgesic effects by binding to opiate receptors located on neuronal processes in which of the following structures?

   (A) Anterior horn

   (B) Dorsal nucleus of Clarke

   (C) Phrenic nucleus

   (D) Intermediolateral cell column

   (E) Substantia gelatinosa

5. The clasp-knife reflex indicates which of the following conditions?

   (A) Lower motor neuron disease

   (B) Upper motor neuron disease

   (C) Spinal shock

   (D) Poliomyelitis

   (E) Normal deep tendon reflexes

6. Activity from muscle spindles is essential for initiating which of the following reflexes?

(A) Babinski's reflex

(B) Crossed extension reflex

(C) Clasp-knife reflex

(D) Myotactic reflex

(E) Flexor reflex

ANSWERS AND EXPLANATIONS

1. The answer is C. Hyperactive tendon reflexes are a characteristic symptom of spinal cord transection after the patient has recovered from spinal shock. Because the spinal cord was completely transected, the patient has no sensations below the lesion and has lost all voluntary motor control. After spinal shock subsides, the muscles become hypertonic, and the deep tendon reflexes are hyperactive.

2. The answer is A. Syringomyelia involves formation of a cavity in the center of the spinal cord where the fibers of the anterolateral system decussate. Hence, pain and temperature sensations from both sides of the body are lost without affecting cutaneous sensations transmitted by the posterior columns. Tabes dorsalis, Brown-Séquard syndrome, or a complete transection of the spinal cord would impair cutaneous sensitivity. In amyotrophic lateral sclerosis, there is a marked loss of motor function, but all somatic sensitivity, including nociception, remains intact.

3. The answer is B. Weakness, fasciculations, and muscle atrophy are all signs indicating degeneration of the lower motor neurons. The lateral horn innervates the autonomic ganglia, and significant weakness or wasting of the muscle would only occur after degeneration of the α-motor neurons. Loss of upper motor neurons in the corticospinal tracts would produce an increase in resting muscle tone. Structures involved in sensory processes, such as the dorsal root ganglia or the posterior horn, would not be implicated in motor degeneration.

4. The answer is E. The substantia gelatinosa uses enkephalin as a neurotransmitter. Opiates act as agonists at enkephalin receptors located on the dendritic processes of neighboring dorsal horn neurons as well as on the presynaptic terminals of the primary afferents entering laminae I and II. Enkephalinergic neurons are not found in any of the other listed areas.

5. The answer is B. The clasp-knife reflex is a pathologic sign resulting from upper motor neuron disease or trauma. None of the reflexes, including the clasp-knife phenomenon, are present during spinal shock or after damage to the lower motor neurons produced by poliomyelitis.

6. The answer is D. The myotactic reflex is elicited by muscle stretch sensed by muscle spindles. Noxious stimulation of free nerve endings elicits the flexor reflex coupled to the crossed extension reflex. Babinski's sign is elicited by gentle tactile stimulation of mechanoreceptors on the sole of the foot. The clasp-knife reflex is a pathologic form of autogenic inhibition elicited by stimulation of the Golgi tendon organs.

ADDITIONAL READING

Brodal A: The somatic afferent pathways. In *Neurological Anatomy in Relation to Clinical Medicine*, 3rd ed. New York, NY: Oxford University Press, 1981, pp 46–147.

Brown AG: *Organization in the Spinal Cord*. New York, NY: Springer, 1981.

Erlanger J, Gasser HS: *Electrical Signs of Nervous Activity*. Philadelphia, PA: University of Pennsylvania Press, 1937.

Melzack R, Wall PD: *The Challenge of Pain*. New York, NY: Basic Books, 1983.

Rexed B: The cytoarchitectonic organization of the spinal cord in the cat. *J Comp Neurol* 96:415–496, 1952.

Sherrington CS: *The Integrative Action of the Nervous System*. New Haven, CT: Yale University Press, 1947 (original copyright 1906).

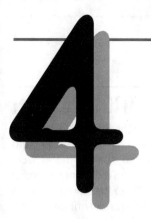

BRAINSTEM AND CRANIAL NERVES

CHAPTER OUTLINE

INTRODUCTION OF CLINICAL CASE

A 60-year-old male stockbroker made an appointment to see his physician after a sudden onset of headache and dizziness. This patient had a long history of smoking cigarettes and consuming three or more alcoholic beverages each day, behavior which undoubtedly contributed to hypertension for which he was prescribed medication. On the morning of the appointment, his right eyelid drooped, and he had difficulty swallowing food at breakfast. During the physical examination, his blood pressure was elevated, but respiration and heart rate were normal. Ptosis was present in the right eye, and when the doctor gently lifted the eyelid, the right pupil was slightly smaller than the left pupil. Both eyes showed pupillary light reflexes and displayed normal eye movements. Facial expression was normal and appeared symmetrical. The right eye had no corneal reflex, and pain sensation was depressed on the right side of the face. The skin on the right side of the face was dry and did not perspire. Hearing was normal for a 60-year-old person, but the man was unable to maintain his balance after closing his eyes. Speech was noticeably hoarse, but there was no inflammation of the nose, throat, or ear canals. The tongue protruded on the midline, the uvula deviated toward the left, and the right palate drooped. Both arms and legs had normal strength, and deep tendon reflexes were intact. The response to pinprick was weaker on the left side of the body although the patient could detect light touch equally well on both sides.

INTRODUCTION

The brainstem lies rostral to the spinal cord and is subdivided into the medulla, pons, and midbrain. Most cranial nerves are attached to the brainstem and transmit sensory and motor information to and from nuclear groups that monitor and control the sensory and motor activities of the head. Extensive interconnections between different regions of the brainstem mediate simple reflexes and regulate more complex functions such as respiration, sleep, and consciousness. The brainstem also contains many fibers of passage that interconnect the spinal cord and brainstem with higher levels of the neuraxis. A large number of functionally diverse neural structures reside in close proximity in the brainstem and, consequently, damage to this region usually produces a constellation of neurologic symptoms and frequently results in death.

GENERAL ORGANIZATION OF THE BRAINSTEM

The brainstem has an organization that follows a pattern similar to the organization of the spinal cord. In both regions, nuclear groups are segregated according to their connections with peripheral nerve fibers. In the spinal cord, afferent nerve fibers project to sensory nuclei in the dorsal horn, and efferent nerve fibers originate from motor nuclei in the ventral horn. A similar pattern is evident in the brainstem, although the relative location of sensory and motor nuclei is different because the sensory nuclei in the brainstem are displaced from their original location during embryologic development.

Transverse Organization

As described in Chapter 2, sensory and motor nuclei in the brainstem are derived, respectively, from the alar and basal plates of the neural tube. During development, the dorsal part of the rostral neural tube becomes thinner and allows the lateral walls of the neural tube to unfold. This process causes the alar plates to move lateral to the basal plates. With further cellular proliferation, the sensory and motor nuclei of the brainstem undergo further differentiation into somatic and visceral subdivisions (Figure 4-1).

Sensory and motor nuclei in the brainstem are classified according to their association with different submodalities of the cranial nerve fibers. Some of these nuclei have the same classification used in the spinal cord (1–4 below). Other cranial nerves and their brainstem nuclei are classified as "special" because of their embryologic origin or their involvement with special sensory functions (5–7 below).

> *Motor brainstem nuclei* are located medially. *Sensory brainstem nuclei* are located laterally.

1. General somatic efferent (GSE) nuclei give rise to cranial nerve fibers that innervate somatic musculature.
2. General visceral efferent (GVE) nuclei give rise to parasympathetic preganglionic fibers that innervate the peripheral parasympathetic ganglia.
3. General visceral afferent (GVA) nuclei receive afferent fibers from receptors located in the thoracic and abdominal viscera.
4. General somatic afferent (GSA) nuclei receive afferent fibers from mechanoreceptors in the skin, muscles, and joints.
5. Special visceral efferent (SVE) nuclei innervate striated muscles of branchiomeric origin such as the muscles of the larynx, pharynx, and face.
6. Special visceral afferent (SVA) nuclei receive projections from taste receptors located in the oral cavity.
7. Special somatic afferent (SSA) nuclei receive afferent projections from fibers concerned with hearing or balance.

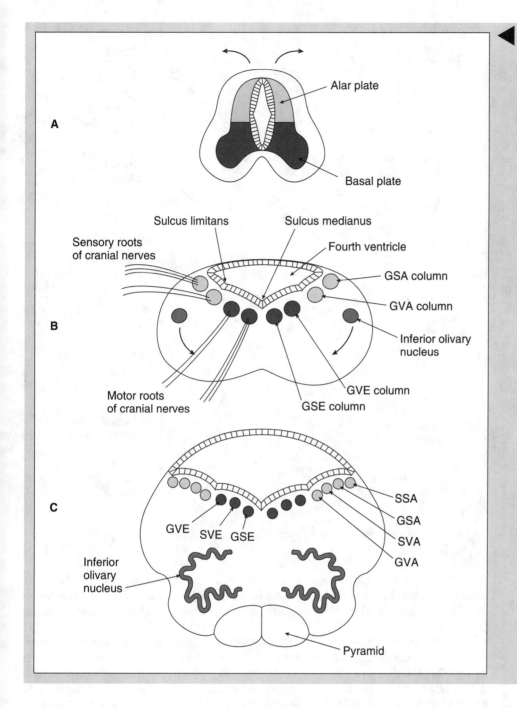

FIGURE 4-1
Location and Development of Cell Columns in the Brainstem. *(A) Relative position of the general afferent and efferent modalities in the embryonic brainstem. (B) During development the lateral walls of the neural tube unfold to form the medulla and other parts of the brainstem. (C) Neuronal proliferation results in further subdivision of the cell columns into general and special cranial nerve nuclei. GSA = general somatic afferent; GVA = general visceral afferent; GVE = general visceral efferent; GSE = general somatic efferent; SSA = special somatic afferent; SVA = special visceral afferent; SVE = special visceral efferent.*

Many brainstem nuclei form neural circuits similar to those seen in the spinal cord that mediate spinal reflexes. Afferent projections from sensory receptors in the head are conveyed by nerve fibers whose cell bodies are located in the cranial ganglia. The cranial ganglia are analogous to the dorsal root ganglia of the spinal cord because they contain pseudounipolar neurons whose proximal axons enter the brainstem and terminate in sensory nuclei located lateral to the sulcus limitans. In turn, the sensory nuclei send projections medially to nearby motor nuclei. These motor nuclei innervate striated muscles in the head, face, and intraoral cavity as well as autonomic ganglia that control glands or smooth muscles. Hence, cranial nerve reflexes are mediated by a series of neuronal connections that resemble the multisynaptic reflex arcs described for the spinal cord (Figure 4-2).

Efferent fibers in the cranial nerves originate from visceral and somatic motor nuclei in the brainstem that are reminiscent of the lateral and ventral horns in the spinal cord. As in the spinal cord, brainstem motor neurons use acetylcholine at their synaptic

Cranial nerve reflexes depend upon connections between sensory and motor nuclei.

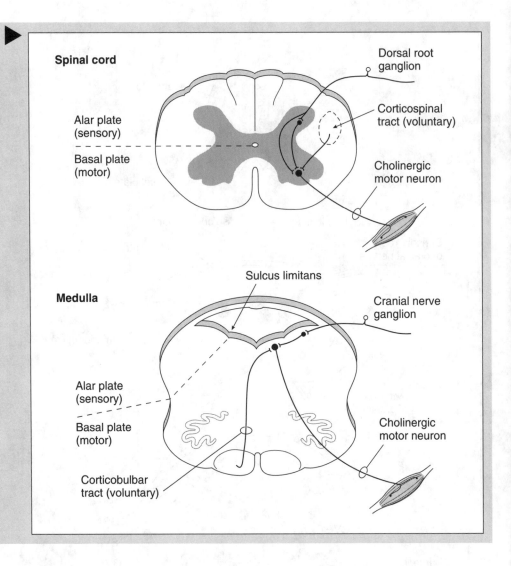

FIGURE 4-2

Comparison of Spinal Cord and Medulla. Sensory and motor nuclei in the spinal cord and brainstem are found in separate regions of the spinal cord and medulla. Similar circuits in the spinal cord and brainstem mediate reflexive movements and execute motor commands issued from the cerebral cortex.

The **corticobulbar tract** consists of all cortical projections to the cranial nerve nuclei. Many fibers in this tract are upper motor neurons that mediate motor activity in the head.

terminals to communicate with peripheral muscles or autonomic ganglia. Similar to the α-motor neurons in the spinal cord, the brainstem motor nuclei represent lower motor neurons, and a lesion of the cranial motor nucleus or its efferent fibers causes muscular paralysis.

In addition to receiving local inputs for mediating reflexive movements, the somatic motor nuclei receive connections from the motor cortex that control voluntary movements. Corticobulbar projections descend through the internal capsule and crus cerebri before synapsing on specific sets of cranial nerve nuclei in the brainstem (Figure 4-3). In cases where corticobulbar fibers innervate motor nuclei, these fibers are analogous to the corticospinal tract because both sets of fibers function as upper motor neurons. In contrast to the corticospinal tract, which projects almost exclusively to the contralateral side, corticobulbar projections are predominately bilateral. Depending on the specific fibers that are affected, corticobulbar lesions may impair voluntary movements of the face, eyes, mouth, tongue, or larynx.

Longitudinal Organization

Cranial nerve nuclei are arranged in longitudinal cell columns extending rostrocaudally as shown in Figure 4-4. In general, sensory nuclei are elongated (up to several millimeters) and contain large numbers of relatively small neurons. By comparison, most motor nuclei in the brainstem contain large neurons that tend to be clustered into smaller, more compact groups. Some motor groups in the medulla, however, extend rostrocaudally for several millimeters and give rise to multiple nerve rootlets that emerge at regular intervals and contribute efferent fibers to cranial nerves IX, X, XI, and XII.

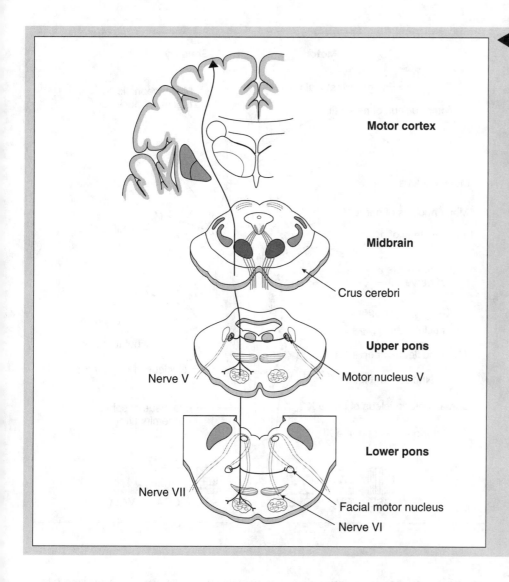

Motor cortex

Midbrain

Crus cerebri

Upper pons

Nerve V

Motor nucleus V

Lower pons

Nerve VII

Facial motor nucleus

Nerve VI

FIGURE 4-3
Corticobulbar and Corticopontine Projections. *Descending fibers from the cerebral cortex traverse the internal capsule and crus cerebri to form corticobulbar and corticopontine connections. Most corticobulbar fibers innervate the motor nuclei in the brainstem directly or indirectly (via the reticular formation) to mediate voluntary control of motor activity in the head. Other corticobulbar fibers project to sensory nuclei in the brainstem to modulate the transmission of sensory information. Corticopontine fibers project ipsilaterally to the pontine nuclei, which, in turn, project to the contralateral cerebellar cortex.*

Many sensory nuclei in the brainstem receive afferent fibers from more than one cranial nerve. Multiple inputs occur in cases where afferents of the same modality enter the brainstem through different cranial nerves and project to different rostral–caudal levels of the same sensory nucleus. By comparison, only the nucleus ambiguus contributes efferent fibers to more than one cranial nerve.

THE MEDULLA

The medulla marks the transition from the spinal cord to the brainstem, and many structures in the spinal cord extend into the medulla. Unlike the spinal cord, the medulla gradually expands in diameter as it acquires additional nuclei and fiber tracts at more rostral levels.

The spinomedullary junction occurs where the pyramidal decussation interrupts the anterior median fissure on the ventral surface (Figure 4-5). Rostral to this decussation, the pyramidal tracts lie adjacent to the midline and extend the entire length of the medulla. In the rostral half of the medulla, each pyramidal tract is flanked by a large protruding mass, the inferior olivary nucleus. The olivary nuclei were so named because of their prominence on the lateral surface of the medulla, which resembles an olive. The olivary nuclei are bounded by the preolivary (or anterolateral) and postolivary sulci. A series of hypoglossal nerve rootlets emerge from the preolivary sulcus lying between the

FIGURE 4-4 ▶
Location of Sensory and Motor Nuclei in the Brainstem. A schematic diagram of the sensory and motor cell columns extending through the brainstem. Each cell column is coded as indicated by the legend. GSE = general somatic efferent; GVE = general visceral efferent; SVE = special visceral efferent; SSA = special somatic afferent; GSA = general somatic afferent; VA = visceral afferent. (Source: Adapted with permission from Brodal A: Neurological Anatomy in Relation to Clinical Medicine. Oxford, England: Oxford University Press, 1981, p 451.)

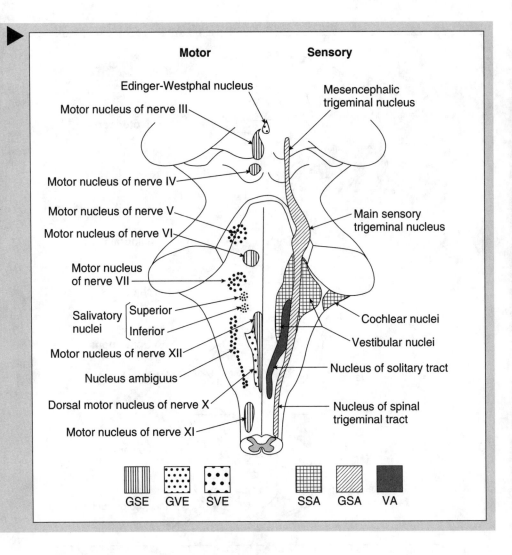

A **tuberculum** is a small lump or elevation.

pyramidal tract and the inferior olive. The postolivary sulcus contains emerging rootlets from the glossopharyngeal (IX), vagal (X), and spinal accessory (XI) nerves.

On the lateral and dorsal surfaces, the longitudinal tracts and sulci of the spinal cord continue into the medulla without interruption (Figure 4-6). The dorsal (or posterior) columns lie on both sides of the posterior median sulcus, which terminates at the obex, a midline point that marks the caudal end of the floor of the fourth ventricle. On each side of the obex lie several small protuberances called the tuberculum gracilis, tuberculum cuneatus, and tuberculum cinereum. These elevations mark the underlying nucleus gracilis, nucleus cuneatus, and spinal trigeminal tract and nucleus. A shallow groove called the posterior intermediate sulcus separates the nucleus gracilis from the more lateral nucleus cuneatus, whereas the posterolateral sulcus separates the tuberculum cuneatus from the tuberculum cinereum.

The dorsal surfaces of the medulla and pons form the floor of the fourth ventricle and contain many structures that can be seen after removing the cerebellum. Rostral to the obex are the hypoglossal trigones, a pair of small bumps that mark the underlying hypoglossal nuclei on each side of the midline. More laterally, the vagal trigone overlies the dorsal motor nucleus of the vagus. Lateral to the sulcus limitans lies the vestibular area and the cerebellar peduncles, which form the lateral wall of the fourth ventricle. More rostrally, the boundary between the medulla and pons occurs where the stria medullares traverse the floor of the fourth ventricle.

Internal Structures of the Medulla

The organization of the medulla is best understood by studying its internal structures as they appear in transverse sections. Figure 4-7 illustrates the position of the major

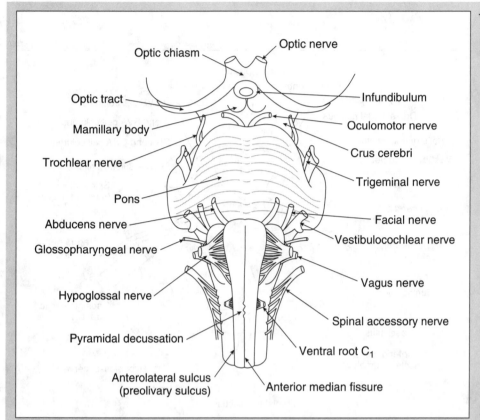

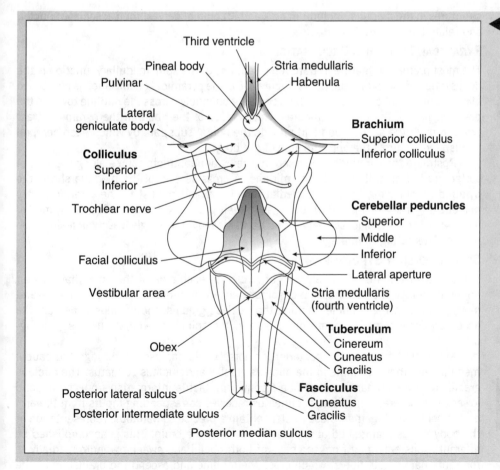

▶ FIGURE 4-7 ▶
Transverse Organization of the Medulla.
This schematic drawing indicates the position of the major nuclei and fiber tracts in the medulla organized according to their functional components. GSE = general somatic efferent; GVE = general visceral efferent; SVE = special visceral efferent; GVA = general visceral afferent; SVA = special visceral afferent; SSA = special somatic afferent; GSA = general somatic afferent.

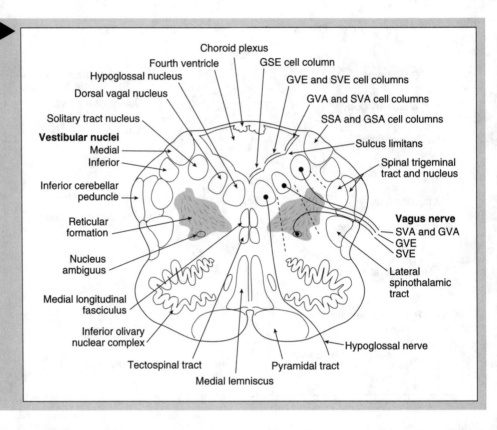

The **pyramidal decussation** allows the motor cortex to control the opposite side of the body.

The **nucleus gracilis** receives tactile information from the leg. The **nucleus cuneatus** receives tactile information from the arm.

structures in the medulla, including the X and XII cranial nerves, their associated nuclei, and related nuclei and fiber tracts.

PYRAMIDAL TRACT AND DECUSSATION

The most prominent feature in transverse sections of the spinomedullary junction is the decussation of the pyramidal tracts (Figure 4-8). The pyramidal decussation is composed of large bundles of corticospinal fibers coursing obliquely across the midline towards the posterior part of the lateral funiculus. Nearly 90% of the fibers in the pyramidal tract cross through the decussation and provide the neural substrate by which each cerebral hemisphere controls the opposite side of the body.

Rostral to the pyramidal decussation, the pyramidal tracts course along the ventral surface of the medulla next to the midline. A cross section of the medulla shows the pyramidal tract lying below the medial lemniscus and medial to the inferior olivary nucleus (Figures 4-9 and 4-10). Because of their proximity, the pyramidal tract, medial lemniscus, and hypoglossal nerve can be damaged by a single vascular lesion (see Inferior Alternating Hemiplegia).

SOMATOSENSORY STRUCTURES

The dorsal medulla contains a group of nuclei on each side of the obex that play an important role in the transmission of somatosensory information. From the midline and moving laterally, these nuclei include the nucleus gracilis, the nucleus cuneatus, the accessory (or external) cuneate nucleus, and the spinal trigeminal nucleus (see Figure 4-9).

Myelinated axons of the posterior (or dorsal) columns ascend through the caudal medulla until they terminate in the nucleus gracilis and nucleus cuneatus. The nucleus gracilis receives primary afferent fibers conveying tactile information from the leg and lower trunk, whereas the nucleus cuneatus receives corresponding inputs from the arm and upper trunk. Together, these nuclei contain a precise somatotopic representation of the body that is maintained at successive levels of the brain. This is accomplished by efferent axons emerging from the base of both nuclei and sweeping ventromedially to form internal arcuate fibers, which cross the midline and ascend the brainstem as the

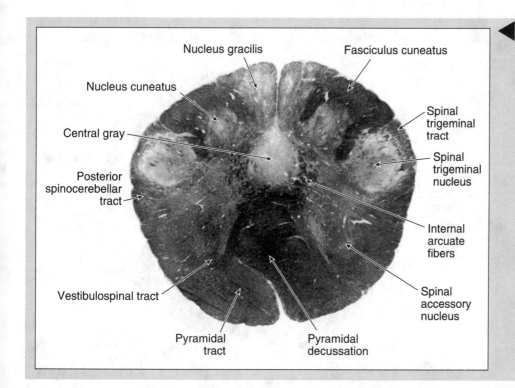

FIGURE 4-8
Tranverse View of the Spinomedullary Junction. This photomicrograph illustrates the pyramidal decussation and several nuclear groups in the caudal part of the medulla.

Nucleus gracilis

Fasciculus cuneatus

Nucleus cuneatus

Central gray

Spinal trigeminal tract

Spinal trigeminal nucleus

Posterior spinocerebellar tract

Internal arcuate fibers

Vestibulospinal tract

Spinal accessory nucleus

Pyramidal tract

Pyramidal decussation

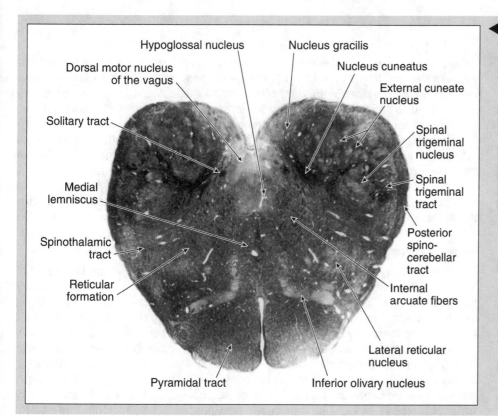

FIGURE 4-9
Transverse View of the Medulla. This photomicrograph illustrates the medulla at the level of the obex and shows the position of several cranial nerve nuclei at their most caudal extent. The internal arcuate fibers and medial lemniscus are apparent in the central portion of the section.

Hypoglossal nucleus

Nucleus gracilis

Dorsal motor nucleus of the vagus

Nucleus cuneatus

External cuneate nucleus

Solitary tract

Spinal trigeminal nucleus

Medial lemniscus

Spinal trigeminal tract

Spinothalamic tract

Posterior spino-cerebellar tract

Reticular formation

Internal arcuate fibers

Lateral reticular nucleus

Pyramidal tract

Inferior olivary nucleus

medial lemniscus. Fibers from the nucleus gracilis are located ventral to those originating in the nucleus cuneatus and impose a topographical representation of the medial lemniscus that resembles a headless, erect body. The decussation of these second-order fibers provides the basis by which cutaneous inputs from the body are transmitted to somatosensory regions in the contralateral thalamus and cerebral cortex.

The accessory cuneate nucleus, located dorsolateral to the main cuneate nucleus, receives primary afferents from muscle spindles and Golgi tendon organs in the hand.

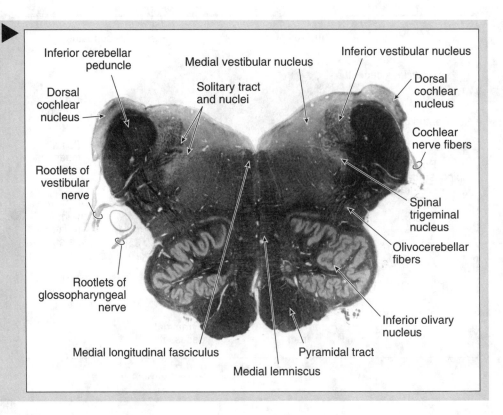

FIGURE 4-10

Transverse View of the Rostral Medulla. *This photomicrograph illustrates the major structures in the rostral medulla. The dorsal surface of the rostral medulla forms the floor of the fourth ventricle and contains the vestibular and cochlear nuclei. The massive inferior cerebellar peduncles consist of several groups of myelinated fibers that project into the cerebellum. The inferior olivary nucleus is seen bulging along the ventrolateral surface of the medulla.*

Labels in figure: Inferior cerebellar peduncle; Medial vestibular nucleus; Inferior vestibular nucleus; Dorsal cochlear nucleus; Solitary tract and nuclei; Dorsal cochlear nucleus; Cochlear nerve fibers; Rootlets of vestibular nerve; Spinal trigeminal nucleus; Olivocerebellar fibers; Rootlets of glossopharyngeal nerve; Inferior olivary nucleus; Medial longitudinal fasciculus; Pyramidal tract; Medial lemniscus

The axonal processes from these mechanoreceptors pass through the posterior columns without synapsing in the dorsal horn of the spinal cord. Hence, the accessory cuneate functions as the forelimb equivalent of the dorsal nucleus of Clarke. The accessory cuneate sends a projection of second-order neurons, the cuneocerebellar tract, into the cerebellar cortex by way of the inferior cerebellar peduncle.

The spinal trigeminal tract conveys primary afferent fibers from four cranial nerves (V, VII, IX, X) to the spinal trigeminal nucleus. The spinal trigeminal nucleus extends into the upper cervical segments (C1–C4) of the spinal cord where it blends into the gray matter. The caudal part of the spinal trigeminal nucleus bears a striking resemblance to the substantia gelatinosa and other laminae of the dorsal horn and, not surprisingly, this part of the spinal trigeminal nucleus is involved in processing pain sensations from the head.

> The **spinal trigeminal nucleus** receives pain inputs from the head. The **substantia gelatinosa** receives pain inputs from the body.

INFERIOR OLIVE AND INFERIOR CEREBELLAR PEDUNCLE

The inferior olivary nucleus is a large convoluted structure in the ventrolateral part of the rostral medulla that is surrounded medially and dorsally by slender accessory olivary nuclei (see Figure 4-10). The inferior olive and its accessory nuclei have strong connections with neurons in the cerebellum, a brain structure considered important for its motor functions. Based on their afferent connections, however, the inferior olivary nuclei and cerebellum can be considered as sensory components in a larger network of nuclei that interact to mediate motor control. Thus, the olivary nuclei receive ascending sensory inputs directly from the spinal cord as well as indirect inputs from the nucleus gracilis, nucleus cuneatus, and the inferior vestibular nucleus. The inferior olivary nuclei also receive descending projections from regions closely identified with motor functions, including the red nucleus and the motor cortex, and these connections suggest the inferior olive may use sensory information to modify motor commands from these higher levels. In turn, the inferior olive sends a large collection of efferent fibers across the midline to course dorsolaterally and merge with other fibers of the inferior cerebellar peduncle. Olivocerebellar fibers are also identified as climbing fibers and provide a major source of excitatory input to the giant Purkinje cells of the cerebellar cortex.

> The **inferior cerebellar peduncle** contains four main fiber groups: olivocerebellar, cuneocerebellar, posterior spinocerebellar, and vestibulocerebellar.

The inferior cerebellar peduncle is a massive fiber tract located in the dorsolateral region of the rostral medulla. Most fibers in the inferior cerebellar peduncle are olivo-cerebellar fibers that originate from the contralateral inferior olive. Other fibers from the posterior spinocerebellar and cuneocerebellar tracts also merge into the inferior cerebellar peduncle and convey information about muscle tone in the upper and lower limbs. The inferior cerebellar peduncle is sometimes called the restiform body; fibers adjacent to the fourth ventricle that interconnect the vestibular nuclei with the cerebellum constitute the juxtarestiform body.

Cranial Nerve Nuclei of the Medulla

The medulla contains several sensory and motor cranial nerve nuclei: the hypoglossal nucleus, the supraspinal (or spinal accessory) nucleus, the dorsal motor nucleus of the vagus, the nucleus ambiguus, the nucleus of the solitary tract, and the spinal trigeminal nucleus (see Figure 4-4).

HYPOGLOSSAL NUCLEUS (GSE—XII)

The hypoglossal nucleus extends the entire length of the medulla and is found near the dorsal midline where it bulges into the floor of the fourth ventricle (see Figure 4-9). Axons of the large cholinergic neurons in the hypoglossal nucleus course ventrally and pass between the inferior olive and pyramidal tract until they emerge as a series of rootlets in the anterolateral sulcus. The hypoglossal nerve innervates the intrinsic and extrinsic muscles of the tongue, which are used for chewing, swallowing, and articulating speech. In addition to receiving inputs from the cerebral cortex (i.e., corticobulbar fibers), the hypoglossal nucleus also receives taste inputs from the nucleus of the solitary tract and tactile inputs from the spinal trigeminal nucleus. These connections are thought to mediate reflexive movements of the tongue during the chewing and swallowing of food.

> *The **hypoglossal nucleus** innervates the extrinsic and intrinsic tongue muscles.*

A unilateral lesion of the hypoglossal nucleus or nerve causes paralysis of the ipsilateral tongue. Consequently, patients with a hypoglossal lesion are unable to stick their tongue out straight. Instead, the tongue deviates toward the side of the lesion. Furthermore, close inspection of their tongue reveals atrophy or fasciculations on the denervated side because a hypoglossal nerve lesion represents degeneration of a lower motor neuron. Hypoglossal nerve fibers are usually damaged in response to occlusion or hemorrhage of the local blood supply.

Inferior Alternating Hemiplegia (Wallenberg's Syndrome). Each tributary from the anterior spinal artery supplies blood to the pyramid, medial lemniscus, and hypoglossal nerve on one side of the medulla (Figure 4-11). Consequently, occlusion of one of these tributaries causes ipsilateral paralysis of the tongue in combination with contralateral paresis of the arm and leg. These symptoms form a distinct syndrome that is called inferior alternating hemiplegia (Wallenberg's syndrome) because it affects opposite sides of the body (alternating) and is the result of a lesion at the caudal end of the brainstem (inferior). Some patients may complain of tactile insensitivity on the contralateral body, but this symptom varies because the medial lemniscus is often spared, and even if it is damaged, other spinal pathways can compensate for the sensory loss.

> ***Wallenberg's syndrome** involves paralysis of the ipsilateral tongue and contralateral body.*

SPINAL ACCESSORY NUCLEUS (GSE—XI)

The spinal accessory (or supraspinal) nucleus is a long column of cells that extends from the caudal medulla through the upper five or six cervical segments of the spinal cord and occupies a position near the ventral horn (see Figure 4-8). Efferent nerve fibers depart ventrolaterally from the spinal accessory nucleus to innervate the ipsilateral sternocleidomastoid and trapezius muscles. The sternocleidomastoid muscles are responsible for turning the head, and a unilateral lesion of the spinal accessory nucleus or nerve causes weakness in turning the head away from the side of the lesion. The shoulder on the lesioned side also droops noticeably because the trapezius muscle is paralyzed (Figure 4-12). These muscles are branchiomeric in origin, and consistent with this view, a few anatomists place the spinal accessory nerve in the SVE category. However, most believe that all nerve fibers exiting the spinal cord to innervate striated muscle should be classified as GSE fibers.

> *The **spinal accessory nucleus** innervates the trapezius and sternocleidomastoid muscles.*

FIGURE 4-11
Location of Vascular Accidents in the Medulla. *This diagram indicates the structures in the medulla that may be damaged in inferior alternating hemiplegia (Wallenberg's syndrome) and in the lateral medullary syndrome.*

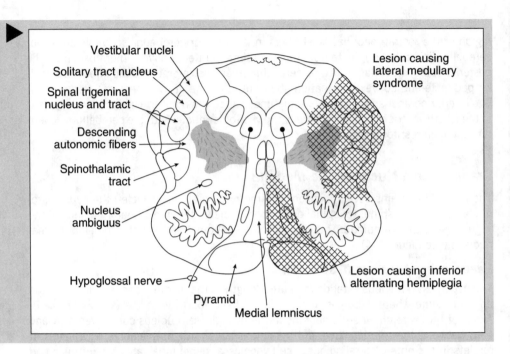

DORSAL MOTOR NUCLEUS OF THE VAGUS (GVE—X)

The dorsal motor nucleus of the vagus is a collection of small cholinergic cells that lie lateral to the hypoglossal nucleus and form the vagal trigone in the floor of the fourth ventricle. Preganglionic parasympathetic fibers depart ventrolaterally from the dorsal motor nucleus and pass below the spinal trigeminal nucleus to emerge from the brainstem with other components of the vagus nerve (see Figure 4-9).

The dorsal motor nucleus is the principal source of parasympathetic preganglionic fibers in the brainstem. These fibers innervate postganglionic neurons that control the glands of the pharyngeal and laryngeal mucosa and the smooth muscles of the thoracic and abdominal viscera. Consistent with the "rest and digest" role of the parasympathetic system, neuronal activity in the dorsal motor nucleus of the vagus slows heart rate, stimulates peristalsis and gastric acid secretion, and causes bronchial constriction. The dorsal motor nucleus of the vagus receives inputs from several brain regions that regulate autonomic functions, including the hypothalamus and the reticular formation. The dorsal motor nucleus also receives input from surrounding sensory nuclei, especially the nucleus of the solitary tract.

*The **dorsal motor nucleus of the vagus** exerts parasympathetic control over pharyngeal and laryngeal glands and over the smooth muscles of the thoracic and abdominal viscera.*

NUCLEUS AMBIGUUS (SVE—IX AND X)

As its name implies, the nucleus ambiguus is difficult to visualize in most histologic preparations of the brainstem. In sections stained for acetylcholinesterase, however, the nucleus ambiguus appears prominently in the lateral reticular formation, approximately halfway between the inferior olive and the spinal trigeminal nucleus. Efferent fibers from the nucleus ambiguus depart ventrolaterally, and some are joined by fibers from the dorsal motor nucleus of the vagus as they give rise to cranial nerves IX and X. The nucleus ambiguus innervates the striated muscles of the pharynx and larynx, which are important for voluntary and reflexive movements involved in swallowing, gagging, vomiting, and speech. The nucleus ambiguus receives inputs from the corticobulbar tract and from surrounding parts of the reticular formation to mediate voluntary movements. The spinal trigeminal nucleus and the nucleus solitarius send second-order projections to the nucleus ambiguus that are important for mediating reflexive movements.

*The **nucleus ambiguus** innervates the striated muscles of the pharynx and larynx.*

NUCLEUS OF THE SOLITARY TRACT

The solitary tract is a compact bundle of SVA and GVA fibers from cranial nerves VII, IX, and X, which extends the entire length of the medulla. The solitary tract is isolated from other brainstem tracts, and its fibers are entirely surrounded by second-order neurons that form the nucleus of the solitary tract. Axons in the solitary tract terminate in different

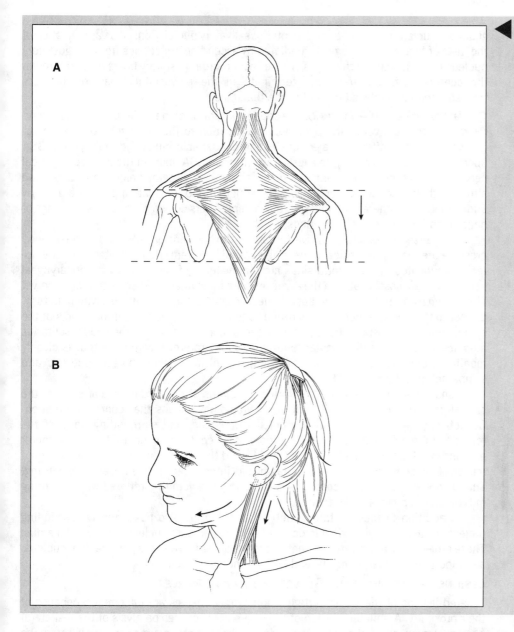

A

B

FIGURE 4-12
Clinical Signs of Accessory Nerve Damage.
(A) The shoulder droops because the trapezius muscle is paralyzed. (B) There is weakness in turning the head away from the side of the lesion because the sternocleidomastoid muscles are paralyzed. (Source: Reprinted with permission from Wilson-Pauwels L, et al: Cranial Nerves—Anatomy and Clinical Comments. *Toronto, Ontario: B. C. Decker, 1988, p 145.)*

parts of the nucleus solitarius according to their functional modality. The rostral third of the nucleus solitarius is called the gustatory nucleus because it receives inputs from SVA fibers innervating taste buds, whereas the caudal solitarius receives inputs from GVA fibers innervating the thoracic and abdominal viscera.

Rostral Solitarius (SVA—VII, IX, and X). The gustatory part of the nucleus solitarius is located in the dorsolateral part of the rostral medulla, ventral to the vestibular nuclei (see Figures 4-7 and 4-10). The gustatory nucleus receives SVA inputs from cranial nerves VII, IX, and X. The intermediate nerve, a branch of cranial nerve VII, contains SVA fibers that innervate taste buds in the rostral two-thirds of the tongue. The SVA fibers derived from taste buds in the caudal third of the tongue travel within cranial nerve IX. Only a few SVA fibers from cranial nerve X terminate in the gustatory nucleus, and these are derived from taste buds on the epiglottis.

The anatomic connections of the gustatory nucleus indicate the variety of functions that rely on taste information. Local projections from the gustatory nucleus mediate reflexes involving the oral cavity, while ascending projections to the diencephalon subserve the cognitive aspects of taste. Thus, the gustatory nucleus projects locally to the nucleus ambiguus and the hypoglossal nucleus to modulate reflexive movements of the tongue and larynx that occur during chewing, swallowing, and coughing. The production of saliva while eating represents a reflex that is mediated by local connections from the

The **rostral solitarius** *receives taste information from the tongue. The* **caudal solitarius** *receives cardiovascular and visceral information from the thoracic and abdominal cavities.*

gustatory nucleus to the superior and inferior salivatory nuclei. Conscious appreciation of the taste of food and beverages is mediated by ascending projections from the gustatory nucleus to the ipsilateral thalamus. These second-order gustatory fibers ascend through the central tegmental tract and terminate in the parvocellular part of the ventroposteromedial nucleus (VPMpc) in the thalamus.

Caudal Solitarius (GVA—IX and X). The caudal two-thirds of the nucleus solitarius extend rostrally from the level of the pyramidal decussation to the entry zone of the glossopharyngeal nerve. Afferent projections to the caudal solitarius arise mainly from GSA fibers in the vagus nerve and, to a lesser extent, from GSA fibers in the glossopharyngeal nerve. These cranial nerves innervate the abdominal viscera, heart, and lungs, and although their mechanisms of sensory transduction and innervation pattern are poorly understood, it is generally agreed that these nerve fibers convey pain, diffuse feelings of nausea, and other visceral sensations.

Specialized receptors sensitive to carbon dioxide tension, pH, and arterial blood pressure are located at critical sites in the vascular system. Baroreceptors and chemoreceptors located in the carotid sinus are innervated by fibers of the glossopharyngeal nerve, whereas those located in the aortic arch are innervated by fibers of the vagus nerve. These primary afferent fibers synapse on neurons in the caudal solitarius, which, in turn, project to the dorsal motor nucleus of the vagus or to thoracic and lumbar levels of the spinal cord (solitariospinal tract). These efferent connections from the caudal solitarius mediate important cardiovascular reflexes and illustrate how cardiac output is closely monitored and controlled by feedback loops involving specific parasympathetic and sympathetic centers.

Consistent with its role in monitoring the status of the cardiovascular system, the caudal solitarius is connected with other brainstem regions that control ventilation. Collectively, the caudal solitarius, nucleus ambiguus, and surrounding parts of the reticular formation form a medullary respiratory center that drives the lower motor neurons of the phrenic nucleus (i.e., C3–C5) and the anterior horn of the thoracic cord responsible for controlling the diaphragm and intercostal muscles used in breathing. This medullary region also coordinates coughing and vomiting reflexes with breathing movements to prevent aspiration.

> *The **medullary respiratory center** is the region around the nucleus ambiguus that projects to the phrenic nucleus and other regions that execute breathing movements.*

In addition to these outputs, the caudal solitarius also has extensive ascending projections to the paraventricular, dorsomedial, and arcuate nuclei of the hypothalamus. These projections, along with connections to the amygdala and the parabrachial nucleus, are important for integrating visceral and autonomic responses.

LESIONS OF THE VAGUS AND GLOSSOPHARYNGEAL NERVES

Isolated lesions of the vagus and glossopharyngeal nerves are uncommon because of their proximity. A unilateral lesion of the vagus nerve causes paralysis of the ipsilateral pharynx, larynx, and soft palate. Damage to the lower motor neurons originating from the nucleus ambiguus results in hoarseness, dysphonia, and difficulty in swallowing. Speech takes on a pronounced nasal character, and fluids enter the nasal cavity during attempted swallowing due to dysfunction of the larynx and pharynx. In these patients, the soft palate is elevated on the normal side, and the uvula deviates away from the side of the lesion. In rare instances where the vagus nerve is affected bilaterally, loss of vagal inhibition causes paralysis of the esophagus and stomach, complete loss of the carotid sinus reflex, and tachycardia. Sudden bilateral damage to vagal fibers entering the recurrent laryngeal nerve causes complete paralysis of the pharynx and larynx. Unless a tracheotomy is performed immediately, the patient will die of asphyxiation.

> *Loss of the gag reflex is a clinical sign indicating a lesion of the glossopharyngeal nerve.*

Symptoms produced by isolated lesions of the glossopharyngeal nerve are due mainly to interruption of its sensory fibers. Glossopharyngeal lesions interfere with the somatosensory innervation of the posterior third of the tongue, the tonsil, the palatal arches, and the pharynx. These deficits are responsible for loss of the gag reflex on the ipsilateral side. In addition, taste is not present on the posterior side of the ipsilateral tongue, although this deficit is usually not noticed by the patient unless it is specifically tested (Figure 4-13).

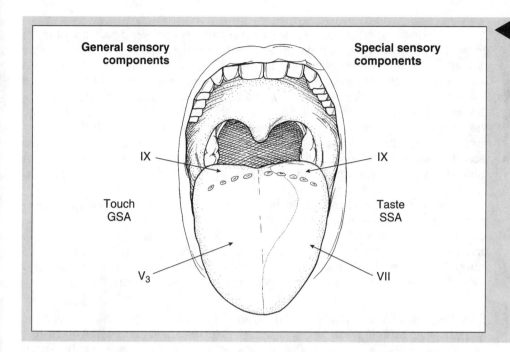

General sensory components

Special sensory components

IX

IX

Touch GSA

Taste SSA

V₃

VII

FIGURE 4-13
Sensory Supply of the Tongue. The anterior and posterior parts of the tongue are innervated by different cranial nerves. (Source: *Reprinted with permission from Wilson-Pauwels L, et al: Cranial Nerves—Anatomy and Clinical Comments. Toronto, Ontario: B. C. Decker, 1988, p 159.*)

TRIGEMINAL SENSORY NUCLEI

Somatosensory innervation of the head is mediated by primary GSA fibers distributed among the trigeminal, facial (or intermediate), glossopharyngeal, and vagus nerves. The somatosensory components of these nerves project to three trigeminal nuclei that extend through the medulla, pons, and midbrain (see Figure 4-4). The spinal trigeminal nucleus extends from the spinal cord through the medulla and the caudal half of the pons. The main (or principal) sensory nucleus forms a compact nucleus at the midpontine level, just caudal to the mesencephalic nucleus, which extends into the midbrain (Figure 4-14).

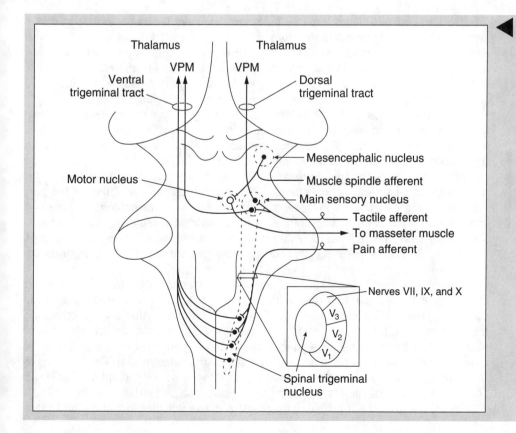

Thalamus

Thalamus

VPM

VPM

Ventral trigeminal tract

Dorsal trigeminal tract

Mesencephalic nucleus

Muscle spindle afferent

Motor nucleus

Main sensory nucleus

Tactile afferent

To masseter muscle

Pain afferent

Nerves VII, IX, and X

V₃

V₂

V₁

Spinal trigeminal nucleus

FIGURE 4-14
Trigeminal Pathways. Tactile and nociceptive fibers in the trigeminal nerve project differentially to the main sensory and spinal trigeminal nuclei, respectively. The inset indicates the somatotopic organization of the spinal trigeminal nucleus in a transverse section. VPM = ventroposteromedial nucleus.

*The **trigeminal nuclei** contain a main sensory nucleus—cutaneous inputs; a spinal trigeminal nucleus—pain and temperature inputs; a motor trigeminal nucleus—muscles of mastication; and a mesencephalic nucleus—muscle spindle inputs.*

Most primary afferent fibers entering the trigeminal nuclei originate from the trigeminal nerve. The trigeminal nerve conveys tactile and nociceptive sensations from the face, the anterior two-thirds of the tongue, the cornea, the dura mater, and the mucous lining of the mouth and nose. As its name implies, the trigeminal nerve consists of three divisions: the ophthalmic, the maxillary, and the mandibular branches. After entering the pons, most first-order trigeminal fibers bifurcate and send a short collateral axon into the main sensory nucleus and a much longer descending axon to the spinal trigeminal nucleus. These descending axons form the spinal trigeminal tract, which is located along the lateral aspect of the spinal trigeminal nucleus. Some trigeminal fibers do not bifurcate but terminate either in the main sensory nucleus or in the spinal trigeminal nucleus.

Only a small proportion of GSA fibers originate from the intermediate, glossopharyngeal, or vagus nerves and join the spinal trigeminal tract before terminating in the spinal trigeminal nucleus. All of these nerves supply GSA fibers to the external ear and to portions of the tympanic membrane. Additional GSA fibers in the glossopharyngeal nerve innervate the posterior third of the tongue, while some GSA fibers in the vagus nerve supply the pharynx, the larynx, and the meninges of the posterior cranial fossa.

Spinal Trigeminal Nucleus (GSA—V, VII, IX, and X). The spinal trigeminal nucleus is the longest cranial nerve nucleus, largely because it receives terminals from GSA fibers from four cranial nerves (i.e., V, VII, IX, X) that span most of the medulla and pons. The spinal trigeminal tract is somatotopically organized with mandibular fibers located dorsally, ophthalmic fibers located ventrally, and maxillary fibers located in between (see Figure 4-14). As the spinal trigeminal tract descends, it becomes narrower as individual fibers depart medially to terminate in the adjacent spinal trigeminal nucleus. The spinal trigeminal tract and nucleus descend into upper cervical segments C2 or C3 of the spinal cord where they merge into Lissauer's tract and the underlying dorsal horn. The trigeminal nucleus is traditionally divided into three parts: (1) a pars caudalis that extends from the spinal cord to the level of the obex, (2) a pars interpolaris that forms the middle third of the nucleus and extends rostrally to the pontomedullary junction, and (3) a pars oralis that lies in the pons and merges into the principal (or main) sensory nucleus of the trigeminal nerve.

The pars caudalis blends into the spinal cord and has a laminar organization that is nearly identical to the cytologic structure of the dorsal horn. The most superficial layer, lamina I, receives synaptic terminals from GSA fibers containing substance P and resembles the posteromarginal layer of the spinal cord. Lamina II is immunoreactive for enkephalin and appears to play a role analogous to the substantia gelatinosa. Laminae III and IV contain larger neurons that form the magnocellular nucleus.

The cytologic organization of the pars caudalis suggests that this nucleus is involved in processing pain and temperature information from the head. Consistent with this view, trigeminal tract fibers projecting to the pars caudalis are small in diameter and resemble the C fibers that convey nociceptive impulses to the spinal cord. Clinical studies have shown that sectioning the spinal trigeminal tract in the medulla (trigeminal tractotomy) reduces chronic pain without interfering with cutaneous sensitivity. Although the pars interpolaris and pars oralis both receive nociceptive and cutaneous inputs, there is a gradual shift towards processing cutaneous information at these more rostral subdivisions. In general, the pars interpolaris is concerned mainly with processing cutaneous inputs from the face, whereas the pars oralis is more concerned with processing intraoral inputs.

Secondary trigeminal fibers depart from all levels of the spinal trigeminal nucleus and cross through the reticular formation without forming an obvious tract. After reaching the contralateral side, these secondary trigeminal fibers form the ventral trigeminothalamic tract and ascend through the brainstem in close association with the spinothalamic tract near the lateral tip of the medial lemniscus. Secondary trigeminal fibers project to several thalamic nuclei but terminate most densely in the ventroposteromedial (VPM) nucleus of the thalamus. The integrity of this pathway is critical for conscious perception of pain and other somatosensory stimuli involving the head, neck, face, and intraoral cavity.

The spinal trigeminal nucleus also projects to the reticular formation, and these

*The **spinal trigeminal nucleus** contains a pars oralis—intraoral and tactile inputs; a pars interpolaris—tactile and nociceptive inputs; and a pars caudalis—nociceptive inputs.*

connections appear to form a multisynaptic connection with the thalamus that is analogous to the spinoreticulothalamic pathways. Other secondary trigeminal fibers project to motor nuclei in the brainstem that mediate a variety of cranial reflexes discussed below (Figure 4-15). Finally, some trigeminal fibers project to the cerebellum via the inferior cerebellar peduncle, and presumably, these fibers serve a function analogous to the spinocerebellar tracts.

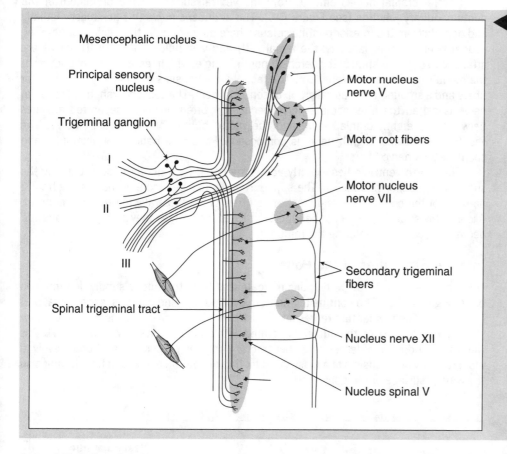

FIGURE 4-15
Local Trigeminal Circuits. *Synaptic connections between primary trigeminal nerve fibers, secondary trigeminal nuclei, and specific motor nuclei mediate the eye blink and jaw jerk reflexes. (Source: Reprinted with permission from Carpenter M: Core Text of Neuroanatomy. Baltimore, MD: Williams & Wilkins, 1991, p 181.)*

Lateral Medullary Syndrome. The posterior inferior cerebellar artery supplies oxygenated blood to several structures in the dorsolateral medulla, including the lateral spinothalamic tract, the spinal trigeminal tract, the spinal trigeminal nucleus, and other nearby structures. Because of the proximity of these structures, interruption of blood flow through the vertebral artery or through one or more tributaries of the posterior inferior cerebellar artery may produce a constellation of symptoms known as the lateral medullary syndrome. This syndrome is characterized most often by a loss of pain and temperature sensitivity on the ipsilateral face (spinal trigeminal lesion) and contralateral body (lateral spinothalamic tract lesion). Opposite sides of the head and body are affected because the spinothalamic tract is a crossed system for the body, whereas the spinal trigeminal tract contains primary afferents from the ipsilateral head. Other symptoms are usually present and may include nausea, vertigo, or dysphonia, depending on whether the damaged area includes the nucleus solitarius, the vestibular nuclei, or the nucleus ambiguus (see Figure 4-11).

Lateral medullary syndrome involves a loss of pain sensitivity on one side of the face and on the contralateral body, accompanied by dysphonia, nausea, or vertigo.

THE PONS

Pons is a Latin word that means "bridge," and this part of the brainstem is called the pons because it forms a functional bridge between the cerebral and cerebellar cortices. Thus, neurons scattered throughout the ventral part of the pons receive descending inputs from the cerebral cortex and relay this information to the cerebellum. Part of this pathway is apparent on the ventral surface of the pons where a mass of transversely oriented fibers are seen coursing laterally and dorsally into the overlying cerebellum. These fibers originate from pontine nuclei and cross the midline before proceeding laterally to form the middle cerebellar peduncle, which enters the cerebellum. On the lateral side of the pons, the middle cerebellar peduncle is perforated by the trigeminal nerve.

Several cranial nerves emerge from the ventral surface of the brainstem at the pontomedullary junction (see Figure 4-5). The abducens nerve (VI) lies most medially and departs from the inferior pontine sulcus where the pyramidal tract emerges from the caudal pons. Further laterally, the facial (VII) and vestibulocochlear (VIII) nerves are attached to the brainstem at the cerebellopontine angle, which represents the junction of the medulla, pons, and cerebellum. The facial nerve consists of a large group of motor fibers and a smaller more lateral group of sensory fibers. The sensory branch of the facial nerve is called the intermediate nerve because it often becomes separated and lies between the eighth cranial nerve and the motor bundle of the seventh nerve. The vestibulocochlear or eighth nerve is composed of separate bundles of vestibular and cochlear SSA nerve fibers.

The fourth ventricle lies directly above the pons, its walls formed, in part, by the superior cerebellar peduncles. The superior cerebellar peduncle is the major efferent pathway of the cerebellum, and most of its fibers project rostrally toward the midbrain. Axons in the superior cerebellar peduncles proceed medially as they ascend the pons and decussate soon after entering the midbrain.

Internal Structures of the Pons

Transverse sections through the pons indicate that this structure is subdivided into two parts (Figure 4-16). The pontine tegmentum evolved first and comprises the dorsal part of the pons. The tegmentum represents a rostral continuation of the medullary reticular formation and contains the nuclei associated with cranial nerves V, VI, VII, and VIII, as well as ascending and descending fiber tracts. The pons proper (or basal pons) evolved more recently and consists of a massive collection of pontine nuclei and fiber bundles on the ventral surface of the pons.

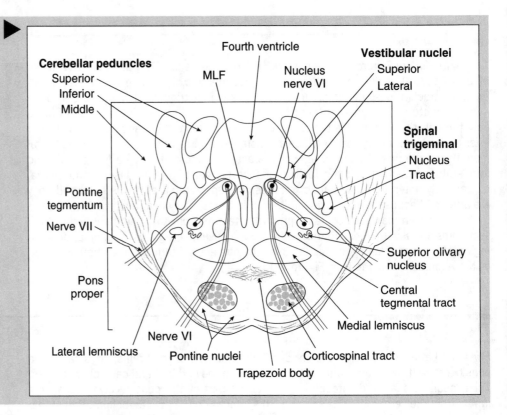

FIGURE 4-16 ▶
Transverse Organization of the Pons. This drawing indicates the position of the major nuclei and fiber tracts in the pontine tegmentum and the ventral pons (or pons proper). The cerebellum lies above the pontine tegmentum and is connected to the brainstem by three fiber bundles called cerebellar peduncles. MLF = medial longitudinal fasciculus.

PONTINE NUCLEI AND THE MIDDLE CEREBELLAR PEDUNCLE

The ventral part of the pons is composed of numerous neurons scattered among fascicles of fibers arranged orthogonally in the transverse and longitudinal directions. The longitudinal fibers are corticofugal projections that eventually terminate in the spinal cord upon numerous nuclei in the brainstem tegmentum or upon the pontine nuclei themselves. Corticopontine fibers from the frontal, temporal, parietal, and occipital lobes terminate ipsilaterally on the scattered neurons comprising the pontine nuclei. The pontine nuclei give rise to pontocerebellar fibers that cross the pons in the transverse plane and project to the contralateral cerebellar cortex via the middle cerebellar peduncle. The pontocerebellar fibers form the second link in the bridge from the cerebral cortex to the cerebellum.

*The **middle cerebellar peduncle** contains pontocerebellar fibers.*

PONTINE TEGMENTUM

At first glance, the medulla and pons appear to contain a bewildering array of fiber tracts and nuclei. Similar principles of organization are evident in both regions, however, and knowledge of the anatomy of the medulla should provide a guide for understanding the organization of the pons.

The central part of the pontine tegmentum is dominated by the reticular formation, a region that appears to lack distinct nuclei but actually contains several identifiable nuclear clusters. In addition, the pontine tegmentum contains a large, distinctive fiber tract called the central tegmental tract (Figure 4-17). The central tegmental tract contains many functional pathways, including fibers that ascend from the reticular formation to the intralaminar nuclei of the thalamus and fibers that descend from the red nucleus to the inferior olive. Fibers from the rostral part of the nucleus solitarius also ascend through the central tegmental tract to convey taste information to the thalamus.

*The **central tegmental tract** contains rubro-olivary, reticulothalamic, and solitariothalamic fibers.*

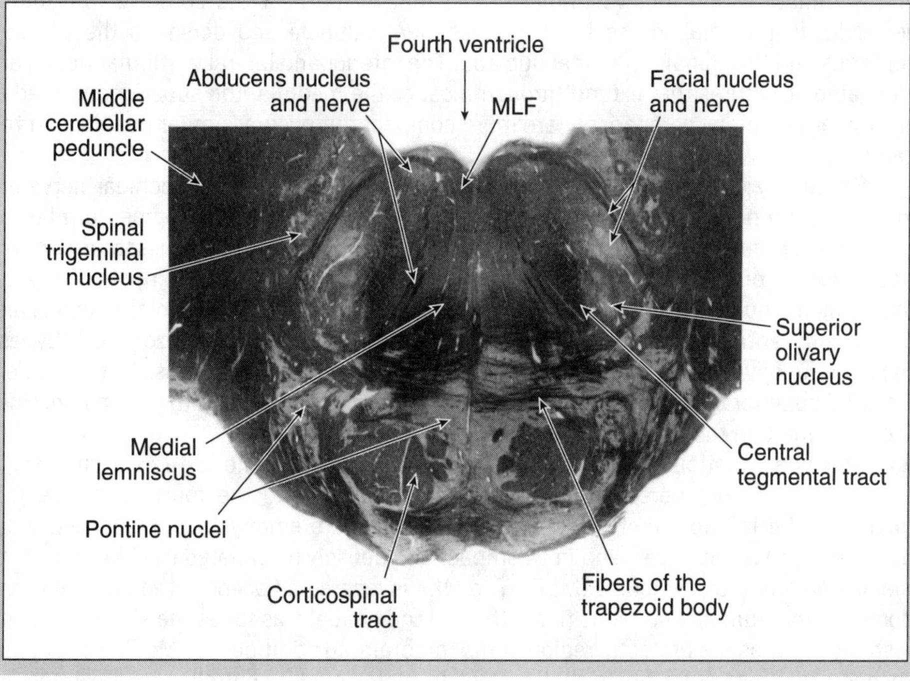

FIGURE 4-17
Transverse View of the Caudal Pons. *This photomicrograph illustrates the abducens and facial nuclei and their cranial nerve fibers in a section through the caudal pons. The ventral portion of the pons contains pontine nuclei that surround the descending fibers of the corticospinal tract. The middle cerebellar peduncles lie laterally and have been partially cropped from view.*

The pontine tegmentum contains several motor nuclei that occupy positions similar to the motor nuclei of the medullary tegmentum. Thus, the nucleus abducens is located near the dorsal midline at a site homologous to the position of the hypoglossal nuclei in the medulla. Like the hypoglossal nerve fibers, axons from motor neurons in the abducens nucleus emerge from the inferior aspect of the nucleus and course ventrally before exiting the brainstem from the pontomedullary junction. Lateral and ventral to the abducens nucleus is the facial nucleus, which resides in approximately the same region as the nucleus ambiguus in the medulla. Facial nerve fibers are unique, however, because they emerge dorsomedially from the facial nucleus and loop around the abducens nucleus (i.e., the facial genu) before assuming a ventrolateral trajectory toward the cerebellopontine angle. More rostrally, at the midpontine level, the motor trigeminal nucleus occupies a position similar to the facial nucleus and sends its efferent fibers laterally through the middle cerebellar peduncle.

SOMATOSENSORY STRUCTURES

As the medial lemniscus enters the pons, its long axis is oriented vertically, and it lies adjacent to the midline. During its ascent through the pons, the medial lemniscus gradually acquires a horizontal orientation at the base of the tegmentum with the arm and upper trunk representations located medially to the leg and lower trunk representations. Consistent with this topography, secondary trigeminal fibers conveying cutaneous sensations from the face and mouth cross the midline and join the medial part of the medial lemniscus. The spinothalamic tract proceeds through the ventrolateral tegmentum of the medulla and continues its ascent through the pons near the lateral tip of the medial lemniscus. The spinal trigeminal tract and nucleus occupy the dorsolateral part of the tegmentum, immediately medial to the middle cerebellar peduncle. More rostrally, the spinal trigeminal nucleus ends and is replaced by the main sensory nucleus of the trigeminal nerve. The motor trigeminal nucleus is located medial to the main sensory nucleus.

AUDITORY AND VESTIBULAR STRUCTURES

The vestibulocochlear nerve enters the brainstem at the pontocerebellar angle where its constituent fibers take separate routes to the vestibular and cochlear nuclei. Auditory fibers enter more laterally and terminate in the dorsal and ventral cochlear nuclei situated, respectively, near the dorsal and ventral edges of the inferior cerebellar peduncle. Vestibular nerve fibers run parallel to the auditory fibers but proceed more medially and terminate within four vestibular nuclei that reside near the corner of the fourth ventricle, just medial to the inferior cerebellar peduncle and dorsal to the nucleus solitarius and the spinal trigeminal nucleus. The inferior and lateral vestibular nuclei are elongated structures that extend through most of the medulla; the superior and medial vestibular nuclei, by comparison, are more compact but occupy similar positions in the caudal pons.

Secondary nuclei and fiber tracts associated with the vestibulocochlear nerve are located in the pons. Immediately ventral to the base of the pontine tegmentum lie the transverse-oriented fibers of the trapezoid body, which contains decussating auditory fibers. Fibers of the trapezoid body project to a number of different nuclear targets, including the nuclei of the superior olivary complex located in the ventrolateral pons just medial and ventral to the facial motor nucleus. Some fibers of the trapezoid body bypass the superior olive and ascend through the pons as the lateral lemniscus. Efferent fibers from the superior olive merge into the lateral lemniscus and ascend the brainstem until they terminate in the inferior colliculus of the dorsal midbrain.

Secondary vestibular fibers project to the cerebellum via the juxtarestiform body, a small collection of fibers that course dorsolaterally around the fourth ventricle just medial to the inferior cerebellar peduncle. Other fibers emerging from the vestibular nuclei either ascend or descend in a compact and densely myelinated tract known as the medial longitudinal fasciculus (MLF). The MLF is located adjacent to the midline in the dorsal tegmentum and contains fibers that extend caudally as far as the spinal cord and rostrally as far as the pretectal region of the midbrain. In addition, the MLF also contains second-order vestibular fibers that project to motor nuclei controlling the extraocular muscles.

Cranial Nerve Nuclei of the Pons

The pons and the pontomedullary junction contain several sensory and motor cranial nerve nuclei: the abducens nucleus, the facial nucleus, the vestibular nuclei, the cochlear nuclei, the trigeminal nuclei, and the salivatory nuclei. The following sections describe the central connections of these nuclei with the exception of the cochlear and vestibular nuclei, which are discussed in Chapters 7 and 8, respectively.

ABDUCENS NUCLEUS (GSE—VI)

The abducens nucleus is a compact structure located adjacent to the midline below the fourth ventricle. One characteristic feature of the abducens nucleus is that it is surrounded by fibers of the facial nerve, which bulge into the fourth ventricle to form the facial colliculus.

The abducens nucleus is composed of two sets of neurons (Figure 4-18). One population of neurons is cholinergic and projects peripherally to innervate the lateral rectus muscle. The other population of neurons, called internuclear neurons, gives rise to efferent fibers that emerge from the medial part of the nucleus and cross the midline before ascending the brainstem through the MLF. The internuclear neurons terminate in specific regions of the oculomotor complex that control the medial rectus muscle. Synchronous activation of both sets of neurons in the abducens nucleus coordinates contraction of the medial and lateral recti muscles to produce conjugate horizontal movements of both eyes toward the ipsilateral side.

> The **abducens nucleus** innervates the lateral rectus muscle.

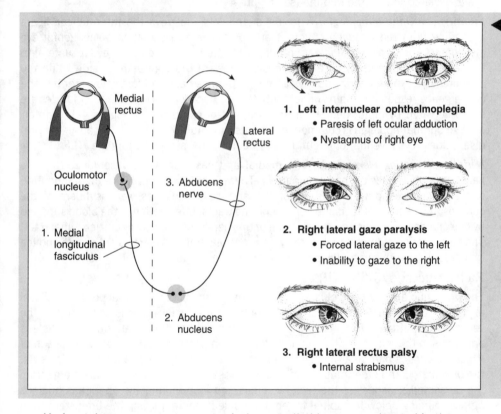

1. Left internuclear ophthalmoplegia
- Paresis of left ocular adduction
- Nystagmus of right eye

2. Right lateral gaze paralysis
- Forced lateral gaze to the left
- Inability to gaze to the right

3. Right lateral rectus palsy
- Internal strabismus

FIGURE 4-18
Connections of the Abducens Nucleus. *The abducens nucleus contains neurons that project to the lateral rectus muscle and to the contralateral oculomotor complex. Activation of the abducens nucleus causes horizontal conjugate eye movements as indicated by the arrows. The drawings to the right indicate deficits in eye movements following selective damage to the numbered neural structures. (Source: Adapted from Carpenter M: Core Text of Neuroanatomy. Baltimore, MD: Williams & Wilkins, 1991, p 167.)*

Horizontal eye movements are precisely controlled by neurons located in the paramedian pontine reticular formation (PPRF). The PPRF receives inputs from the frontal eye fields, a specialized region of the motor cortex, as well as from the superior colliculus, the vestibular nuclei, and the cerebellum. The PPRF contains different functional classes of neurons that integrate information from these regions to control the velocity and direction of conjugate eye movements. In addition to its local connections with the abducens nucleus, the PPRF also sends projections directly through the MLF to coordinate the activities of the abducens with the trochlear and oculomotor nuclei. Similar projections from the vestibular system to the abducens and oculomotor nuclei coordinate eye movements that compensate for rotary or linear movements of the head.

Lesions of the Abducens Nucleus. The clinical symptoms produced by a lesion of the abducens nucleus are significantly different from those produced by damage to the abducens nerve because each lesion affects a different population of neurons (see Figure 4-18). Following a lesion of the abducens nucleus, there is paralysis of the ipsilateral lateral rectus due to loss of the lower motor neurons and paresis of the contralateral medial rectus due to loss of the internuclear neurons. Neither eye can be directed to the lesioned side, and the imbalance of muscular activity causes both eyes to turn toward the intact side. This set of symptoms is called lateral gaze paralysis because both eyes are forcefully turned in the same direction. The convergence response (ability to look at one's nose) remains intact, however, because the medial rectus muscle is not directly paralyzed but still receives oculomotor commands that are controlled by brain regions other than the abducens nucleus.

Lesions of the Abducens Nerve. The abducens nerve has the longest intracranial course of the cranial nerves and, consequently, is the most commonly injured cranial nerve. Paralysis of the lateral rectus muscle alone results in horizontal diplopia (double vision). Diplopia results when a point in the visual field falls on noncorresponding parts of the two retinas and occurs whenever both eyes are not fixated on the same focal point. Following a lesion of the abducens nerve, diplopia is minimal when the patient looks straight ahead or toward the intact side but becomes maximal on attempted gaze toward the lesioned side. The affected eye is adducted because tonic activity in the intact medial rectus is unopposed, and this muscular imbalance produces an internal strabismus in which the eye is deviated toward the midline (see Figure 4-18).

Internuclear Ophthalmoplegia. A lesion of the MLF destroys the internuclear fibers ascending from the abducens nucleus and produces a dissociation of horizontal eye movements known as internuclear ophthalmoplegia. In this event, the eye ipsilateral to the lesion fails to adduct on attempted gaze toward the contralateral side while the abducted eye exhibits horizontal nystagmus (repetitive back and forth movements). The convergence response remains intact for both eyes because the medial recti muscles are still innervated by motor neurons in the oculomotor complex (see Figure 4-18). Internuclear ophthalmoplegia is common in patients with multiple sclerosis because this viral disease destroys myelination around many neural pathways, including the MLF.

Middle Alternating Hemiplegia. The medial and basal pons are vascularized by the paramedian branches of the basilar artery. These tributaries supply the medial pontine nuclei, the descending root fibers of the abducens nerve, as well as fibers of the corticospinal, corticobulbar, and corticopontine tracts. Interruption in the blood supplied by one of these tributaries causes a lesion of this nerve and the nearby corticospinal tract. The combination of lateral rectus palsy and contralateral hemiparesis of the arm and leg that results from this vascular event is referred to as middle alternating hemiplegia.

FACIAL NUCLEUS (SVE—VII)

The facial nucleus is a large cluster of cholinergic neurons in the caudal pons at the level of the abducens nucleus. In transverse sections, the facial nucleus is located in the ventrolateral reticular formation, a position equivalent to the location of the nucleus ambiguus in the medulla. The facial nucleus is composed of several subnuclei, each of which innervates particular muscles such as the stapedius, the digastric, the platysma, the buccinator, and other muscles of facial expression. Facial motor fibers emerge from the dorsomedial aspect of the facial nucleus and loop around the abducens nucleus before coursing below the spinal trigeminal nucleus and departing the brainstem from the cerebellopontine angle. The close relationship between the abducens nucleus and the genu of the facial nerve indicates that a focal lesion in the dorsal part of the pons can simultaneously damage both structures (see Figure 4-17).

The facial nucleus receives connections from the trigeminal system that enable it to mediate the clinically significant corneal reflex (see Figure 4-15). The ophthalmic division of the trigeminal nerve provides the cornea with the densest sensory innervation of any peripheral structure, making it exquisitely sensitive to specks of dust and other foreign objects. When the cornea is lightly touched, sensory impulses are transmitted along trigeminal nerve fibers to the main sensory nucleus and to the pars caudalis of the spinal trigeminal nucleus. These trigeminal nuclei project bilaterally to the facial nucleus, which controls the orbicularis oculi. Hence, both eyes blink automatically in response to corneal stimulation of either eye.

The facial nucleus also receives descending connections from the motor cortex to mediate voluntary facial movements. Corticobulbar fibers originating from the motor cortex convey impulses directly to the facial nucleus. Additional projections from the motor cortex to neighboring parts of the reticular formation may also convey impulses multisynaptically to the facial nucleus. In most individuals, the motor cortex sends

Diplopia is double vision resulting from loss of conjugate eye movements.

Middle alternating hemiplegia consists of lateral rectus palsy in combination with contralateral hemiparesis.

The facial nucleus innervates the muscles of facial expression.

projections bilaterally to those parts of the facial nuclei that control the frontalis and other muscles of the upper face (Figure 4-19). By contrast, the remaining parts of the facial nucleus, which control the lower face, receive only unilateral projections from the contralateral hemisphere. This explains why most individuals raise both eyebrows simultaneously but control the lower facial muscles independently.

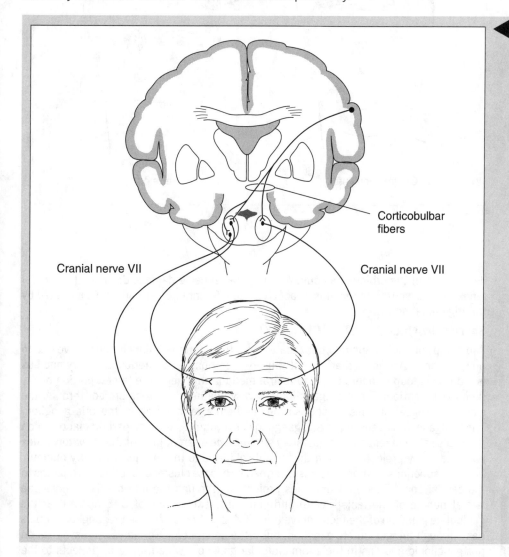

Corticobulbar fibers

Cranial nerve VII

Cranial nerve VII

FIGURE 4-19
Corticobulbar Projections to the Facial Nucleus. *Each cortical hemisphere sends bilateral projections to regions of the facial nucleus controlling the upper face muscles but sends contralateral projections to those regions controlling the lower face muscles.*

Central Facial Palsy. Arteriosclerosis or a small stroke that affects corticobulbar fibers passing through the internal capsule may produce a central facial palsy. When descending fibers to the facial nucleus are damaged by unilateral lesions in the internal capsule, there is significant weakness of the lower facial muscles contralateral to the lesion and a loss of voluntary facial movements (Figure 4-20). Although central facial palsies are sometimes associated with hemiplegia, there is no loss of the corneal reflex, lacrimation, or salivation because the lower motor neurons of the facial nerve are intact and continue to innervate the peripheral muscles and glands. Interestingly, a patient with a central facial palsy can smile spontaneously on the weakened side because the connections that mediate facial responses to emotional stimuli are separate from the corticobulbar pathways, although the exact route of this projection is not known.

Central facial palsy involves an upper motor neuron lesion of the corticobulbar tract. **Bell's palsy** *involves a lower motor neuron lesion of the facial nerve.*

Bell's Palsy. A lesion of the facial nucleus or nerve causes ipsilateral paralysis of all facial muscles (see Figure 4-20). This condition, known as Bell's palsy, is characterized by complete atrophy of the ipsilateral facial muscles as indicated by a flattening of the nasolabial fold, a widening of the palpebral fissure, and a droop in the corner of the mouth. Patients with Bell's palsy experience difficulty in chewing food because the buccinator muscle is paralyzed, and they are unable to close their ipsilateral eye because of

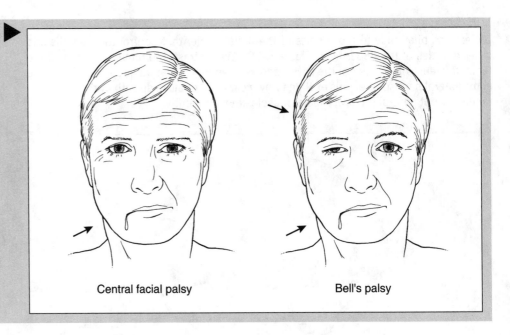

FIGURE 4-20 ▶
Comparison of Central Facial Palsy and Bell's Palsy. Central facial palsy is caused by a lesion of the corticobulbar projections. As the upper facial muscles receive bilateral innervation, only the lower facial muscles lose voluntary control. Bell's palsy affects lower motor neurons and causes paralysis of both upper and lower facial muscles.

Central facial palsy   Bell's palsy

denervation of the orbicularis oculi. Although facial nerve damage disables the corneal reflex, corneal sensation remains intact because afferent impulses are still conducted by the trigeminal nerve.

SALIVATORY NUCLEI (GVE—VII AND IX)

Two groups of cholinergic neurons located near the pontomedullary junction give rise to preganglionic GVE fibers that control salivary secretions. The inferior salivatory nucleus is a diffuse group of neurons in the rostral medulla that lie in the lateral portion of the reticular formation. These preganglionic parasympathetic neurons project through the glossopharyngeal and lesser petrosal nerves before terminating in the otic ganglion. The postganglionic cells of the otic ganglion convey impulses to the parotid gland, which produces saliva in response to gustatory stimuli. The afferent limb of the salivatory reflex is mediated by projections from the rostral solitarius to the inferior salivatory nucleus.

The superior salivatory nucleus is formed by a loose cluster of cholinergic neurons in the caudal pons. This nucleus sends projections through the intermediate nerve (the lateral bundle of the facial nerve) and splits into two groups of GVE fibers near the geniculate ganglion of the facial nerve (Figure 4-21). Some of these preganglionic fibers pass through the geniculate ganglion, enter the chorda tympani nerve, and synapse on postganglionic neurons in the submandibular ganglion, which, in turn, projects to the submandibular and sublingual glands to control salivation. The remaining GVE fibers enter the greater petrosal nerve and terminate in the pterygopalatine ganglion where two groups of postganglionic neurons are responsible for innervating the lacrimal gland or the mucous lining of the mouth and nose. The superior salivatory nucleus receives inputs from secondary trigeminal fibers, and this reflex arc mediates the secretion of tears in response to corneal irritation. Both the inferior and superior salivatory nuclei are controlled by descending pathways from the hypothalamus, the major brain region for coordinating the activities of the autonomic nervous system.

Lesions of the Facial Nerve Fibers. The superior salivatory nucleus and other brainstem nuclei contribute fibers to the facial nerve. Consequently, damage to the facial nerve or its peripheral branches produces different constellations of symptoms that vary according to the precise location of the lesion (see Figure 4-21). A lesion near the stylomastoid foramen, for example, results in Bell's palsy but does not produce other symptoms because only SVE fibers originating from the facial nucleus are affected at this location. If the lesion occurs just distal to the geniculate ganglion, however, the chorda tympani is likely to be damaged, and Bell's palsy would be accompanied by hyperacusis due to paralysis of the stapedius, impaired salivation due to loss of GVE fibers innervating

*The **inferior salivatory nucleus** controls the parotid gland. The **superior salivatory nucleus** controls the submandibular, sublingual, and lacrimal glands.*

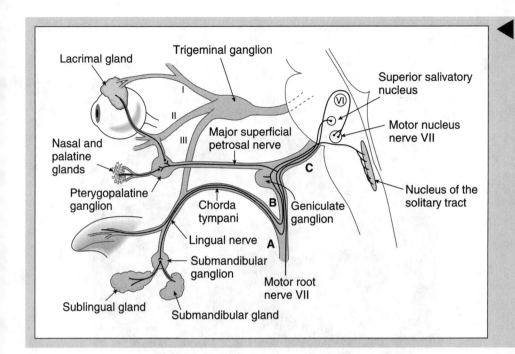

FIGURE 4-21
Functional Components of the Facial Nerve. *The facial nerve contains fibers connected to the facial nucleus, the nucleus fasciculus solitarius, and the superior salivatory nucleus. Lesions at the stylomastoid foramen (site A), distal to the geniculate ganglion (site B), or near the cerebellopontine angle (site C) produce different constellations of symptoms as described in the text. (Source: Adapted from Carpenter M: Core Text of Neuroanatomy. Baltimore, MD: Williams & Wilkins, 1991, p 171.)*

the submandibular ganglion, and loss of taste sensation from the anterior two-thirds of the tongue. If a lesion occurred near the entry of the facial nerve into the brainstem, the lacrimal reflex would be lost due to interruption of GVE fibers innervating the pterygopalatine ganglion, and this disturbance would accompany all of the symptoms described above.

MAIN SENSORY NUCLEUS OF THE TRIGEMINAL NERVE (GSA—V)

The main (or principal) sensory nucleus of the trigeminal nerve lies rostral to the spinal trigeminal nucleus and is seen in transverse sections of the pons where the trigeminal nerve passes through the middle cerebellar peduncle (Figure 4-22). The main sensory nucleus receives cutaneous information from the face and, functionally, is considered the cranial equivalent to the posterior column nuclei. Large diameter, heavily myelinated axons from all three divisions of the trigeminal ganglion enter the pons and terminate on second-order neurons of the main sensory nucleus. The somatotopic organization of the main sensory nucleus follows the same inverted pattern as the spinal trigeminal nucleus where the ophthalmic representation is located ventrally, the mandibular representation is located dorsally, and the maxillary representation is intermediate in position.

Secondary trigeminal projections from the main sensory nucleus ascend in two separate pathways to the thalamus (see Figure 4-14). Axons from the ventral part of the main sensory nucleus cross the midline and join the cervical representation of the medial lemniscus as it proceeds to the VPM nucleus of the contralateral thalamus. These secondary fibers are identified as the ventral trigeminothalamic tract even though they are separate from the ventral pain-conveying fibers originating in the spinal trigeminal nucleus. The dorsal part of the main sensory nucleus sends a small projection, the dorsal trigeminothalamic tract, to the ipsilateral VPM nucleus so that cutaneous sensations of the mouth and tongue are in register with gustatory sensations that proceed to adjacent regions of the thalamus. The VPM nucleus projects to the parietal operculum where the conscious sensations of touch and pressure of the face and intraoral cavity are mediated.

Tic Douloureux. Sometimes called trigeminal neuralgia, tic douloureux is characterized by repetitive, transient attacks of severe pain afflicting one or more subdivisions of the trigeminal nerve. The etiology of tic douloureux is unknown, but in susceptible individuals, it may be triggered by touching specific parts of the face or by eating. Tic douloureux is usually treated by cauterizing or chemically destroying the branches of the trigeminal nerve that are prone to such attacks. Depending on the site of the surgical lesion, the patient loses tactile sensation in the face, mouth, and cornea (along with loss of the

FIGURE 4-22 ▶
Transverse View of the Mid Pons. This photomicrograph shows the midpontine region of the brainstem surrounded by the cerebellum dorsally and the middle cerebellar peduncles laterally. Fascicles of the trigeminal nerve can be seen in proximity to the motor trigeminal and main sensory nuclei.

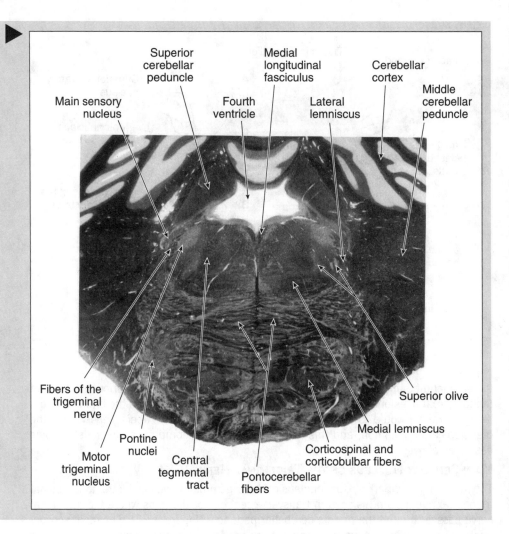

FIGURE 4-22 ▶
Transverse View of the Mid Pons. This photomicrograph shows the midpontine region of the brainstem surrounded by the cerebellum dorsally and the middle cerebellar peduncles laterally. Fascicles of the trigeminal nerve can be seen in proximity to the motor trigeminal and main sensory nuclei.

corneal blink reflex) or may experience difficulty chewing food if the motor component of the trigeminal nerve is affected. In some cases, a medullary tractotomy is performed to destroy the descending pain fibers of the spinal trigeminal tract without affecting tactile sensitivity.

MOTOR TRIGEMINAL NUCLEUS (SVE—V)

The motor trigeminal nucleus is a compact structure located immediately medial to the main sensory trigeminal nucleus. Cholinergic fibers from the motor trigeminal nucleus emerge as a separate motor root that travels with the mandibular division to innervate the muscles of mastication (i.e., masseter, anterior digastric, mylohyoid) and the tensor tympani of the middle ear. Voluntary movements of the mandible are mediated by corticobulbar fibers that project bilaterally from the motor cortex to the motor trigeminal nuclei (see Figure 4-3). Most inputs to the motor trigeminal nucleus, however, are primary afferent fibers of the trigeminal nerve or secondary fibers from the spinal trigeminal nucleus (see Figures 4-14 and 4-15). Other collateral projections from the mesencephalic trigeminal nucleus relay proprioceptive information from the masseter to the motor trigeminal nucleus. This pathway enables muscle spindles in the masseter to activate the motor trigeminal nucleus and execute the jaw jerk reflex, a monosynaptic stretch reflex elicited by tapping the jaw. The motor trigeminal nucleus also receives auditory inputs to activate the tensor tympani during loud sounds to dampen movements of the malleus and the other bony ossicles of the middle ear.

THE MIDBRAIN

The midbrain is the smallest subdivision of the neuraxis. The dorsal surface of the midbrain contains a series of paired elevations that form the superior and inferior colliculi (or tectum). The trochlear (IV) nerves emerge immediately posterior to the caudally located inferior colliculi. The superior colliculi, located further rostrally, are situated immediately posterior to the pineal gland, a structure that marks the junction between the mesencephalon and diencephalon.

The ventral surface of the midbrain is marked by a massive pair of myelinated fiber tracts, the crus cerebri, which contain descending corticospinal, corticopontine, and corticobulbar fibers. The crus cerebri is also known as the cerebral peduncle and, therefore, the space between the cerebral peduncles is the interpeduncular fossa. The oculomotor (III) nerves emerge from the interpeduncular fossa as indicated by Figure 4-23.

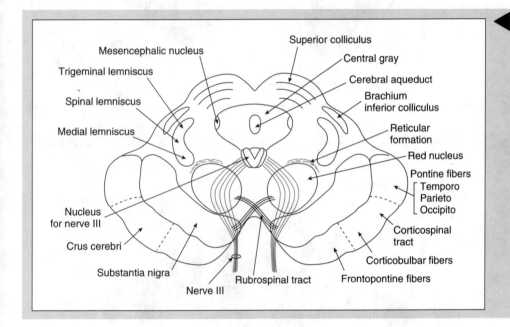

FIGURE 4-23
Transverse Organization of the Midbrain. *This drawing indicates the position of the major nuclei and fiber tracts in the midbrain at the level of the superior colliculus.*

Internal Structures of the Midbrain

Due to its short length, transverse sections through the midbrain are capped by either the inferior or the superior colliculi (Figures 4-24 and 4-25). The cerebral aqueduct perforates the midbrain below these tectal regions and is surrounded by a pale, homogeneous zone called the periaqueductal gray region. At the level of the inferior colliculus, the tegmentum is dominated by fiber tracts such as the lateral and medial lemnisci, the superior cerebellar peduncles, the central tegmental tract, and the MLF. At the level of the superior colliculus, the tegmentum contains prominent nuclei, including the red nucleus, the substantia nigra, and the oculomotor nuclear complex.

TECTAL REGION

The midbrain tectum is sometimes called the quadrigeminal plate after its paired nuclear tenants, the inferior and superior colliculi. Located on the dorsal midbrain, the inferior colliculus receives ascending inputs from the cochlear nuclei, the superior olives, and other auditory nuclei located in the pons. These ascending projections travel through the lateral lemniscus and literally engulf the ventral aspect of the inferior colliculus (see Figure 4-24). The inferior colliculus contains tonotopic representations of the cochlea and plays an important role in sound localization. The inferior colliculus sends most of its output to the medial geniculate nucleus of the thalamus, which, in turn, projects to the primary auditory cortex in the temporal lobe.

The superior colliculus lies rostral to the inferior colliculus and has a distinctive laminated structure when viewed in transverse sections (see Figure 4-25). Afferent

FIGURE 4-24 ▶

Transverse View of the Caudal Midbrain.
This photomicrograph illustrates the cau-
dal half of the midbrain, which contains
the inferior colliculus and the ascending
fibers of the lateral lemniscus. The de-
cussating fibers of the superior cerebellar
peduncles are prominent in the central
part of the tegmentum.

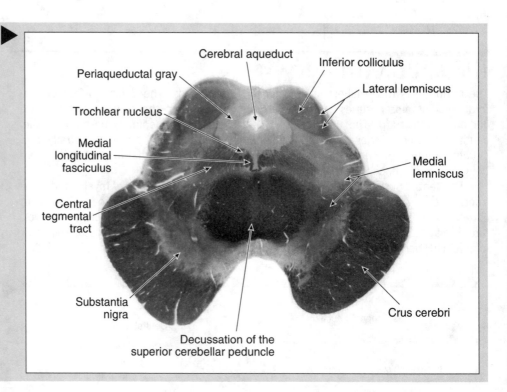

Cerebral aqueduct
Periaqueductal gray
Inferior colliculus
Lateral lemniscus
Trochlear nucleus
Medial longitudinal fasciculus
Medial lemniscus
Central tegmental tract
Substantia nigra
Crus cerebri
Decussation of the superior cerebellar peduncle

FIGURE 4-25 ▶

Transverse View of the Rostral Midbrain.
This photomicrograph illustrates the ros-
tral half of the midbrain, which contains
the superior colliculus, the red nucleus,
the substantia nigra, and the crus cerebri.
The oculomotor complex gives rise to ocu-
lomotor nerve fibers that pass through the
red nucleus before exiting through the in-
terpeduncular fossa.

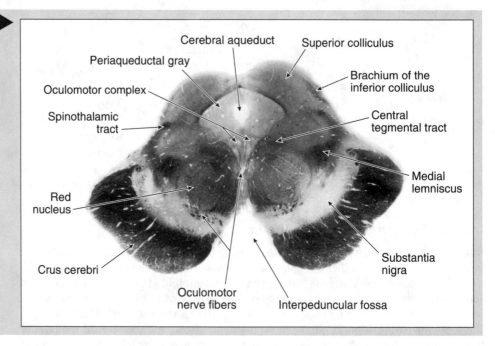

Cerebral aqueduct
Periaqueductal gray
Superior colliculus
Oculomotor complex
Brachium of the inferior colliculus
Spinothalamic tract
Central tegmental tract
Red nucleus
Medial lemniscus
Crus cerebri
Substantia nigra
Oculomotor nerve fibers
Interpeduncular fossa

projections to the superior colliculus come mainly from the retina (via the optic nerve and tract) and from the primary visual (striate) cortex of the occipital lobe. The upper layers of the superior colliculus are concerned with detecting moving targets and other stimuli of visual interest, whereas the lower layers initiate and maintain tracking responses of the eyes and head. Consistent with its role in vision, the major outputs of the superior colliculus are to visual nuclei in the thalamus, such as the lateral geniculate and the pulvinar, and to the prestriate visual cortex. Tracking movements of the head and eyes are mediated by efferent projections from the superior colliculus to the cervical spinal cord (via the tectospinal tract) and to neurons comprising the PPRF.

SUPERIOR CEREBELLAR PEDUNCLE

With few exceptions, nearly all efferent projections from the cerebellum ascend through the brainstem via the superior cerebellar peduncle. The superior cerebellar peduncle forms the lateral wall of the fourth ventricle in the rostral pons and continues its ascent through the lateral part of the midbrain tegmentum (see Figures 4-22 and 4-24). In the caudal midbrain, the superior cerebellar peduncle is bordered by other ascending fiber tracts, including the lateral lemniscus, the medial lemniscus, and the central tegmental tract. Further rostrally, at the level of the inferior colliculus, the fibers of the superior cerebellar peduncle decussate within the tegmentum and continue their ascent towards the red nucleus. Nearly a third of the crossed fibers of the superior cerebellar peduncle terminate in the red nucleus while the remainder proceed further rostrally to the ventrolateral thalamus, which, in turn, projects to the motor cortex. Hence, the superior cerebellar peduncle represents the pathway by which sensory information from the cerebellum reaches the red nucleus and motor regions of the thalamus.

*The **superior cerebellar peduncle** contains cerebellorubral, cerebellothalamic, and anterior spinocerebellar fibers.*

PERIAQUEDUCTAL GRAY REGION

The periaqueductal gray region consists of densely packed cells surrounding the cerebral aqueduct. Although the periaqueductal gray region has a uniform appearance in myelin-stained sections, it actually contains distinct clusters of neurons that are grouped according to the presence of serotonin, enkephalin, endorphins, and other neuropeptides. Opiate receptors are densely distributed in specific regions of the periaqueductal gray region and underscores the importance of this area in processing nociceptive information. The periaqueductal gray region projects to the raphe magnus and the paragigantocellular nucleus of the reticular formation, regions that send descending projections to the dorsal horn of the spinal cord to modulate nociceptive transmission in the spinothalamic system. These descending connections may provide the anatomic substrate for the clinical finding that electrical stimulation of the periaqueductal gray region ameliorates chronic pain.

RED NUCLEUS

The red nucleus is named after its ruddy appearance in a freshly cut brain. Located dorsal to the substantia nigra, the red nucleus is virtually encapsulated by the myelinated fibers of the superior cerebellar peduncle, the central tegmental tract, and the medial lemniscus. The red nucleus is an important part of the motor system that receives inputs from the motor cortex and sends descending projections to the ventral horn of the spinal cord via the rubrospinal tract. In addition, the red nucleus receives ascending projections from the deep cerebellar nuclei and sends descending projections to the inferior olivary nucleus via the central tegmental tract. Thus, the red nucleus is part of a larger network of feedforward and feedback pathways involved in motor control. Lesions of the red nucleus produce tremor and ataxia (lack of motor coordination) in the contralateral body, which are usually expressed by irregular movements of the lower limbs, especially during walking.

SUBSTANTIA NIGRA

The substantia nigra is located in the rostral half of the midbrain where it forms a thick nucleus along the dorsal margin of the crus cerebri. The substantia nigra is composed of two distinct layers: a ventral pars reticulata and a dorsal pars compacta. The pars reticulata contains small neurons that project to the superior colliculus and parts of the thalamus. The pars compacta is a darkly pigmented region that contains large dopaminergic neurons, which project almost exclusively to the basal ganglia, a forebrain region involved in sensorimotor integration and other aspects of motor control. The dopaminergic neurons of the substantia nigra degenerate during Parkinson's disease, a serious motor disorder characterized by rigidity, tremor at rest, and the inability to initiate movements.

CRUS CEREBRI

Located on the ventral surface of the midbrain are a massive bundle of corticofugal fibers that descend through the internal capsule and terminate in the brainstem or the spinal cord. Known as the crus cerebri, these corticofugal projections consist of corticospinal, corticobulbar, and corticopontine fibers. Corticospinal fibers originate mainly from motor and parietal cortical areas and travel through the central portion of the crus cerebri before collecting into the more compact pyramidal tract as they enter the caudal pons and medulla. Corticobulbar fibers are also located in the central portion of the crus cerebri but leave this bundle as they reach the brainstem level where they terminate within specific nuclei. Some corticobulbar fibers innervate sensory nuclei, but most innervate the motor nuclei that control movements of the eyes, face, mouth, tongue, and larynx.

The corticopontine fibers are located on the medial and lateral extremes of the crus cerebri and depart from this bundle when it enters the pons.

Cranial Nerve Nuclei of the Midbrain

The midbrain contains two sensory cranial nerve nuclei: the trochlear nucleus and the oculomotor complex. Both of these nuclei are concerned with controlling muscles associated with the eye.

TROCHLEAR NUCLEUS (GSE—IV)

> The **trochlear nucleus** innervates the superior oblique muscle.

The trochlear nucleus is a small oval-shaped nucleus that lies embedded in the MLF at the level of the inferior colliculus. Cholinergic fibers of the trochlear nerve exit the nucleus dorsally and cross the midline through the superior medullary velum before emerging from the dorsal surface of the midbrain immediately posterior to the inferior colliculus. Each trochlear nerve innervates the contralateral superior oblique muscle, which produces intortion (top of eye rotates towards the nose) and downward-lateral movements of the eyeball (Figure 4-26). To mediate voluntary contraction of the superior oblique muscle, corticobulbar fibers synapse on neurons in the adjacent reticular formation, which, in turn, project to the trochlear nucleus. The trochlear nucleus also receives vestibular inputs that ascend through the MLF to coordinate contractions of the superior oblique muscle with respect to head movements.

The trochlear nerve passes around the lateral aspect of the midbrain and emerges, with the oculomotor nerve, between the posterior cerebral and superior cerebellar arteries. Consequently, aneurysms of those blood vessels may compress or stretch the trochlear nerve. Such insults cause the eyeball to extort and impair the ability to look downward. This explains why patients with trochlear nerve damage invariably report difficulty in climbing down a stairway. These patients usually compensate for ocular extortion by tilting their head toward the unaffected eye to bring the denervated eye into proper alignment (Figure 4-27).

OCULOMOTOR COMPLEX (GSE AND GVE—III)

> The **oculomotor complex** innervates the medial rectus, inferior rectus, superior rectus, inferior oblique, and levator palpebra muscles and controls the pupillary sphincter.

The oculomotor complex is a collection of paired nuclei that form a V-shaped cell column straddling the midline of the rostral midbrain. The oculomotor nuclei send both crossed and uncrossed cholinergic GSE fibers ventrally into the tegmentum and through large portions of the red nucleus before emerging from the interpeduncular fossa. Separate nuclei in the oculomotor complex innervate the medial, superior, and inferior recti and the inferior oblique muscles to produce eye movements in several directions (Figures 4-28 and 4-29). The central nucleus, located on the midline, innervates the levator palpebrae bilaterally, which explains why both eyes usually blink simultaneously.

One part of the oculomotor complex, the Edinger-Westphal nucleus, is composed of preganglionic parasympathetic neurons whose GVE fibers project to the ciliary ganglion. Postganglionic projections to the ciliary body and pupillary sphincter control the shape of the lens and size of the pupil, respectively. Activation of the ciliary body increases the

FIGURE 4-26 ▶

Actions of the Superior Oblique. The superior oblique muscle passes through a bony loop, the trochlea, and attaches to the superior surface of the eyeball. Contraction of the superior oblique causes the top of the eye to rotate (or intort) towards the nasal side while simultaneously moving downward and slightly lateral. (Source: Adapted with permission from Wilson-Pauwels L, et al: Cranial Nerves—Anatomy and Clinical Comments. Toronto, Ontario: B. C. Decker, 1988, p 46.)

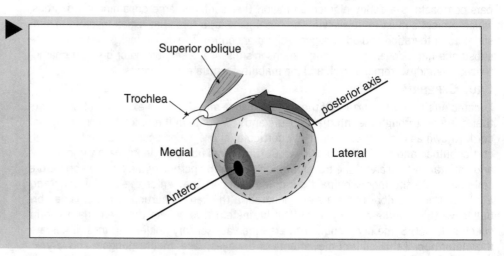

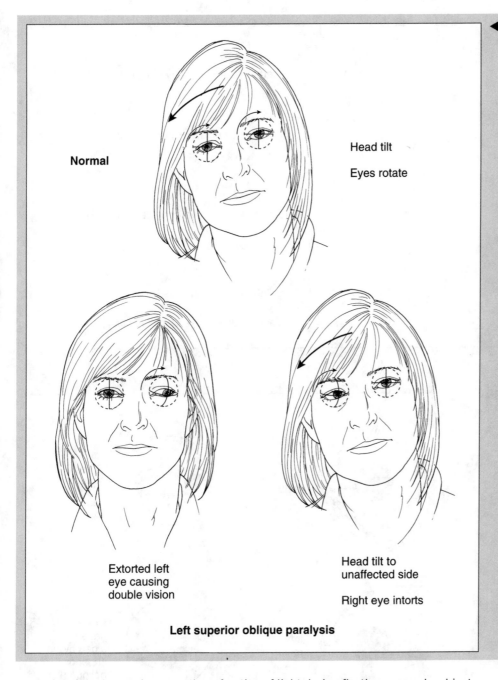

Normal

Head tilt

Eyes rotate

Extorted left
eye causing
double vision

Head tilt to
unaffected side

Right eye intorts

Left superior oblique paralysis

◄ FIGURE 4-27
Effects of Trochlear Nerve Damage. When
the head is tilted, both eyes rotate around
the anteroposterior axis to maintain a vertical image on the retina. Paralysis of the superior oblique muscle causes ocular extortion, and the patient compensates by tilting
the head in the opposite direction. (Source:
Adapted with permission from Wilson-
Pauwels L, et al: Cranial Nerves—Anatomy
and Clinical Comments. Toronto, Ontario:
B. C. Decker, 1988, p 47.)

convexity of the lens to increase the refraction of light during fixation on nearby objects.
Contraction of the annular muscle of the pupillary sphincter causes pupillary constriction, which decreases the amount of light entering the eye. These processes occur
automatically as part of the accommodation-convergence reaction when ocular fixation is
shifted from distant to nearby objects. Other components of the visual system are
responsible for contracting the medial recti of both eyes to produce ocular convergence.

Oculomotor Ophthalmoplegia. A complete lesion of the oculomotor nerve produces a
well-defined constellation of neurologic symptoms called oculomotor ophthalmoplegia
(Figure 4-30). First, oculomotor nerve damage causes ptosis (drooping eyelid) due to
paralysis of the levator palpebral muscle. A patient may attempt to compensate for ptosis
by contracting the frontalis muscle to help raise the eyelid. Second, if the eyelid is gently
raised during a clinical examination, the patient's eye is strongly abducted and directed
downward by the lateral rectus and superior oblique muscles because those muscles are
unopposed after the remaining extraocular muscles have been paralyzed. Although
external strabismus is present in oculomotor ophthalmoplegia, patients might not experience diplopia if the affected eye is covered by the drooping eyelid. Finally, damage to the

FIGURE 4-28 ▶

The Oculomotor Complex. *The oculomotor complex is a collection of subnuclei that innervate specific sets of extraocular muscles. (A) Horizontal view of the subnuclei within the oculomotor complex and their peripheral targets. (B) Coronal view of the oculomotor complex at a section indicated by the* dashed line *in part A.*

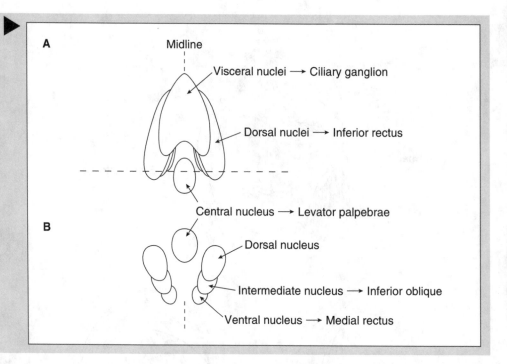

FIGURE 4-29 ▶

Eye Movements Controlled by the Oculomotor Complex. *This diagram shows four extraocular muscles, innervated by the oculomotor nerve, that cause the eye to adduct, gaze downward or upward, or extort.* (Source: *Reprinted with permission from Wilson-Pauwels L, et al:* Cranial Nerves— Anatomy and Clinical Comments. *Toronto, Ontario: B. C. Decker, 1988, p 33.)*

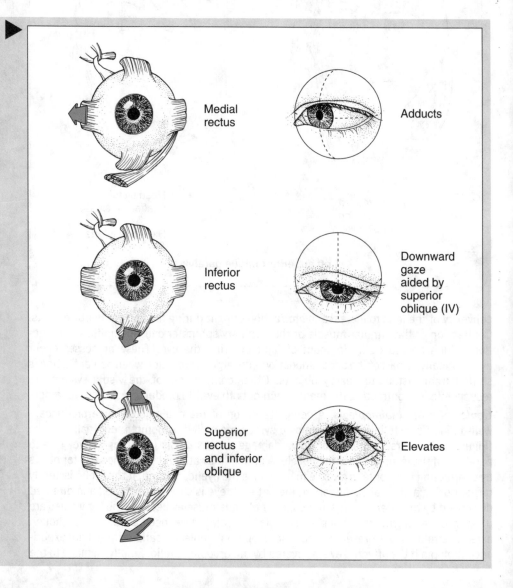

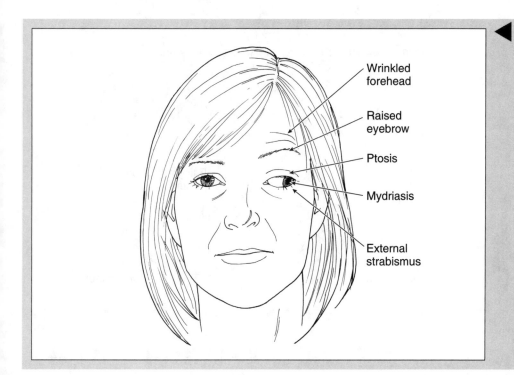

Wrinkled
forehead

Raised
eyebrow

Ptosis

Mydriasis

External
strabismus

FIGURE 4-30
Oculomotor Ophthalmoplegia. *A lesion of the oculomotor nerve causes ptosis, mydriasis, and external strabismus. (*Source: Reprinted with permission from Wilson-Pauwels L, et al: Cranial Nerves—Anatomy and Clinical Comments. *Toronto, Ontario: B. C. Decker, 1988, p 39.)*

GVE fibers projecting from the Edinger-Westphal nucleus causes mydriasis (pupillary dilation) due to loss of muscle tone in the pupillary sphincter and the unopposed action of the dilator muscles in the iris. Ocular ophthalmoplegia is often caused by compression of the oculomotor nerve, resulting from aneurysms of the posterior cerebral or superior cerebellar arteries.

Pupillary Light Reflex. The Edinger-Westphal nucleus and its neuronal connections are essential for constricting both pupils during increased illumination. This response, known as the pupillary light reflex, is demonstrated by flashing a light in one eye and observing the immediate constriction of the pupil in that eye (direct light reflex) and in the contralateral eye (consensual light reflex). These responses are mediated by serial connections from the retina to the midbrain and back to the periphery. Although most retinal projections terminate in the thalamus, some retinal ganglion neurons project to the pretectal olivary nucleus, which lies rostral and *lateral* to the superior colliculus (Figure 4-31). Reciprocal connections through the posterior commissure link the pretectal regions on each side of the midbrain. The pretectal olivary nuclei also project bilaterally to the Edinger-Westphal nuclei, which project to the ciliary ganglia. Postganglionic neurons in the ciliary ganglion innervate the pupillary sphincter, which constricts the diameter of the pupil. Hence, the pupillary light reflex is clinically significant because it provides a simple method for testing the integrity of the optic and oculomotor nerves and their central connections.

Loss of **pupillary light reflex** indicates an insult to the optic nerve, the pretectal region, the Edinger-Westphal nucleus, or the oculomotor nerve.

A lesion of the optic nerve causes blindness in the affected eye and abolishes the direct and consensual pupillary light reflexes if light is flashed into the affected eye. Assuming both optic nerves are intact, damage to the visceral motor fibers innervating the ciliary ganglion on one side causes an ipsilateral loss of the direct light reflex but does not interfere with the consensual reflex in the contralateral eye.

Loss of the pupillary light reflex is often produced by an increase in intracranial pressure resulting from a tumor, an abscess, or a subdural hematoma caused by a blow to the head. In these cases, the uncus of the temporal lobe herniates into the tentorial notch and compresses or stretches the third cranial nerve as it travels along the medial side of the uncus and parahippocampal gyrus (Figure 4-32).

Argyll-Robertson Pupil. An Argyll-Robertson pupil is characterized by a small pupil that does not respond to light directed into the eye. Despite the loss of the pupillary light reflex, the pupil exhibits an accommodation-convergence reaction and becomes smaller

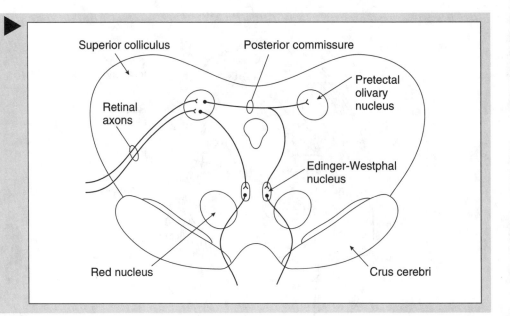

FIGURE 4-31 ▶

The Pretectal Nuclei. *The pretectal nuclei receive direct connections from retinal ganglion cells and send projections bilaterally to the Edinger-Westphal nuclei, which, in turn, send fibers through the oculomotor nerve to the ciliary ganglion.*

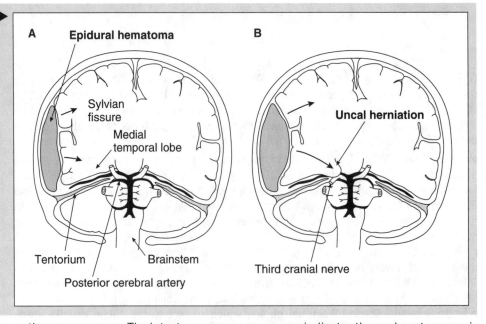

FIGURE 4-32 ▶

Epidural Hematoma. *(A) Trauma to the head may cause intracranial bleeding, which compresses the underlying brain. (B) Eventually, the uncus herniates through the tentorial notch and causes compression of the oculomotor nerve. (Source: Reprinted with permission from Lawrence P: Essentials of Surgical Specialties. Baltimore, MD: Williams and Wilkins, 1993, p 302.)*

as the eyes converge. The intact convergence response indicates the oculomotor nerve is intact and suggests that loss of the pupillary light reflex is caused by damage to the afferent limb of the reflex circuit, not the GVE fibers emerging from the Edinger-Westphal nucleus. Although the exact site of damage is not known, it is thought that an Argyll-Robertson pupil is produced by lesions in the pretectal region surrounding the posterior commissure.

Horner's Syndrome. Horner's syndrome is characterized by miosis (small pupil), enophthalmos (sunken eye), pseudoptosis (a partially drooping eyelid due to loss of innervation of the superior and inferior tarsal muscles), and anhidrosis (dryness of the skin on the ipsilateral side of the face). Lesions that cause Horner's syndrome may occur at many locations but involve damage either to the peripheral autonomic nervous system or to the central autonomic pathways that course through the brainstem and spinal cord. In the brainstem, Horner's syndrome can be caused by damage to descending autonomic fibers from the hypothalamus that pass through the dorsolateral part of the tegmentum. Further caudally, damage to the lateral horn of the cervical spinal cord or to peripheral sympathetic preganglionic and postganglionic fibers of the superior cervical ganglion may also cause Horner's syndrome.

Horner's syndrome is caused by a loss of sympathetic innervation and results in miosis, pseudoptosis, enophthalmos, and anhidrosis.

Superior Alternating Hemiplegia (Weber's Syndrome). Vascular lesions involving the medial part of the cerebral peduncle may destroy oculomotor nerve root fibers (lower motor neuron) together with the corticospinal and corticobulbar fibers (upper motor neuron) descending through the crus cerebri (Figure 4-33). Thus, occlusion of the paramedian branches of the posterior cerebral or superior cerebellar arteries causes contralateral hemiparesis of the limb and facial muscles accompanied by ipsilateral oculomotor ophthalmoplegia. This set of symptoms is known as superior alternating hemiplegia or Weber's syndrome.

> ***Weber's syndrome*** *is a combination of ophthalmoplegia and contralateral hemiparesis.*

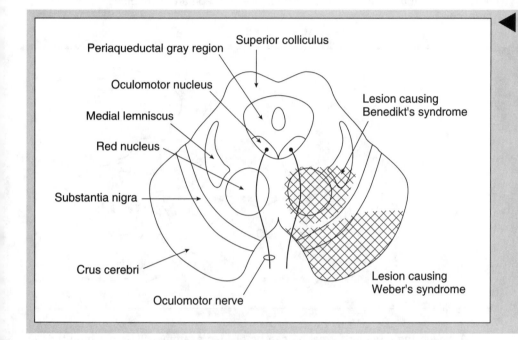

◀ **FIGURE 4-33**
Lesion Sites in the Midbrain. *The crosshatching indicates sites that are damaged in Benedikt's syndrome and in superior alternating hemiplegia (Weber's syndrome).*

Benedikt's Syndrome. In Benedikt's syndrome, the lesion site involves the red nucleus and surrounding fibers of the superior cerebellar peduncle (see Figure 4-33). Nearby fibers of the medial lemniscus and spinothalamic tracts are usually affected as well, and in some instances, the lesion may damage descending fibers of the oculomotor nerve. Benedikt's syndrome is characterized by contralateral hyperkinesia, tremor, and ataxia. All of these symptoms are associated with cerebellar dysfunction and occur in Benedikt's syndrome because the lesion interrupts the ascending fibers of the superior cerebellar peduncle. Patients with this disorder may experience loss of cutaneous and deep sensations if the medial lemniscus is damaged or show ophthalmoplegia if the oculomotor nerve is affected.

THE RETICULAR FORMATION

The reticular formation is an extensive network of cells and poorly differentiated nuclei located throughout the brainstem tegmentum. Its location in the central core of the brainstem allows the reticular formation to monitor and integrate information from different sensory, visceral, and limbic systems. Unlike most systems in the brainstem, however, the reticular formation is not topographically organized but has diffuse ascending and descending projections that influence all levels of the neuraxis. Substantial evidence indicates that the reticular formation plays a critical role in the control of autonomic functions, the modulation of pain and muscular reflexes, and the regulation of consciousness, sleep, and behavioral arousal.

Anatomic Organization of the Reticular Formation

Initially, the term reticular formation was used to indicate the diffuse network of interconnections formed by neurons in the brainstem tegmentum that lie outside the well-defined cranial nerve nuclei. Many neurons in the reticular formation have long dendrites that extend radially from the soma, often in a plane that is orthogonal to the longitudinal axis of the brainstem. This spatial configuration enhances the ability of these neurons to sample neural inputs across a wide region of the brainstem and is consistent with electrophysiologic recordings showing that these neurons respond to many sensory modalities. In addition, reticular formation neurons exhibit considerable divergence as their axons ascend or descend long distances and send collateral projections into numerous regions of the brainstem and thalamus. As shown by Figure 4-34, axons of some reticular formation neurons may even bifurcate into separate ascending and descending branches.

FIGURE 4-34 ▶

Cellular Connections in the Reticular Formation. An example of a neuron in the reticular formation of a young rat. Axonal collaterals project to the nucleus gracilis, the nucleus gigantocellularis, the periaqueductal gray region, several nuclei in the thalamus, the hypothalamus, and the zona incerta. NG = nucleus gracilis; NGC = nucleus gigantocellularis; PGR = periaqueductal gray region; Pf = parafascicular nucleus; PC = paracentral nucleus; MD = mediodorsal nucleus; H = hypothalamus; Z = zona incerta; TN = thalamic nuclei. (Source: Adapted with permission from Kandel E, et al: Principles of Neural Science. New York, NY: Elsevier, 1991, p 693.)

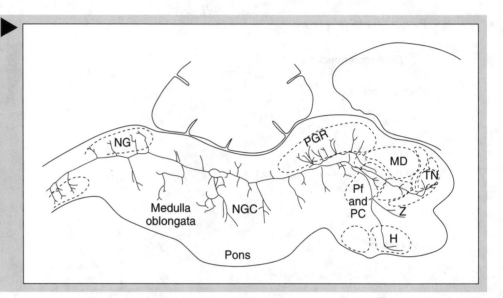

Although the reticular formation can be divided anatomically into a multitude of nuclei, conceptually it can be organized into three major cell columns extending longitudinally through the brainstem and a fourth set of nuclei that have common projections to the cerebellum (Figure 4-35). The columnar organization of the reticular formation is represented by the following groups: (1) a midline group of raphe nuclei, (2) nuclei in the parasagittal medial zone, and (3) nuclei in the parasagittal lateral zone.

RAPHE NUCLEI

*The **raphe nuclei** lie on the midline of the brainstem tegmentum.*

*The **raphe nuclei** consist of serotonergic and peptidergic neurons that project to widespread regions of the neuraxis to regulate pain, arousal, and sleep.*

The raphe nuclei form a thin group of cells that lie in and around the midline seam of the tegmentum. Most raphe nuclei are composed of serotonergic cells, although some contain neuropeptides such as cholecystokinin. Many raphe neurons have long projections that ascend as far as the cerebral cortex or descend the length of the spinal cord. The raphe nuclei are divided into a rostral group located in the rostral pons and midbrain and a caudal group located in the caudal pons and medulla.

The caudal raphe nuclei contain three separate neuronal populations: the raphe obscurus, the raphe pallidus, and the raphe magnus. These groups receive ascending somatosensory inputs from the spinal cord, the dorsal column nuclei, and the trigeminal nuclei as well as receiving descending inputs from the periaqueductal gray region. Most of the ascending inputs convey information related to the nociceptive qualities of a somatosensory stimulus. The raphe magnus sends an important projection to the spinal cord that terminates in the dorsal horn and probably plays a major role in reducing the transmission of nociceptive impulses into the spinothalamic tract. This view is based on physiologic studies, which demonstrate that the application of serotonin inhibits the responses of dorsal horn neurons to nociceptive inputs conveyed by C and Aδ fibers.

The rostral raphe nuclei are composed of the raphe pontis, the superior central nucleus, the dorsal tegmental nucleus, and the dorsal nucleus of the raphe. These nuclei are involved in regulating forebrain activity, although their functions are not entirely understood. The raphe pontis sends projections to the cerebellum, whereas the other raphe nuclei project rostrally through the median forebrain bundle to the hippocampus, limbic cortex, substantia nigra, thalamus, neostriatum, and cerebral cortex. The neuro-

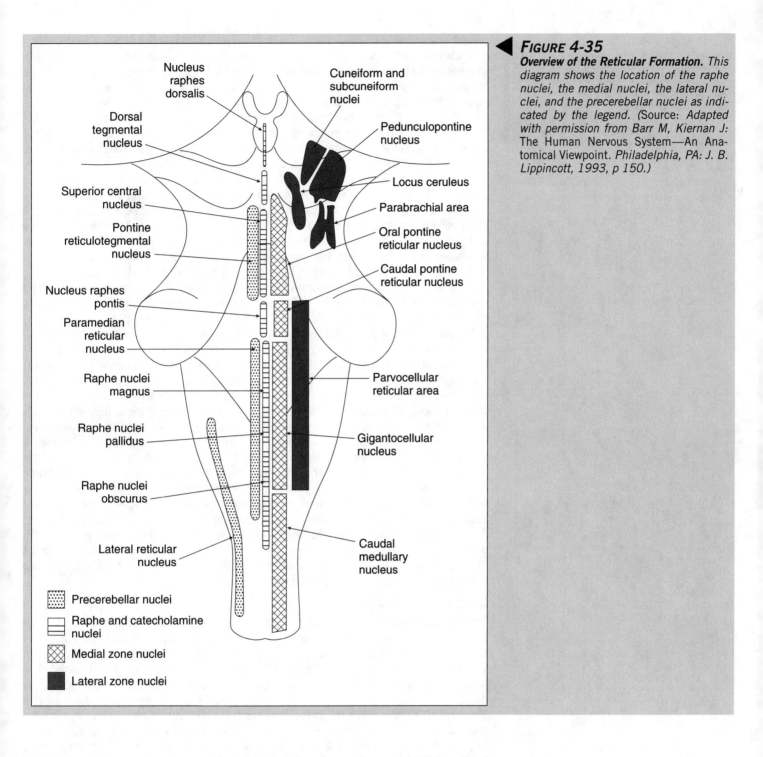

FIGURE 4-35
Overview of the Reticular Formation. *This diagram shows the location of the raphe nuclei, the medial nuclei, the lateral nuclei, and the precerebellar nuclei as indicated by the legend. (Source: Adapted with permission from Barr M, Kiernan J: The Human Nervous System—An Anatomical Viewpoint. Philadelphia, PA: J. B. Lippincott, 1993, p 150.)*

nal activity of the rostral raphe nuclei exhibit distinct patterns that are highly correlated with different stages of sleep and arousal.

MEDIAL RETICULAR ZONE

Adjacent to the raphe nuclei are a group of reticular nuclei that comprise the medial zone of the reticular formation. The medial zone includes the medial two-thirds of the reticular formation and provides most of the ascending and descending projections from the reticular formation. The medial zone of the reticular formation includes the nucleus gigantocellularis (in the medulla), the nucleus reticularis pontis (subdivided into oral and caudal parts in the pons), and the cuneiform and subcuneiform nuclei (in the midbrain). Most neurons in the medial nuclei are large and have extensive dendritic and axonal arborizations. The medial reticular zone receives its input mainly from the lateral reticular zone, which is activated largely by sensory modalities of a somatic or visceral origin. Medial zone neurons have long ascending and descending axons that give off collateral

*The **medial reticular zone** is the effector or motor part of the reticular formation. The **lateral reticular zone** is the afferent or sensory part of the reticular formation.*

projections to other parts of the reticular formation, the cranial nerve nuclei, the intralaminar nuclei of the thalamus, and the spinal cord. These connections, especially those to specific motor nuclei in the spinal cord and brainstem, have prompted a conceptual view of the medial zone as the "effector" or motor part of the reticular formation.

Ascending projections from the medial zone of the reticular formation contribute most of the fibers that form the ascending reticular activating system. This system ascends through the central tegmental tract and terminates in the intralaminar nuclei of the thalamus. The intralaminar nuclei do not receive inputs from a single sensory modality and are the only group of thalamic nuclei that have diffuse projections to all lobes of the cerebral cortex. Electrical stimulation of the intralaminar nuclei or of the reticular activating system causes a sleeping animal to awake. Conversely, bilateral damage to the central tegmental tract or to the intralaminar thalamic nuclei produces a state of coma. This does not mean that consciousness is located within the reticular activating system but rather that the conscious activities of the cerebral cortex depend upon excitatory influences from the thalamus and other subcortical regions.

There are two descending projections from the medial reticular zone that exert a powerful influence on spinal reflexes, muscle tone, and motor activity. The medullary reticulospinal tract arises from the gigantocellular reticular nucleus, descends bilaterally in the ventral part of the lateral funiculus, and terminates on interneurons in laminae VII and IX. The medullary reticulospinal system inhibits muscle tone and decreases the amplitude of myotactic reflexes. By comparison, the pontine reticulospinal system arises from the nucleus reticularis pontis, descends through the MLF in the anterior funiculus, and terminates on interneurons in laminae VII and VIII. In animals, electrical stimulation of the pontine reticulospinal system increases the muscle tone of the antigravity muscles and facilitates spinal reflexes. Together, these findings indicate that the medullary and pontine reticulospinal systems have antagonistic roles whose function is to provide a balance of inhibitory and excitatory influences on spinal circuits. Furthermore, the reticulospinal tracts receive direct innervation from the cerebral cortex and may provide an alternative to the pyramidal tract for sending motor commands to spinal motor neurons. Thus, infants born without cerebral hemispheres (anencephaly) are capable of executing simple movements that include yawning, suckling, and orienting behaviors. Animals whose brainstems have been transected at the midcollicular level can still display certain motor activities, such as postural changes or periodic limb movements that resemble walking. It is assumed that pathways descending from the reticular formation are critical for executing these behaviors.

LATERAL RETICULAR ZONE

The lateral zone of the reticular formation receives sensory information used to mediate cranial nerve reflexes and basic visceral functions. The lateral zone of reticular nuclei is located in the lateral third of the tegmentum, just medial to the spinal trigeminal system (in the medulla and pons) and the superior cerebellar peduncle (in the midbrain). The lateral reticular zone includes the parvocellular nucleus (in the medulla and pons), the parabrachial nucleus (in the pons and midbrain), and the pedunculopontine nucleus (in the pons). The parvocellular region is composed of small neurons that receive inputs from secondary sensory nuclei and from axonal collaterals of the ascending spinothalamic, trigeminothalamic, auditory, and vestibular pathways. The parvocellular region projects to the medial reticular zone and to the raphe nuclei, which, in turn, have descending projections that modulate sensory transmission and ascending projections that maintain arousal. The parabrachial nuclei receive afferent projections from nuclei, such as the nucleus of the solitary tract, which are concerned with limbic and visceral functions. Finally, the pedunculopontine nucleus has major projections to the substantia nigra, subthalamic nucleus, motor cortex, and raphe nuclei, all of which play a role in motor functions.

CEREBELLAR RELAY NUCLEI

Some nuclei in the reticular formation, such as the paramedian and lateral reticular nuclei in the medulla and the reticulotegmental nucleus in the pons, project almost exclusively to the cerebellum. The lateral reticular nucleus lies dorsal to the inferior olivary nuclei and receives input from spinoreticular fibers, spinothalamic collaterals, and the red nucleus. The lateral reticular nucleus projects to the cerebellum via the inferior cerebellar peduncle and forms a portion of the mossy fiber projection system. The paramedian nucleus is located near the medullary midline and receives input from the cerebellum and cerebral cortex. The reticulotegmental nucleus is located in the paramedian region of the pons (between the medial lemnisci) and also receives input from the cerebral cortex and the deep cerebellar nuclei. Because all of these nuclei project to the cerebellum, it is assumed that they play an important role in controlling movements, but their exact roles are unclear.

LOCUS CERULEUS

A group of pigmented neurons located in the ventrolateral part of the periaqueductal gray region appear as a bluish spot in freshly cut sections through the pons. Known as the locus ceruleus (or blue spot), this nucleus contains a homogeneous group of neurons that use norepinephrine as a neurotransmitter and innervate every level of the neuraxis from the spinal cord to the cerebral cortex. Ascending axons from the locus ceruleus contribute fibers to the dorsal tegmental bundle and to the medial forebrain bundle. Some neurons in the locus ceruleus project to a single target such as the hippocampus, whereas other neurons have divergent axons with widely distributed terminations in the diencephalon and cerebral cortex. The diffuse distribution of noradrenergic terminals from the locus ceruleus bears a resemblance to the serotonergic innervation pattern of the raphe nuclei and some evidence indicates that these neurotransmitter systems complement each other. Because its efferent projections are so widely distributed, the locus ceruleus is unlikely to be involved in relaying specific information but may increase the overall excitability of its postsynaptic targets, perhaps to modulate attention and general arousal.

> The **locus ceruleus** contains noradrenergic neurons located in the lateral part of periaqueductal gray and is involved in regulating arousal and attention.

RESOLUTION OF CLINICAL CASE

When conducting a neurologic examination, it is important to pay special attention to symptoms affecting opposite sides of the body because such signs are invaluable for determining the precise location of a lesion, tumor, or other event affecting the nervous system. In the clinical case presented in this chapter, decreased pain sensitivity on the right side of the face and left side of the body suggests a lesion of the spinothalamic tract (contralateral body) and adjacent spinal trigeminal nucleus (ipsilateral face). Damage to the spinal trigeminal nucleus would also cause an ipsilateral loss of the corneal reflex. These symptoms are classic signs of the lateral medullary syndrome and, based on the patient's high blood pressure and other medical history, indicate that the patient has experienced a stroke affecting the right posterior inferior cerebellar artery. This artery supplies blood to many nuclei and fiber tracts in the lateral medulla, and a decrease in the blood supply to these structures can produce a constellation of symptoms. Hence, dizziness was caused by damage to the vestibular nuclei, whereas dysphonia and a drooping soft palate indicate the nucleus ambiguus was affected. Pseudoptosis (a partially drooping eyelid), miosis (small pupil), and anhidrosis (lack of perspiration) on one side of the face indicate a loss of sympathetic innervation caused by the interruption of descending autonomic pathways in the lateral medulla.

REVIEW QUESTIONS

Directions: For each of the following questions, choose the **one best** answer.

1. The presence of ptosis, mydriasis, and external strabismus on one side of the face indicates a lesion of which cranial nerve?
    (A) Abducens nerve
    (B) Trochlear nerve
    (C) Oculomotor nerve
    (D) Facial nerve
    (E) Optic nerve

2. Which of the following conditions is characterized by symptoms involving only one side of the body?
    (A) Lateral gaze paralysis
    (B) Bell's palsy
    (C) Weber's syndrome
    (D) Wallenberg's syndrome
    (E) Lateral medullary syndrome

3. A unilateral lesion of the medial longitudinal fasciculus (MLF) produces
    (A) lateral gaze paralysis
    (B) internal strabismus
    (C) impairment of convergent eye movements
    (D) dissociation of conjugate eye movements
    (E) ptosis

4. Which of the following nerves is most likely to be damaged if the gag reflex is absent?
    (A) Glossopharyngeal nerve
    (B) Trigeminal nerve
    (C) Facial nerve
    (D) Spinal accessory nerve
    (E) Hypoglossal nerve

5. Which of the following medullary structures would remain intact following occlusion of the posterior inferior cerebellar artery?
    (A) Spinothalamic tract
    (B) Spinal trigeminal nucleus
    (C) Hypoglossal nerve
    (D) Nucleus ambiguus
    (E) Nucleus solitarius

6. Which of the following functions is mediated primarily by the caudal nucleus solitarius?
    (A) Sense of taste
    (B) Saliva production
    (C) Arterial baroreception
    (D) Peristalsis of the esophagus
    (E) Reflexive movements of the larynx during swallowing

ANSWERS AND EXPLANATIONS

1. The answer is C. The oculomotor nerve innervates the levator palpebrae, the pupillary sphincter, and all extraocular muscles except the lateral rectus and the superior oblique. Hence, oculomotor nerve damage results in a drooping eyelid, pupillary dilation, and lateral deviation of the eyeball. A lesion of the abducens nerve produces internal strabismus, not external strabismus. A lesion of the trochlear nerve impairs the ability to look downward. A lesion of the facial nerve causes Bell's palsy, whereas a lesion of the optic nerve causes blindness.

2. The answer is B. Bell's palsy is a unilateral facial paralysis caused by damage to the lower motor neurons of the facial nerve. Lateral gaze paralysis causes both eyes to be directed to one side. Weber's and Wallenberg's syndromes are both alternating hemiplegias that involve a unilateral paralysis of the body that is associated with contralateral paralysis of muscles controlling the eye or the tongue, respectively. Lateral medullary syndrome is characterized by a loss of pain and temperature sensation on the ipsilateral face and the contralateral body.

3. The answer is D. The MLF contains fibers interconnecting the abducens and oculomotor nuclei. Damage to the MLF impairs the ability to coordinate horizontal eye movements. Lateral gaze paralysis is produced by an abducens nucleus lesion, whereas internal strabismus is produced by an abducens nerve lesion. Convergent eye movements are not impaired by MLF lesions because the medial recti are still innervated by both oculomotor nerves and the motor command for convergent eye movements is not transmitted through the MLF. Ptosis is usually a sign of oculomotor nerve damage.

4. The answer is A. The glossopharyngeal nerve contains GSA fibers that innervate the posterior third of the tongue and mediate the afferent limb of the gag reflex. The trigeminal nerve contains GSA fibers that innervate the anterior two-thirds of the tongue, but only stimulation of the posterior tongue elicits gagging. The nucleus ambiguus and its SVE fibers mediate the motor limb of the gag reflex, but these fibers do not emerge from the facial, spinal accessory, or hypoglossal nerves.

5. The answer is C. Occlusion of the posterior inferior cerebellar artery causes loss of pain sensitivity on the ipsilateral face and contralateral body that is often seen with dysphonia and nausea. These symptoms correspond to the lateral medullary syndrome, which is associated with damage to the spinal trigeminal nucleus, the spinothalamic tract, the nucleus ambiguus, and the nucleus solitarius. The hypoglossal nucleus and its emerging nerve are supplied by the anterior spinal artery.

6. The answer is C. The caudal solitarius receives afferent information concerning blood pressure from baroreceptors located in the aortic arch and the carotid sinus. The rostral part of the nucleus solitarius is concerned with taste information from the tongue. The production of saliva is controlled by the inferior and superior salivatory nuclei and their connections to specific parasympathetic ganglia. Vagal nerve fibers emerging from the dorsal motor nucleus of the vagus and the nucleus ambiguus control peripheral movements of the esophagus and the larynx, respectively.

ADDITIONAL READING

Brodal A: *Neurological Anatomy in Relation to Clinical Medicine*, 3rd ed. New York, NY: Oxford University Press, 1981, pp 448–577.

Dubner R, Bennett GJ: Spinal and trigeminal mechanisms of nociception. *Ann Rev Neurosci* 6:381–418, 1983.

Moore RY, Bloom FE: Central catecholamine neuron systems: anatomy and physiology of the norepinephrine and epinephrine systems. *Ann Rev Neurosci* 2:113–168, 1979.

Sears ES, Franklin GM: Diseases of the cranial nerves. In *The Science and Practice of Clinical Medicine*, vol 5. New York, NY: Grune & Stratton, 1980, pp 471–494.

Wilson-Pauwels L, Akesson EJ, Stewart PA: *Cranial Nerves: Anatomy and Clinical Comments*. Toronto, Ontario: B. C. Decker, 1988.

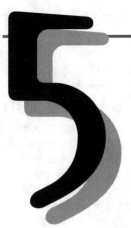

THALAMOCORTICAL ORGANIZATION

INTRODUCTION OF CLINICAL CASE

The emergency medical service was called to the home of P. S., a 79-year-old woman who had fallen and was unable to get up. The paramedics determined that P. S. was paralyzed on the left side; preliminary diagnosis was an infarct of the right middle cerebral artery. With the patient's condition stable, she was transported to the emergency room of the local hospital. A full series of computed tomography (CT) scans was ordered before P. S. was admitted to the hospital; carotid and vertebral angiograms were performed the following day. When the staff neurologist began his neurologic examination of P. S., he found her to be clearheaded and cooperative. After checking her vital signs, the physician asked P. S. to move her left arm. P. S. began to protest that she had no left arm, and no movement was observed. The physician encountered the same reaction when he asked P. S. to move her left leg. P. S. obligingly moved her right arm and leg when asked. Testing the patient's sense of fine touch met with similar results: cooperative and accurate reports when stroking the right limbs and obstinate denial that either of her left limbs existed.

THALAMIC ORGANIZATION

*The **dorsal thalamus** is typically referred to simply as the thalamus.*

The dorsal thalamus, which is typically referred to simply as the thalamus, contributes to motor, sensory, limbic, and vegetative functions. Given its diverse functions, the thalamus receives afferent projections from many areas of the brain; most of its efferent projections, however, are to the cerebral cortex (Table 5-1). The nuclei of the thalamus can be classified according to their cortical projections, functions, or relative location. Based on their cortical projections, the thalamus is divisible into specific sensory relay nuclei, cortical relay nuclei, association nuclei, nonspecific nuclei, and intrinsic nuclei.

TABLE 5-1 ▶
Afferent and Efferent Projections of the Major Thalamic Nuclei

	Afferent Projections	Efferent Projections	Function
Specific sensory relay			
VPL	Dorsal column nuclei Spinothalamic tract	Postcentral gyrus	Somesthesis
VPM	Principal trigeminal nucleus	Postcentral gyrus	Somesthesis
VPMpc	Solitary nucleus	Anterior insula	Gustation
MGN	Inferior colliculus	Temporal lobe	Audition
LGN	Retina	Occipital cortex	Vision
Cortical relay nuclei			
VL	Cerebellum Globus pallidus Globus pallidus	Precentral gyrus Frontal cortex	Movement Motor planning Motor planning
VA	Substantia nigra	Frontal eye fields	Directed eye movements
Association nuclei			
Anterior	Hypothalamus	Cingulate gyrus	Memory
MD	Amygdala Pontine parabrachial nucleus Substantia nigra Frontal cortex	Frontal cortex Frontal eye fields	Emotion and affect Olfaction Pain
LD	Hypothalamus	Cingulate gyrus	Autonomic correlates of emotion
LP	Superior colliculus	Parietal association cortex	Vision
Posterior nucleus	Spinothalamic tract	Insula Cingulate gyrus Parietal and temporal association cortices	Pain
Pulvinar	Superior colliculus	Parietal, occipital, and temporal cortices	Vision
Nonspecific nuclei			
Midline nuclei	Reticular formation	Entire cortex	Arousal
CM-Pf complex	Motor and premotor cortices Basal ganglia Reticular formation	Striatum	Motor integration
Intrinsic nucleus			
Reticular	Cortex	Thalamus	Gating cortical input

Note. VPL = ventroposterolateral nucleus; VPM = ventroposteromedial nucleus; VPMpc = parvocellular division of the VPM nucleus; MGN = medial geniculate nucleus; LGN = lateral geniculate nucleus; VL = ventral lateral nucleus; VA = ventral anterior nucleus; MD = medial dorsal nucleus; LD = lateral dorsal nucleus; LP = lateral posterior nucleus; CM-Pf = centromedian-parafascicular nuclei.

The specific sensory relay nuclei receive ascending projections from the somatosensory, auditory, visual, and gustatory systems and project to their respective primary cortical areas. The cortical relay nuclei link nonsensory regions such as the cerebellum and hypothalamus with circumscribed cortical areas. The thalamic association nuclei project to widespread areas of the frontal and parietal association cortex. The diffuse cortical projections of the nonspecific thalamic nuclei play a vital role in attention; other subcortical projections of these nuclei contribute to integration of motor control. The reticular nucleus is classified as an intrinsic thalamic nucleus because its projections remain within the thalamus. The afferent and efferent projections of the major thalamic nuclei are summarized in Table 5-1.

Location and Organization of the Thalamus

The thalamus is a pair of egg-shaped nuclei located at the rostral end of the brainstem. The thalamus forms the wall of the third ventricle dorsal to the hypothalamic sulcus between the interventricular foramen rostrally and the posterior commissure caudally. Its dorsal surface forms the floor of the lateral ventricle. Laterally, the thalamus is bounded by the internal capsule and the body of the caudate nucleus. The caudal pole of the thalamus is formed by the medial and lateral geniculate nuclei. In 80% of the population, the left and right thalami are joined by a narrow cellular bridge, the massa intermedia.

The key landmark for understanding the internal organization of the thalamus is the internal medullary lamina, which divides the thalamus into anterior, medial, and lateral parts. The lateral division of the thalamus is further divided into dorsal and ventral parts. Within the caudal third of the thalamus the internal medullary lamina splits and encapsulates several nuclei collectively known as the intralaminar nuclei (Figure 5-1).

> The **massa intermedia** also is called the interthalamic adhesion.

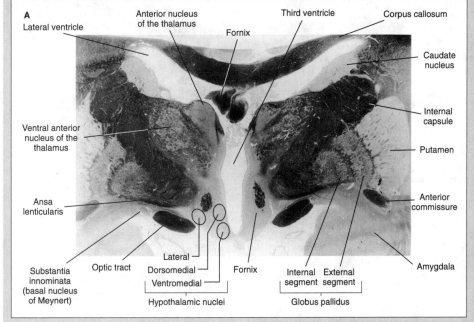

◀ **FIGURES 5-1A–5-1E**
Photomicrographs of the Human Thalamus (Weigert Stain). Figure 5-1F shows the plane of section for the slides shown in Figures 5-1A–5-1E.

◀ **FIGURE 5-1A**
Coronal Section through the Rostral Thalamus at the Level of the Anterior Thalamic Nuclei.

FIGURE 5-1B ▶
Coronal Section through the Thalamus at the Level of the Medial Dorsal Nucleus.

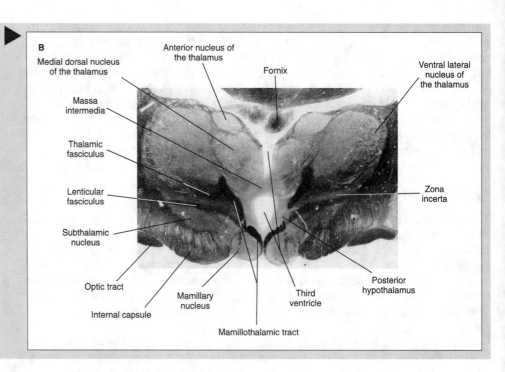

B

Medial dorsal nucleus of the thalamus
Anterior nucleus of the thalamus
Fornix
Ventral lateral nucleus of the thalamus
Massa intermedia
Thalamic fasciculus
Lenticular fasciculus
Subthalamic nucleus
Zona incerta
Optic tract
Mamillary nucleus
Internal capsule
Mamillothalamic tract
Third ventricle
Posterior hypothalamus

FIGURE 5-1C ▶
Coronal Section through the Thalamus near the Rostral Limit of the Ventroposteromedial Nucleus.

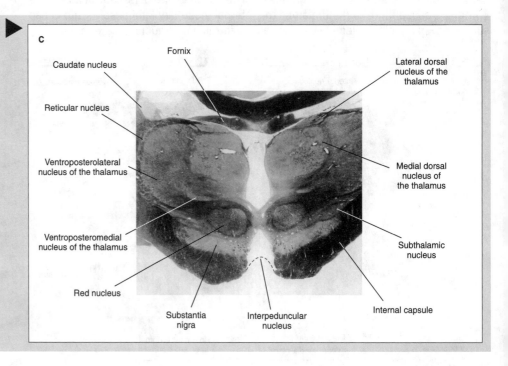

C

Caudate nucleus
Fornix
Lateral dorsal nucleus of the thalamus
Reticular nucleus
Medial dorsal nucleus of the thalamus
Ventroposterolateral nucleus of the thalamus
Ventroposteromedial nucleus of the thalamus
Subthalamic nucleus
Internal capsule
Red nucleus
Substantia nigra
Interpeduncular nucleus

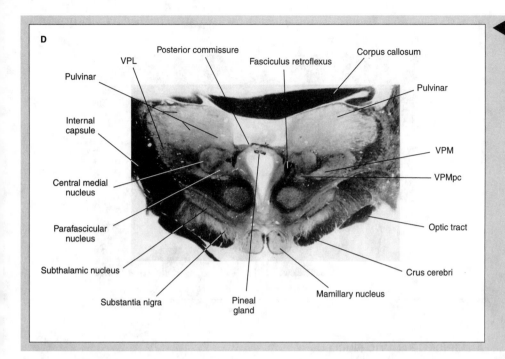

D

Pulvinar

VPL

Posterior commissure

Fasciculus retroflexus

Corpus callosum

Pulvinar

Internal capsule

VPM

VPMpc

Central medial nucleus

Parafascicular nucleus

Optic tract

Subthalamic nucleus

Crus cerebri

Substantia nigra

Pineal gland

Mamillary nucleus

FIGURE 5-1D
Coronal Section through the Caudal Thalamus. VPM = ventroposteromedial nucleus; VPMpc = parvocellular division of the VPM nucleus.

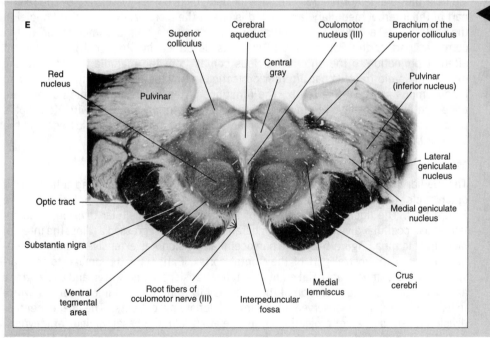

E

Red nucleus

Superior colliculus

Cerebral aqueduct

Oculomotor nucleus (III)

Brachium of the superior colliculus

Pulvinar

Central gray

Pulvinar (inferior nucleus)

Optic tract

Lateral geniculate nucleus

Medial geniculate nucleus

Substantia nigra

Crus cerebri

Ventral tegmental area

Root fibers of oculomotor nerve (III)

Interpeduncular fossa

Medial lemniscus

FIGURE 5-1E
Coronal Section through the Diencephalic-Mesencephalic Junction.

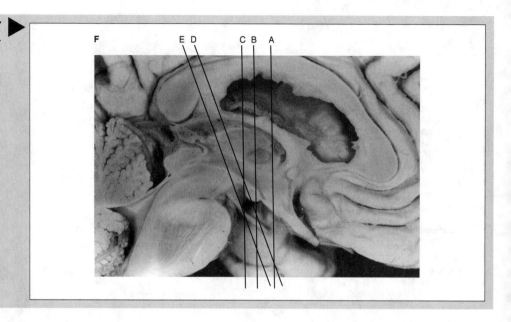

ANTERIOR THALAMIC NUCLEUS

*The **thalamic tubercle** is the bulge of the anterior thalamic nuclei into the lateral ventricle.*

The anterior nucleus forms the anterior tubercle, which protrudes into the lateral ventricle near the foramen of Monro. The anterior nucleus is partially enclosed by the rostral part of the internal medullary lamina and is one of the more easily recognized nuclei in the thalamus (see Figure 5-1). The anterior nucleus relays limbic information to the cortex as part of the Papez circuit, which is described in Chapter 13. The largest afferent projection to the anterior nucleus comes from the mamillary nuclei via the mamillothalamic tract. Other afferent projections from the medial temporal lobe and hippocampus arrive via the fornix. The functions of the anterior thalamic nucleus are uncertain but are believed to involve memory and attention. Patients with Korsakoff's psychosis show degeneration of the mamillary nuclei, the mamillothalamic tract, and the anterior thalamic nucleus.

*The **anterior thalamic nuclei** form the thalamic link of the limbic system.*

MEDIAL THALAMIC NUCLEI

*The **medial thalamic nuclei** project heavily to the frontal lobe.*

The medial thalamic nuclei include the medial/dorsal (MD) nucleus and a half dozen other nuclei located on the midline, some of which form the massa intermedia (see Figure 5-1). The nucleus MD consists of the medial magnocellular division, a dorsolateral parvocellular division, and a thin paralaminar division pressed against the internal medullary lamina (Figure 5-2). The parvocellular division has extensive reciprocal connections with the rostral part of the frontal cortex. Patients with damage to the parvocellular MD demonstrate a flat emotional tone, transient memory loss, and anterograde amnesia. Surgical disconnection of the nucleus MD from the frontal lobe causes symptoms similar to those observed in prefrontal lobotomy patients. The magnocellular division receives afferent projections from the amygdala, the basal nucleus of Meynert, and the primary and secondary olfactory cortices located in the temporal lobe. The magnocellular division of nucleus MD is the thalamic relay for olfactory information bound for the orbitofrontal cortex. The orbitofrontal cortex, unlike the olfactory areas located on the temporal lobe, consists of neocortex. The paralaminar nucleus MD receives ascending projections from the substantia nigra and the pontine parabrachial nucleus and has been implicated in eye movement and pain perception.

Other nuclei in the medial part of the thalamus are much smaller and less prominent than the nucleus MD. These nuclei represent a rostral continuation of the brainstem central gray. Like the central gray, these small and poorly differentiated regions of the medial thalamus are involved in vegetative functions. The midline thalamic nuclei receive afferent projections from numerous brainstem nuclei including the nucleus of the solitary tract, the pontine parabrachial nuclei, the periaqueductal gray, the raphe nuclei, and the locus ceruleus. The midline nuclei have weak but widespread projections

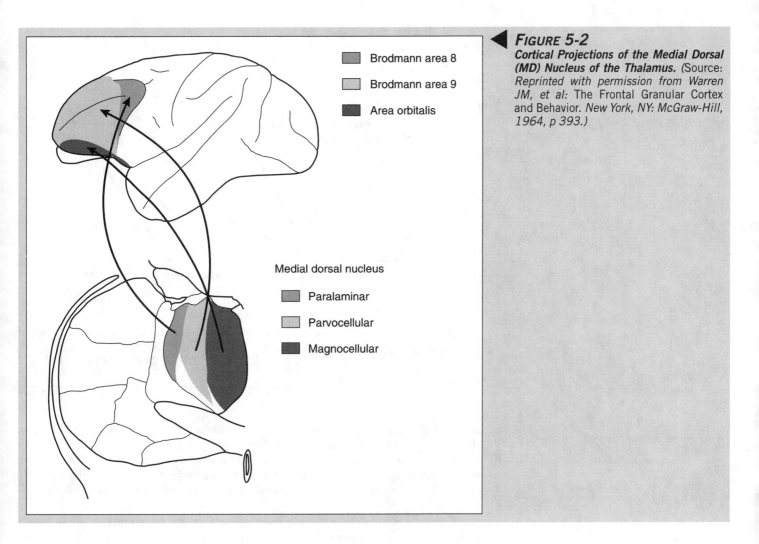

Brodmann area 8

Brodmann area 9

Area orbitalis

Medial dorsal nucleus

Paralaminar

Parvocellular

Magnocellular

FIGURE 5-2
Cortical Projections of the Medial Dorsal (MD) Nucleus of the Thalamus. *(Source: Reprinted with permission from Warren JM, et al:* The Frontal Granular Cortex and Behavior. *New York, NY: McGraw-Hill, 1964, p 393.)*

to the cerebral cortex; some of their projections to the amygdala and the basal ganglia suggest that they link the autonomic nervous system with emotion, memory, and movement.

LATERAL THALAMIC NUCLEI

The lateral thalamus consists of dorsal and ventral tiers. While the dorsal tier nuclei are among the least understood nuclei in the thalamus, the ventral tier consists of specific sensory relay nuclei whose functions are among the best understood.

Dorsal Tier Nuclei. The dorsal tier of the thalamus, from rostral to caudal, includes the lateral dorsal (LD), the lateral posterior (LP), and pulvinar nuclei (see Figure 5-1). The nucleus LD, like its rostral neighbor the anterior nucleus, is encapsulated, receives afferent projections from the mamillary nuclei, temporal lobe, and hippocampal formation, and projects to the cingulate gyrus. The nucleus LP, which lies immediately caudal to the nucleus LD, is more closely aligned with its caudal neighbor, the pulvinar. The pulvinar, the largest thalamic nucleus, is wedged between the medial and lateral geniculate nuclei at the junction between the diencephalon and mesencephalon. The pulvinar receives its afferent projections from the superficial layers of the superior colliculus and projects to visual association areas in the occipital, parietal, and temporal lobes. The pulvinar is the thalamic relay in the extrageniculate visual pathway, which reaches its pinnacle of development in primates (see Chapter 10).

Ventral Tier Nuclei. The ventral tier nuclei include, from rostral to caudal, the ventral anterior (VA), the ventral lateral (VL), and the ventral posterior (VP) nuclei. The rostrocaudal sequence of the ventral tier nuclei is preserved at the cortical level (Figure 5-3).

The nucleus VA, which receives afferent projections from the basal ganglia and

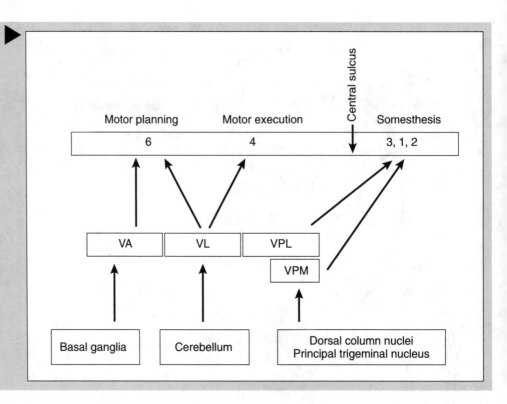

FIGURE 5-3

Ventral Tier Nuclei of the Thalamus and the Cerebral Cortex Have the Same Rostrocaudal Organization. VA = ventral anterior nucleus; VL = ventral lateral nucleus; VPL = ventroposterolateral nucleus; VPM = ventroposteromedial nucleus.

*The **VA nucleus** is involved in motor planning and initiation.*

*The **VL nucleus** refines motor execution.*

*The **VPL** and **VPM nuclei** are somatosensory relays.*

*The **posterior nucleus** is involved with pain.*

substantia nigra, initiates movement through its projections to the premotor cortex (Brodmann area 6). The nucleus VL not only links the basal ganglia with the premotor cortex, but also connects the cerebellum with the primary motor cortex (Brodmann area 4). Feedback from the cerebellum to the primary motor cortex improves fine motor control. The contributions of the VA and VL to movement are discussed in more detail in Chapter 11.

Somatosensory and nociceptive information from the body ascends in the medial lemniscus and spinothalamic tract, respectively, and terminates in the ventroposterolateral (VPL) nucleus. A smaller and more medially located region, the ventroposteromedial (VPM) nucleus, receives similar information from the face and oral cavity via the dorsal and ventral trigeminothalamic tracts. Together, the VPL and VPM nuclei contain a topographical representation of the entire body. The orderly projection of these ventral posterior nuclei to the postcentral gyrus provides the basis for the topographical organization of the primary somatosensory cortex (Figure 5-4). The most medial aspect of the nucleus VPM is the parvocellular relay for gustatory information, whose primary cortical area lies at the crest of the insula. The somatosensory and gustatory systems are described in more detail in Chapters 6 and 9, respectively.

POSTERIOR NUCLEUS

The posterior thalamic nucleus is located between the VPL nucleus and the pulvinar. Although not as well understood as its neighbors, the posterior nucleus receives nociceptive input from the anterolateral system and projects to the insula, cingulate gyrus, and association cortices in the parietal and temporal lobes. The peripheral and central pain pathways are described in Chapter 6.

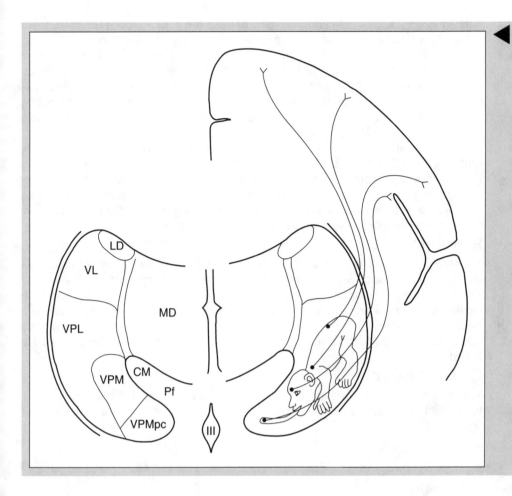

◀ *FIGURE 5-4*
Schematic Diagram of the Projections from the Somatosensory and Gustatory Thalamic Nuclei to the Cerebral Cortex. LD = lateral dorsal nucleus; VL = ventral lateral nucleus; VPL = ventroposterolateral nucleus; VPM = ventroposteromedial nucleus; VPMpc = parvocellular division of the VPM nucleus; CM = centromedian nucleus; Pf = parafascicular nucleus; MD = medial dorsal nucleus.

LATERAL AND MEDIAL GENICULATE NUCLEI

The lateral and medial geniculate nuclei, which together form the metathalamus, are the thalamic relays for vision and audition, respectively. The lateral geniculate nucleus (LGN) is located at the caudal pole of the thalamus, lateral to the crus cerebri and medial geniculate nucleus (MGN), and ventral to the pulvinar (see Figure 5-1). In transverse sections, the LGN is horseshoe-shaped and consists of six layers. Crossed and uncrossed axons of the optic tract enter the LGN at the hilus and terminate in separate lamina. Axons from the contralateral eye terminate in layers 1, 4, and 6; the ipsilateral eye projects to layers 2, 3, and 5. There is no interocular integration within the LGN. The LGN projects to the primary visual cortex located along the banks of the calcarine sulcus. The central organization of the visual system is described in more detail in Chapter 10.

MGN is located at the caudal pole of the thalamus, medial to the LGN, dorsal to the crus cerebri, and ventral to the pulvinar. The lamination of the MGN, though present, is not readily apparent because the interlaminar bands are unmyelinated. Ascending projections to the MGN originate in the inferior colliculus; efferent projections of the MGN ascend to the auditory cortex along the auditory radiations. The MGN is described in more detail in Chapter 7.

> The **MGN** and **LGN** together are known as the metathalamus.

INTRALAMINAR NUCLEI

In the caudal third of the thalamus, the internal medullary lamina splits and forms an oval pocket that contains the intralaminar nuclei (see Figure 5-1). The largest of the

*The **parafascicular nucleus** is named for its proximity to the fasciculus retroflexus.*

intralaminar nuclei are the centromedian (CM) and the parafascicular (Pf) nuclei. The CM nucleus receives descending projections from the primary motor cortex, the basal ganglia, and the brainstem reticular formation. The afferent projections of the Pf nucleus originate in the premotor cortex. Both nuclei have light, widespread projections to the cerebral cortex as well as dense projections to restricted areas of the basal ganglia (CM → putamen; Pf → caudate nucleus). These projections along with others to the subthalamic nucleus, substantia nigra, and the globus pallidus suggest that CM and Pf nuclei integrate cortical and subcortical aspects of movement.

The central lateral (CL) nucleus is one of the small intralaminar nuclei located further rostrally. The CL nucleus is a sliver-shaped cluster of cells in the seam between the dorsomedial nucleus and the VPL nucleus. Input to the CL nucleus comes from the spinothalamic tract, the deep cerebellar nuclei, and the pontine parabrachial nucleus. Its projections to the cerebral cortex and the striatum suggest that the CL nucleus may play a role in state-dependent arousal of the cerebral cortex.

RETICULAR NUCLEUS

The reticular nucleus forms a thin shell between the external medullary lamina and the internal capsule along the lateral and rostral surfaces of the thalamus (see Figure 5-1). The reticular nucleus forms part of a feedback loop that enables the cerebral cortex to modulate its own afferent input from the thalamus as a function of arousal and as a mechanism for selective attention (Figure 5-5). Despite its intimate relationship with the dorsal thalamus, the reticular nucleus is, in fact, an embryologic derivative of the ventral thalamus.

*Because the efferent projections of the reticular nucleus are restricted to the thalamus, it is classified as an **intrinsic** or **subcortical thalamic nucleus**.*

INTERNAL CAPSULE

The internal capsule consists of reciprocal connections between the thalamus and cortex as well as descending projections from the cerebral cortex to the brainstem and

FIGURE 5-5 ▶

Afferent and Efferent Projections of the Reticular Nucleus. *The reticular nucleus receives afferent projections from the cerebral cortex and the thalamus, but projects only to the thalamus. The thalamus and cerebral cortex may use the reticular nucleus to screen information bound for the cerebral cortex.*

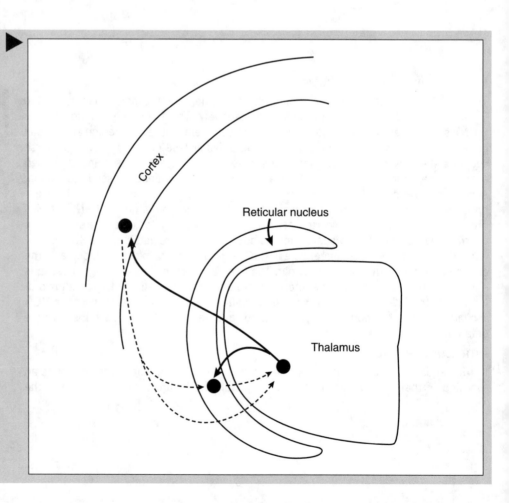

spinal cord. In horizontal sections, the internal capsule resembles a boomerang with its two long limbs joined at the genu located near the foramen of Monro (Figure 5-6). The anterior limb of the internal capsule consists of thalamic projections to the frontal cortex and descending frontopontine fibers. The posterior limb contains the superior thalamic radiations, which connect the motor and somatosensory nuclei of the thalamus with the precentral and postcentral gyri of the cerebral cortex. The caudal part of the posterior limb contains corticospinal projections, which control the arms, trunk, and legs. Corticobulbar fibers that project to the facial and oral motor nuclei of the brainstem pass through the genu of the internal capsule.

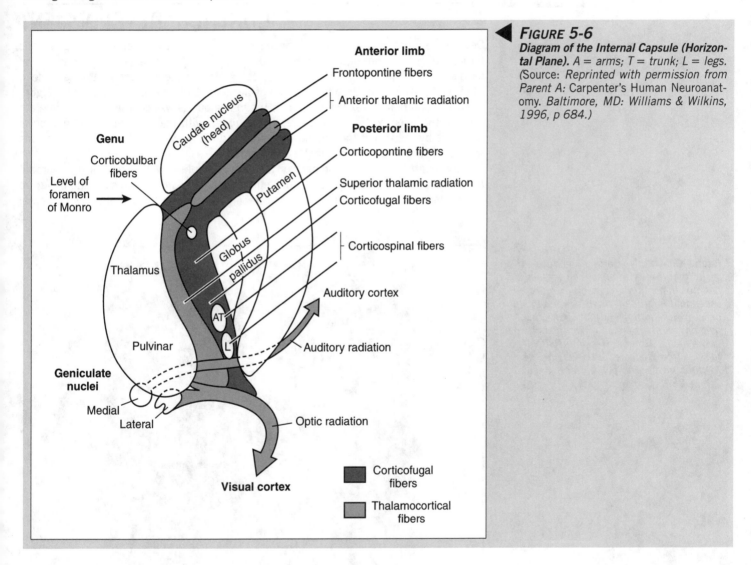

◀ *FIGURE 5-6*
Diagram of the Internal Capsule (Horizontal Plane). *A = arms; T = trunk; L = legs.* (Source: *Reprinted with permission from Parent A:* Carpenter's Human Neuroanatomy. *Baltimore, MD: Williams & Wilkins, 1996, p 684.)*

CEREBRAL CORTEX

The cerebral cortex is the laminated shell of neurons, glia, axons, and dendrites that forms the surface of the telencephalon. The cerebral cortex represents the crowning achievement of the central nervous system (CNS) and is widely believed to be the structure that distinguishes humans from other animals. Large parts of the cerebral cortex are dedicated to personality, strategic planning, sensory perception, volitional movement, and language.

Two different classes of cortex are found in the telencephalon: allocortex and neocortex. Allocortex, an early evolutionary development, is found in the hippocampal formation (archicortex) and the olfactory cortex (paleocortex). Neocortex, which covers the remainder of the telencephalon, is described in this chapter.

Because the organization of the cerebral cortex is linked so closely to that of the thalamus, the key to understanding the cerebral cortex lies in the thalamus. The entire cerebral cortex is connected to the thalamus, and in some cases, to multiple nuclei of the thalamus.

CORTICAL DEVELOPMENT

Development of the cerebral cortex proceeds from the inside out.

Development of the cerebral cortex begins during the first trimester as radial glial cells form a lattice from the ventricular zone to the perimeter of the telencephalon. Radial glial cells act as scaffolding for postmitotic neuroblasts to migrate from the ventricular zone to their final position on the outer surface of the immature telencephalic vesicle (Figure 5-7). The cerebral cortex develops from the inside out as waves of neuroblasts migrate through the deep cortical layers already populated with mature neurons. Migration is complete by the end of the second trimester, and with few exceptions, no new neurons will be added to the cortical mantle afterwards.

Although the full complement of neurons is in place well before birth, neuronal maturation continues until adulthood. Neurons gradually increase in size, add dendritic spines and synapses, and develop more elaborate dendritic trees. Both environmental

FIGURE 5-7 ▶

Radial Glial Cells. Cortical neurons migrate from the ventricular zone to their final positions in the cerebral cortex by ascending a lattice formed by radial glial cells. n = neuron; gf = glial fiber. Embryonic day numbers are shown at the bottom of the figure. (Source: Reprinted with permission from Rockefeller University Press: At the horizon: The cell surface. Search: 29, 1996.)

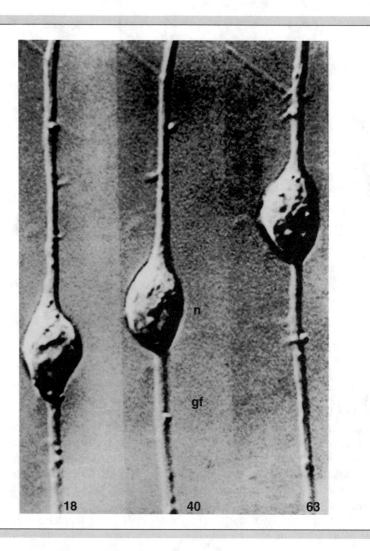

and genetic factors affect maturation of the cerebral cortex. Impoverished environments or sensory loss caused by denervation may reduce the number of synapses in the cerebral cortex. The importance of genetic factors is evident in children with Down's syndrome. Histologic examination of the brains of patients with Down's syndrome shows dendritic trees with fewer dendritic spines and a less complex branching pattern than found in normal brains.

The surface of the cerebral cortex is initially flat and featureless but gradually develops dozens of folds called gyri. The earliest landmarks to appear on the cortical surface are the central (Rolando) and lateral (Sylvius) sulci, which flank the primary somatosensory, auditory, and motor areas. Folding of the cerebral cortex maximizes the amount of neocortex within the limited confines of the calvarium. The success of this design is striking. If the human brain lacked gyri and sulci as many species do (e.g., mice), the total surface area of the cerebral cortex would be about 190 mm². Folding of the cortex has increased its surface area approximately 13 times to 2,500 mm², most of which is buried within the sulci.

Gyrencephalic brains have gyri and sulci. Lissencephalic brains are featureless.

CORTICAL CYTOARCHITECTURE

Cell Types

Pyramidal and granule (stellate) cells are the most common neurons in the cerebral cortex. Pyramidal cells have a pyramid-shaped soma (10–70 µm in diameter), a prominent apical dendrite, small basal dendrites, and a lone basal axon (Figure 5-8). Unlike other neurons, pyramidal cells have a consistent orientation in the cortex. The single apical dendrite of the pyramidal cell arborizes through more superficial cortical layers while the numerous, short basal dendrites ramify within the deeper cortical layers. The lone basal axon may ramify locally or project to remote cortical and subcortical targets. Granule cells, by comparison, have much smaller (5-15 µm in diameter), star-shaped somas and shorter processes, which rarely project beyond the cortical mantle. Spiny granule cells are excitatory while nonspiny granule cells are inhibitory; both have short axonal and dendritic processes that form local cortical circuits.

Pyramidal cells are the efferent neurons of the cerebral cortex.

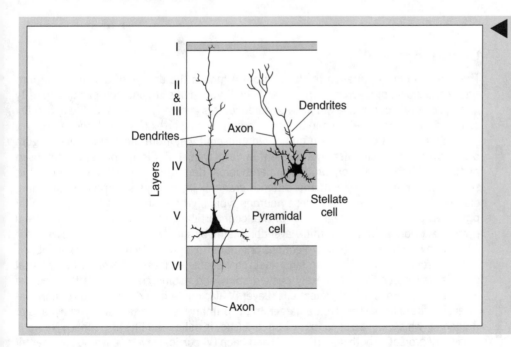

◄ **FIGURE 5-8**
Cross Section of the Cerebral Cortex. *Pyramidal and stellate (granule) cells are the most common neurons within the cerebral cortex.*

Neurotransmitters

Cortical neurons contain an assortment of inhibitory and excitatory neurotransmitters. The inhibitory neurotransmitter γ-aminobutyric acid (GABA) is found in nonspiny granule cells, which are the most common inhibitory neurons in the cerebral cortex. The two most common excitatory neurotransmitters in the cerebral cortex, glutamate and aspartate, are found in the synaptic terminals of pyramidal and spiny granule neurons. Pyramidal neurons are the cells of origin for the long intracortical and subcortical (e.g., corticostriate, corticopontine, corticospinal) projections. Glutamate and aspartate also are found within the axon terminals of thalamocortical neurons.

Glutamate and *aspartate* are the two most common neurotransmitters in the cerebral cortex

Other neurotransmitters in the cerebral cortex arise from neurons located in remote locations such as the raphe nuclei (serotonin), the locus ceruleus (norepinephrine), the nucleus of Meynert (acetylcholine), and the mesolimbic system (dopamine). These neurotransmitters do not have direct actions on cortical neurons but rather modulate the actions of other neurotransmitters in the cerebral cortex. Serotonergic projections from the raphe nuclei terminate primarily in cortical layers III and IV, which receive thalamic input. For this reason, serotonin is believed to act as an alerting mechanism that sharpens sensory processing by the cerebral cortex. Serotonin also has been implicated in sleep and pain perception. The noradrenergic projections from the locus ceruleus also may play a role in the sleep–wake cycle, but because most noradrenergic terminals are located in the deeper layers of the cerebral cortex system, they are believed to modulate cortical output as well. Widespread regions of the cerebral cortex receive cholinergic projections from the basal nucleus of Meynert, a group of medium and large neurons located beneath the anterior commissure. Because the basal nucleus of Meynert degenerates in patients with Alzheimer's disease, it is possible that acetylcholine plays an important role in higher order processes like learning and memory. Dopaminergic projections from the ventral tegmental area are important for normal cognitive function. Because excessive levels of dopamine may be partly responsible for affective disorders such as schizophrenia, the most effective antipsychotic drugs are dopamine antagonists.

Cortical neurons also contain a variety of neuroactive peptides, including cholecystokinin, vasoactive intestinal polypeptide, neuropeptide Y, somatostatin, substance P, and corticotropin-releasing factor. These peptides, like many of the neurotransmitters described above, modulate the activity of other neurotransmitters in the cerebral cortex.

Lamination

The cerebral cortex varies in thickness from 4 mm in the depths of a sulcus to 2 mm across the crown of a gyrus. Differences in cell type, cell size, and cell-packing density give the cerebral cortex a laminated appearance. It is generally agreed that the neocortex contains six layers of cells while the more primitive allocortex has only three layers.

The **neocortex** consists of six layers.

The six layers of cortex are numbered consecutively from the pial surface (Figure 5-9). Layer I, the molecular layer, is the thin, largely acellular fringe of tissue composed primarily of horizontally oriented axons and apical dendrites derived from cortical and subcortical neurons. Layer II, the external granular layer, consists primarily of small, closely packed granule cells. These neurons typically have short dendritic and axonal processes that form an integral part of the local cortical circuits. Layer III, the external pyramidal layer, is a relatively thick layer dominated by small and medium-size pyramidal cells. Many local intracortical projections originate from layer III while the longer subcortical projections derive from the larger neurons located in layer V. Layer IV, the internal granular layer, consists of densely packed spiny and aspiny granule cells that receive ascending thalamocortical projections. Layer IV also contains a dense plexus of horizontal axons, the external band of Baillarger. In the primary visual cortex the external band of Baillarger, which can be seen in unstained tissue, is called the line of Gennari. Neurons in layer IV project to both superficial (II) and deep (V) cortical layers. Layer V, the internal pyramidal layer, is the primary output layer of the cerebral cortex. Layer V is composed of medium and large pyramidal neurons, including the large Betz cells located in the primary motor cortex. Layer V also is noted for the internal band of Baillarger, a prominent

In the **visual cortex**, the external band of Baillarger is known as the line of Gennari.

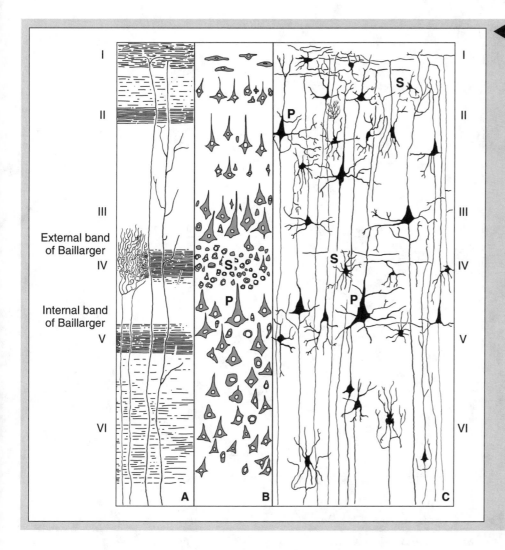

External band
of Baillarger

Internal band
of Baillarger

FIGURE 5-9
Cross Section of the Cerebral Cortex. (A) A myelin stain shows the horizontally and vertically oriented fibers that connect different parts of the cerebral cortex. The internal and external layers of Baillarger are the largest bands of horizontal fibers in the cerebral cortex. (B) A cresyl violet stain binds to the endoplasmic reticulum of the cell bodies. (C) The Golgi stains by permeating the entire neuron, highlighting cell bodies, axons, and dendrites. P = pyramidal neuron; S = stellate neuron. (Source: Reprinted with permission from Ranson SW, et al: The Anatomy of the Nervous System. Philadelphia, PA: W. B. Saunders, 1966, p 437.)

swath of horizontally oriented axon collaterals. Layer VI, the multiform layer, contains an assortment of cell types including pyramidal, granule, and spindle-shaped fusiform cells. Pyramidal cells in layer VI project to the thalamus.

Regional Differences

Despite the general agreement that the cerebral cortex consists of six layers, regional variations in the laminar pattern are common and represent the basis for subdividing the cortex into separate areas. The cytoarchitectonic map of the cerebral cortex proposed by Brodmann in 1909 remains the most widely used partition of the cerebral cortex (Figure 5-10). The underlying assumption of Brodmann was that regional variation in cortical lamination reflects functional heterogeneity. Among the 47 anatomically distinct cortical areas described by Brodmann, about one dozen are used routinely by physicians and scientists to designate areas of the brain whose functions are generally agreed upon (see Table 5-2). Brodmann's classification system has been supplemented but not displaced by more recent descriptions of the connectional, functional, and histochemical organization of the cerebral cortex.

*Some **Brodmann areas** are synonymous with a specific function.*

Columnar Organization

Abundant research has shown that cortical neurons also are arranged into vertical columns. The presence of cortical columns was first revealed in the sensory systems because sensory stimulation is easy to administer and the cortical responses to peripheral stimulation are readily interpretable. It is unclear, however, whether columns are peculiar to sensory cortices or represent a neural blueprint for the entire brain.

*The **cortical column** is the functional unit of the cerebral cortex.*

FIGURE 5-10 ▶

Brodmann Areas. Major cytoarchitectural divisions of the lateral (A) and medial (B) surfaces of the cerebral cortex based on the divisions of Brodmann (1909).

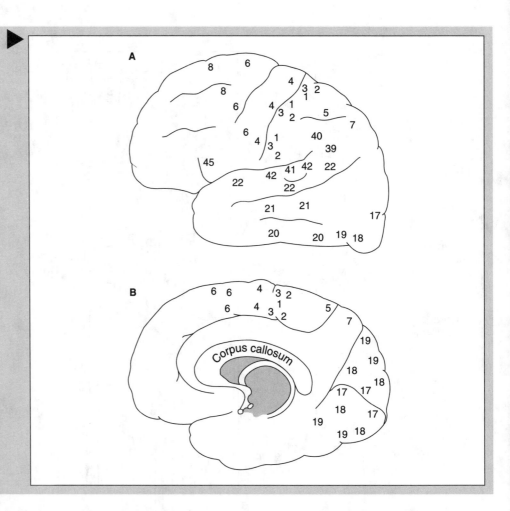

TABLE 5-2 ▶

Selected Brodmann Areas of the Cerebral Cortex

Brodmann Area	Location	Function
17	Banks of calcarine sulcus	Primary visual cortex
18, 19	Medial aspect of occipital lobe	Secondary visual cortex
5, 7	Posterior parietal cortex	Sensory association cortex
3, 1, 2	Postcentral gyrus	Primary somatosensory cortex
4	Precentral gyrus	Primary motor cortex
6	Superior and middle frontal gyri	Premotor cortex
44, 45	Inferior frontal gyri	Speech
41, 42	Superior temporal gyrus	Auditory cortex

The first description of cortical columns was made by Mountcastle, who recorded the stimulus-induced activity of single neurons in the primary somatosensory cortex. Mountcastle discovered that successive neurons encountered by an electrode usually respond to stimulation of one body area (e.g., a single finger) if the electrode is inserted perpendicularly to the pial surface. Electrode penetrations parallel to the pial surface encounter neurons whose receptive fields gradually shift across the periphery. Subsequent research by Hubel and Wiesel in the visual system and Abeles and Goldstein in the auditory system confirmed the generality of this concept. Columns in the primary visual cortex contain neurons that respond to the same part of the visual field and have similar response properties (e.g., eye dominance or orientation). Cortical columns have not been identified in the gustatory or olfactory system, but neither sensory system has been studied thoroughly enough to rule out their existence. In the senses known to have columns, the cerebral cortex contains a map of the peripheral receptor sheet (i.e., the skin, the retina, or inner ear).

Conceptually, a cortical column represents a processing module interposed between specific sets of input and output connections. The complexity of an individual column is astounding, however, because multiple inputs may be integrated and multiple outputs generated. Inputs for a single column may arrive from the thalamus, various brainstem areas (e.g., the raphe nuclei), or other cortical areas. The outputs from an individual cortical column terminate in a variety of subcortical regions while others project to neighboring areas of the cerebral cortex or to corresponding areas of the opposite hemisphere.

Cortical Projections

A high horizontal transection through each hemisphere reveals that the gray matter of the cerebral cortex lies above a thick layer of white matter, the corona radiata (see Chapter 2, Figure 2-7). The myelinated axons of the corona radiata form the interface between the cerebral cortex and the rest of the nervous system. The most superficial fibers of the corona radiata contribute to local intracortical circuits. Fibers located more deeply generally are longer and project greater distances (Figure 5-11). Some interconnect

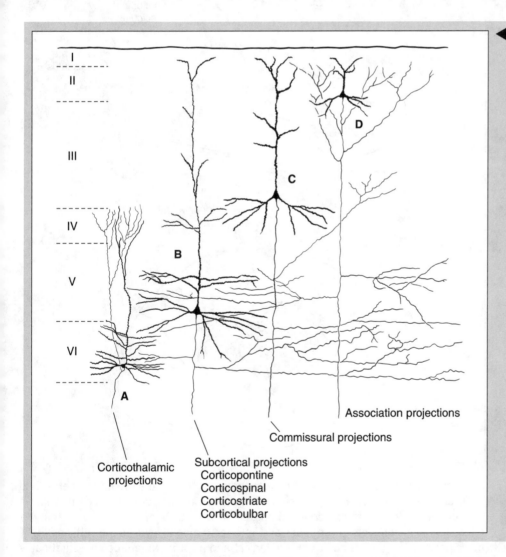

FIGURE 5-11
Laminar Origins of Corticofugal Projections. (Source: *Reprinted with permission from Jones EG: Connectivity of the primate sensory-motor cortex. In* Cerebral Cortex: Sensory-Motor Areas and Aspects of Cortical Connectivity. *Edited by Jones EG, Peters A. New York, NY: Plenum Press, 1986, p 146.)*

different cortical lobes or the two hemispheres; the longest fibers project to subcortical structures as distant as the spinal cord. Based on these projection patterns, cortical projections are classified as association fibers, commissural fibers, or subcortical projection fibers.

Association fibers provide intracortical connections and, depending on their length, are classified as either short or long. Short association fibers are U-shaped because they

*Association fibers are **intra**hemispheric.*

connect adjacent gyri (Figure 5-12). Long association fibers connect different lobes within the same hemisphere. Five of the more notable long association pathways are the uncinate fasciculus, the arcuate fasciculus, the superior and inferior longitudinal fasciculi, and the cingulum. The uncinate fasciculus is a short, curved pathway that connects the inferior and middle temporal gyri with the orbital gyri of the frontal lobe. The arcuate fasciculus projects from the superior temporal gyrus to the middle and inferior frontal gyri. Whereas the uncinate fasciculus carves out a relatively direct pathway between the insula and the temporal lobe, the arcuate fasciculus takes a longer, sweeping trajectory around the insula. The fibers of the superior and inferior longitudinal fasciculi lie close to the arcuate fasciculus but interconnect the parietal and occipital lobes with the frontal and temporal lobes, respectively. The cingulum, which lies buried within the cingulate gyrus, is the primary efferent pathway from the frontal and parietal lobes to the parahippocampal gyrus and adjacent temporal lobe.

FIGURE 5-12 ▶

Intracortical Pathways. *(A) Phantom of the cerebral cortex showing the superior and inferior longitudinal fasciculi, the arcuate fasciculus and the U-shaped fibers of the intracortical pathways. (B) Phantom showing the location of the cingulum relative to the corpus callosum.*

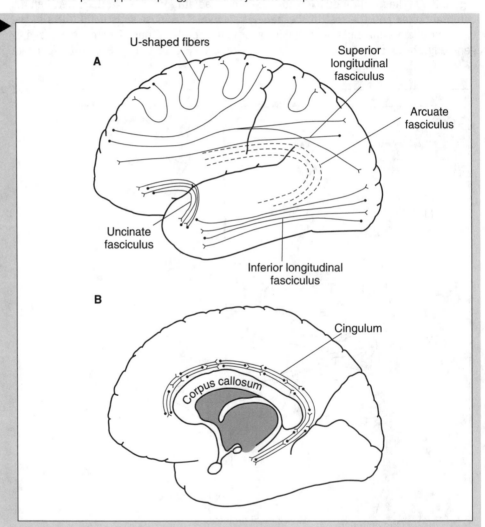

*Commissural fibers are **inter**hemispheric.*

*The **corpus callosum** consists of the rostrum, genu, body, and splenium.*

Commissural pathways connect corresponding regions of the two hemispheres. It is believed that commissural pathways enable the two hemispheres to share information and function as a unit. The anterior commissure, a small band of fibers buried within the telencephalon, connects the middle and inferior temporal gyri of the left and right hemispheres. The corpus callosum, the largest and most important commissural pathway, forms the floor of the longitudinal fissure and the roof of the lateral ventricles (Figure 5-13; see Chapter 2, Figure 2-6). The corpus callosum consists of four parts, the rostrum, genu, body, and splenium. Because the corpus callosum does not extend to the rostral or caudal pole of the brain, callosal fibers from these areas retreat from the poles and cross in the rostrum and splenium, respectively. In horizontal sections these commissural fibers resemble arcs, called the anterior and posterior forceps. The specialized functions of the right and left cerebral hemispheres have been elucidated in patients

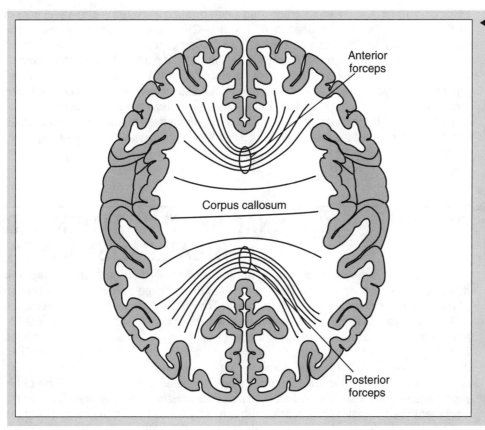

FIGURE 5-13
Anterior and Posterior Forceps of the Corpus Callosum.

whose commissural pathways were severed in order to contain epileptiform activity within one hemisphere.

Projection fibers exit the cerebral cortex and descend to subcortical structures, including the thalamus, the basal ganglia, the brainstem, and the spinal cord. Projection fibers pass through the corona radiata and the internal capsule, a massive tract that descends through the telencephalon before forming the lateral boundary of the diencephalon (Figure 5-14). After the internal capsule passes through the diencephalon, it

Projection fibers *project to subcortical targets.*

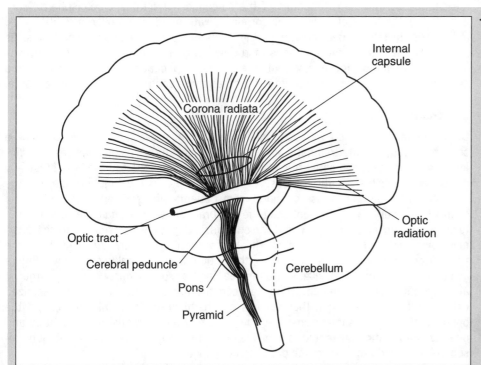

FIGURE 5-14
Corticofugal Pathways. Dissection of the telencephalon reveals the fibers of the corona radiata. As the fibers of the internal capsule exit the telencephalon, it forms the crus cerebri, passes through the mesencephalon, and then forms the pyramidal tract on the ventral surface of the medulla. (Source: Reprinted with permission from Williams PL: Gray's Anatomy, 38th ed. Philadelphia, PA: W. B. Saunders, 1995, p 1177.)

assumes a new name, the crus cerebri, and a new position along the ventrolateral margin of the mesencephalon (see Chapter 4, Figure 4-24). At the caudal boundary of the mesencephalon, the crus cerebri divides into numerous fascicles that burrow through the ventral pons (see Chapter 4, Figure 4-22). During their passage through the pons, the number of these fascicles decreases as projections depart to the pontine (corticopontine) and cranial nerve nuclei (corticobulbar). Near the caudal pons the remaining fascicles coalesce into the compact pyramidal tracts located on the ventral surface of the medulla (see Chapter 4, Figure 4-9). After this arduous trip through the brainstem, the only fibers left in this once majestic pathway are those of the corticospinal tract (see Chapter 4, Figure 4-8).

FUNCTIONAL SPECIALIZATION AND BILATERAL SYMMETRY

The concept of functional specialization within the cerebral cortex dates to antiquity, but it lacked empirical support until 1861 when Paul Broca linked damage to a small region of the frontal cortex with an inability to speak. The concept of functional specialization within the cortex was bolstered by the discovery of specific sensory and motor areas related to the contralateral side of the body. It would be a mistake, however, to view the cerebral cortex as a patch quilt of compartments dedicated to minute motor skills, sensory attributes, or personality traits.

Broca's rule states that language is located in the left hemisphere of right-handed individuals.

Broca's discovery that speech functions were located in the left hemisphere of his right-handed patient suggested that the two cerebral hemispheres are not functionally equivalent despite their apparent anatomic similarity. While the differences between the two hemispheres are striking for language, for most other skills the two hemispheres are essentially the same.

The discovery of functional asymmetries between the two hemispheres naturally led to one hemisphere being designated as the dominant one. To this day, handedness is used to designate the dominant hemisphere. According to Broca, the left hemisphere controls the right hand and language. Despite its widespread use, the notion of a dominant hemisphere is antiquated, inadequate, and often inaccurate. The concept of hemispheric dominance arose when neuroscientists lacked the sophistication to identify the subtle but important functions of the so-called nondominant hemisphere. More importantly, the locus of language is correlated with handedness only in right-handed individuals; in left-handed individuals the relationship approaches chance levels. As more is learned about the functions of the so-called nondominant hemisphere, this nomenclature may disappear along with the obvious implication that the functions of the nondominant hemisphere are less important than those controlled by the dominant side.

Split-Brain

Our understanding of how various functions are lateralized in the cerebral cortex have come from patients with traumatic brain injury, clinical studies using noninvasive brain-imaging techniques, and patients whose left and right hemispheres have been surgically disconnected for therapeutic reasons. All three have provided valuable insight but the most definitive data are those obtained from patients with severed interhemispheric connections. Surgical disconnection of the cerebral hemispheres, called a commissurotomy, is the procedure of last resort for epileptic patients whose seizures resist pharmacologic control. A commissurotomy involves sectioning the corpus callosum and the anterior and hippocampal commissures; the optic chiasm typically is not cut. While a commissurotomy prevents seizures from spreading from one hemisphere to the other, it also prevents neural communication between the hemispheres. In a commissurized patient, sensory information that reaches one hemisphere is unable to cross to the opposite side. Thus, somatosensory, visual, auditory and perhaps even gustatory and olfactory information presented to one side of the body would reach one cerebral hemisphere but would not cross to the opposite hemisphere.

Roger Sperry, whose pioneering work on commissurized patients earned him the Nobel Prize, has given us tremendous insight into how different skills are lateralized within the brain. In a typical experiment, a visual image is projected onto the half of a patient's visual field, which projects to the opposite hemisphere (Figure 5-15A). In order for the patient to describe that image verbally, the information must be transmitted to the language areas, which in most right-handed individuals, are located in the left hemisphere. When the commissural fibers are intact, the two hemispheres readily share this visual information. Following section of the corpus callosum, images presented to the lateral part of the visual field of the left eye reach the right hemisphere but not the left hemisphere, which leaves the patient unable to describe the object verbally (Figure 5-15B). If the same image were presented to the medial part of the visual field of the right eye, the commissurotomy would be irrelevant because this visual information does not pass through the corpus callosum on its way to the visual and language areas of the left hemisphere (Figures 5-15C and D).

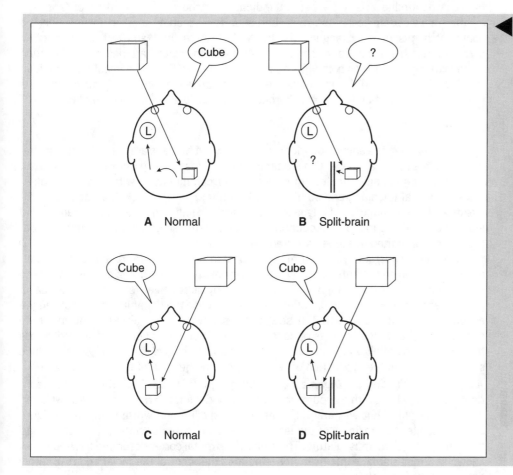

A Normal   **B** Split-brain   **C** Normal   **D** Split-brain

◀ *FIGURE 5-15*
Hemispheric Transfer Following Commissurotomy. *(A) The visual image of a cube shone into the nasal half of the left eye is processed by the right occipital lobe. After the information is transferred to the left hemisphere, the patient is able to report verbally that the object was a cube. (B) Following a commissurotomy, visual information that ascends to the right hemisphere does not reach the language areas in the left hemisphere. In this case, the commissurized patient is unable to describe the stimulus verbally. (C), (D) When the visual image of a cube is shone into the nasal half of the right eye, both the normal and commissurized patient are able to identify the stimulus verbally.*

Hemispheric Dominance

Studies on commissurized patients have shown that the most profound interhemispheric differences are in the association areas rather than in the primary sensory or motor areas of the cortex. In addition, the degree to which skills are lateralized to one hemisphere is related to handedness. Most skills in right-handed individuals are strongly, but not completely, lateralized; in left-handed and ambidextrous individuals, on the other hand, there is better balance between the two hemispheres. For this reason, accurate generalizations about hemispheric specialization can be made only for right-handed individuals (approximately 88% of the population).

As a rule, the left hemisphere in right-handed persons is specialized for the comprehension and production of language, analysis of temporal order and duration, and symbolic representation. Thus, the left hemisphere is better-suited for sequential analysis of sensory information that retains its importance as discrete items. For example, words retain their individuality, even when embedded in a stream that forms a sentence. The right hemisphere, by comparison, is more holistic. The right hemisphere is specialized for perception of space, synthesis of sensory information into a new unified form (e.g., music, form, color, faces), and perception and expression of emotion. The motor aspects of language (i.e., speech, writing) are strongly lateralized to the left hemisphere, while its emotive components are located primarily in the corresponding area of the right hemisphere. Cerebral dominance is determined by genetic and environmental (i.e., in utero) factors.

In right-handed individuals, there is a strong but not perfect relationship between handedness and language. In non–right-handed individuals (i.e., those who are left-handed or ambidextrous) predictions about the location of language approach chance levels. Despite this uncertainty, the locus of language expression must be determined prior to neurosurgical procedures involving the temporal lobe or inferior frontal cortex. Because handedness is not a perfect indicator for the cortical location of language another more certain technique must be used. The accepted method for locating the dominant hemisphere for language is the Wada test. In the Wada test, a short-acting barbiturate such as amobarbital is injected into one of the carotid arteries. As the injection is made, the patient raises both arms and begins counting. When the injection is made in the artery ipsilateral to the language area, the contralateral arm falls and counting is interrupted; an injection in the other carotid artery has no effect on the verbal task.

Language

Communication in the animal kingdom is common, but humans are the only species that communicates with language. Other animals such as insects (e.g., bees, termites), fish, birds, and nonhuman primates (monkeys, apes) communicate with chemical (pheromones), visual (display), and auditory (barks, chirps, calls) signals that lack the complexity of human language. Language is creative, virtually unlimited in its range, and independent of the mode of production and comprehension; animal communication, besides being limited in scope, is stereotypic in form.

Without a satisfactory animal model, research on the central organization of language has relied on patients who have suffered some type of neurologic accident. These studies have shown that language is controlled by subcortical (e.g., thalamus, basal ganglia) and cortical structures. Patients with damage to the thalamus and basal ganglia are often mute, but the roles that these structures play in language are not known. At the cortical level, language consists of cognitive and motor components distributed across the temporal, parietal, and frontal lobes. Focal cortical lesions in these regions produce specific deficits in the production of language, comprehension of language, or both.

Aphasias and the Cortical Organization of Language. In 1863, Paul Broca described a right-handed patient with a circumscribed lesion in the left inferior frontal gyrus who had difficulty speaking but was able to comprehend spoken and written language (Figure 5-16). Despite the proximity of the lesion to the primary motor cortex, this patient had full control of his oral musculature. The area in the frontal cortex described by Broca, now known as Broca's area, contains motor templates that control the facial and respiratory components of speech.

In 1874, Carl Wernicke separated language into motor and cognitive components. Wernicke reported that damage to the temporal lobe interferes with language comprehension but not the ability to speak. The language comprehension area, now known as Wernicke's area, includes the posterior aspect of the temporal lobe and part of the inferior parietal lobule (see Figure 5-16). Projections from the visual, auditory, and somatosensory cortices to Wernicke's area enable written, spoken, and tactile (e.g., Braille) signals to be interpreted for linguistic content. Wernicke's area interprets sensory symbols that have linguistic meaning. For example, the symbols "B-U-G" should conjure up images and definitions of insects. Other areas of the brain that associate insects with descriptive (brown, crawly) and emotional (disgusting, infectious) labels create a detailed image laced with the appropriate emotional tone. Other arbitrary symbols (e.g., ☺ , ♦ , ⌂ , ↗) that have no meaning, do not generate images or stir memories. Following damage to Wernicke's area, words and sounds that should have meaning lie stranded within the sensory cortex along with other meaningless symbols.

The language deficits associated with damage to Broca's area and Wernicke's area

Hemispheric specialization, even in right-handed individuals, is relative rather than absolute.

*We speak with the **left hemisphere.***

Broca's area is located on the inferior frontal gyrus of most right-handed individuals.

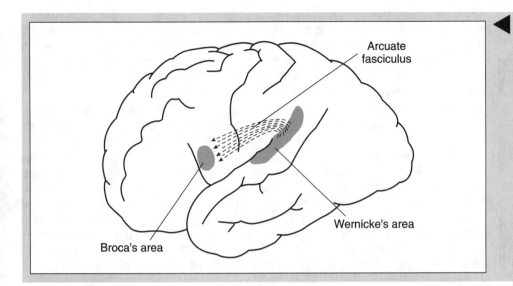

FIGURE 5-16
Cortical Organization of Language. The arcuate fasciculus, which courses around the perimeter of the insula, connects the language areas in the parietal (Wernicke's area) and frontal (Broca's area) lobes.

are strikingly different. Broca's aphasia is characterized by slow, labored, and poorly articulated speech. Sentences are telegraphic, that is, they include nouns and attributes of objects at the expense of small words such as "is" and "if." Patients with Broca's aphasia also have difficulty writing. Because their speech is labored and technically poor, Broca's aphasia is considered a nonfluent aphasia.

Broca's aphasia is a nonfluent aphasia.

In Wernicke's aphasia, speech is effortless with well-preserved rhythm and melody. Speech may be a little more rapid than normal and have normal grammatical structure, but comprehension is poor and accompanied by severe reading and writing disabilities. Patients who have trouble finding the right word may compensate by making up words (neologisms), substituting one word for another (paraphasia), or creating a meaningless word salad (jargon aphasia). Patients with Wernicke's aphasia are noteworthy for their fluent speech but lack of comprehension.

Wernicke's aphasia is a fluent aphasia.

Damage to the arcuate fasciculus, the pathway that connects Wernicke's area with Broca's area, causes a conduction aphasia. Patients with conduction aphasias are fluent and comprehension is good because both Broca's area and Wernicke's area are intact. Naming is severely impaired, and there is some word substitution; writing, spelling, reading aloud are severely impaired (see Figure 5-16).

Wernicke's description of language as a serial process is both simplistic and incomplete, but nevertheless, remains credible because it accounts for many of the language and speech disorders observed in the clinic.

Central Correlates of Language. The constellation of symptoms described by Broca have been described previously; Broca's lasting contribution to this field was the link he forged between left hemispheric control of language and right-handedness. The lateralization of language has several neuroanatomic correlates, but the most pronounced is the size of the planum temporale (PT). The PT is a wedge-shaped area at the caudal end of the superior temporal gyrus that includes part of Wernicke's area (Figure 5-17). The PT is

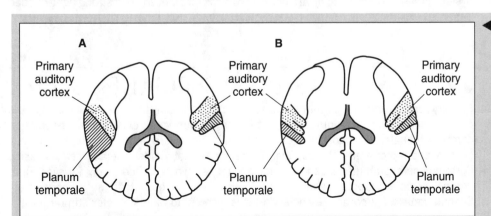

FIGURE 5-17
Superior Surface of the Temporal Lobe Exposed by Dissection. The planum temporale (PT) is located posterior to the primary auditory cortex. (A) In the normal brain, the left PT is significantly larger than the right PT. (B) In dyslexic patients, the PTs of the left and right hemispheres are nearly equal in size.

larger on the left side in 89% of the population and, on average, is 40% larger than the right side; in extreme cases, the left PT may be 10 times larger. Enlargement of the PT in the left hemisphere is accompanied by lengthening of the Sylvian fissure. The larger size of the left PT is accompanied by a higher concentration of choline O-acetyltransferase, which suggests a high level of neural activity. Broca's area and the angular gyrus (Brodmann area 39) also are larger on the left side.

Dyslexia. The hallmarks of developmental dyslexia are an inability to read proficiently and an impaired directional sense. Developmental dyslexia is a diagnosis of exclusion, which means that a reading disorder is attributed to dyslexia after all other neurologic, motivational, and sociologic causes have been ruled out. The incidence of developmental dyslexia is about 3%. Postmortem examination of the brains of dyslexic individuals has shown both gross and microscopic abnormalities within the PT and auditory cortex on the left side. At the gross level, the left and right PTs are symmetrical in size, unlike normal brains where the left PT is noticeably larger. The PT of dyslexic patients also may show micropolygyria and thinning of the parietal corpus callosum, which connects the left and right PTs. At the microscopic level, the planum temporale and inferior frontal gyrus (Broca's area) have dysplasic (abnormal) lamination and ectopic (misplaced) cell groups.

Albert Galaburda of Harvard has suggested that dyslexia, left-handedness, cortical symmetry, and certain immune disorders are caused by in utero mutagenesis induced by endogenous testosterone. Although the evidence for this view is circumstantial, it is appealing because it explains the high correlation of these seemingly unrelated phenomena, which are more prevalent in males. According to Galaburda, testosterone prevents the left hemisphere from reaching its normal, exaggerated size by delaying its maturation. This delay also makes the left hemisphere vulnerable to in utero mutagenic agents, such as testosterone. The right hemisphere, by maturing earlier, would have a briefer period of vulnerability. Dyslexic patients have a higher incidence of micropolygyria and microscopic abnormalities in left hemispheric language areas than in corresponding areas in the right hemisphere. These pathologic changes are seldom observed in nondyslexic patients.

Plasticity of Language. Recovery of language function following an infarct of the middle cerebral artery or resection of a tumor varies tremendously between individuals. Because language in most right-handed individuals is strongly lateralized, a stroke in the dominant hemisphere is likely to produce a severe and irreversible language deficit.

Although a bilateral representation for language may predispose otherwise healthy people to dyslexia, it may provide a neural substrate for recovery of language function following damage to the dominant hemisphere. Normally, language functions resident in the nondominant hemisphere are suppressed by the dominant side. Following damage to the dominant side, however, the normally silent hemisphere is released from this suppression and begins to "speak." This interpretation is consistent with the observation that dyslexic and non–right-handed stroke patients, whose language skills are often represented bilaterally, show better recovery following a stroke than right-handed patients. Because the tendency for language to be located bilaterally extends to right-handed individuals who either are dyslexic or have relatives who are non–right-handed or dyslexic, these patients also have a better prognosis for recovery than strong right-handed patients.

> *Cortical asymmetry* is the norm, not the exception.

> *Dyslexia* is defined as left-right confusion and a failure to read with normal proficiency.

> *Micropolygyria* are numerous pathologically small gyri that lack normal lamination.

> *Dyslexia* is associated with **left-handedness, diabetes, rheumatoid arthritis,** and **ulcerative colitis**.

> *Left-handed* and *dyslexic individuals* have better recovery of language function than *right-handed, nondyslexic* individuals.

ASSOCIATION CORTEX

Primary sensory and motor cortices constitute about 25% of the total surface area of the cerebral cortex; the remaining 75% of the cortical surface is classified as association cortex. Although tremendous strides have been made toward understanding the primary sensory and motor areas, the association areas have not yielded their secrets as easily. Certain general statements can be made about the association cortices, however. First, cortical association areas receive and elaborate on the output of the primary areas. Second, neurons in cortical association areas respond to more complex stimuli. Lastly, damage to association cortex produces more complex deficits than seen following damage to primary sensory or motor areas. For example, damage to association cortex may not interfere with sensory processing per se but rather with the ability to use that information to interact with the environment. These deficits, which take many forms, are classified as agnosias and apraxias. An agnosia is an inability to recognize or attach meaning to an object despite the patient having normal intellect, memory, and visual, auditory, and somesthetic abilities. An apraxia is an inability to engage in purposeful movement that cannot be attributed to motor paralysis or sensory loss, per se.

*An **agnosia** is an inability to recognize familiar objects through the senses of touch, vision, or hearing.*

Parietal Lobe

The parietal lobe can be divided on functional grounds into anterior and posterior parts. The anterior part, which is located along the postcentral gyrus, contains the primary somatosensory cortex (Brodmann areas 3, 1, and 2; see Chapter 6). The association areas within the posterior parietal lobe are located in the inferior and superior parietal lobules. The inferior parietal lobule, which consists of the supramarginal (Brodmann area 40) and angular (Brodmann area 39) gyri, forms part of Wernicke's area, whose role in language comprehension was discussed in the previous section. The superior parietal lobule, Brodmann areas 5 and 7, is located immediately posterior to the primary somatosensory cortex and superior to the inferior parietal lobule. The superior parietal lobule assembles somatosensory, auditory, and visual information from the adjacent regions of the parietal, temporal, and occipital lobes, respectively, into complex multimodal percepts of our immediate extrapersonal space. Ultimately, this spatial map is used by the motor system to coordinate movement within our extrapersonal space. Although both lobules are responsible for higher order processing of sensory information, their projections to the frontal cortex help initiate motor behavior.

*The **inferior parietal lobule** has a role in language comprehension.*

*The **superior parietal lobule** organizes extrapersonal space.*

Neurophysiologic experiments in monkeys and clinical observations in human patients have provided a two-tiered understanding of the function of the parietal association cortex. Single neurons in the superior parietal lobule respond when a monkey actively engages objects within the environment. For example, neurons respond when a monkey reaches for or grasps an object or visually tracks a moving object. Passive manipulation of the hand or arm, which would activate neurons in the primary somatosensory cortex, is ineffective in the superior parietal cortex. Thus, neurons within the superior parietal lobule respond to behaviorally relevant stimuli that are actively engaged within the immediate extrapersonal space. The data from human patients suggest that the superior parietal lobule acts as a liaison between sensory perception and motor execution. In general, patients with damage to the superior parietal lobule on the nondominant side not only fail to engage the local environment, but also ignore it. Patients with sensory neglect ignore objects that enter the contralateral space and, in extreme cases, will deny ownership of their contralateral limbs. Not surprisingly, these patients have trouble dressing themselves (dressing apraxia) and copying pictures (constructional apraxia). Their portrayals of other inanimate objects such as clocks and flowers are similarly affected (Figure 5-18). Some patients with apraxias are able to identify an object (e.g., a comb or spoon), but they are unable to use the object properly. Sensory neglect of the contralateral body space, or asomatognosia, occurs more often following damage to the right (i.e., nondominant) hemisphere. For this reason, it is believed that the right parietal lobe may attend to the environment on both the left and right sides while the left hemisphere attends only to the contralateral side.

*Patients with damage to the **superior parietal lobule of the right hemisphere** may not interact with their immediate extrapersonal space.*

Gerstmann's syndrome, characterized by damage to the angular gyrus in the dominant hemisphere, is marked by left-right confusion, an inability to perform simple arithmetic calculations (acalculia), an inability to write down thoughts (agraphia), and an inability to name fingers (finger agnosia; Table 5-3). Damage further posteriorly at the parieto-occipital border produces Balint's syndrome in which patients are unable to use visual guidance to grasp an object. These patients retain their ability to make spontaneous or reflexive eye movements, but lack the ability to gaze at a target on command. Balint's syndrome also illustrates how the parietal lobe allows us to engage our immediate extrapersonal space.

***Gerstmann's syndrome** is caused by damage to the supramarginal gyrus.*

FIGURE 5-18 ▶
Drawings of a Clock Face and Flower by a Patient with Sensory Neglect. *The model appears on the left and the patient's copy on the right. Note that the patient has squeezed all twelve numbers of the clock face onto the right side. Similarly, the patient's drawing of the flower has petals only on the right side.*

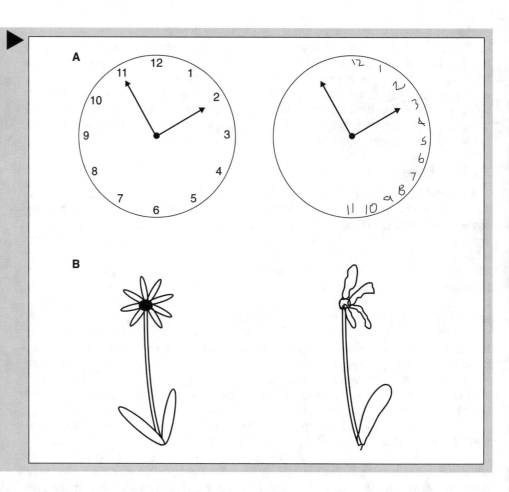

TABLE 5-3 ▶
Association Cortex Deficits

Disorder	Deficit
Abulia: from the Greek meaning "no will or drive"	General slowing of the intellect
Acalculia: from the Latin meaning "no calculations"	Simple arithmetic calculations
Achromatopsia: from the Greek meaning "no color"	Color discrimination
Agnosia: from the Greek meaning "lack of knowledge"	Object recognition
Agraphia: from the Greek meaning "no writing"	Writing letters or words
Alexia: from the Greek meaning "no reading"	Reading
Anosognosia: from the Greek meaning "no knowledge of disease"	Denial of disease
Apraxia: from the Greek meaning "lack of action"	Familiar, purposeful movements
Asomatognosia: from the Greek meaning "no knowledge about the body"	Sensory and motor neglect
Prosopagnosia: from the Greek meaning "no knowledge of faces"	Facial recognition

Temporal Lobe

The temporal lobe contains the primary auditory cortex, higher order auditory and visual cortices, and primitive cortical areas that work in conjunction with the hippocampal formation in memory acquisition.

The higher order visual association areas of the temporal lobe represent a rostral extension of the visual areas located in the occipital lobe. The analysis of the visual images, which began in the retina, is completed in the visual association areas of the temporal and parietal lobes. Both laboratory and clinical data demonstrate that sophisticated visual analysis takes place in the temporal lobe. For example, neurons located in the inferior temporal lobe of the monkey respond when the subject is shown a picture of a face. These "face-neurons" are less responsive to other visual stimuli whose shape or luminance resembles the effective face stimulus. Similarly, the effectiveness of a stimulus is reduced if the facial features are inverted, obscured, or scrambled. The faces that prove to be most effective stimuli are "generic faces," that is, they have all of the features of a face but do not depict specific or familiar people. If neurons in the temporal lobe play a role in facial recognition, one might predict that temporal lobe damage in humans would interfere with the ability to recognize faces. This disorder, known as prosopagnosia, is a form of object agnosia caused by damage to Brodmann areas 20 and 21, which include the lateral aspect of the temporal lobe and the occipitotemporal gyrus on the ventral surface of the brain. Although prosopagnosia usually is caused by a lesion in the right temporal lobe, it may accompany unilateral damage to the left hemisphere. Patients with prosopagnosia are unable to recognize their own friends and family; in extreme cases, they may not recognize themselves. In other forms of object agnosia patients may experience difficulty distinguishing among the members of other classes, such as groups of houses, cars, or boats. Some patients with object agnosias can compensate for their specific deficit if cues from other sensory modalities are available. A patient unable to recognize the face of a friend, for example, may be able to identify that person by voice, clothes, or gait. Another agnosia associated with damage to the occipitotemporal region is achromatopsia, an inability to discriminate between colors. Achromatopsia should not be confused with color blindness, which is caused by lack of one or more visual pigments in the retina. Patients with achromatopsia are unable to attribute meaning to color and thus are unable to utilize color cues.

> *Prosopagnosia* is an inability to recognize faces.

The medial inferior aspect of the temporal lobe, which includes the parahippocampal gyrus, acts as a staging area for sensory information bound for the underlying hippocampal formation. Damage to these areas impairs acquisition of new memories but leaves retrieval of existing memories relatively unimpaired. The role of the parahippocampal gyrus and the hippocampal formation is discussed in Chapter 13.

Frontal Lobe

As the previous sections have shown, the parietal, temporal, and occipital cortices are concerned with the reception and interpretation of sensory information. The frontal lobe defies simple descriptive labels, in part, because it has such a complex pattern of reciprocal connections with the rest of the brain. In general, the frontal lobe is intimately involved with higher order thought processes, personality, and planning and execution of behavior.

On functional grounds, the frontal lobe consists of motor and association areas. The smaller motor region is located within Brodmann areas 4, 6, and 8 in the caudal half of the frontal lobe. These motor areas are critically important for initiation and execution of skilled movements (see Chapter 11). The association areas, by comparison, contribute to distinctly human activities such as planning, memory, problem-solving ability, and proper social conduct. Although research on nonhuman primates has provided some insight into the function of prefrontal cortex, the most revealing data have come from clinical cases involving traumatic injury, disease, or neurosurgical intervention.

The association areas of the frontal lobe, known as prefrontal cortex, consist of ventromedial, superomedial, and dorsolateral parts.

The ventromedial area encompasses all of the orbital cortex and part of the medial surface of the frontal lobe. Damage to the ventromedial area produces profound changes in mood and affect and may trigger impulsive and improper behavior. The first major insight into the function of the prefrontal area was provided by Phineas T. Gage, a railroad worker whose unfortunate accident in 1848 has earned him a permanent position in the annals of neurology. Mr. Gage was a railroad foreman entrusted with setting the charge used to blast the right of way through the stony Vermont countryside. Setting the charge involved pouring gunpowder into a predrilled hole, covering it with sand, and compressing it with the flat end of a tamping iron. One day as Mr. Gage bent over a blasting hole and tamped the powder into place, the charge ignited prematurely, propelling the tamping iron

> Damage to the *ventromedial part of the frontal lobe* causes changes in mood and affect.

out of the hole. The tamping rod pierced Mr. Gage's face just below the cheek bone, drove through the left eye orbit and into the cranial vault before exiting the top of his skull (Figure 5-19). Mr. Gage survived this accident, but his personality was permanently altered. Prior to the accident Mr. Gage was serious, intelligent, conscientious, and polite; afterwards, he was impatient, childish, crude, and irresponsible.

FIGURE 5-19 ▶
Drawing of Phineas Gage's Skull with the Tamping Iron Shown as It Passed Through His Skull. The most severe damage was sustained by the left frontal lobe and the orbital gyri. Because Mr. Gage's language functions remained unimpaired, it would appear that Broca's area was not seriously damaged.

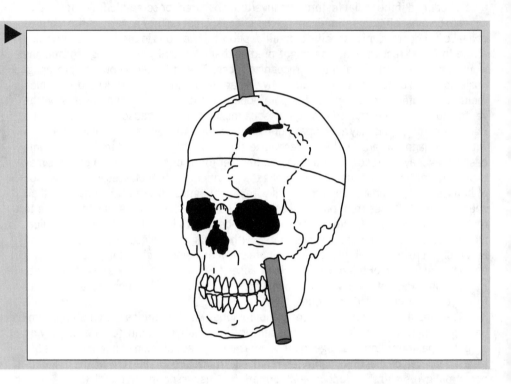

*Damage to the **superior medial part of the frontal lobe** impairs recognition of emotional tone.*

Other clinical cases since have confirmed that damage to the frontal lobe causes flattened affect as well as a loss of social inhibition and initiative. In addition to these changes in personality, patients with frontal lobe damage typically are unable to plan a course of action, despite having normal intellect, memory, and sensory-motor function. Frontal lobe damage neutralizes pain, that is, patients report that they can feel pain, but they are relieved of the suffering. This constellation of symptoms is now referred to as the frontal lobe syndrome.

These clinical data, together with several lesion experiments in nonhuman primates, prompted Egas Moniz to suggest that frontal lobotomies could be used to treat psychiatric disorders (e.g., depression, anxiety) and intractable pain in human patients. The first frontal lobotomies were performed in the 1940s. Later, a less radical surgery, the prefrontal leucotomy was introduced, which severed the afferent and efferent connections between the frontal cortex and the MD nucleus of the thalamus and the cingulate gyrus. Both surgeries achieved the desired effects but left the patients withdrawn and without sufficient initiative and drive to lead independent and productive lives. The use of lobotomies and leucotomies waned in the late 1950s, in part because newly discovered tranquilizers proved to be safer, more effective, and more acceptable treatments for psychiatric disorders.

The superior medial area is an important site for personal characteristics such as introversion and extroversion. Our ability to comprehend the emotional tone of others and generate appropriate emotions of our own reside in the superior medial region. Patients with damage to this area may lack the proper level of arousal and alertness to initiate behavior, a condition referred to as abulia. Patients with damage to the superior medial area also may be unable to adapt their behavior to changing task conditions. This phenomenon, called perseveration, has been studied extensively in monkeys with focal lesions in the superior medial prefrontal cortex. These monkeys are taught a task, lesioned, and then retested with the same task. Their performance on the task is not affected by the lesion, but if the task is changed so that the monkeys must adopt a new strategy, they perseverate with the old, now maladaptive strategy. The dorsolateral pre-frontal cortex is poorly understood, but damage in this area is known to impair creative thinking.

RESOLUTION OF CLINICAL CASE

The paramedics' diagnosis of a stroke involving the right middle cerebral artery was correct, but they incorrectly concluded that the patient was paralyzed. In fairness to the paramedics, a correct diagnosis in this case would have required much more time with the patient than typically available in the field. This patient exhibited the classic symptoms of asomatognosia or sensory neglect. Patients with asomatognosia are unable to move their limbs on one side of the body, not because they are paralyzed but because they do not recognize that the limbs are theirs. Similarly, they do not report somatosensory stimulation applied to that side of their body. In this case the patient suffered a stroke of the right middle cerebral artery, which supplies the posterior parietal cortex. Sensory neglect of the left side of the body ensued.

REVIEW QUESTIONS

Directions: For each of the following questions, choose the **one best** answer.

1. Patients with damage in Wernicke's area can be expected to

    (A) demonstrate a nonfluent aphasia because they are unable to select the proper words

    (B) be unable to hum a melody

    (C) demonstrate a fluent aphasia if Broca's area is intact

    (D) maintain their ability to comprehend words spoken or read but are unable to arrange a sentence and speak smoothly

    (E) have labored, telegraphic speech

2. A neurosurgeon is considering neurosurgical intervention on a 31-year-old right-handed male epileptic patient. Which of the following results from the Wada test would allow the surgeon to conclude that language in this patient is not located in the hemisphere that controls his preferred hand?

    (A) The patient is unable to speak following injection of the right carotid artery

    (B) The patient is unable to speak following injection of the left carotid artery

    (C) Injection of the left carotid artery produces paralysis of the right arm

    (D) Injection of the left carotid artery produces paralysis of the left arm

    (E) The patient is unable to sing following injection of the right carotid artery

3. Patients with damage to the prefrontal cortex

    (A) have flattened affect

    (B) are unable to recognize faces of familiar people

    (C) are color blind

    (D) neglect objects in their immediate extrapersonal space

    (E) may recognize a nail file but be unable to use it

4. The most important structure for understanding the spatial organization of the various thalamic nuclei is the

    (A) pulvinar

    (B) reticular nucleus

    (C) ventroposteromedial nucleus (VPM)

    (D) internal medullary lamina

    (E) anterior thalamic nucleus

5. Which of the following pathways connects corresponding areas of the left and right hemispheres?

    (A) Superior longitudinal fasciculus

    (B) Uncinate fasciculus

    (C) Internal capsule

    (D) Anterior commissure

    (E) Cingulum

6. Which of the following disorders is characterized by an inability to recognize faces?

(A) Gerstmann's syndrome

(B) Broca's aphasia

(C) Prosopagnosia

(D) Asomatognosia

(E) Balint's syndrome

ANSWERS AND EXPLANATIONS

1. The answer is C. The hallmark of Wernicke's aphasia is that the patient remains fluent, provided the damage does not spread into Broca's area. Patients with Wernicke's aphasia lose their ability to comprehend spoken or written language. The ability to hum a tune is not related to damage in Wernicke's area.

2. The answer is A. Because language functions are located in the left hemisphere of most right-handed individuals, a patient with crossed language dominance would have language located in the right hemisphere. An inability to speak following injection of the right carotid artery would indicate that language was located in the right hemisphere. Paralysis of the right arm would take place following injection of the left carotid artery, but it would not indicate the presence of a crossed language dominance. An inability to speak following injection of the left carotid artery would refute the assertion of a crossed language dominance, not support it. Injection of the left carotid artery would not paralyze the left arm under any circumstances. An inability to sing following injection of the right carotid artery also would suggest that language was located in the left hemisphere.

3. The answer is A. Patients with damage to the prefrontal cortex have flattened affect as well as poor problem-solving skills, memory, and social graces. Patients with prosopagnosia have trouble identifying faces following damage to the lateral and ventral surfaces of the temporal lobe. Cortically mediated color blindness (achromatopsia) also may be caused by damage to the ventral aspect of the temporal lobe. Parietal lobe damage in the nondominant hemisphere may cause sensory neglect or apraxias.

4. The answer is D. The internal medullary lamina is the most useful thalamic landmark because it divides the thalamus into medial and lateral sections and serves as a landmark for estimating the anterior-posterior position. The pulvinar, nucleus VPM, and the anterior thalamic nuclei are local landmarks that do not organize the thalamus along any dimension. The reticular nucleus is not a very useful landmark because its shape remains virtually unchanged from one end of the thalamus to the other.

5. The answer is D. The superior longitudinal fasciculus, uncinate fasciculus, and cingulum are intrahemispheric association pathways. The internal capsule links the cerebral cortex to multiple subcortical areas located on the same side of the brain.

6. The answer is C. Prosopagnosia is an inability to recognize familiar faces. Patients with Gerstmann's syndrome are unable to perform simple arithmetic calculations, cannot write down their thoughts or name their fingers, and have left-right confusions. Broca's aphasia is a nonfluent aphasia caused by damage to the inferior frontal gyrus of the dominant hemisphere, usually the left. Lesions of the parietal lobe of the nondominant hemisphere cause asomatognosia—sensory neglect of the left side of the body. Patients with Balint's syndrome are able to make spontaneous eye movements but cannot direct their gaze to a target on command.

ADDITIONAL READING

Abeles M, Goldstein MH Jr: Functional architecture in cat primary auditory cortex: columnar organization and organization according to depth. *J Neurophysiol* 33:172–187, 1970.

Annett M: Laterality and types of dyslexia. *Neurosci Biobehav Rev 20*: 631–636, 1996.

Brodmann K: Vergleichende Lokalisation lehre der Grosshirnrinde in *ihren Prinzipien dargestellt auf Grund des Zellenbaunes.* Leipzig, Germany: J. A. Barth, 1909, p 324.

Damasio H: The return of Phineas Gage: clues about the brain from the skull of a famous patient. *Science* 264:1102–1105, 1994.

Hubel DH, Wiesel TN: Receptive fields, binocular interaction, and functional architecture in the cat's visual cortex. *J Physiol* 160:106–154, 1962.

Mountcastle VB: Modality and topographic properties of single neurons of cat's somatic sensory cortex. *J Neurophysiol* 20:408–434, 1957.

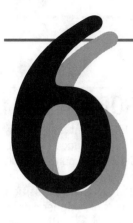

6 SOMESTHESIS

CHAPTER OUTLINE

INTRODUCTION OF CLINICAL CASE

A 45-year-old woman with severe face pain was examined at the pain clinic. She experienced recurrent episodes of intense, stabbing pain in the center of her left cheek. These attacks usually occurred three or four times a day, and each episode would last for at least 10 minutes. The pain had a sharp, searing quality and was accompanied by involuntary twitching movements in the maxillary part of her face. These attacks had a sudden onset and could be triggered by eating or by touching the center of her cheek. She was careful not to touch this part of her face and would not let the physician touch this area either. To prevent triggering these attacks, the woman minimized her facial movements by not smiling and would skip meals to avoid chewing movements. In fact, she had lost 25 lbs in the last 6 months, and her weight was in the bottom quartile for someone of her age and height. Despite this significant loss of weight, the woman was generally healthy, and a dental examination indicated that her teeth and gums were free of disease.

INTRODUCTION TO THE SOMATOSENSORY SYSTEM

The somatosensory system is responsible for detecting all stimuli that contact the body. Thus, it mediates the sensations of touch and temperature that are produced by innocuous stimuli contacting the skin. It also mediates the sensations of pain that are produced by injury or disease. Finally, the somatosensory system also responds to skeletal movements and mediates the kinesthetic sensations that signal limb position.

To perform these tasks, the somatosensory system has thousands of peripheral nerve fibers that convey somatic information into the central nervous system (CNS). The peripheral components of the somatosensory system include all of the general somatic afferent nerves that innervate the skin, muscles, and joints. Somatosensory nerve fibers also supply the meninges, the surfaces of the nasal and oral cavities, and many organs in the thoracic and abdominal viscera. These afferent nerve fibers project to specific nuclei in the spinal cord and brainstem that, in turn, project to the forebrain.

The dorsal column–medial lemniscal system conveys tactile and kinesthetic information, and it is segregated from the anterolateral system, which conveys pain and temperature information. These two systems were described in Chapters 3 and 4. This chapter completes the discussion of these systems and their relationship to cutaneous sensation and pain. Although the peripheral receptors and nerves and the central pathways that convey information from the muscles and tendons to the cerebellum are considered part of the somatosensory system, the cerebellar pathways and their inputs do not mediate conscious sensations and are not discussed here.

SKIN FUNCTIONS

The skin, or integument, is a major organ of the body. The skin has an area ranging from 1.5 to 2.5 m² in a typical adult and a thickness that varies from 1.5 to 4.0 mm, thus forming approximately 8% of total body mass.

The skin has many important functions that are essential for life. It is a formidable barrier against microbes and protects the organism from a variety of mechanical, chemical, thermal, and photic stimuli in the environment. Although the skin prevents dehydration, it also excretes and absorbs limited amounts of fluid. The skin is highly vascularized, and changes in blood flow through the skin are important for regulating body heat. Many aspects of health and aging are reflected in skin appearance, and it serves as an indicator for certain pathologic conditions (e.g., chicken pox, shingles, jaundice).

The skin contains a high density of free nerve endings and specialized cutaneous receptors, which supply the brain and spinal cord with a rich source of sensory information. Tactile information acquired by active touch is essential for making skilled hand movements and for discriminating the size, shape, and texture of objects. The sense of touch also provides a subtle means of social communication and is critical for establishing intimacy or for engaging in sexual behavior. Furthermore, the skin is a versatile sensory organ that may substitute for loss of other sensory modalitites; blind or deaf individuals learn to rely on the somatosensory system to acquire information that, otherwise, would be unavailable to them.

Some of the afferent fibers innervating the skin and the deeper tissues are responsible for detecting noxious events capable of producing tissue damage. These nociceptive fibers mediate painful sensations produced by intense mechanical, thermal, or chemical stimuli. Nociceptive fibers also innervate the visceral organs and mediate the painful sensations associated with myocardial infarction, arthritis, or other diseases.

INNERVATION OF THE SKIN

The skin is formed by two tightly opposed layers of tissue: epidermis and dermis. The epidermis is located superficially and is composed of stratified epithelial cells. Directly below the epidermis is the dermis, which is composed of moderately dense connective tissue. Most peripheral fibers innervating the skin terminate in the dermis or in the lower part of the epidermis (Figure 6-1).

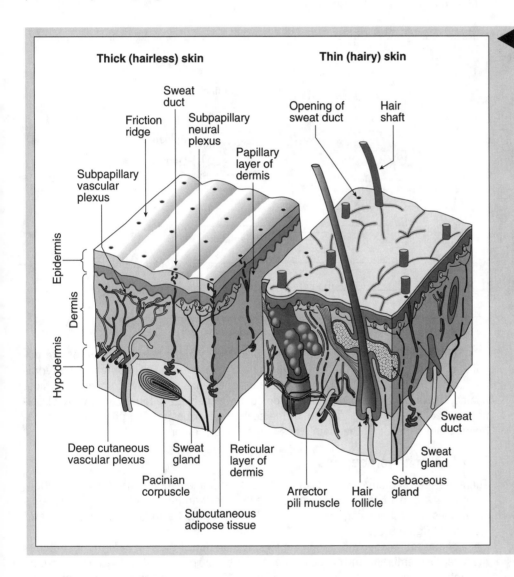

FIGURE 6-1
Structure of the Skin. *Diagram illustrating the organization of glabrous and hairy skin. The sensory innervation of the glabrous skin is shown in more detail in Figure 6-3.*

When discussing the neural innervation of the skin, it is useful to distinguish between glabrous skin and hairy skin. Glabrous skin is devoid of hairs and covers the surface of the palm, the sole of the foot, and the flexor surfaces of the digits and toes; the remainder of the body is covered by hairy skin. Glabrous skin has a distinct texture imparted by a series of papillary ridges or grooves, which provide friction for manipulating objects or traction during locomotion. Glabrous skin is thicker than hairy skin and has a greater density of sweat glands to cool the skin. Although sensory endings in both the glabrous and hairy skin are extremely sensitive to cutaneous stimulation, only the glabrous skin on the hand is used for fine tactile discrimination.

Afferent fibers in the skin are categorized according to the physical stimulus that optimally activates their receptive endings. Thus, somatosensory nerve fibers have generally been classified as mechanoreceptive, thermoreceptive, or nociceptive. These terms provide an indication of the sensory quality that is conveyed by a given fiber, but their usefulness is limited because many fibers respond to more than one sensory modality.

Sensory fibers in the skin are also categorized by their adaptive properties to a constant stimulus (Figure 6-2). Fibers that respond continuously to steady indentation are called slowly adapting fibers. Rapidly adapting fibers, by comparison, respond to changes in stimulus position or during the onset and offset of a stimulus. Rapidly adapting mechanoreceptors respond best to vibrations or to the phasic components of a stimulus, whereas static stimuli are better represented by slowly adapting mechanoreceptors.

Rapidly adapting fibers respond to vibrations. Slowly adapting fibers respond to constant indentations.

FIGURE 6-2

Sensory Adaptation. Peripheral mechanoreceptors and their nerve fibers show different rates of adaptation to a maintained indentation of the skin. Rapidly adapting mechanoreceptors adapt quickly to changes in skin position; slowly adapting mechanoreceptors continue to respond during the plateau portion of the skin indentation.

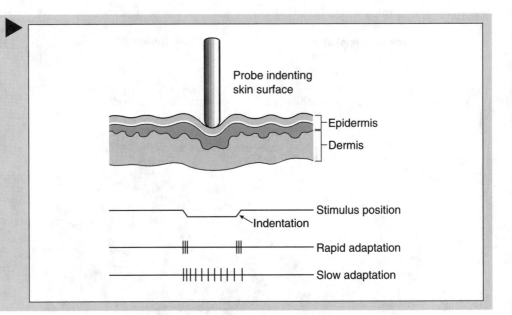

Somatosensory fibers are also classified according to the morphology of their terminal endings. Most mechanoreceptive fibers have an encapsulated ending or their terminals are juxtaposed against other cellular specializations. By comparison, most nociceptive and thermoreceptive fibers do not have specialized terminals and are classified as free nerve endings. The following section describes the morphologic and functional characteristics of the main types of mechanoreceptors.

Tactile Mechanoreceptors

There are several distinct classes of cutaneous mechanoreceptors that vary in location, morphology, and in their responses to mechanical stimulation of the skin: Merkel's corpuscles, Meissner's corpuscles, Ruffini's corpuscles, Pacini's corpuscles, and hair receptors (Figure 6-3).

For most cutaneous mechanoreceptors, stimulation of the skin deforms or stretches the receptor membrane and causes a change in its ionic permeability. The flow of positive ions into the receptor produces a depolarizing potential, which spreads passively along the nerve ending until it reaches a trigger site and evokes an action potential. The process of converting external mechanical energy into a series of neural impulses is known as sensory transduction. Different categories of mechanoreceptors vary in their ability to transduce certain forms of mechanical energy because of the structure of their encapsulated endings. Despite these differences, all cutaneous mechanoreceptors are innervated by large diameter Aβ fibers, which conduct impulses rapidly to the CNS.

Sensory transduction is the process of converting physical energy into neural impulses.

Merkel's Corpuscles. Merkel's corpuscles are located in the epidermis immediately under the papillary ridges of the glabrous skin. Merkel's corpuscles consist of expanded disk-shaped nerve terminals, Merkel's disks, that are closely apposed to the basal membrane of small Merkel's cells (see Figure 6-3). A cluster of 5–10 Merkel's cells are innervated by a single myelinated nerve fiber, which branches into a corresponding number of disk-like endings. Merkel's cells lie in the basal epidermis and have spike-shaped processes,

Merkel's Corpuscles
Slowly adapting, small receptive fields.

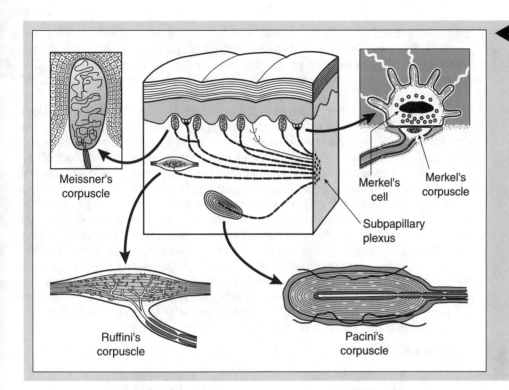

FIGURE 6-3
Innervation of the Glabrous Skin. The glabrous skin is innervated by a plexus of nerve fibers that terminate in a variety of cutaneous mechanoreceptors, including Meissner's corpuscles, Ruffini's corpuscles, Pacini's corpuscles, and Merkel's corpuscles.

which protrude into the surrounding epithelium. Large dense-core vesicles (80–120 μm) in Merkel's cells are gathered near their junction with the nerve terminal, and these vesicles may release neuropeptides that modulate the activity of the nerve ending.

Merkel's corpuscles comprise at least one-fourth of the mechanoreceptors of the hand and are densest in the fingertips, lips, and external genitalia. The high density of Merkel's corpuscles in these regions is closely related to their tactile sensitivity. Consistent with their close proximity to the papillary ridges in the glabrous skin, the receptive fields of fibers innervating Merkel's corpuscles are small, perhaps 2–4 mm in diameter. Merkel's corpuscles exhibit slowly adapting responses to punctuate indentations of the skin and mediate sensations of light pressure required to code local form, edges, and other surface features of objects manipulated by the hand.

Meissner's Corpuscles. Meissner's corpuscles are large receptors (30 μm by 80 μm), which occupy the groove between the dermal papillae of the glabrous skin (see Figure 6-3). They have a cylindrical shape with their long axis oriented perpendicular to the surface of the skin. The corpuscle is comprised of an outer capsule surrounding a central core of arborized nerve fibers. The outer capsule is formed by a layer of connective tissue that is continuous with the perineurium of the afferent nerve fibers. Usually two or three myelinated nerve fibers invade the interior of the capsule to form a coiled bundle of processes among a dense collection of flattened cells known as lemmocytes.

The dense layers of connective tissue and lemmocytes surrounding the nerve terminals endow Meissner's corpuscles with specific filtering properties. Meissner's corpuscles are rapidly adapting mechanoreceptors, which discharge during vibratory stimulation in the range of 10–50 hertz (Hz). Like Merkel's corpuscles, Meissner's corpuscles have small receptive fields because they are located close to the surface of the epidermis. Meissner's corpuscles account for the largest proportion (40%) of mechanoreceptors in the hand and, consistent with their sensitivity to low frequency vibrations, are important for discriminating the texture of objects moved across the fingertips.

Pacini's Corpuscles. Pacini's corpuscles are located in the subcutaneous tissue directly underneath the dermis and in deeper regions of the body, including the interosseous membranes, the joints, and the mesentery. Pacini's corpuscles are oval or spherical in shape and may extend up to 2 mm along the axis of the nerve terminal. The encapsulated ending of Pacini's corpuscle consists of one nerve terminal surrounded by a concentric

Meissner's Corpuscles
Rapidly adapting (10–50 Hz), small receptive fields.

Pacini's Corpuscles
Rapidly adapting (100–300 Hz), large receptive fields.

arrangement of flattened cells or lamellae, which give it an onion-like appearance (see Figure 6-3). The lamellae are separated from each other by a thin layer of fluid that flows between the lamellae as the corpuscle is deformed by external mechanical forces. The lamellae and the afferent nerve terminal are enclosed within an external capsule of elastic fibrous tissue.

Pacini's corpuscles are exceedingly sensitive and may respond to skin deformations of a few microns. Pacini's corpuscles are rapidly adapting mechanoreceptors, and they are noted for their ability to exhibit phase-locked discharges during high frequency (100–300 Hz) sinusoidal vibrations of the skin. Phase-locked responses are the product of the multiple layers of cells and fluid, which surround the nerve terminal and dampen the effects of steady pressure or other slow perturbations of the skin. When the layers of encapsulation are removed, the naked nerve fiber exhibits a much slower rate of adaptation. Because of their exquisite sensitivity and their deep location in the skin, Pacini's corpuscles respond to small vibrations transmitted through the subcutaneous tissue. The construction and location of Pacini's corpuscles endows them with large receptive fields, which may span an entire digit or a large part of the palm (Figure 6-4). Pacini's corpuscles in the hand and fingertips are essential for tactile discrimination and probably serve a function similar to Meissner's corpuscles but at higher frequencies. Pacini's corpuscles located in the joints or mesentery detect vibrations transmitted to the skeleton and serve to detect vibrations of the ground or other substrate supporting the body.

FIGURE 6-4

Cutaneous Receptive Fields. *Comparison of receptive fields for different classes of rapidly and slowly adapting mechanoreceptors in the glabrous skin. Meissner's corpuscles and Merkel's corpuscles, which are located superficially, have very small receptive fields. Pacini's corpuscles, which are located in the subdermal layers, have highly sensitive receptive fields (small dots), which are surrounded by larger regions of reduced sensitivity (shading). Ruffini's corpuscles are located in the deep part of the dermis and respond to stretching large areas of skin (arrows).*

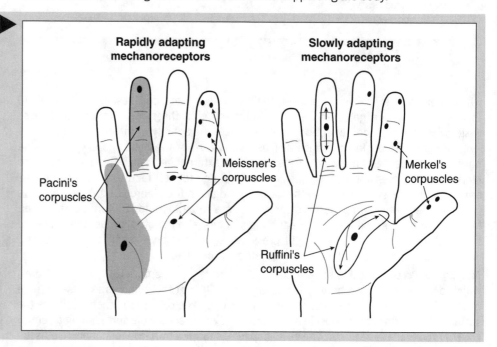

Ruffini's Corpuscles
Slowly adapting, large receptive fields.

Ruffini's Corpuscles. Ruffini's corpuscles are spindle-shaped encapsulated structures that are located in the lower part of the dermis and resemble the Golgi tendon organs in the musculotendinous junction (see Chapter 3). Ruffini's corpuscles contain bundles of collagenous fibers enclosed by a fibrous sheath that is continuous with the perineurium of the afferent nerve. The capsule is innervated by a single myelinated fiber, which forms a network of branched processes throughout the collagen bundles (see Figure 6-3).

The long axis of Ruffini's corpuscle is oriented parallel to the skin surface and, for this reason, the receptor responds best to stretching of the skin. Ruffini's corpuscles may respond to stimulation over large areas of skin, and sustained deformation of their receptive fields evokes a slowly adapting response. The exact function of Ruffini's corpuscles is not clear because they may respond to external stimulation or to internal stimulation generated by muscle contraction. Ruffini-like receptors are also found in joint capsules, where they appear to serve a kinesthetic function.

Hair Receptors. Several hair types have been classified according to thickness, length, and the structure of the hair follicle. Most hairs are innervated by free nerve endings, which enter the hair follicle and encircle the hair either at its base, at an intermediate level, or at superficial levels just below the epidermis (Figure 6-5). Some nerve fibers form a collection of palisade endings, which run along the length of the follicle. In addition, many nerve terminals associated with Merkel's corpuscles surround the neck of the hair follicle, just below the epidermis where the hair emerges from the skin.

Depending on the type of hair that is innervated and the morphology of the afferent ending, the fiber may exhibit rapidly adapting or slowly adapting responses. Most nerve fibers that terminate around hairs respond to lever-like movements of the hair. Although some animals possess extremely large whiskers or vibrissal hairs that are actively moved during exploration, human skin hairs are passive detectors that help determine the part of the body being stimulated.

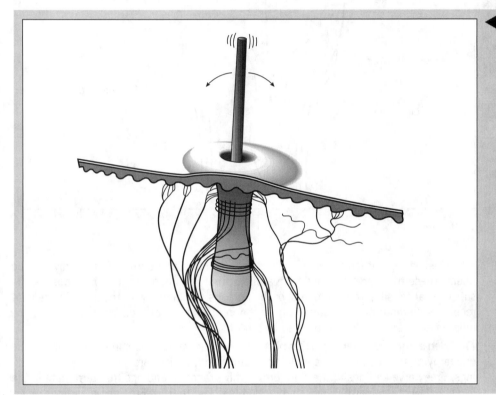

◀ *FIGURE 6-5*
Innervation of a Hair Follicle. Free nerve endings encircling the follicle are activated by lever-like movements of the hair.

Kinesthetic and Nociceptive Endings

Some receptors in the somatosensory system are specialized to detect stimuli affecting the muscles, joints, or other deep tissues of the body. Most of these receptors are responsible for the perception of kinesthesia or pain.

Joint Receptors. Four types of joint receptors have been identified in various parts of the joint capsule and are innervated by a dedicated set of nerve fibers or by branches of afferent nerves that innervate nearby muscles. Three of these receptors are derived from myelinated nerve fibers whose endings terminate in specialized encapsulated endings that resemble Ruffini's corpuscles, Pacini's corpuscles, or Golgi tendon organs (Figure 6-6). The different types of encapsulated joint receptors vary somewhat in their distribution and are located in the fibrous joint capsule or in the intrinsic and extrinsic ligaments.

Encapsulated joint endings are basically tension receptors that respond to stretching of the tissues in the joint. Some joint receptors are slowly adapting and their rate of activity indicates the angle of the joint. Other joint receptors are rapidly adapting and their activity encodes the speed or acceleration of joint movement. These populations of slowly and rapidly adapting joint receptors work together and allow individuals to recognize the position of their limbs at rest or during motor activity.

Slowly adapting joint receptors signal limb position. *Rapidly adapting joint receptors* signal limb movement.

FIGURE 6-6 ▶

Joint Receptors. Schematic diagram of a joint and its sensory innervation. Joint capsules are innervated by free nerve endings and nerve terminals that resemble Pacini's and Ruffini's corpuscles. Ligaments are innervated by free nerve endings and nerve terminals that resemble Golgi tendon organs.

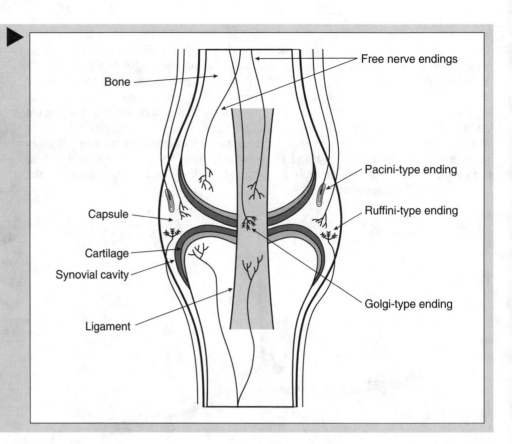

The last type of joint receptor is not encapsulated and derives from unmyelinated fibers. These free nerve endings form a plexus that terminates in the joint capsule, the subsynovial capsule, the ligaments, or the fat pads associated with the joint. These joint receptors mediate pain sensations from the joint that are caused by trauma or by the inflammation and swelling produced by arthritis.

Free Nerve Endings. A large portion of the afferent nerve terminals in the skin and in the deeper lying tissues lack encapsulated endings and, hence, are called free nerve endings. Free nerve endings in the skin form highly branched endings that terminate in the layers below the epidermal–dermal junction (see Figure 6-3). Free nerve endings innervate ligaments, tendons, blood vessels, the meninges, the periosteum, the cornea, the respiratory tracts, and the capsules enclosing organs in the thoracic and visceral cavities. Free nerve endings also terminate in all types of muscles (i.e., striated and smooth), including the myocardium.

Regardless of the tissue in which they terminate, almost all free nerve endings convey impulses related to the perception of pain or temperature. The axons of free nerve endings have small diameters and conduct impulses more slowly than the fibers that innervate tactile mechanoreceptors. Some free nerve endings are classified as thermoreceptors because they convey innocuous sensations of warmth or cold. Other free nerve endings have relatively high thresholds and respond only to noxious mechanical stimulation or to extreme temperatures. These nociceptive fibers are subdivided further depending on whether they respond best to mechanical tissue damage, to extreme temperatures, or to chemical stimulation. All nociceptive fibers have free nerve terminals and the morphologic basis for these different submodalities is not clear.

Tactile Discrimination

Tactile sensitivity increases with the density of nerve fibers that innervate a given area of skin.

The surface of the body is not uniformly sensitive to tactile stimulation, and this property is easily demonstrated in a two-point discrimination task. In this task, a pair of calipers is used to stimulate two points on the skin simultaneously, and subjects are asked to report whether they detect one or two stimuli. The distance between the two points is varied from one trial to the next trial until the minimum distance required to distinguish a pair of stimuli has been determined. In normal individuals, the skin of the digits, palm, or face can resolve the presence of stimuli that are separated by a few millimeters (Figure 6-7). By comparison, separate sites on the leg or trunk cannot be distinguished unless they are separated by several centimeters.

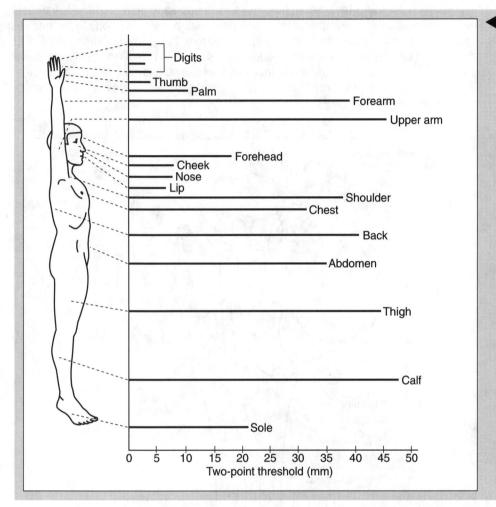

FIGURE 6-7
Distribution of Tactile Sensitivity. *Different parts of the body vary in their sensitivity as measured by the two-point discrimination task.*

The threshold for two-point discrimination varies directly with the density of afferent fibers that supply a given region of skin. For example, a large number of dorsal root ganglion neurons innervates the skin on the tip of a finger and every peripheral fiber that supplies the fingertip only innervates a few papillary ridges. By comparison, the same area of skin on the trunk is supplied by a small number of dorsal root ganglion neurons, and each of their fibers innervates a much larger area of skin. Indentation of two adjacent sites on a digit is likely to evoke neural activity in two distinct populations of peripheral fibers. When the same stimuli are applied to the trunk, however, only a single population of peripheral fibers is likely to be activated.

The ability to recognize different textures depends on several factors besides the high density of nerve endings in the digits. To discriminate silk from velvet, for example, most people rub the material with their fingertips to acquire a unique sensory impression of each fabric. By actively touching the fabric with their fingertips, people simultaneously activate several populations of different mechanoreceptors (i.e., Meissner's, Pacini's, Merkel's, Ruffini's) and produce a continuous flow of neural impulses in their peripheral fibers. This activity ascends the neuraxis and produces a complex pattern of activity within multiple cortical areas. Although the mechanism of texture discrimination is not completely understood, the perception of smoothness and other textural qualities depends on the ability to associate particular stimulus features with the specific patterns of neural activity in the cerebral cortex.

DORSAL COLUMN–MEDIAL LEMNISCAL AND TRIGEMINOTHALAMIC SYSTEMS

The spinal nerves and their ascending axons in the dorsal columns of the spinal cord convey cutaneous and kinesthetic information from all parts of the body to the nucleus gracilis and nucleus cuneatus (Figure 6-8). Axons from these dorsal column nuclei cross the midline and ascend through the medial lemniscus until they terminate in the lateral part of the ventroposterior thalamus (nucleus ventroposterolateral, VPL). The nucleus VPL projects ipsilaterally through the internal capsule and terminates in the postcentral gyrus of the cerebral cortex.

FIGURE 6-8 ▶

Cutaneous Pathways. *Summary of the pathways that convey cutaneous sensations to the thalamus and cerebral cortex. The trigeminothalamic system and the dorsal column–medial lemniscal system conduct cutaneous information from the face and body, respectively. VPL = ventroposterolateral nucleus; VPM = ventroposteromedial nucleus.*

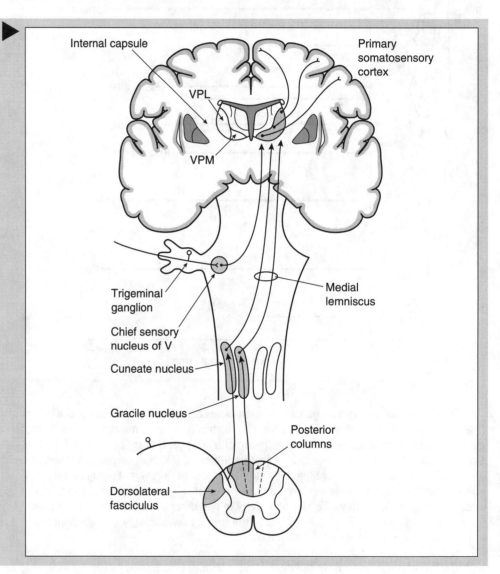

Cutaneous information from the face and mouth is conveyed by the ophthalmic, maxillary, and mandibular divisions of the trigeminal nerve to the principal (or chief) sensory nucleus and the rostral part of the spinal trigeminal nucleus. These trigeminal nuclei project across the midline and ascend the brainstem as the ventral trigeminothalamic tract. This tract is associated with the medial part of the medial lemniscus and terminates in the medial part of the ventroposterior thalamus (nucleus ventroposteromedial, VPM). Like the nucleus VPL, the nucleus VPM projects to the postcentral gyrus of the cerebral cortex.

The dorsal column–medial lemniscal system and the trigeminothalamic pathways convey cutaneous information from the periphery to the cerebral cortex by a series of three neurons (two synapses). Because these pathways consist of large diameter fibers that are heavily myelinated, cutaneous information is transmitted rapidly into consciousness with a high degree of fidelity.

Topographical Organization

Each neuron in the somatosensory system responds to external stimulation within a discrete peripheral region known as the receptive field. The dorsal column nuclei and the trigeminal nuclei are topographically organized so that adjacent neurons have neighboring receptive fields on the body. This somatotopic organization is preserved at subsequent levels of the somatosensory system by a precise point-to-point pattern of projections to the thalamus and cortex. Thus, the topography of neurons in each region forms a complete representation, or neural map, of the head and body. Somatotopic maps are not isomorphic representations of the body; they contain prominent distortions that reflect the differential distribution of peripheral receptors throughout the body. For example, the thalamic and cortical representations of the hand and mouth occupy a disproportionally large part of the neural map because these body regions are more densely innervated than other parts of the body.

Somatosensory Thalamus

The somatosensory thalamus is subdivided into medial (VPM) and lateral (VPL) nuclei that form the ventrobasal complex. This region is somatotopically organized such that the leg representation lies in the lateral part of nucleus VPL, the arm representation lies in the medial part of nucleus VPL, and the head representation occupies all of the nucleus VPM. Within nucleus VPM, cutaneous inputs from the face are represented more laterally than cutaneous inputs from the tongue and intraoral cavity.

Different parts of the ventrobasal complex respond to specific submodalities. Neurons in the central core region of the ventrobasal complex respond to gentle, cutaneous stimulation. The central cutaneous area is surrounded by a shell of neurons that respond to joint movement or to manipulation of the muscles and other deep tissues. The segregation of cutaneous and proprioceptive submodalities indicate that information from Merkel's, Meissner's, Pacini's, or Ruffini's receptors is transmitted predominately to the central core region, whereas information from muscle spindles, Golgi tendon organs, and encapsulated joint receptors terminate in the shell of the ventrobasal complex.

Cutaneous mechanoreceptors project to the central core region of VPM and VPL nuclei. *Joint* and *muscle receptors* project to the surrounding shell region of VPM and VPL nuclei.

Primary Somatosensory (SI) Cortex

The principal neurons in the ventrobasal thalamus send topographically organized projections to the SI cortex, which is located in the postcentral gyrus. The SI cortex contains a complete somatotopic map of the body such that the medial part of the postcentral gyrus represents the lower limb and lower trunk, the middle third of the gyrus represents the upper trunk and arm, and the lateral third of the gyrus represents the face and head. Intraoral structures are represented near the parietal operculum (Figure 6-9).

The SI cortex is subdivided into four cytoarchitectonic regions known as Brodmann areas 3a, 3b, 1, and 2. Each of these areas contains a complete neural map of the body, which is based on differential projections from the central core and superficial shell of the ventrobasal thalamus (Figure 6-10). Some projections from the shell region convey information about the muscles to area 3a; other neurons in this region convey information about the joints to area 2. Neurons in the core region convey cutaneous information to areas 3b and 1. Consistent with these projection patterns, cortical lesions restricted to areas 3b and 1 produce deficits in texture discrimination. Lesions of area 2, on the other hand, impair the ability to discriminate size or shape because these skills depend on information from encapsulated joint receptors.

Cutaneous mechanoreceptors project to Brodmann areas 3b and 1. *Joint* and *muscle receptors* project to Brodmann areas 2 and 3a, respectively.

FIGURE 6-9

Map of Primary Somatosensory (SI) Cortex. The somatotopic organization of the SI cortex is determined by the pattern of projections from the ventroposteromedial (VPM) and ventroposterolateral (VPL) nuclei of the thalamus.

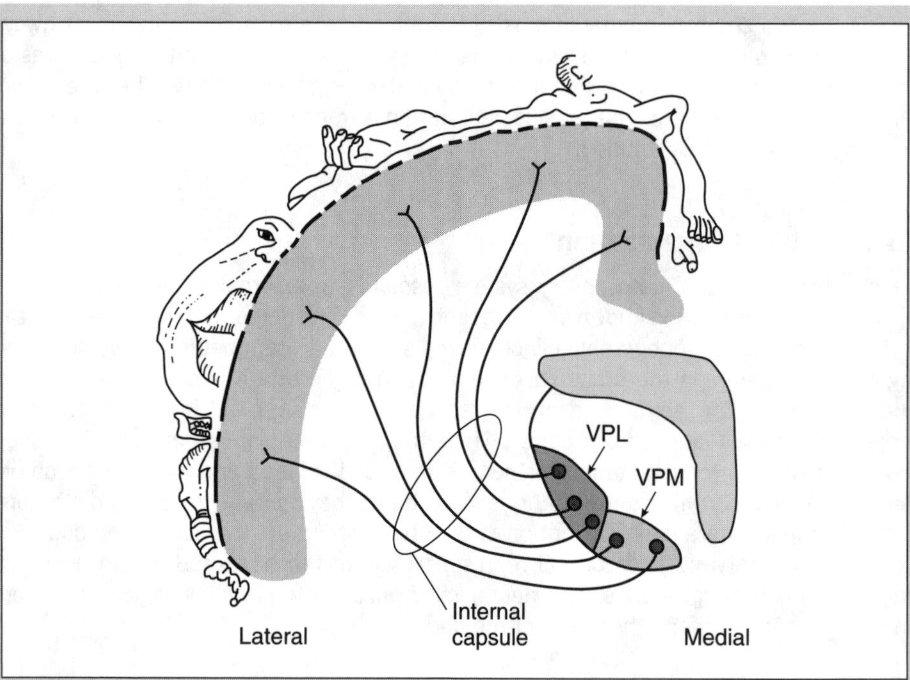

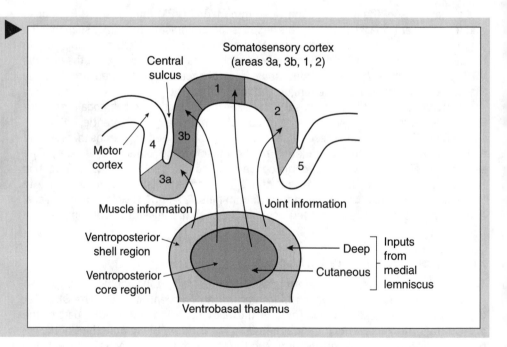

Lateral   Internal capsule   Medial

FIGURE 6-10

Deep and Cutaneous Submodalities. Cutaneous information is transmitted from a central core region in nucleus ventroposterolateral (VPL) to Brodmann areas 3b and 1 in the primary somatosensory cortex. Information from deep tissues (i.e., muscles and joints) is transmitted from the superficial part of nucleus VPL to areas 3a and 2.

Secondary Somatosensory (SII) Cortex

The SII cortex is located in the upper bank of the Sylvian sulcus. Substantial evidence indicates that somatosensory information is processed in the SI cortex before it is transmitted to the SII cortex. Although neurons in the ventral part of the ventrobasal complex project directly to the SII cortex, the majority of somatosensory projections from the thalamus terminate in the SI cortex. Most of the somatosensory projections to the SII cortex originate from the SI cortex, not the thalamus. In addition, selective lesions of the SI cortex cause SII neurons to become unresponsive to tactile stimulation; similar lesions of the SII cortex, however, have little effect on the responsiveness of SI neurons. These findings suggest a hierarchical organization in which somatosensory information is processed sequentially by the ventrobasal thalamus, SI cortex, and SII cortex.

The hierarchical organization of the somatosensory cortex suggests that the SII cortex is involved in higher order processing of somatosensory information. Consistent with this view, SII neurons have larger receptive fields than SI neurons representing similar parts of the body. Furthermore, SII neurons are more responsive to peripheral stimulation if attention is directed to the part of the body receiving stimulation. Neurons in the SII cortex project to the insula, which, in turn, projects to limbic structures such as the amygdala and hippocampus. This serial pathway suggests that the SII cortex plays a role in forming tactile memories, perhaps for recognizing textures and other features of hand-held objects.

Somatosensory Connections to the Motor Cortex

The posterior part of the SI cortex (Brodmann areas 1 and 2) sends dense projections to motor and premotor cortical areas (Brodmann areas 4 and 6, respectively). The primary motor cortex sends feedback connections to somatosensory cortical areas 1, 2, and 3a. These corticocortical projections interconnect topographically matched regions in the somatosensory and motor cortical areas. Thus, the digit representations in sensory and motor areas are reciprocally connected. These cortical interconnections allow tactile information to modulate efferent signals from the motor cortex and strongly suggest that somatosensory information is used to guide hand movements during object manipulation.

NEURAL BASIS OF PAIN

The treatment of pain is an important aspect of clinical practice, which requires an understanding of the pain pathways and their neural mechanisms. The presence of pain indicates that specific sets of peripheral nerve fibers have been activated by tissue damage or by irritating stimuli that produce inflammation. In many cases, the cause of pain is easily identified. Pain caused by toothache, earache, sore throat, or skin trauma, for example, are well localized. The intensity and sensory qualities of pain vary widely and may depend on several factors. Pain originating from the musculoskeletal system has a dull, aching character and is poorly localized. Visceral pain sensations are often diffuse and radiate away from the affected organ. Although visceral pain may reflect irritation or disease at a specific site, determining the cause of such pain may require several diagnostic tests.

Nociceptive Afferents

Pain is considered a specific sensory modality in the somatosensory system because all noxious sensations are conveyed by specific classes of nociceptive fibers. Peripheral nociceptive fibers are classified into two groups on the basis of axon diameter and conduction velocity. One class of fibers, the thinly myelinated Aδ fibers, have conduction velocities of 10–40 meters per second (m/s) and respond to excessive mechanical or thermal stimulation. Activation of Aδ fibers causes immediate sensations of intense, sharp pain. Another class of nociceptive fibers, the C fibers, also respond to mechanical tissue damage, extreme temperatures, or noxious chemicals. The C fibers conduct impulses at a much slower velocity (1–2 m/s) and convey pain sensations that are characterized by a dull throbbing or burning quality. Pain sensations conveyed by C fibers are called slow pain because they occur after a noticeable time delay.

C fibers convey slow pain of a burning or throbbing character. Aδ fibers convey fast pain of a sharp, stabbing character.

Tissue damage causes a cascade of local chemical changes that sensitize nociceptors to subsequent stimulation (Figure 6-11). Following trauma, the surrounding tissue releases many substances, including bradykinin, histamine, and prostaglandins. These chemicals excite nearby nociceptive fibers and cause them to release substance P, a chemical that activates mast cells. In turn, the mast cells release histamine, and this chemical causes further activation of the nociceptive fibers. Substance P also causes local capillaries to dilate; the resultant increase in blood flow leads to edema, which causes another release of bradykinin. Collectively, these chemical mechanisms tend to excite nociceptive nerve fibers and lower their threshold to external stimulation. Conse-

FIGURE 6-11 ▶

Peripheral Sensitization. Tissue damage causes local cells to release bradykinin and prostaglandins, which excite nociceptive fibers and cause them to release substance P and other neuropeptides. Substance P causes histamine release and promotes vasodilation, effects that cause additional release of bradykinin. These chemical changes increase the sensitivity of nociceptive fibers to subsequent stimulation.

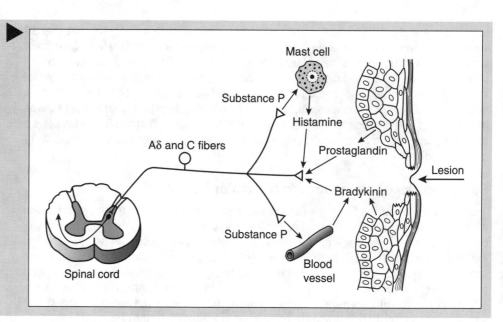

Allodynia is increased sensitivity to stimuli that normally are innocuous. Hyperalgesia is increased sensitivity to stimuli that cause moderate pain.

quently, normally innocuous stimuli are perceived as painful (allodynia) and more intense stimuli are extremely noxious (hyperalgesia). Although these local responses increase the intensity of pain and may prolong its duration, they are essential for the healing process and improve recovery by encouraging the patient to protect the injured area from additional trauma.

Anterolateral and Trigeminothalamic Systems

As discussed in Chapters 3 and 4, the central pathways that conduct pain and temperature information are segregated from those that conduct cutaneous information. Most nociceptive information coming from the body is conducted through the spinal cord and brainstem by the fibers of the anterolateral system. Unlike the dorsal column–medial lemniscal system, the anterolateral system has several groups of fibers (i.e., spinothalamic, spinoreticular, spinomesencephalic, and spinotectal) that terminate in multiple regions of the brainstem and thalamus (Figure 6-12).

The anterolateral system is the collection of spinothalamic, spinoreticular, spinomesencephalic, and spinotectal fibers.

Nociceptive and thermoreceptive nerve fibers from the body enter the spinal cord through the dorsal roots and terminate on neurons in the dorsal horn. The anterolateral system originates mainly from projection neurons in laminae I, IV, V, and, to a lesser extent, from laminae VI and VII. Neurons in these laminae send axons through the white commissure and up the spinal cord through the ventrolateral part of the lateral funiculus. As the anterolateral system ascends through the lateral part of the brainstem, many fibers peel away from the main tract to terminate in the reticular formation, the periaqueductal gray (PAG) region, or the superior colliculus. The remaining fibers in the anterolateral system eventually terminate in the nucleus VPL of the thalamus. This latter group of fibers, known as the lateral spinothalamic tract, conveys thermal and nociceptive information mainly from Aδ fibers. Most nociceptive information conducted by C fibers is sent to the reticular formation, which sends polysynaptic projections to the intralaminar nuclei of the thalamus.

The trigeminothalamic system conveys nociceptive information from one side of the brainstem to the contralateral thalamus. Noxious sensations from the face and head enter the brainstem primarily through the trigeminal nerve. A few fibers of cranial nerves VII, IX, and X also innervate the ear, tongue, throat, and the meninges. All of these primary afferent fibers descend through the spinal trigeminal tract and synapse on neurons in the spinal trigeminal nucleus of the medulla. Second-order neurons in the spinal trigeminal nucleus send axons across the midline and ascend through the trigeminothalamic tract (or trigeminal lemniscus) until they terminate in the nucleus VPM of the thalamus.

Referred pain is visceral pain that appears to originate from surrounding areas.

Referred Pain Sensations. Deep pain sensations arising from the viscera are difficult to localize and frequently produce sensations that are associated with the cutaneous parts of the body. Visceral pain that seems to originate from sites other than the affected organ

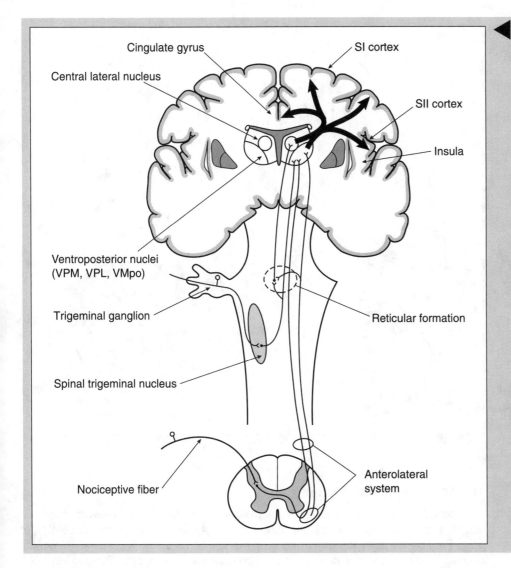

Cingulate gyrus

Central lateral nucleus

SI cortex

SII cortex

Insula

Ventroposterior nuclei
(VPM, VPL, VMpo)

Trigeminal ganglion

Reticular formation

Spinal trigeminal nucleus

Nociceptive fiber

Anterolateral
system

FIGURE 6-12
Ascending Pain Pathways. *Summary of the pathways that convey pain and temperature information to the brainstem, thalamus, and cerebral cortex. The fibers of the anterolateral system terminate in the ventrobasal complex and the posterior part of the ventral medial nucleus (VMpo). Other fibers terminate in the reticular formation, which, in turn, sends ascending projections to the central lateral nucleus. Pain sensitive regions in the thalamus project to a variety of cortical regions, including the anterior cingulate gyrus, the insula, and the primary (SI) and secondary (SII) somatosensory cortices.*

is known as "referred" pain. Referred pain occurs because the projection neurons in the anterolateral system receive convergent inputs from cutaneous fibers innervating the skin and from nociceptive fibers innervating visceral organs such as the heart or stomach (Figure 6-13). In this situation, the brain is unable to identify the exact source of the pain because the projection neurons are normally activated by cutaneous stimulation. In making a clinical diagnosis, it is helpful to know that different types of visceral pain produce well-defined patterns of referred sensations. For example, insufficient blood flow to the myocardium produces angina, a form of referred pain characterized by the sensation of extreme pressure on the upper chest that is often accompanied by pain radiating into the left arm. Referred pain is also produced by nociceptive fibers innervating the gallbladder (pain in the scapula), the kidney (pain in the lower abdominal wall), the appendix (pain in the anterior abdominal wall around the umbilicus), or the prostate gland (pain in the abdominal wall, lower back, or upper legs).

Forebrain Structures Involved in Pain

Many parts of the thalamus and cerebral cortex receive ascending projections from the anterolateral system and the reticular formation to mediate the perception of pain. The exact mechanisms by which pain is processed in the forebrain are not understood but appear to involve a complex network of thalamic and cortical regions that control the autonomic and affective responses to pain.

FIGURE 6-13

Referred Pain Sensations. Nociceptive fibers innervating organs in the thoracic and visceral cavities often terminate on neurons of the anterolateral system, which receive convergent inputs from cutaneous sources. Activation of these nociceptive fibers may give rise to cutaneous sensations.

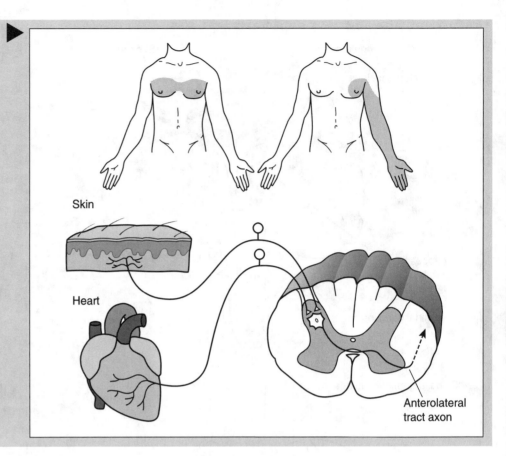

Skin

Heart

Anterolateral tract axon

Thalamic Representation of Pain

The ascending fibers of the lateral spinothalamic tract terminate in several thalamic nuclei, and there is controversy regarding the role of these nuclei in the perception of pain. Projections from the dorsal horn of the spinal cord and the spinal trigeminal nucleus have dense terminations in the ventrobasal complex (nuclei VPM and VPL) and the posterior part of the ventral medial nucleus (VMpo), which lies immediately caudal to nucleus VPM and medial to the posterior part of nucleus VPL. Nucleus VMpo is a major pain processing center in the thalamus, and neurons in this region respond specifically to noxious stimulation. By comparison, neurons in nucleus VPM or VPL are activated by cutaneous or noxious stimulation, and their discharge rate is directly related to the intensity of the stimulation. This response pattern resembles the wide dynamic responses in the dorsal horn of the spinal cord (see Chapter 3) and underscores the view that cutaneous and noxious information are both conveyed in the anterolateral system. These responses in nuclei VPM and VPL also suggest that the rate of neuronal activity may encode the intensity of pain. Neurons in the ventral posterior parts of the thalamus, including nucleus VMpo, are topographically organized, and this probably mediates the ability to localize noxious stimulation.

Spinothalamic fibers also terminate in nonspecific regions of the thalamus that lack topographic organization. Ascending spinothalamic projections from the deeper layers of the dorsal horn terminate in the intralaminar complex of the thalamus, especially in the central lateral nucleus. This direct route to the intralaminar complex of the thalamus may also be supplemented by a second, indirect pathway. Thus, some anatomists contend that nociceptive neurons in the reticular formation send polysynaptic projections to the intralaminar nuclei. There is little evidence, however, to suggest that these pathways are involved in mediating the discriminative aspects of pain perception. Neurons in the central lateral nucleus and other parts of the intralaminar complex respond to noxious stimulation but have large receptive fields, which make them unsuitable for localizing pain. The intralaminar nuclei receive convergent inputs from many brain regions and

*The **ventrobasal complex** is involved in discriminitive aspects of pain. The **central lateral nucleus** is involved in affective components of pain.*

send diffuse projections to the cerebral cortex. The diffuse nature of thalamocortical projections from the intralaminar nuclei suggest that any nociceptive information received from the reticulothalamic pathways would be used to regulate cortical excitability and behavioral arousal. More specifically, the intralaminar nuclei might be concerned with modulating the emotional aspects of suffering and other affective components of pain perception.

Thalamic Pain Syndrome. Lesions in the ventral posterior thalamus may produce a form of central pain that is associated with abnormal and unpleasant somatic sensations. The thalamic pain syndrome is characterized initially by analgesia that, after several weeks or months, is replaced by paresthetic sensations (burning, prickling, or lacerating pain). Thalamic pain and other central pain syndromes are also associated with allodynia (i.e., pain evoked by gentle stimulation of a hypersensitive region).

Although the exact mechanism of central pain is unknown, the sequence of analgesia followed by paresthesia suggests that a lesion-induced loss of neurons is followed by sprouting of inappropriate neuronal connections or by other events that increase the activity of nociceptive neurons. Central pain is not alleviated by morphine or other opiate-based narcotics because the syndrome is produced by lesions in brain regions that do not contain high concentrations of opiate receptors. Pharmacologic agents that suppress overall neuronal activity (e.g., antiepileptic drugs) are the most successful agents for treating central pain.

> *Central pain is produced by lesions that lead to abnormal neural activity in the nociceptive pathways of the CNS.*

Cortical Representation of Pain

The importance of the cerebral cortex in pain perception was disputed for many years because few physiologic studies found nociceptive neurons in the SI or SII cortex. By comparison, many neurons in the ventral posterior thalamus respond to intense thermal or noxious stimulation. Moreover, electrical stimulation of the thalamus produces pain responses in humans and animals. In addition, electrical stimulation of the SI cortex rarely caused human patients to perceive pain, and removal of the SI cortex did not prevent the perception of pain. For many years, this and other evidence prompted the widely held view that pain sensations were mediated by the thalamus and its nociceptive inputs.

Although the exact cortical mechanisms for perceiving pain remain elusive, evidence from studies using noninvasive imaging techniques clearly demonstrates a substantial increase in blood flow to specific cortical areas during intense thermal or noxious stimulation. The largest increases in cortical blood flow were observed in the insula and the anterior part of the cingulate gyrus. These results are consistent with anatomical studies showing that the ventrobasal and intralaminar regions of the thalamus project to anterior parts of the cingulate gyrus, while the nucleus VMpo projects to the insula (see Figure 6-12). The insula and anterior cingulate gyrus are part of the limbic system, and pain-induced activation of these regions indicates their involvement in the affective components of pain. The anterior cingulate cortex also plays a role in directing attention to a variety of sensory stimuli and may serve a similar function in response to pain.

The somatosensory cortex is activated by noxious stimulation, but to a lesser degree than the insula or the anterior cingulate cortex. SI and SII cortices receive direct and indirect projections from the ventrobasal complex, and these connections mediate the discriminative aspects of pain perception. Indeed, removal of SI and SII cortices impairs the ability to localize painful stimulation but does not completely prevent the perception of pain because other cortical areas (i.e., insula, anterior cingulate gyrus) also receive substantial inputs from the ventroposterior thalamus.

Phantom Limb Pain. Following removal of an arm or leg, nearly all patients report sensations from the missing limb. The most vivid sensations arising from the missing or phantom limb usually involve the distal structures (e.g., hand, foot) that received the highest density of innervation (Figure 6-14). For some patients, the phantom limb seems normal in size; while other patients perceive the distal hand or foot extending directly from the proximal stump. Phantom sensations, though commonly associated with limbs, may arise following denervation of any part of the body. Thus, phantom breasts are reported sometimes by women after mastectomy, and paralyzed individuals may perceive phantom sensations from parts of the body below the level of the transected spinal cord.

FIGURE 6-14 ▶

Phantom Sensations. Illustration of phantom sensations in patients whose arm or leg has been amputated. The dashed line indicates the outline of the missing limb and the cross-hatching indicates the part of the missing limb that has phantom sensations. (Source: Reprinted with permission from Solonen FI: The phantom phenomenon in amputated Finnish war veterans. Acta Ortho Scand Suppl: 1–37, 1962.)

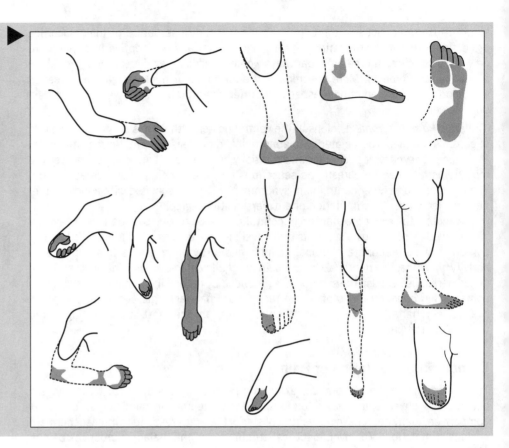

Phantom sensations are managed, in part, by prosthetic devices.

Phantom sensations can also be induced by local anesthesia, and patients undergoing arm surgery frequently report false impressions of their limb during anesthetic block of the brachial plexus.

Phantom sensations can be relatively benign or can be characterized by serious debilitating pain. Nearly 70% of all limb amputees experience burning or cramping pain. Phantom limb pain is a common cause of chronic pain and cannot be managed with narcotic drugs because it is not specifically caused by activity in brain regions that contain high concentrations of opiate receptors. Instead, phantom pain appears to originate from distorted and unregulated signal patterns in the somatosensory cortex. When the somatosensory cortex is deprived of normal sensory inputs, the cortical map becomes reorganized, and the spatiotemporal pattern of activity may resemble those patterns underlying the perception of burning pain. Current speculation holds that cramping pain arises because the somatosensory cortex sends the motor cortex a signal to move the phantom limb and, in the absence of a true limb, the message to move the limb becomes progressively stronger until cramping sensations occur.

Phantom limb sensations and pain can be managed to some degree by fitting the patient with a prosthetic limb. In time, patients acquire the feeling that the prosthetic limb is real or "fleshed out." This occurs, in part, because deep and cutaneous mechanoreceptors in the stump retain sensibility and are activated whenever the prosthetic limb is moved or perturbed. The perception of the phantom limb should eventually correspond to the visual image of the artificial limb, and this may help to reduce the pain that often accompanies phantom limb sensations.

Migraine Headache. Severe recurring headaches that are preceded by sensory, motor, or visual symptoms denote the features of a classic migraine headache. In most cases, premonitory symptoms are visual and appear to be correlated with paroxysms of neuronal discharges followed by inhibition, or spreading depression, in the visual cortex. Thus, visual scotomas or hallucinations are common before the onset of headache pain and may expand from one part of the visual field to another as the dysfunctional zone moves across the visual cortex. In addition, migraine headache is often correlated with a decrease in cerebral vascular perfusion that occurs in the occipital lobe before progressing rostrally. Current speculation, however, holds that decreased vascular perfusion occurs secondary to a depression in neuronal activity.

The exact cause of migraine headache is unknown, but several findings suggest that serotonergic projections from the brainstem play a critical role. Thus, migraine headache is alleviated by sleep, and sleeping is correlated with a reduction in the activity of serotonergic neurons in the dorsal raphe nuclei. By contrast, electrical stimulation of the dorsal raphe nuclei can produce migraine-like headaches. Ascending projections from the dorsal raphe nuclei terminate in the lateral geniculate nucleus, the superior colliculus, the visual cortex, and on cerebral arteries. Any of these projections could provide a basis for the visual or circulatory symptoms associated with migraine headaches.

Like other forms of central pain, migraine headache is not associated with elevated activity in the peripheral nociceptive fibers or in the ascending pathways of the anterolateral system. Although narcotics can relieve chronic headaches, they are employed only as a last resort. Migraine headache is most effectively treated by drugs (e.g., sumatriptan or ergotamine) that act selectively at certain types of serotonergic receptors to inhibit the firing of dorsal raphe neurons.

Central Modulation of Pain

The perception of pain depends on the context of events surrounding an injury as well as the cultural and social experiences of the individual. Perhaps the most striking example of nonsensory influences on the response to pain is illustrated by soldiers in the midst of a battle. During these situations, many soldiers ignore their wounds and deny having any pain until they are out of danger. The ability to inhibit pain during a crisis is highly adaptive because the individual must attend to other stimuli and make appropriate behavioral responses for survival. Higher order regions in the CNS, including the frontal cortex, can interact with nociceptive pathways to reduce the perception of pain under certain conditions.

The existence of neural systems for modulating pain was long suspected because small quantities of morphine or opium exert powerful analgesic effects that are mediated by specific receptors in the brain. The presence of opiate receptors in the CNS was confirmed in the 1970s and prompted the view that some neural systems must contain endogenous compounds to regulate the perception of pain. This view was supported by studies showing that opiate receptors were highly concentrated in parts of the brainstem, and that electrical stimulation of these areas caused analgesia by inhibiting neurons in the dorsal horn of the spinal cord. The discovery of neural systems that contain enkephalins, endorphins, and other opiate neuropeptides suggests that these systems are important for modulating pain signals.

"Endorphin" means endogenous morphine.

Descending Modulatory Systems. Several descending pathways from the brainstem and forebrain are involved in suppressing the transmission of nociceptive information from the periphery (Figure 6-15). These descending projections include serotonergic fibers originating from the nucleus raphe magnus and noradrenergic fibers originating from the nucleus paragigantocellularis of the reticular formation. Both neurochemical pathways descend through the dorsolateral funiculus of the spinal cord and terminate in Rexed's laminae II and III of the dorsal horn where they activate enkephalinergic neurons in the substantia gelatinosa. Other serotonergic projections terminate in the spinal trigeminal nucleus and activate enkephalinergic neurons that inhibit the transmission of nociceptive information from the face and head.

The raphe magnus and ventrolateral medulla are regulated by descending projections from neurons in the PAG region of the midbrain. The PAG region contains a variety of neurotransmitters, including serotonin, glutamate, and many neuropeptides. Consistent with its role in modulating pain, the PAG region contains high concentrations of opiate receptors and all three classes of opioid neuropeptides (i.e., enkephalins, endorphins, dynorphins). Descending projections from the PAG region can activate the serotonergic projections from the nucleus raphe magnus. Hence, electrical stimulation of the PAG region or the nucleus raphe magnus have similar analgesic effects. Other neurons in the PAG region project to the spinal trigeminal nucleus or to the spinal dorsal

Periaqueductal gray region contains a high concentration of opioid neuropeptides and projects to regions that control pain transmission.

FIGURE 6-15 ▶

Pain Modulating Pathways. *The peri-aqueductal gray (PAG) region can be engaged by ascending fibers of the anterolateral system or by descending inputs from the hypothalamus and the cerebral cortex. Descending projections from the PAG region activate serotonergic neurons in the nucleus raphe magnus or noradrenergic neurons in the nucleus paragigantocellularis. Descending projections from these regions activate enkephalinergic neurons in the dorsal horn of the spinal cord and the spinal trigeminal nucleus.*

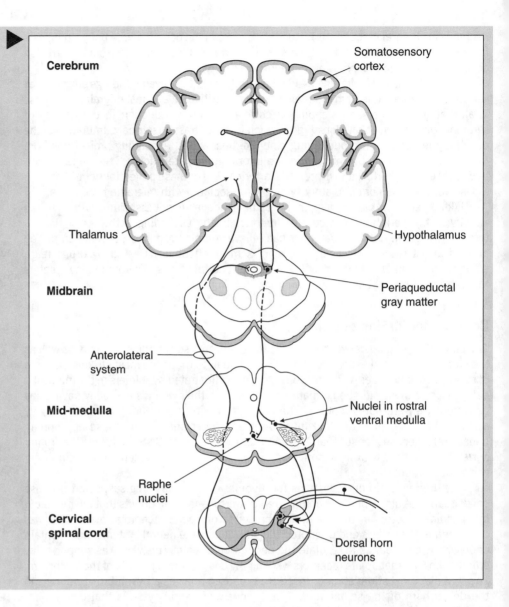

Cerebrum

Somatosensory cortex

Thalamus

Hypothalamus

Midbrain

Periaqueductal gray matter

Anterolateral system

Mid-medulla

Nuclei in rostral ventral medulla

Raphe nuclei

Cervical spinal cord

Dorsal horn neurons

horn; these projections use substance P and cholecystokinin to activate enkephalinergic interneurons in lamina II of those nociceptive regions.

The descending modulatory systems can be activated directly to produce analgesia. Some patients obtain relief from chronic pain by electrically stimulating the PAG region or the nucleus raphe magnus. After electrodes are chronically implanted into these brain regions, the patient determines when brief pulses of electrical current are sent through the electrodes to produce brief periods of analgesia.

In the absence of direct electrical stimulation, the descending modulatory systems can be engaged by several neural mechanisms. Fibers in the ascending anterolateral system that terminate in the ventrolateral medulla or in the PAG region provide one mechanism by which ascending pain impulses can excite these modulatory systems. In addition, the periventricular region of the hypothalamus sends enkephalinergic projections to the PAG region, and activation of this pathway during autonomic arousal may provide another mechanism for suppressing pain during emergency conditions. Furthermore, the prefrontal and somatosensory cortical areas also send descending projections to the PAG region. These corticofugal pathways may engage the PAG region and, although these pathways are not fully understood, it is well known that pain perception is influenced by social experience, personality, and other psychological factors.

RESOLUTION OF CLINICAL CASE

This case illustrates trigeminal neuralgia, a pain disorder that affects one or more branches of the trigeminal nerve. Also known as tic douloureux, this disorder is characterized by recurring paroxysms of sharp, penetrating pain in the lips, cheek, or other parts of the face. The pain typically affects one side of the face, usually within the territory of the maxillary division of the trigeminal nerve. The pain is often accompanied by involuntary facial movements or ipsilateral lacrimation. The frequency of the attacks may vary, and their periodic nature distinguishes them from the steady throbbing pain that accompanies tooth disease or sinus infection. The painful attacks produced by trigeminal neuralgia can be provoked by touching trigger zones on the face or by facial movements (e.g., smiling or chewing). For this reason, patients suffering from trigeminal neuralgia often skip meals to avoid triggering an attack and may become undernourished.

Trigeminal neuralgia is attributed to excessive neuronal activity in the spinal trigeminal nucleus, but the cause of the pain remains unknown. Trigeminal neuralgia may occur secondary to brainstem lesions produced by multiple sclerosis, yet it is unusual to detect noticeable damage in the trigeminal nerve or in the trigeminothalamic pathways. Some have argued that trigeminal neuralgia is the result of anomalous blood vessels compressing the fifth cranial nerve, but there is little evidence to support or refute this view.

Trigeminal neuralgia is treated with anticonvulsant agents, such as carbamazepine, phenytoin, or baclofen. These drugs are not analgesics and are ineffective in treating most types of pain. Relief from attacks can also be gained by surgical techniques that destroy the nociceptive fibers innervating the face. Thus, it is common practice to employ radiofrequency stimulation to destroy the small diameter pain fibers while sparing the less vulnerable large diameter fibers.

REVIEW QUESTIONS

Directions: For each of the following questions, choose the **one best** answer.

1. Vibratory sensations are mediated by which of the following mechanoreceptors?
    (A) Pacini's corpuscles
    (B) Ruffini's corpuscles
    (C) Merkel's corpuscles
    (D) Encapsulated joint receptors
    (E) Muscle spindles

2. Which of the following types of pain are best treated with opiate narcotics?
    (A) Phantom limb pain
    (B) Trigeminal neuralgia
    (C) Childbirth pain
    (D) Central (thalamic) pain
    (E) Migraine headache

3. Cutaneous information and nociceptive information are processed by which of the following neural structures?
    (A) Anterior cingulate gyrus
    (B) Periaqueductal gray (PAG) region
    (C) Substantia gelatinosa
    (D) Secondary somatosensory (SII) cortex
    (E) Nucleus raphe magnus

4. Which of the following sites would be most suitable for implanting stimulating electrodes to alleviate chronic pain sensations?
    (A) Primary somatosensory (SI) cortex
    (B) Spinal trigeminal nucleus
    (C) Nucleus raphe magnus
    (D) Intralaminar nucleus of the thalamus
    (E) Dorsal horn of the spinal cord

5. Which of the following tracts conveys cutaneous information to the ventro-posteromedial (VPM) nucleus?
    (A) Spinal trigeminal tract
    (B) Trigeminothalamic tract
    (C) Medial lemniscus
    (D) Central tegmental tract
    (E) Lateral spinothalamic tract

ANSWERS AND EXPLANATIONS

1. The answer is A. Only Pacini's and Meissner's corpuscles respond continuously to vibrotactile stimulation. Afferent fibers from Pacini's corpuscles may discharge at frequencies as high as 100–300 hertz (Hz) and become entrained to vibrations in that frequency range. Meissner's corpuscles become entrained to vibrations at frequencies of 10–30 Hz. Mechanoreceptors such as Ruffini's corpuscles and Merkel's corpuscles are best activated by punctuate indentations. Joint receptors and Golgi tendon organs respond to limb movements.

2. The answer is C. Narcotics administered into the lumbar cistern during childbirth activate enkephalin receptors in the dorsal horn of the spinal cord, which suppress the transmission of pain from the lower body. Opiate narcotics are ineffective in alleviating phantom limb pain or central pain syndromes because these are produced by abnormal patterns of activity in the thalamus and cortex, brain regions that do not have high concentrations of opiate receptors. Trigeminal neuralgia is probably mediated by excessive activity in the trigeminal nerve or spinal trigeminal nucleus and is treated by anticonvulsant drugs that inhibit neuronal activity without activating opioid receptors. The exact cause of migraine headache is not well understood but appears to be mediated by paroxysms of cortical activity that are evoked by ascending inputs from the dorsal raphe nuclei. Antimigraine drugs act by modulating serotonergic transmission; they do not activate opioid receptors.

3. The answer is D. The SII cortex processes cutaneous and nociceptive information. The anterior cingulate gyrus, the PAG region, the substantia gelatinosa, and the nucleus raphe magnus are mainly concerned with processing pain information.

4. The answer is C. Electrical stimulation of the nucleus raphe magnus has been used successfully in patients suffering from chronic pain. Activation of the descending serotonergic fibers from the nucleus raphe magnus can activate enkephalinergic neurons in multiple levels of the spinal cord. By comparison, electrical stimulation of the somatosensory cortex, the spinal trigeminal nucleus, or the intralaminar nuclei do not alleviate chronic pain. In some instances, electrical stimulation of the ventral posterior nuclei of the thalamus may alleviate pain by disrupting the transmission of pain signals through the thalamus. Stimulation of the dorsal horn of the spinal cord is likely to activate neurons giving rise to the anterolateral system and would cause more pain, not less.

5. The answer is B. The trigeminothalamic tract conveys cutaneous and nociceptive information to the nucleus VPM of the thalamus. The spinal trigeminal tract terminates in the spinal trigeminal nucleus, not in the thalamus. The medial lemniscus conveys cutaneous information from the body to the ventroposterolateral (VPL) nucleus. The central tegmental and lateral spinothalamic tracts convey nociceptive information from the body to nucleus VPL and the intralaminar nuclei.

ADDITIONAL READING

Craig AD, Bushnell MC, Zhang ET, et al: A thalamic nucleus specific for pain and temperature sensation. *Nature* 372:770–772, 1994.

Darian-Smith I: The sense of touch: performance and peripheral neural processes. In *Handbook of Physiology: The Nervous System*, vol III. Edited by Brookhart JM, Mountcastle VB. Bethesda, MD: American Physiological Society, 1984, pp 739–788.

Pons TP, Garraghty PE, Friedman DP, et al: Physiological evidence for serial processing in the somatosensory cortex. *Science* 237:417–420, 1987.

Talbot JD, Marrett S, Evans AC, et al: Multiple representations of pain in human cerebral cortex. *Science* 251:1355–1358, 1991.

Wall PD, Melzack R: *Textbook of Pain*. New York, NY: Churchill Livingstone, 1989.

7

AUDITORY SYSTEM

CHAPTER OUTLINE

INTRODUCTION OF CLINICAL CASE

A. D., a 50-year-old man, had been home from work for several days with flu-like symptoms: dizziness, headache, nausea, and vomiting. There was little improvement in A. D.'s condition during this time. After A. D. began showing signs of an unsteady gait, his wife scheduled an appointment with the physician. The patient was still unsteady when he arrived in the office. As the patient's history was being taken, he admitted that he had been having more headaches than usual over the last 6 months. Examination of the patient revealed *nystagmus* to the right side and mild weakness of the left facial musculature, accompanied by mild facial anesthesia. The corneal reflex was diminished only on the left side, and there was mild *papilledema* bilaterally. The patient disputed his wife's claim that his hearing had deteriorated over the last few years, but admitted that he had had trouble understanding people over the telephone. An examination of taste showed perception of a saline solution to be weaker on the left side of the anterior tongue.

OVERVIEW

The importance of hearing derives from the fact that speech is the most common medium for language and communication. Severe hearing deficits isolate patients from both family and friends and exert a tremendous impact on their quality of life. As the material in this chapter is presented, it should be borne in mind that identification of a hearing loss is a sign of a disease and not a diagnosis. The key to diagnosis is having a solid understanding of the physics of sound as well as the anatomy and physiology of the auditory system. Once the correct diagnosis is made and the proper treatment initiated, most types of hearing loss can be corrected.

PHYSICAL PROPERTIES OF SOUND

Frequency *is measured in hertz and is perceived as pitch.*

Sound consists of oscillations or vibrations of a medium, such as air or bone. For pure tones, the oscillations are both periodic and sinusoidal, but most sounds, including speech, involve complex, aperiodic fluctuations in pressure that the auditory system decomposes into simple sine waves (Figures 7-1 and 7-2). Because these sinusoidal increases (compression) and decreases (rarefaction) in pressure represent a form of vibration, the adequate stimulus for audition is mechanical energy; this explains why a vibrating tuning fork placed on the base of the mastoid process of the temporal bone produces an audible sound. The perceived *pitch* of a sound is related to the frequency of the pressure oscillations each second, expressed in hertz (Hz).

Sound intensity *is measured in decibels and is perceived as loudness.*

The range of human hearing is usually cited as 20–20,000 Hz, but this is true only for children. The upper frequency limit recedes at the rate of 300 Hz per year, beginning at age 20. *Loudness*, the perceptual correlate of sound intensity, is measured as the peak-to-trough difference in sound pressure level. Loudness is expressed on a logarithmic scale devised by Alexander Graham Bell, appropriately named the decibel (dB) scale.

FIGURE 7-1

Compression and Rarefaction of Air Molecules Associated with a Pure Tone. *Vibrations from a tuning fork are transmitted through the media (e.g., air, water, bone) adjacent to the ear as a series of oscillatory molecular compressions and rarefactions. The frequency of these oscillations determines the perceived pitch of the tone; the magnitude of the pressure wave is correlated with loudness. Loudness is independent of pitch. (Source: Adapted with permission from Yin TCT: Audition. In* Neuroscience in Medicine. *Edited by Conn PM: Philadelphia, PA: J. B. Lippincott, 1995, p 486.)*

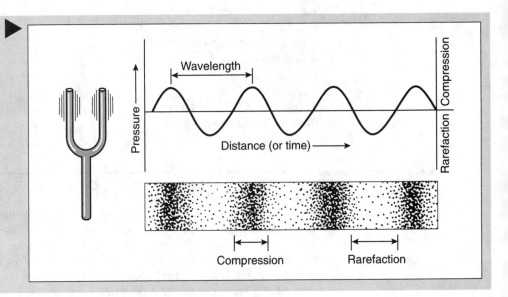

The dynamic range for hearing spans almost 12 logarithmic units or 120 dB, from a lower limit close to the physical background of thermal energy (brownian movement) up to the point of pain where physical injury may occur. Despite this tremendous operating range, human subjects can distinguish between two sounds that differ by as little as 0.5 dB. Figure 7-3 illustrates the decibel rating of some familiar sounds. As Figure 7-4 shows, threshold sensitivity varies significantly across the audio spectrum. The ear is most sensitive to frequencies between 2000 and 4000 Hz and becomes progressively less sensitive to lower and higher frequencies. Most conversational speech is based on frequencies from 250 to 4000 Hz, a range within which our sensitivity is good.

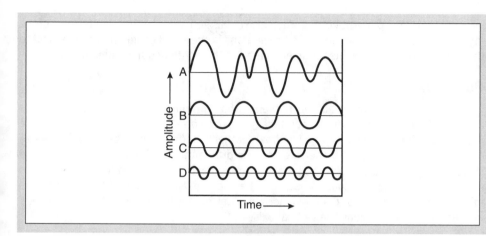

FIGURE 7-2
Relationship Between Complex Sounds and Pure Tones. *Most natural sounds, including speech, consist of complex pressure waves (panel A) rather than periodic, sinusoidal oscillations. However, complex waves can be decomposed into a series of sine waves that vary in amplitude, frequency, and phase through a process that is not well understood but is reminiscent of Fourier analysis (panels B, C, and D).*

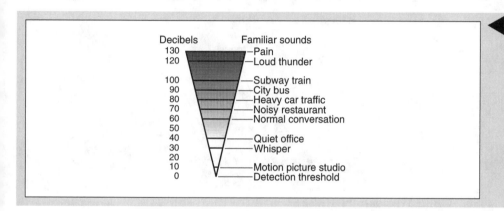

FIGURE 7-3
Decibel Ratings of Familiar Sounds

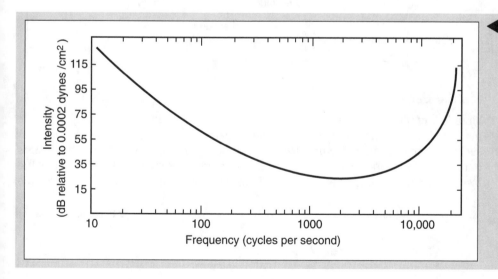

FIGURE 7-4
Human Detection Thresholds. *Monaural detection thresholds expressed as a function of frequency. (Source: Adapted with permission from Gulick WL, et al: Hearing: Physiological Acoustics, Neural Coding and Psychoacoustics. New York, NY: Oxford University Press, 1989, p 110.)*

GENERAL ORGANIZATION OF THE TRANSDUCTIVE APPARATUS

The peripheral auditory apparatus can be divided into three parts: the outer ear, the middle ear, and the inner ear. The outer ear collects and funnels sound waves to the eardrum, whose movements are transmitted directly to the ossicles of the middle ear. The ossicles transmit vibrations of the tympanic membrane to the inner ear, where sound transduction takes place. Electrophysiologic signals generated in the receptor cells of the inner ear are conducted to the first-order neurons in the spiral ganglion, which project to the dorsal and ventral cochlear nuclei located at the pontomedullary junction.

Outer Ear

The *outer ear* consists of the auricle, or pinna, whose primary function is to gather sounds and funnel them into the external auditory meatus and onto the *tympanic membrane* (see Figure 7-5). The efficacy with which animals gather sounds varies, depending on the size of their ears and on whether they are capable of orienting their ears toward the sound source. Although the pinna acts as a passive receptacle for sound in humans, it makes other important contributions to hearing. The complex architecture of the pinna favors midrange frequencies that dominate normal vocalization. In addition, the pinna assists in sound localization along the vertical axis.

FIGURE 7-5 ▶
The Peripheral Auditory Apparatus. The constituent parts of the outer, middle, and inner ear are shown. The cochlea is "unfolded" to illustrate the continuity of the scala vestibuli between the oval and round windows.

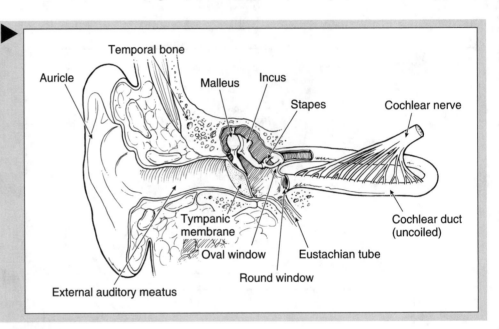

Middle Ear

Hammer → anvil → stirrup.

Vibrations of the tympanic membrane are transmitted across the middle ear by a chain of three *ossicles* or bones. The first bone, the *malleus* (hammer), is attached to the inner surface of the eardrum (Figure 7-6; see Figure 7-5). Movement of the malleus is transmitted to the *incus* (anvil) and then to the *stapes* (stirrup), which is attached to the *oval window* of the fluid-filled inner ear. Transmission of the acoustic signal across the

FIGURE 7-6 ▶
The Ossicles of the Middle Ear. The three ossicles of the middle ear are the malleus, incus, and stapes. The tympanic membrane (not shown) would be located to the left of the figure.

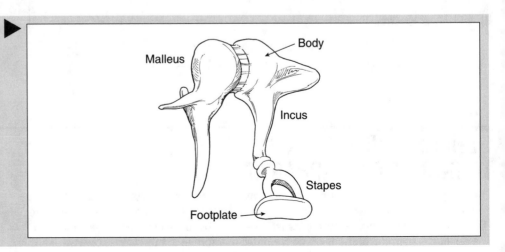

middle ear is a critical step in sound transduction because normally 99.9% of a sound conducted in air is reflected at a transition to a fluid medium. Partial compensation for this potential loss is achieved by the ossicular chain, which matches the impedance between the outer ear and the inner ear. The basis for the impedance match is the 22:1 ratio between the area of the tympanic membrane and the area of the oval window that allows the ossicles to act like an "energy funnel." A smaller contribution to the *impedance matching* is the lever action created by movement of the ossicles.

> **Ossicles** provide impedance matching.

Patients with otosclerotic restriction of stapedic motion experience a 20–30 dB loss of sensitivity, which is clinically significant. Even though transmission through the middle ear is severely impeded, these patients continue to hear sounds conducted to the inner ear through the bones of the skull. Two diagnostic tests (Rinne's test and Weber's test) used to distinguish between hearing loss resulting from middle ear dysfunction and hearing loss of sensorineural origin are discussed at the end of this section.

The middle ear is filled with air, and it communicates with the nasopharynx through the eustachian tube. The eustachian tube is usually closed but opens during swallowing to prevent or dissipate pressure gradients that may develop between the middle ear and the outside world. Obstruction of airflow through the eustachian tube creates a pressure differential between the middle and outer ear that not only impedes the movement of the eardrum, thereby muffling sounds, but also causes discomfort and may rupture the eardrum in severe cases. This explains why airline passengers hear better after "popping their ears" to equalize pressure across the eardrum.

At the other extreme are loud sounds capable of damaging the delicate structures of the inner ear. Two muscles within the middle ear, the *tensor tympani* and *stapedius*, protect the inner ear: the tensor tympani, by limiting the excursions of the tympanic membrane and the stapedius, by limiting the movement of the stapes. The tensor tympani muscle is innervated by neurons in the trigeminal motor nucleus of the pons. The stapedius, on the other hand, is innervated by neurons in the facial nucleus. One of the presenting symptoms of damage to the facial nerve is hyperacusis, the perception that sounds of normal intensity are too loud. Like the pupillary reflex, contractions of the tensor tympani and the stapedius muscles are consensual. The response latency for the stapedius and tensor tympani muscles is on the order of 10 msec, making these protective reflexes more effective for sustained, rather than for brief, percussive sounds. Both of these muscles also play a role in the suppression of auditory transmission during self-vocalization.

Inner Ear

The inner ear consists of membranous sacs and ducts encased in bony chambers and canals within the petrous bone of the temporal lobe. Based upon anatomic and functional considerations, the inner ear is divisible into two parts: the *cochlea*, which is concerned with hearing, and the *semicircular canals* and *otolith organs*, which are concerned with balance (Figure 7-7). The partitioning of hearing and balance into dedicated areas is preserved during the approach to and ascent through the central nervous system (CNS). Separate nerve fibers of the *vestibulocochlear nerve* (cranial nerve VIII) convey auditory and vestibular information to different nuclei in the brainstem. Accordingly, the senses of hearing and balance are treated in separate chapters in this book.

Cochlea

The cochlea is a fluid-filled tube coiled two and one-half times around itself to resemble a snail shell (see Figure 7-7). The *vestibular (Reissner's)* and *basilar membranes* partition the cochlea into three chambers (Figure 7-8). The *scala vestibuli* and *scala tympani* flank an inner chamber, the *scala media* (or cochlear duct), which contains the specialized epithelium of the *organ of Corti* where sound transduction takes place. The scalae vestibuli and tympani are filled with a cerebrospinal-like fluid called *perilymph* and are continuous with one another at the *helicotrema*, a small opening located at the apex of the cochlear coil. The scala media is filled with *endolymph*, a clear fluid with a high potassium (K^+) concentration that is formed by the *stria vascularis*, a layer of vascular

> *"Cochlea"* is Latin for snail.

FIGURE 7-7 ▶

Auditory and Vestibular Components of the Inner Ear. The cells of origin of the cochlear nerve are located in the spiral ganglion, which is distributed along the length of the cochlea. The bones of the middle ear, which are not shown in this figure, would be located to the left of the cochlea. The inset illustrates the in situ location and orientation of the inner ear. (Source: Reprinted with permission from Brodel M: Three unpublished drawings of the anatomy of the human ear. Phila-delphia, PA: W. B. Saunders, 1946.)

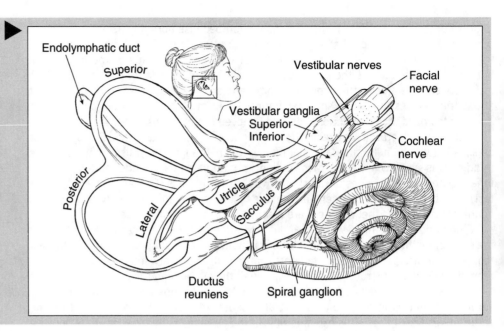

FIGURE 7-8 ▶

Cross Section of the Cochlea. A full appre-ciation of the three main chambers of the cochlea—the scala vestibuli, the scala tympani, and the scala media—can be achieved when the cochlea is viewed in cross section. Sound transduction takes place at the hair cells of the organ of Corti, which is located along the basilar mem-brane.

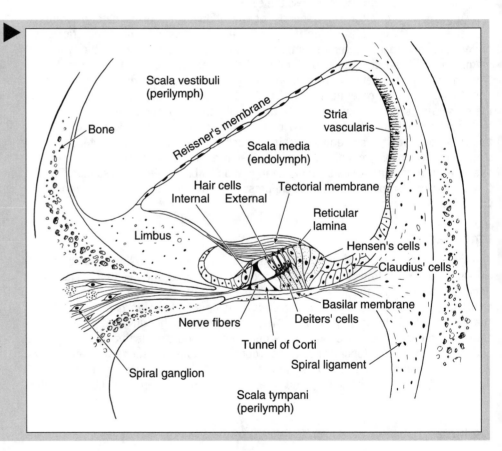

tissue located on the outer wall of the cochlea duct. Endolymph perfuses the scala media as well as the semicircular canals and otolith organs of the inner ear. The piston-like action of the footplate of the stapes against the oval window creates a pressure wave in the perilymph of the scala vestibuli that travels through the helicotrema into the scala tympani. Compliance of the round window at the basal end of the scala tympani enables the pressure wave to traverse the cochlea rather than being reflected at the oval window by the incompressible perilymph. As these pressure waves distort the vestibular and basilar membranes, movement is transmitted, in turn, to the endolymph of the scala media, the organ of Corti, and the *tectorial membrane* suspended above the organ of Corti from its point of attachment at the limbus.

Organ of Corti

The organ of Corti within the scala media is a region of almost bewildering mechanical complexity. The basilar membrane stretches between the modiolus and the spiral ligament and serves as the platform for the organ of Corti where sound transduction takes place (see Figure 7-8). The most important components of the organ of Corti are the inner and outer hair cells. The *inner hair cells* form a single row on the basilar membrane adjacent to the modiolus while the *outer hair cells* form three rows on the opposite side of the tunnel of Corti. The *stereocilia* of the outer hair cells are arranged in the form of a chevron (Figure 7-9). Both inner and outer hair cells have a tuft of 30–200 stereocilia of graded height emerging from a tough cuticular plate at the apical surface of the cell body (Figure 7-10). Because the tips of the stereocilia contact the overlying tectorial mem-

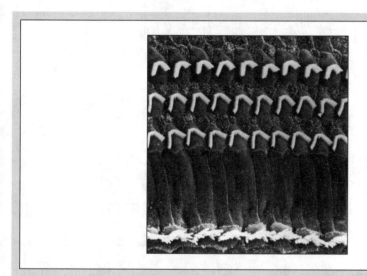

◀ **FIGURE 7-9**
Scanning Electron Micrograph of the Organ of Corti. *The organ of Corti contains a single row of inner hair cells and three rows of outer hair cells. In this photomicrograph, the tectorial membrane has been removed. (Source: Reprinted with permission from Lewis ER, et al:* The Vertebrate Inner Ear. *Boca Raton, FL: CRC Press, 1985, p 21.)*

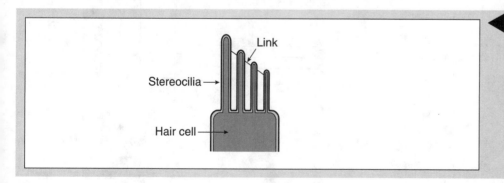

Link
Stereocilia
Hair cell

◀ **FIGURE 7-10**
Linkage of Adjacent Hair Cells of the Inner Ear. *Adjacent stereocilia on each hair cell are linked by thin fibers. This linkage enables movement of taller cilia to distort the apical tips of adjacent cilia, which, in turn, opens K$^+$ channels and initiates the electrochemical cascade of sound transduction.*

brane, pressure waves within the cochlea displace the basilar and tectorial membranes and bend the stereocilia. The different pivotal points of the tectorial and basilar membranes on the limbus produce a shearing force on the stereocilia that amplifies the generator potential of the hair cells (Figure 7-11; see also Figure 7-8). Both inner and outer hair cells, like receptor cells in other sensory systems, communicate with the distal dendritic processes of the first-order neurons (Figure 7-12).

Differences in the innervation patterns of inner and outer hair cells suggest that each cell type plays a unique role in sound transduction. Roughly 3000 inner hair cells synapse onto 20,000 cochlear nerve fibers (Figure 7-13). By comparison, approximately 20,000 outer hair cells converge onto 3000 cochlear nerve fibers. The high degree of signal preservation at the synapses between the inner hair cells and the first-order neurons suggests that inner hair cells are the primary receptor cells of the auditory system.

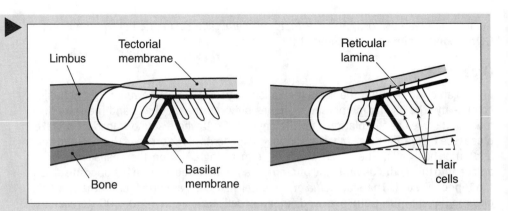

FIGURE 7-11

Shearing Force within the Organ of Corti. *Diagrammatic representation of the shearing force applied to the tips of the hair cell cilia. The shearing force is caused by the different pivotal points of the basilar and tectorial membranes on the bony modiolus. (Source: Reprinted with permission from Davis H: Transmission and transduction in the cochlea. Laryngoscope 68:359–383, 1958.)*

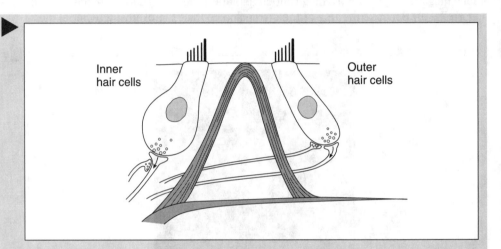

FIGURE 7-12

Afferent and Efferent Innervation of the Inner and Outer Hairs. *Electrical activity in both inner hair cells and outer hair cells is transmitted to the cochlear nerve across synapses located at the base of these cells. Axosomatic synapses located at the base of outer hair cells may enable neurons located within the periolivary nuclei to sharpen sound transduction within local regions of the organ of Corti. Afferent information from the inner hair cells may be modulated by efferent axodendritic synapses located near the distal end of the cochlear nerve fibers.*

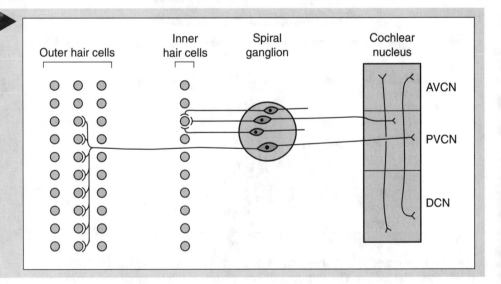

FIGURE 7-13

Innervation Patterns of the Inner and Outer Hair Cells. *The divergent innervation pattern of the inner hair cells ensures redundancy and reliable transmission to the CNS. Outer hair cells, by comparison, show tremendous convergence onto single spiral ganglion cells, causing the identity of individual cells to be lost. Afferent information arising from both inner and outer hair cells projects to all three divisions of the cochlear nucleus. AVCN = anterior ventral cochlear nucleus; PVCN = posterior ventral cochlear nucleus; DCN = dorsal cochlear nucleus.*

Outer hair cells differ from inner hair cells in several key ways. First, outer hair cell stereocilia do not merely contact the tectorial membrane, they penetrate it. Second, outer hair cells may increase or decrease their length by as much as 5% during mechanical or electrical stimulation. Although the mechanism for the kinetic ability of the outer hair cells is uncertain, it has been hypothesized that vibrations of the outer hair cells during sound reception induce an electrokinetic resonance in the outer hair cells that reinforces basilar membrane movement. This hypothesis not only justifies the large number of outer hair cells and their highly convergent synaptic arrangement but also explains why these cells act as a unit.

The cochlear nerve, in addition to its large population of afferent fibers, contains a significant contingent of efferent fibers that project from the *superior olivary complex* of the pons to the cochlea (see Figure 7-12). These efferent *olivocochlear projections* may gate incoming information. The cholinergic olivocochlear projections synapse directly on the distal processes of the cochlear nerve near the base of the inner hair cells, apparently to modulate the afferent activity en route to the brain. By comparison, olivocochlear projections to the outer hair cells synapse directly on the basolateral surface of the cell body, suggesting that their role in sound transduction is likely to be different. With the recent demonstration that outer hair cells have motile properties, these axosomatic synapses may enable the outer hairs to act as effectors to restrict movements of the basilar and tectorial membranes and thus protect the inner hair cells from overstimulation. This is consistent with research showing that electrical stimulation of the cochlear nerve hyperpolarizes outer hair cells and that removal of outer hair cells raises the auditory threshold.

Sound Transduction

Displacement of the basilar and tectorial membranes causes hair cells of the organ of Corti to bend at their point of attachment at the cuticular plate. The stereocilia move as a unit because the tip of each stereocilium is linked to the side of its taller neighbor (Figure 7-14; see also Figure 7-10). Bending the stereocilia in one direction stretches the cross-links between adjacent stereocilia and distorts a channel protein (see Figure 7-14), allowing K^+ in the endolymph to flow down its concentration gradient into the stereocilia. Passive spread of the depolarization to the hair cell soma activates an inward calcium (Ca^{2+}) current and drives an outward K^+ current that releases neurotransmitter from the base of the hair cell. Bending the stereocilia in the opposite direction releases the tension on the cross-links and allows the K^+ channels to close (see Figure 7-14). The interplay of the K^+ and Ca^{2+} cycles produces an electrochemical resonance in the stereocilia that reinforces the mechanical action of the tectorial membrane and produces sharper tuning along the basilar membrane.

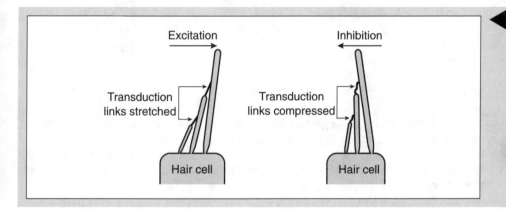

FIGURE 7-14
Ciliary Cross-Links. The cross-links between adjacent stereocilia may provide the trigger mechanism for the electrochemical events associated with sound transduction. This diagram illustrates how movement of the hair cell stereocilia in one direction may stretch the cross-links secured to adjacent stereocilia, thus enabling its K^+ channels to open. Movement of the stereocilia in the opposite direction allows the cross-links to relax and the ion channels to close.

Coding of Pitch

Despite active discussion and debate for over a century, there is still no consensus regarding the mechanisms responsible for pitch perception. Presently, there is partial support for place and frequency theories of pitch perception. *Place theories* maintain that perception of pitch varies according to the locus of excitation along the basilar membrane. The earliest place theory dates to the mid-nineteenth century when Helmholtz suggested that the fibers of the basilar membrane resonate like a harp. According to Helmholtz's resonance theory, high tones stimulate the basal region of the basilar membrane while low tones are effective near the apex (Figures 7-15 and 7-16). Experiments conducted decades later by von Bekesy demonstrated that the resonance theory was untenable because the fibers of the basilar membrane are cross-linked to one another and lack sufficient tension to resonate as suggested by Helmholtz. Furthermore,

Bass is not at the base; it is at the apex.

FIGURE 7-15 ▶

Tonotopic Organization of the Cochlea. *Transduction of high frequencies takes place near the oval window; cells that respond to low frequencies are located near the helicotrema at the apex of the cochlea. Note that as the width of the basilar membrane progressively increases from the base to the apex, the thickness and tension of the basilar membrane decreases.*

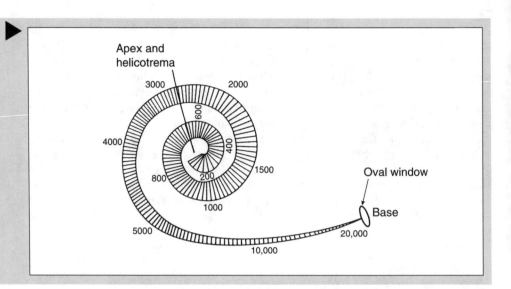

FIGURE 7-16 ▶

Tonotopic Organization of the Cochlea. *(A) Vibrations conducted from the oval window to the cochlea produce deflections in the basilar membrane that travel from the base to the apex. Maximal displacement of the basilar membrane occurs within a restricted region that varies as a function of auditory frequency. (B) High tones produce maximal displacement near the oval window, where the basilar membrane is relatively narrow. Maximal displacement of the basilar membrane takes place near the apex during stimulation with low tones.*

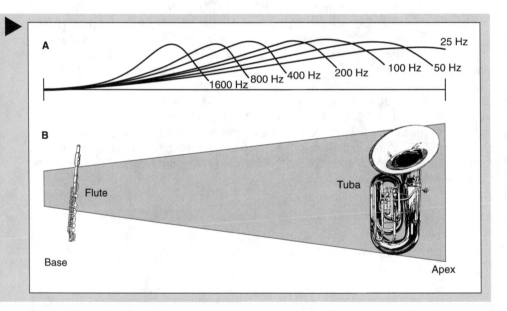

Tonotopic *is to hearing as* **somatotopic** *is to touch.*

auditory stimuli distorted large portions of the basilar membrane, not focal areas as required by the resonance theory. Although the mechanical properties postulated by Helmholtz were wrong, the general concept of the place theory was correct and today forms the basis for the tonotopic organization that begins in the cochlea and is observed at every level of the auditory system up to and including the cerebral cortex.

Von Bekesy showed that auditory stimulation produces a traveling wave that spreads from the base to the apex with one region of maximal displacement. The locus of maximal displacement is determined by the mechanical characteristics of the basilar membrane, the fluid dynamics of the cochlea, and the frequency of the auditory stimulus. Basilar membrane displacement is largest near the base of the cochlea for high-pitched tones; low tones preferentially distort the apex of the basilar membrane near the helicotrema (see Figures 7-15 and 7-16). The crest of the traveling wave, however, is too broad to allow fine discriminations of pitch, especially at low frequencies. Von Bekesy suggested that the peak displacement may be sharpened by lateral inhibition, but a more recent and as yet unproven hypothesis seems more appealing. This hypothesis holds that oscillations of the generator potential may enable the cochlear hair cells to change length in phase with the motion of the tectorial membrane, thereby amplifying the peak displacement.

The competing theory of pitch perception is the *frequency theory*, or the "telephone theory," first devised by Rutherford in the late nineteenth century. As originally conceived, the telephone theory postulates that the basilar membrane vibrates as a whole and translates the vibration frequency into a neural discharge frequency. As the field of neurophysiology matured, it became apparent that neurons are unable to follow frequencies above 800–1000 Hz. The frequency theory fell into disfavor but received a partial reprieve when Wever suggested that auditory neurons respond to every second, third, or nth beat of the basilar membrane to keep pace with auditory frequencies in excess of 1000 Hz. The demonstration that neurons in the cochlear nerve fire in synchrony with the basilar membrane movement has provided support for Wever's "volley theory," at least for tones up to 5000 Hz. At present, it is thought that the frequency and place theories combine to span the entire auditory spectrum. According to this duplex theory, low tones (i.e., < 5000 Hz) are encoded by the frequency of action potentials while high tones (i.e., > 5000 Hz) are encoded by the location of the active neurons.

CENTRAL ANATOMY

Cochlear Nuclei

The cell bodies of the vestibulocochlear nerve (cranial nerve VIII) are located within the spiral ganglion of the inner ear (see Figure 7-7 and 7-8). The distal processes of these bipolar neurons synapse on the basolateral surface of the inner and outer hair cells while the central processes course through the internal auditory meatus before entering the brain at the cerebellopontine angle just lateral, dorsal, and caudal to the root of the vestibular branch of cranial nerve VIII (see Chapter 4, Figure 4-10). All fibers of the vestibulocochlear nerve bifurcate upon entering the brain and terminate in the anterior and posterior divisions of the ventral cochlear nucleus (AVCN and PVCN) and the dorsal cochlear nucleus (DCN) [Figure 7-17]. The dorsal and ventral cochlear nuclei are located on the lateral aspect of the inferior cerebellar peduncle and form a distinct bulge called the acoustic tubercle. Primary auditory fibers that issue from the apex of the basilar membrane transduce low frequency tones and terminate in the ventrolateral quadrant of each cochlear nucleus. Fibers emanating from the base of the cochlea, where higher frequency tones are represented, project to the dorsomedial quadrant of the cochlear nuclei. In this manner, the *tonotopic organization* established within the organ of Corti is preserved in the cochlear nuclei.

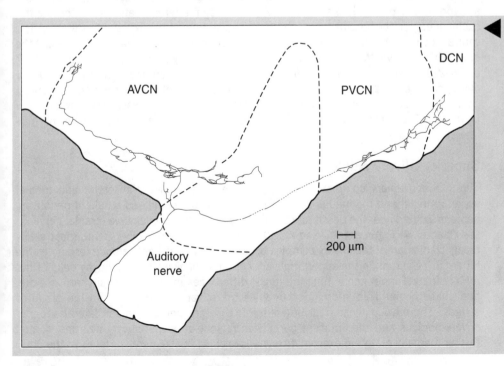

FIGURE 7-17
Reconstruction of an Individual Auditory Nerve. *As this auditory fiber enters the brainstem, the root branch bifurcates to form ascending and descending branches that terminate in the anterior ventral cochlear nucleus (AVCN), the posterior ventral cochlear nucleus (PVCN), and the dorsal cochlear nucleus (DCN) [horseradish peroxidase stain].* (Source: Reprinted with permission from Ryugo DK, Rouiller EM: The central projections of intracellularly labeled auditory fibers. J Comp Neurol 271:132, 1988.)

Among the different neuron types in the cochlear nuclei, bushy cells are particularly noteworthy. Bushy cells have short, thick dendritic trees and are distributed throughout the AVCN. Primary auditory neurons have extensive terminations with large synaptic endings on the soma and proximal dendrites of spherical bushy cells. These very secure synaptic configurations, called the end-bulbs of Held (Figure 7-18), are believed to create the high-fidelity links that the auditory system uses to locate sound sources in the environment.

FIGURE 7-18 ▶
An End-bulb of Held. The end-bulbs of Held located in the anterior ventral cochlear nucleus provide the secure links in the ascending auditory pathway necessary for localization of sound.

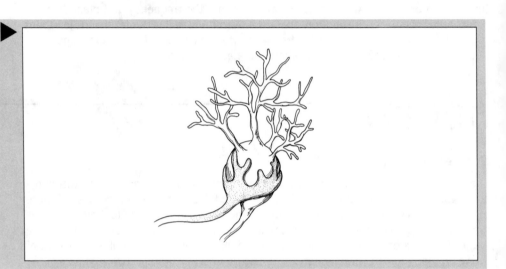

As auditory information leaves the cochlear nuclei, its ascent through the neuraxis becomes bilateral, but the contralateral pathway predominates. There are three efferent pathways from the cochlear nuclei: the dorsal, intermediate, and ventral acoustic striae (Figure 7-19). The *dorsal acoustic stria* exits the dorsal aspect of the dorsal cochlear nucleus, curves around the inferior cerebellar peduncle, and courses medially through the pontine tegmentum before ascending to the midbrain via the lateral lemniscus. The *intermediate acoustic stria* exits from the dorsal tip of the ventral cochlear nucleus and crosses the tegmentum ventral to the dorsal stria. The intermediate stria sends a small projection to the periolivary nuclei, but most of this tract merges with the other ascending auditory fibers of the lateral lemniscus. The major efferent pathway of the ventral cochlear nuclei, the *ventral acoustic stria*, arises primarily from axons of bushy cells. The ventral acoustic stria projects to the ipsilateral *superior olivary nuclei* before crossing the brain within the ventral tegmentum as the *trapezoid body* (see Chapter 4, Figures 4-17 and 4-22). Small groups of fibers from the trapezoid body terminate within the superior olivary complex, the nuclei of the trapezoid body, and the reticular formation; the largest contingent, however, joins the contralateral *lateral lemniscus* and ascends to the *inferior colliculus*. The ventral cochlear nucleus does not have a direct projection to the ipsilateral inferior colliculus.

Superior Olivary Nuclei

The superior olivary complex consists of three main nuclei (the lateral and medial superior nuclei and the medial nucleus of the trapezoid body) and a halo of periolivary neurons located near the descending root fibers of the abducens nerve (cranial nerve VI; see Chapter 4, Figures 4-17 and 4-22). The lateral superior olive is the most easily recognizable part of the olivary complex because its "folded" appearance resembles the letter "S." Neurons in the superior olivary complex receive from the bushy cells of the AVCN binaural input concerning interaural differences in sound intensity, arrival time, and phase angle. This information enables the olivary nuclei to locate the origin of sounds. The olivocochlear tract originates from other neurons in the lateral superior olivary nucleus and the adjacent periolivary region; other periolivary neurons located further medially maintain axosomatic synapses on the basolateral surfaces of the outer

Sound localization is based on interaural differences in loudness, phase angle, and time of arrival.

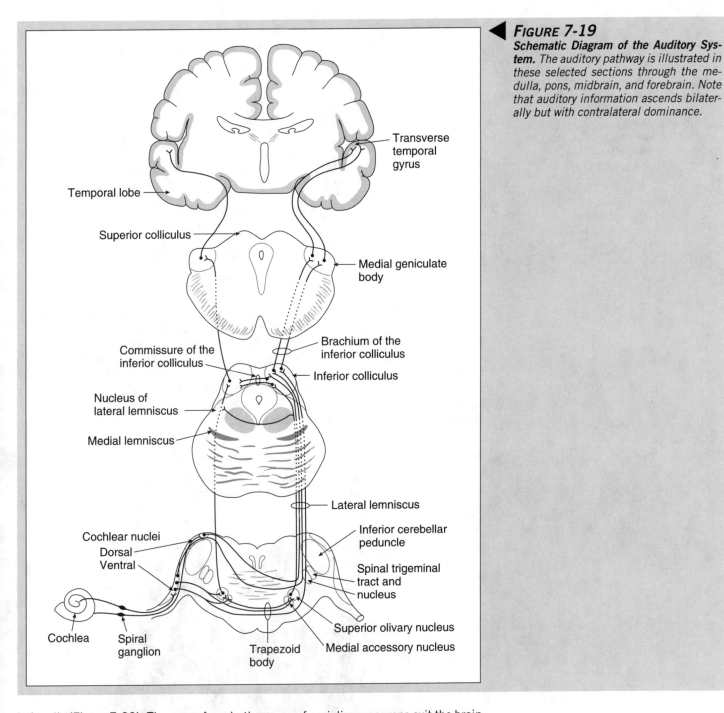

FIGURE 7-19
Schematic Diagram of the Auditory System. The auditory pathway is illustrated in these selected sections through the medulla, pons, midbrain, and forebrain. Note that auditory information ascends bilaterally but with contralateral dominance.

Labels in figure:
Transverse temporal gyrus
Temporal lobe
Superior colliculus
Medial geniculate body
Commissure of the inferior colliculus
Brachium of the inferior colliculus
Inferior colliculus
Nucleus of lateral lemniscus
Medial lemniscus
Lateral lemniscus
Inferior cerebellar peduncle
Cochlear nuclei
Dorsal
Ventral
Spinal trigeminal tract and nucleus
Cochlea
Spiral ganglion
Trapezoid body
Superior olivary nucleus
Medial accessory nucleus

hair cells (Figure 7-20). The axons from both groups of periolivary neurons exit the brain within the vestibular portion of cranial nerve VIII before joining the cochlear division at the vestibulocochlear anastomosis. After the olivocochlear tract passes through the spiral ganglion, it enters the organ of Corti by perforating the bony capsule of the modiolus. Other neurons with the superior olivary complex act as interneurons in the *stapedial reflex*. The stapedial reflex is mediated by projections from the bushy cells of the AVCN to the superior olivary complex, which, in turn, projects to the facial motor nucleus, where lower motor neurons complete the reflex.

Neurons in the superior olivary complex, along with many in the dorsal cochlear nucleus and PVCN, project to the inferior colliculus via the lateral lemniscus. The lateral lemniscus contains axons that originate from all three divisions of the contralateral cochlear nucleus, the lateral superior olive bilaterally, and the ipsilateral medial superior olive. The lateral lemniscus originates near the lateral border of the superior olivary complex, where these second-, third-, and fourth-order auditory efferent fibers coalesce.

FIGURE 7-20 ▶

Efferent Projections to the Cochlea. The cells of origin for the efferent projections to the inner and outer hair cells of the cochlea are located in the periolivary nuclei. (Source: Reprinted with permission from Warr WB: Organization of olivocochlear efferents in mammals. In The Mammalian Auditory Pathway: Neuroanatomy. Edited by Webster DB, et al. New York, NY: Springer-Verlag, 1992, p 413.)

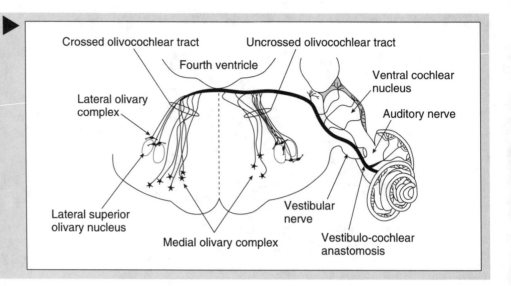

During its ascent through the pons, the lateral lemniscus migrates laterally with the anterolateral system. As the lateral lemniscus enters the midbrain, it resembles a flattened ribbon lying lateral to the parabrachial nucleus and the superior cerebellar peduncle. The continuity of the lateral lemniscus is interrupted by the nuclei of the lateral lemniscus, a series of small relay nuclei that receive minor projections from ascending auditory fibers bound for the inferior colliculus. Further rostrally, the lateral lemniscus assumes a goblet-like appearance that embraces the base of the inferior colliculus as the axons terminate within its central nucleus (Figure 7-21).

FIGURE 7-21 ▶

The Caudal Mesencephalon. The lateral lemniscus, which resembles a narrow ribbon during its ascent through the pons, has a broader appearance as it begins to terminate within the inferior colliculus. (Weigert stain)

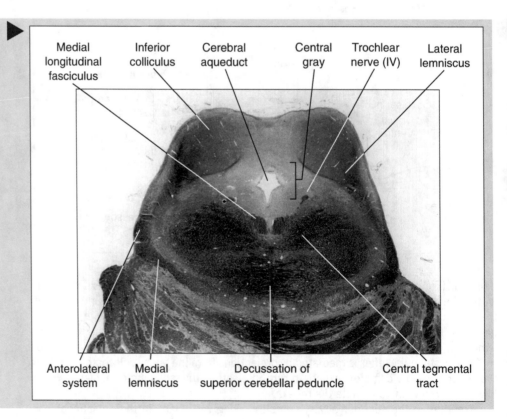

Inferior and Superior Colliculi

The inferior and superior colliculi receive projections from auditory relays of the lower brainstem, but each processes this information for a different end. The inferior colliculus serves as the primary mesencephalic relay for pitch and loudness information bound for the forebrain. The superior colliculus has two parts, a superficial region devoted exclusively to processing visual information and a deeper region that receives multimodal sensory input required for volitional eye and head movements. The inferior and superior colliculi warrant separate discussion.

The inferior colliculus is organized into core and belt regions, but only the core region contains a precise tonotopic organization. The inferior colliculus is divided into three parts based upon cytologic, connectional, and functional criteria: the central nucleus, the dorsal cortex, and the pericentral nucleus. The central nucleus, the core region of the inferior colliculus, receives direct, tonotopically organized projections from all three subdivisions of the contralateral cochlear nucleus. Other projections to the central nucleus from the superior olivary complex contain both ipsilateral and contralateral components, but only some of these have a tonotopic arrangement. Neurons responsive to high frequencies are located more superficially than neurons that respond to low frequencies. The dorsal cortex, part of the belt region, receives monaural input from the cochlear nuclei and a strong descending projection from both primary and secondary auditory cortices. The remaining belt area, the pericentral nucleus, receives some auditory projections, but it gets many more from nonauditory sources such as the spinal cord, the dorsal column nuclei, and the parietal cortex. This pattern of afferent and efferent projections and the fact that weak electrical stimulation produces orientation of the head, eyes, and pinna to the contralateral side suggest that the pericentral nucleus mediates acousticomotor functions.

> Every auditory station beginning with the inferior colliculus has both core and belt regions.

The superior colliculus (see Chapter 4, Figures 4-23 and 4-25) consists of a superficial shell that is devoted exclusively to the visual system and a multisensory core that receives convergent information from the visual, auditory, and somatosensory systems. The role of the superficial layers of the superior colliculus and the remainder of the extrageniculate pathway in the acquisition and tracking of moving objects by the fovea will be discussed in the chapter on the visual system (see Chapter 10). Auditory information ascends to the deep layers of the superior colliculus from the rostral pole of the inferior colliculus as well as from parts of the periolivary nuclei, auditory cortex, and the frontal eye fields. Most of the efferent projections from the deep layers of the superior colliculus descend to regions of the brainstem and spinal cord involved with control of head and eye movements. For example, projections to the pretectum, paramedian pontine reticular formation (PPRF), and the rostral interstitial nucleus of the medial longitudinal fasciculus engage oculomotor reflexes triggered by auditory, visual, or somatosensory stimuli. The tectospinal tract, which also originates in the deep layers of the superior colliculus, descends to the cervical spinal cord and mediates reflexive postural movements of the head and neck. The origin, course, and distribution of the tectospinal tract was described in Chapter 3.

Medial Geniculate Nucleus

Axons originating from the central nucleus of the inferior colliculus form the *brachium of the inferior colliculus*, a robust tract perched on the outside of the midbrain that terminates in the ventral division of the medial geniculate nucleus (MGN) of the thalamus (see Chapter 4, Figure 4-23; see Chapter 5, Figure 5-1E). The MGN is located in the caudal diencephalon ventral to the pulvinar and medial to the lateral geniculate nucleus (LGN). The MGN consists of ventral, dorsal, and medial subdivisions. The ventral division is the largest subdivision and the core projection area for ascending projections from the central nucleus of the inferior colliculus. Like the central nucleus of the inferior colliculus, the ventral MGN is composed of concentric lamellae with a precise tonotopic organization. High frequencies are located in the medial quadrant of the ventral nucleus; low frequencies are located further laterally. The ventral MGN is a key link in the core projection to the primary auditory cortex that plays an important role in auditory discrimination. The dorsal and medial divisions, on the other hand, are considered components of the belt region because they receive significant afferent projections from the pericentral and external nuclei of the inferior colliculus as well as from nonauditory sources such as the lateral tegmentum of the midbrain and the spinal cord. Auditory information ascending through the belt areas may direct attention to auditory cues in the environment or link auditory cues with objects detected by the visual or somatosensory systems.

Auditory Cortex

Auditory cortex is located in the transverse gyri of Heschl and the adjacent regions along the dorsomedial and dorsolateral aspects of the temporal lobe (see Chapter 2, Figure 2-7; see Chapter 5, Figure 5-19). Like the midbrain and thalamic auditory relays, the auditory cortex is organized into core and belt regions. The core region, located in Brodmann area 41 (see Chapter 5, Figure 5-10), represents the primary auditory cortex (AI) and receives ascending projections from the ventral division of the MGN. The higher-order auditory cortex resides in the belt region (Brodmann area 42) around AI and receives most of its input from the dorsal and medial subnuclei. Both sets of corticopetal projections exit the MGN laterally and pass through the sublenticular part of the internal capsule on their way to the temporal lobe.

Neurophysiologic experiments conducted largely in cats have identified several types of columns within AI. Isofrequency columns contain neurons that respond best to a narrow range of frequencies. The orderly arrangement of isofrequency columns creates a tonotopic organization similar to the subcortical auditory relays. In the marmoset, a New World monkey, low frequencies originating near the apex of the cochlea are represented further rostrally in AI than the higher frequencies from the cochlear base (Figure 7-22).

FIGURE 7-22 ▶
Tonotopic Organization of Primary Auditory Cortex. Electrophysiologic recordings in the monkey have enabled scientists to determine that the tonotopic organization initiated in the cochlea extends all of the way to the primary auditory cortex.

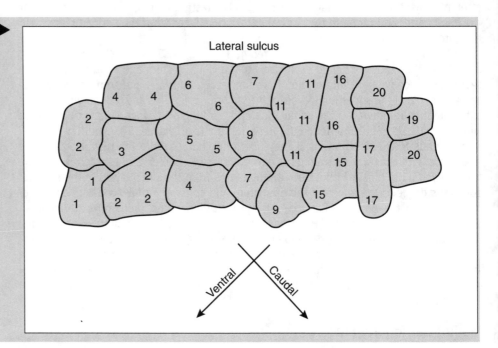

Although human data are limited, the results of positron emission tomography indicate a similar organization. *Binaural columns* are classified as suppression or summation columns. Neurons within *suppression columns* respond better to monaural stimulation of the contralateral ear than to binaural stimulation. Neurons within *summation columns* respond better to binaural stimulation than to monaural stimulation of either ear. Alternating bands of suppression and summation columns are superimposed upon, but oriented perpendicularly, to the isofrequency columns of AI. Because neurons in AI receive binaural input, unilateral cortical damage does not produce deafness in either ear.

Part of the belt region of the left hemisphere includes the *planum temporale* or *Wernicke's area* (Brodmann area 22), whose role in spoken language was discussed in Chapter 5. Damage to Wernicke's area produces word deafness, a type of sensory aphasia characterized by an inability to interpret the meaning of sounds.

CLINICAL ASPECTS

Despite the wide range of causative factors, hearing loss can be classified as either conductive or sensorineural in origin. *Conductive hearing loss* is due to mechanical interference of sound transmission through the outer or middle ear. Otitis media, when accompanied by effusion, is caused by decreased pressure within the middle ear that impedes tympanic membrane movement, resulting in hearing loss. Chronic cases of otitis media in children should be treated aggressively to ensure that normal speech and language development continue during this critical period. Otosclerotic deposits that immobilize the stapes are more commonly observed in adults but can be corrected surgically or with a hearing aid.

Sensorineural hearing loss is caused by damage either to the transduction apparatus within the cochlea, the cochlear nerve, or auditory areas within the CNS. Common causes of damage to the cochlea include ototoxic drugs, age, prolonged exposure to excessive noise, and viral labyrinthitis. Transient episodes of *tinnitus*, vertigo, or deafness can be caused by aminoglycoside antibiotics (e.g., gentamycin), antineoplastic agents (e.g., cisplatin), various heavy metals, and overdoses of quinine and even aspirin. While the mechanisms by which these drugs affect hearing is not known in each case, there is less uncertainty about how loud sounds achieve their deleterious effects; excessively loud sounds bend and break stereocilia and ultimately destroy hair cells within the organ of Corti. For sounds with a narrow frequency spectrum, the damage is usually concentrated in the region along the basilar membrane where transduction of those frequencies takes place. Sensorineural hearing loss also may be caused by compression of the cochlear nerve by acoustic neuromas, which are benign, slow-growing schwannomas or neurinomas that form at the cerebellopontine angle. Because these tumors may become quite large before they are diagnosed, hearing loss may be accompanied by ataxia, vertigo, and loss of taste as a result of involvement of the facial nerve, the vestibular branch of VIII, and the inferior cerebellar peduncle. Unilateral destruction of the cochlear nuclei produces complete deafness in the ipsilateral ear, but damage further centrally produces only partial deafness in the contralateral ear because auditory information ascends bilaterally. Damage to AI, which may have little effect on detection thresholds or identification of pure tones, is more likely to affect processing of brief sounds and perception of temporal sequences of sound, which play an important role in sound localization and the perception of language.

> Auditory deficits are either conductive or sensorineural in nature.

Diagnostic Tests

The distinction between conduction deafness and sensorineural deafness can be made in the clinic with two simple tests that exploit the fact that sound is conducted more efficiently by air than by bone. In *Rinne's test*, a vibrating tuning fork is held against the mastoid process until the patient signals that the sound is no longer audible. Moving the tuning fork to the outside of the pinna reinstates the sound of the tuning fork in individuals with normal hearing and sensorineural deafness. Patients with conduction deafness, however, can hear the tuning fork better when it is applied to the mastoid process because sound transmission through the middle ear is poor. In patients with unilateral deafness, the distinction between conduction and sensorineural deafness also can be distinguished with *Weber's test*. Patients with conduction deafness report that the sound of a vibrating tuning fork held against the forehead is louder in the affected ear; in patients with sensorineural deafness, the sound lateralizes to the normal ear. Auditory threshold deficits greater than 40 dB are almost always of sensorineural origin. Sensorineural deafness caused by damage to the cochlear nerve or lower brainstem can be identified by analyzing the early components of the brainstem auditory evoked potential, but lesions in forebrain auditory areas are best identified with conventional imaging techniques such as magnetic resonance imaging (MRI) or computerized axial tomography (CAT) scan.

RESOLUTION OF CLINICAL CASE

Acoustic neuromas usually present with nonauditory symptoms.

The patient described at the beginning of the chapter demonstrated many of the classic symptoms of an acoustic neuroma. *Acoustic neuromas* are slow-growing tumors that begin on the vestibular division of cranial nerve VIII at the cerebellopontine angle, infiltrate the internal auditory meatus, and gradually envelop both the auditory and vestibular divisions of cranial nerve VIII, the facial nerve (cranial nerve VII), and, in more extreme cases, the trigeminal nerve (cranial nerve V). Because these tumors usually grow to be quite large before they become symptomatic, displacement of the pons and cerebellum is common. The headaches were caused by increased intracranial pressure as indicated by papilledema in both eyes. This patient had a progressive loss of hearing but failed to recognize (or admit) the deficiency. Some patients do recognize, however, that they hear conversations over the telephone better if they hold the receiver to one ear rather than the other. It is not uncommon for patients with acoustic neuromas to seek medical treatment initially for symptoms other than hearing loss. The patient's dizziness and ataxia were caused by entrapment of the vestibular division of cranial nerve VIII and physical displacement of the inferior cerebellar peduncle and the cerebellum itself. Focal testing revealed a taste deficit on the front of the tongue, which is innervated by the chorda tympani, a branch of the facial nerve. Because taste is subserved by three different cranial nerves, few patients ever report gustatory deficits. Involvement of the facial nerve produced a diminished corneal reflex and weak facial musculature on the left side. Spread of the tumor rostrally affected the root of the trigeminal nerve with a resultant facial anesthesia on the ipsilateral side.

REVIEW QUESTIONS

Directions: For each of the following questions, choose the **one best** answer.

1. The ossicles are best described by which of the following statements?

    (A) They conduct sound from the eardrum to the inner ear with remarkable fidelity

    (B) Their movements are modulated by contracting the tensor tympani and stapedius muscles, both of which are innervated by neurons located within the dorsal and ventral cochlear nuclei

    (C) They match the impedance between the air in the auditory meatus and the perilymph of the inner ear

    (D) They connect the tympanic membrane to the round window of the cochlea

    (E) They attach to the oval window which leads into the scala media, where the hair cells are stimulated by a shearing action against the tectorial membrane

2. Which of the following auditory relays receives monaural input?

    (A) The ventral cochlear nucleus

    (B) The inferior colliculus

    (C) The superior olivary nucleus

    (D) The medial geniculate nucleus

    (E) The auditory cortex

3. Hyperacusis is caused by

    (A) paralysis of the tensor tympani muscle

    (B) faulty modulation of the inner and outer hair cells by the olivocochlear tract

    (C) obstruction of the eustachian tube

    (D) damage to the facial nerve

    (E) fusion of the ossicles

4. The tonotopic organization of the dorsal cochlear nucleus

    (A) is related to the spatial organization of pitch along the basilar membrane

    (B) reflects the differential distribution of hair cells along the basilar membrane

    (C) bears no resemblance to the nucleus of the cochlea

    (D) resembles the nucleus of the inferior colliculus

    (E) contributes to our ability to pinpoint the location of sounds in our extrapersonal space

5. Which of the following symptoms is most likely to be observed in a patient with an acoustic neuroma on the right side?

    (A) Paresis of the left leg

    (B) Weakness on the right side of the face

    (C) Paresis of the left arm

    (D) Loss of sensation from the right side of the face

    (E) Loss of the gag reflex

ANSWERS AND EXPLANATIONS

1. The answer is C. The ossicles of the middle ear enable vibrations to make the transition from the compressible medium of air to the incompressible fluid medium of the inner ear. This process, which transmits vibrations at the tympanic membrane to the scala vestibuli via the oval window, is known as impedance matching. As such, audio fidelity is less important than matching the impedance between the outer ear and the inner ear. The transmission of sound along the ossicles may be modulated by contractions of the tensor tympani and stapedius muscles, but the cells of origin for these muscles are located in the facial and trigeminal motor nuclei, not in the cochlear nuclei.

2. The answer is A. The ventral cochlear nucleus receives projections exclusively from the ipsilateral ear. All of the other nuclei listed process binaural input.

3. The answer is D. Hyperacusis, the perception that sounds are excessively loud, is caused by paralysis of the stapedius muscle coincident with facial nerve damage. Patients with paralysis of the tensor tympani muscle caused by damage to the trigeminal nerve or nucleus do not report an enhancement of auditory stimuli. Obstruction of the eustachian tube or fusion of the ossicles would impair hearing, not enhance it.

4. The answer is A. The tonotopic organization of all central auditory relays is related to the projection of the auditory spectrum onto the basilar membrane. The tonotopic organization present in the auditory system has no bearing on our ability to locate sounds in the environment. High frequencies such as those of the flute stimulate the hair cells located near the base of the basilar membrane. The tonotopic organization of the cochlea derives from the mechanical properties of the basilar membrane, not the distribution of hair cells along the membrane.

5. The answer is B. When an acoustic neuroma involves the motor branch of the facial nerve, there may be an ipsilateral, in this case a right-sided, weakness of the face. Choices A and C would accompany damage to the pyramidal tract, an unlikely result of an acoustic neuroma. Choices D and E would accompany damage to the fifth and ninth nerves, respectively; neither exits the brainstem at the cerebellopontine angle and thus are less likely to be affected than cranial nerve VII (choice B).

ADDITIONAL READING

Helfert RH, Snead CR, Altschuler RA: The ascending auditory pathways. In *Neurobiology of Hearing: The Central Auditory System.* Edited by Altschuler RA, Bobbin RP, Clopin BM, et al. New York, NY: Raven Press, 1991, pp 1–25.

Hudspeth AJ: How the ear's works work. *Nature* 341:397, 1989.

Pickles JO: *An Introduction to the Physiology of Hearing,* 2nd ed. New York, NY: Academic Press, 1988, pp 163–204.

Shepherd GM: *Neurobiology,* 2nd ed. New York, NY: Oxford University Press, 1988, pp 304–325.

Webster DB: An overview of mammalian auditory pathways with an emphasis on humans. In *The Mammalian Auditory Pathway: Neuroanatomy.* Edited by Webster DB, Popper AN, Fay RR. New York, NY: Springer-Verlag, 1992, pp 1–22.

Winer JA: The functional architecture of the medial geniculate body and the primary auditory cortex. In *The Mammalian Auditory Pathway: Neuroanatomy.* Edited by Webster DB, Popper AN, Fay RR. New York, NY: Springer-Verlag, 1992, pp 222–409.

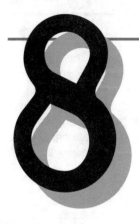

VESTIBULAR SYSTEM

INTRODUCTION OF CLINICAL CASE

M. L., a 68-year-old woman, scheduled an appointment with her primary care physician, complaining of brief but recurrent episodes of vertigo. Most of these attacks were triggered by either rolling over in bed, bending down, or getting up quickly. Several episodes that began when she rolled over in bed ended abruptly when she rolled back to the first side. None of the attacks lasted longer than 1 minute. Physical examination showed an otherwise healthy woman whose physical and mental condition was appropriate for her age. Visual examination of the auditory meatus and the tympanic membrane was unremarkable; hearing appeared normal. During the examination, the physician was able to trigger a vertigo attack by having M. L. sit on the examination table, turn her head to the right side, and quickly lie down on her left side. Confident of his diagnosis, the physician suggested that M. L. perform a series of head and neck exercises each day and predicted that these attacks would stop within a few weeks.

OVERVIEW

Unlike small movements of the hands and fingers, larger movements that involve the arms, legs, or torso often change the body's center of balance and force a repositioning of the head. Reflexive, compensatory adjustments of the musculoskeletal system initiated by the vestibular apparatus prevent a loss of balance. The vestibular system also coordinates head and eye movements to stabilize images on the retina. In the absence of movement, the vestibular system contributes to muscle tone and maintenance of posture. Normally, the actions of the vestibular system do not enter the conscious sphere; following injury, however, symptoms may emerge that are obvious and disabling, at least in the short-term. The importance of the vestibular apparatus should not be gauged by its small size (Figure 8-1).

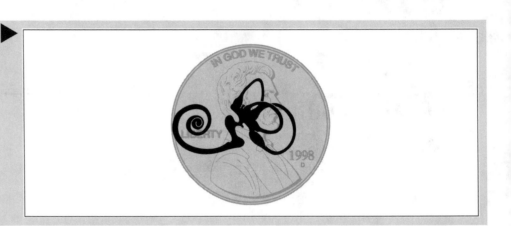

FIGURE 8-1
Vestibular Apparatus in Perspective. The size of the membranous labyrinths and cochlea can be appreciated by superimposing these delicate structures on a sketch of a penny.

PERIPHERAL ORGANIZATION

The auditory and vestibular parts of the inner ear are connected with one another through the ductus reuniens.

The *vestibular apparatus* consists of a series of fluid-filled membranous cavities suspended within the bony labyrinths of the petrous portion of the temporal bone. Though continuous with and in many ways similar to the auditory component of the inner ear, the vestibular apparatus is anatomically and functionally independent.

The vestibular apparatus consists of two parts, the *otolith organs* and the *semicircular canals*. Receptors located within the otolith organs respond to linear acceleration in the vertical or horizontal plane or tilting of the head. Receptors in the semicircular canals (see Chapter 7, Figure 7-7) respond to turning of the head, that is, angular acceleration. The otolith organs and the semicircular canals, like the *cochlea*, are bathed in *endolymph* and have sheets of specialized *hair cells* that respond to mechanical stimulation. Unlike the auditory system, the adequate stimulus for vestibular transduction is the inertial flow of endolymph caused by movement of the head.

Otolith Organs

The *utricle* and the *saccule* are located within the *vestibule*, the large chamber that separates the semicircular canals and the cochlea (see Chapter 7, Figure 7-7). With the head in the upright position, the utricle is oriented horizontally and responds to head tilt and movement along the horizontal plane (Figure 8-2). The vertical orientation of the saccule on the medial wall of the vestibule enables it to respond preferentially to dorsoventral excursions. Sensory transduction in both otolith organs takes place at the hair cells of the *macula*, a 1 mm^2 patch of sensory neuroepithelium. Vestibular hair cells have a tuft of 40–110 apical *stereocilia* arranged like a pipe organ against a single kinocilium (Figure 8-3). The arrangement of stereocilia along one side of the *kinocilium* gives these cells an asymmetrical appearance. The tips of the hair cell cilia are embedded in the overlying otolithic membrane, a gelatinous matrix that contains dense crystals of calcium carbonate called otoconia or *otoliths* (Figure 8-4). The otoconia make the otolithic membrane top-heavy. As the head position changes during rest or linear acceleration, the otolithic membrane tilts and provides additional leverage on the underlying stereocilia.

The orderly arrangement of hair cells within the maculae gives the appearance of a curved equatorial line called the *striola*. In the utricular macula, the hair cells are

"Otoconia" is a Latin word meaning "ear stones."

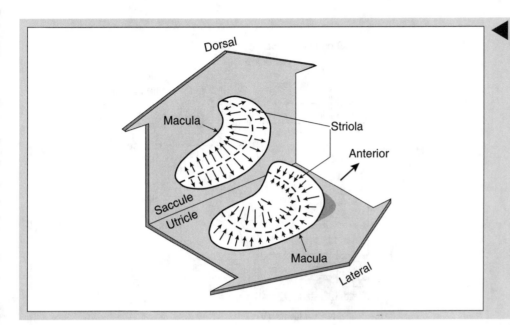

FIGURE 8-2
Orientation of the Otolith Organs. *The saccule and utricle are oriented perpendicularly to one another in the vestibule of the inner ear. The utricle, which is located on the floor of the vestibule, responds to head tilt or linear acceleration in the horizontal plane. The saccule, which forms part of the medial wall of the vestibule, responds to motion in the dorsoventral plane.* (Source: *Adapted with permission from Barber HO, Stockwell CW:* Manual of Electronystagmography. *St. Louis, MO: Mosby, 1976 p 27.*)

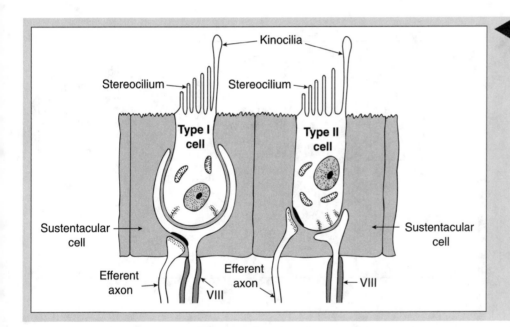

FIGURE 8-3
Vestibular Receptor Cells. *Vestibular hair cells are classified as either type I or type II cells. Type I cells are goblet-shaped and have large chalice-type synapses with the primary afferent neurons. Efferent modulation of afferent activity is suggested by the presence of axodendritic synapses at the distal end of the afferent process. Type II cells are columnar in shape and have multiple, small synapses at the basal end of the cell. Efferent projections to type II cells terminate on the basal surface of the hair cell. Responses of type I hair cells are phasic while those of type II cells are tonic.*

arranged with the kinocilium oriented toward the striola. In the saccule, the hair cells are polarized away from the striola (see Figure 8-2). This anatomic polarity enables linear acceleration to affect the hair cells differentially on each side of the striola. The pronounced curvature of the two striolae and the orthogonal arrangement of the maculae ensure that the two otolith organs are capable of responding to linear acceleration or head tilt in any direction.

Semicircular Canals

There are three semicircular canals oriented perpendicularly to one another so that head rotation in either the x-, y-, or z-axis causes inertial flow of the endolymph through at least one canal (Figure 8-5). One end of each canal contains an enlarged region, the *ampulla*, where the flow of endolymph serves as a mechanical stimulus for sensory transduction (Figure 8-6). The floor of the ampulla contains a ridge of specialized hair cells, the *crista ampullaris*, which is topped by a towering mass of gelatin, the *cupula*. Endolymph flowing through the ampulla pushes the cupula, whose lever action bends the underlying

Roll is rotation around the x-axis (log rolling). Pitch is rotation around the y-axis (leaning forward). Yaw is rotation around the z-axis (scanning the horizon).

FIGURE 8-4 ▶

Otolith Organs. *The hair cells of the otolith organs are covered by a gelatinous substance called the otolithic membrane. The top surface of the otolithic membrane is studded with calcium carbonate crystals, which make the membrane top-heavy. The inherent instability of the otolithic membrane makes the system more responsive to small changes in either tilt or motion.*

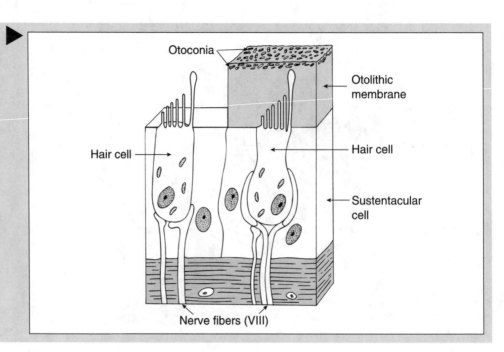

Otoconia

Otolithic membrane

Hair cell

Hair cell

Sustentacular cell

Nerve fibers (VIII)

FIGURE 8-5 ▶

Orientation of the Semicircular Canals. *The three semicircular canals are oriented perpendicularly to one another. The left and right horizontal canals are mirror images of one another. Each anterior canal is the functional opponent of the contralateral posterior canal. (Source: Adapted with permission from Barber HO, Stockwell CW: Manual of Electronystagmography. St. Louis, MO: Mosby, 1976, p 22.)*

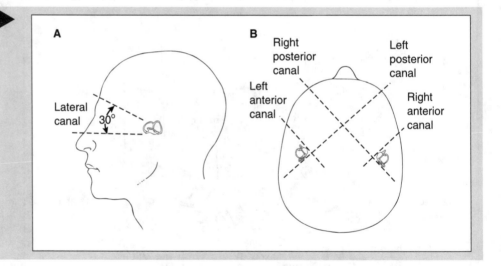

A

Lateral canal

30°

B

Right posterior canal

Left posterior canal

Left anterior canal

Right anterior canal

FIGURE 8-6 ▶

Flow of Endolymph through the Ampulla. *The cupula, by almost completely blocking the lumen of the ampulla, bends as endolymph flows past it. Movement of the cupula provides a mechanical advantage for bending the hair cells of the crista ampullaris, which are located on the floor of the ampulla.*

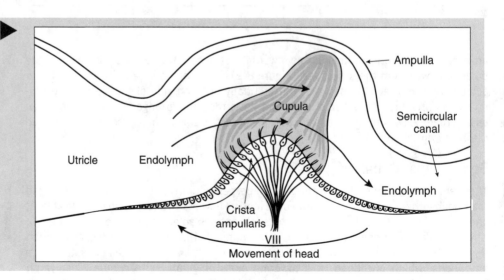

Ampulla

Cupula

Semicircular canal

Utricle

Endolymph

Endolymph

Crista ampullaris

VIII

Movement of head

stereocilia of the hair cells. The hair cells of the crista ampullaris have the same structure as those of the otolith organs and are arranged in a polarized fashion with respect to the utricle. All hair cells in the horizontal canal are polarized toward the utricle; those in the anterior and posterior canals are polarized away from the utricle.

Transduction

The adequate stimulus for transduction is deflection or bending of the stereocilia. Bending of the stereocilia toward the kinocilium depolarizes the cell, while bending away from the kinocilium causes hyperpolarization (Figure 8-7). Thus, deflection of the stereocilia signals direction and intensity of movement. As in the auditory system, fine links between taller stereocilia and their shorter neighbors trigger the flow of ions that generate the hair cell receptor potential. Movement of the stereocilia toward the kinocilium distorts the apical membrane, which increases the influx of potassium ions (K^+). The increase in K^+ current depolarizes the hair cell, which creates a secondary influx of calcium ions (Ca^{2+}) and neurotransmitter release from the basal surface of the cell (Figure 8-8). Movement of the stereocilia away from the kinocilium hyperpolarizes the cell by reducing the influx of K^+. The high spontaneous firing rate of these cells enables them to increase or decrease their activity accordingly.

Turn left, depolarize left; turn right, depolarize right.

Bending toward the kinocilium is excitatory. Bending away from the kinocilium is inhibitory.

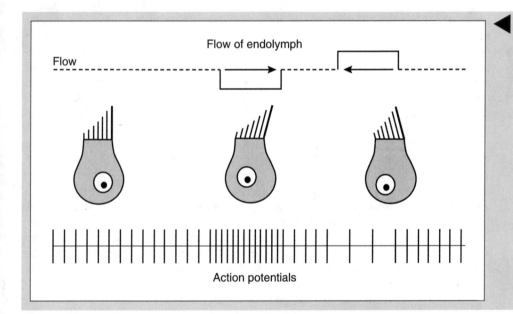

Flow of endolymph

Flow

Action potentials

◀ **FIGURE 8-7**
Functional Polarity of the Vestibular Hair Cells. *Bending of the stereocilia toward the kinocilium depolarizes the receptor cell and increases the firing rate of first-order vestibular fibers. The firing rate of primary vestibular fibers decreases when endolymph flows away from the kinocilium.*

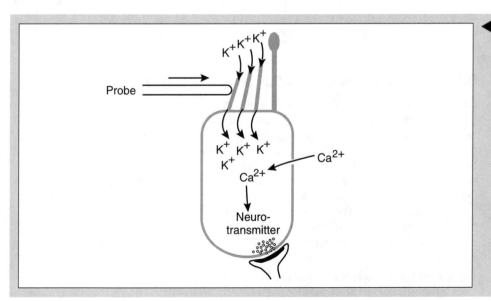

$K^+ K^+ K^+$

Probe

$K^+ K^+ K^+$
K^+
Ca^{2+} ← Ca^{2+}

Neuro-transmitter

◀ **FIGURE 8-8**
Transduction of Vestibular Movement. *Transduction begins when bending of the stereocilia causes a mechanical distortion of the apical surface of the hair cell. When the stereocilia bend toward the kinocilium, the potassium (K^+) channels open, and K^+ flows down its concentration gradient and into the cell. Depolarization of the hair cell causes an influx of calcium ions (Ca^{2+}), which triggers neurotransmitter release. Repolarization begins as the intracellular concentration of Ca^{2+} rises to such a level that K^+ begins to exit through the base of the cell.*

CENTRAL ORGANIZATION

Central Projections of the Vestibular Apparatus

The hair cells of the crista ampullaris and the maculae are innervated by the peripheral processes of bipolar neurons located in *Scarpa's ganglion*, which resides in the internal auditory meatus. The central processes of these cells form the vestibular branch of cranial nerve VIII, which enters the brainstem at the cerebellopontine angle immediately caudal to the auditory fibers (see Chapter 4, Figure 4-10). Vestibular fibers, after coursing dorsomedially between the inferior cerebellar peduncle and the spinal trigeminal tract, bifurcate into ascending and descending branches and terminate in the *vestibular nuclei*.

There are four vestibular nuclei clustered along the floor of the fourth ventricle (Figure 8-9; see Chapter 4, Figure 4-10). The lateral vestibular nucleus is a spherical nucleus located in the lateral tegmentum at the pontomedullary junction. The lateral vestibular nucleus consists of a ventral part that receives projections from the utricle and semicircular canals and a dorsal part whose afferent projections originate in the spinal cord and cerebellum. At its caudal end near the entry level of the vestibular nerve, the lateral vestibular nucleus abuts the rostral pole of the inferior vestibular nucleus. The inferior vestibular nucleus descends almost as far as the dorsal column nuclei. In transverse sections, the inferior vestibular nucleus has a distinctive "salt and pepper" appearance caused by descending fibers of the lateral vestibulospinal tract and the uncinate fasciculus (see Chapter 4, Figure 4-10). The medial vestibular nucleus is located along the medial flank of the inferior and lateral vestibular nuclei. Unlike the other vestibular nuclei, the medial nucleus is composed of small cells and has few myelinated fibers, which gives it a distinctly pale appearance in myelin-stained sections. The superior vestibular nucleus is tucked into the dorsolateral corner of the pontine tegmentum where it forms part of the ventrolateral wall of the fourth ventricle.

Functionally, the vestibular complex can be divided into a rostral part that plays a vital role in coordination of head and eye movements and a caudal part that modulates posture and muscle tone. The rostral part, which includes the superior vestibular nucleus, the ventral part of the lateral nucleus, and the rostral portions of the medial and inferior nuclei, receives projections from the semicircular canals (see Figure 8-9). The caudal part, which includes the caudal aspects of the medial and inferior vestibular nuclei, receives afferent projections from the saccule and utricle.

A small contingent of primary vestibular projections bypasses the vestibular complex and projects directly to the cerebellum. These fibers, along with other secondary vestibulocerebellar and cerebellovestibular fibers, form the juxtarestiform body which is located along the medial aspect of the inferior cerebellar peduncle (see Chapter 4, Figures 4-16 and 4-22).

Other Afferent Projections to the Vestibular Nuclei

Cerebellovestibular Projections. The cerebellum is the largest source of afferent projections to the vestibular nuclei. Inhibitory projections from cerebellar Purkinje cells project to the vestibular nuclei via the juxtarestiform body. Other neurons located in the fastigial nucleus, one of the deep cerebellar nuclei, project bilaterally to the vestibular nuclei and the adjacent reticular formation. The ipsilateral projection from the fastigial nucleus descends within the juxtarestiform body while the contralateral pathway forms the uncinate fasciculus. Neurons in the fastigial nucleus, like those in the other deep cerebellar nuclei, use either glutamate, aspartate, or both as their neurotransmitters and thus are presumed to facilitate the activity in the vestibular nuclei. Postural feedback and vestibular feedback relayed through the cerebellum allow the vestibular nuclei to adjust their output continually to the axial musculature (Figure 8-10).

Corticovestibular Projections. Descending projections from the cerebral cortex normally inhibit the activity of the vestibular nuclei. Damage to this corticovestibular projection

> The lateral vestibular nucleus is also known as Deiters' nucleus.

> The inferior vestibular nucleus is also referred to as the spinal or descending nucleus.

> Purkinje cells are GABAergic.

> The uncinate fasciculus (the hooked tract) exits the cerebellum along the dorsal surface of the superior cerebellar peduncle.

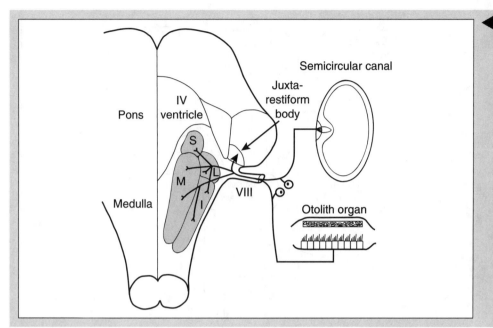

FIGURE 8-9
Vestibular Nuclei. *The four vestibular nuclei line the floor of the fourth ventricle. In this diagram, the fibers of the vestibulocochlear nerve enter the brainstem at the cerebellopontine angle, traverse the lateral vestibular nucleus, and distribute to all four vestibular nuclei. S = superior vestibular nucleus; M = medial vestibular nucleus; L = lateral vestibular nucleus; I = inferior (spinal or descending) vestibular nucleus.*

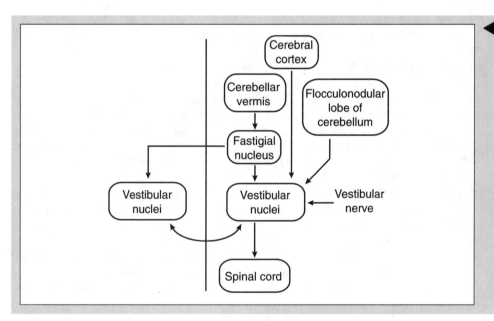

FIGURE 8-10
Block Diagram Illustrating the Afferent Projections of the Vestibular Nuclei.

disinhibits the vestibular nuclei, which causes extensor posturing (i.e., decerebrate rigidity).

Second-Order Vestibular Projections

Ascending, commissural, and descending projections originate from the vestibular nuclei (Figure 8-11).

ASCENDING PROJECTIONS

Thalamocortical Projections. Ascending projections from the medial and inferior vestibular nuclei reach the ventral posterolateral, ventral lateral, and posterior thalamic nuclei before projecting to the vestibular cortex. Several different regions of the cerebral cortex have been implicated in vestibular function, but most of the evidence supports a circumscribed area on the postcentral gyrus close to the face representation.

FIGURE 8-11 ▶

Block Diagram Illustrating the Efferent Projections of the Vestibular Nuclei.

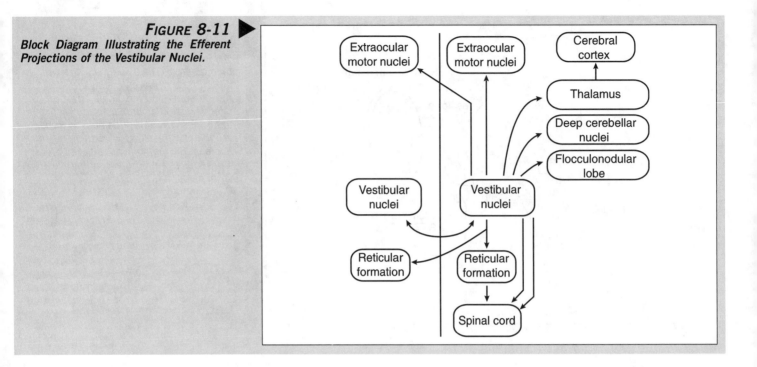

Vestibular sensation may enter the conscious sphere, but in healthy individuals, this seldom happens.

Vestibulocerebellar Projections. The cerebellum uses sensory input to refine movements of the axial and appendicular musculature. The small contingent of primary vestibular fibers that projects to the cerebellum is supplemented by a larger set of second-order projections from the vestibular nuclei. All of the vestibular nuclei except the lateral nucleus project to the cerebellum, but the heaviest projections arise from the caudal portions of the medial and inferior vestibular nuclei. These projections to the cerebellar cortex and the deep cerebellar nuclei relay information about head tilt and linear acceleration from the otolith organs.

Projections to the Extraocular Motor Nuclei. Extensive projections from the vestibular nuclei to the abducens, trochlear, and oculomotor nuclei enable a moving observer to maintain visual fixation on a stationary object. These projections form the basis for the *vestibulo-ocular reflex* (VOR).

The VOR mediates compensatory eye movements that stabilize visual images on the retina during visual tracking. As with other reflexes, the VOR is executed by a three-neuron pathway. The sensory limb of the VOR consists of the primary afferent neurons of the vestibulocochlear nerve that signal rotation of the head. Neurons in the medial and superior vestibular nucleus act as the interneurons that project via the medial longitudinal fasciculus to the efferent limb of the reflex: the motor neurons of the extraocular muscles. In general, vestibular projections to the contralateral extraocular nuclei are excitatory while ipsilateral projections are inhibitory. Motor nuclei that move the eyes to the right receive afferent projections from the vestibular neurons that respond to leftward head rotation and vice versa. The VOR operates in all three planes as well as at intermediate angles, but it can be demonstrated most easily in the horizontal plane (Figure 8-12). Because head rotation typically activates more than one semicircular canal, compensatory eye movements usually involve several extraocular muscles.

The VOR is the basis for the *doll's eye maneuver*, the diagnostic test used to evaluate the integrity of the brainstem in an unconscious patient. The doll's eye maneuver tests most of the vestibulo-ocular circuitry from the periphery to the midbrain as well as the efferent pathways to the extraocular eye muscles. A significant brainstem lesion would likely affect the vestibular pathway in some way. The test is performed with the patient in the supine position. After confirming that the patient has not sustained an injury to the

In the absence of injury, the patient's eye movements resemble those of a doll with glass eyes that roll in their sockets as the head is moved back and forth.

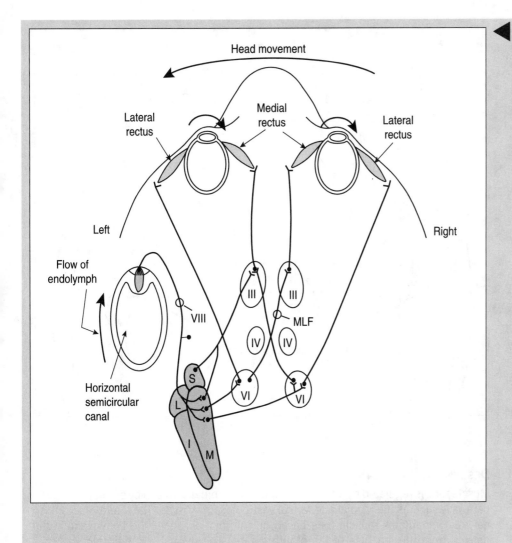

Head movement

Lateral rectus

Medial rectus

Lateral rectus

Left

Right

Flow of endolymph

VIII

III

III

MLF

IV

IV

Horizontal semicircular canal

S

L

VI

VI

I

M

FIGURE 8-12

Vestibulo-Ocular Reflex (VOR). The VOR stabilizes the eyes during head movements, which would otherwise destabilize images on the retina and degrade visual acuity. This diagram shows that rotation of the head to the left initiates compensatory eye movements to the right. Movement of the head to the left causes the endolymph in the left horizontal semicircular canal to flow to the right toward the utricle. As the endolymph flows through the ampulla, the cupula and the underlying stereocilia bend toward the utricle. The resultant depolarization of the receptors causes an increase in the firing rate of the vestibular branch of cranial nerve VIII. The situation is reversed in the right ampulla: fluid movement away from the utricle and kinocilium causes hyperpolarization, which decreases the firing rate in cranial nerve VIII. Activity in the vestibular nerve reaches the vestibular nuclei, which, in turn, project to the motor nuclei of the extraocular muscles. Projections to the abducens nucleus initiate contraction of the right lateral rectus muscle, while those to the oculomotor nucleus contract the left medial rectus muscle. The corresponding antagonist muscles relax. The VOR interconnects all 12 extraocular muscles with the vestibular apparatus to operate in all three planes. MLF = medial longitudinal fasciculus; III = oculomotor nuclei; IV = trochlear nuclei; VI = abducens nuclei; S = superior vestibular nucleus; M = medial vestibular nucleus; L = lateral vestibular nucleus; I = inferior vestibular nucleus. Solid cell bodies are excitatory; open cell bodies are inhibitory.

cervical spine, the head is rotated from side to side. If all vestibulo-ocular pathways are intact, both eyes will move together in the direction opposite to that of the head movement, as if fixed on a stationary object in the center of the visual field.

COMMISSURAL PROJECTIONS

Commissural projections coordinate vestibular activity derived from the left and right sides. At the synaptic level, this coordination differs for the semicircular canals and the otolith organs. Excitatory connections typically are found between the nuclei that receive afferent projections from the otolith organs, while inhibitory connections are associated with neurons that respond to stimulation of the semicircular canals. The difference in synaptic polarity between the linear and rotatory systems is based on how the receptors on the left and right sides of the head are displaced during head movement. During linear acceleration, the otolith organs on both sides of the head move as a unit through space; excitatory commissural projections reinforce neural activity derived from the contralateral side. During head rotation, however, one side of the head moves forward while the other side moves backward. Turning the head to the right should increase the firing rate in the vestibular nerve on the right side of the head and decrease the firing rate on the left side (Figure 8-13). Inhibitory commissural projections accentuate the signal difference already present in the left and right vestibular nerves during head rotation. Commissural connections also assist in vestibular compensation, the restoration of balance between the left and right vestibular nuclei that takes place following unilateral damage to the vestibular nerve or end organ.

Doll's Eye Maneuver.
Turn head left, eyes turn right.

Left and right semicircular canals inhibit one another; left and right otolith organs reinforce each other.

FIGURE 8-13 ▶

Commissural Vestibular Projections. If the head is turned to the left, the endolymph in the left semicircular canal flows to the right toward the utricle, depolarizes the hair cells in the crista ampullaris, and increases the firing rate of vestibular fibers in cranial nerve VIII. The endolymph within the right horizontal canal flows away from the utricle causing hyperpolarization of the hair cells and a lower firing rate in the cranial nerve and nuclei on that side. The firing rate within the right vestibular nuclei is reduced further by the inhibitory commissural connections from the contralateral side.

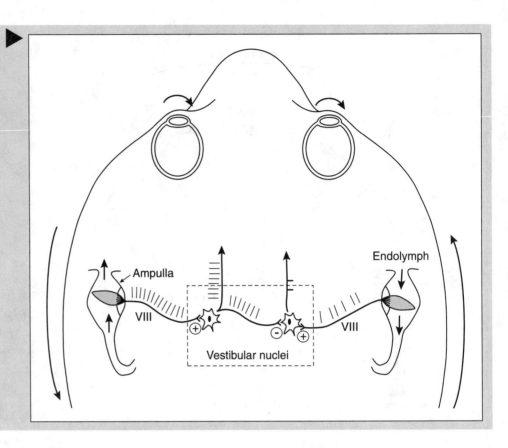

DESCENDING PROJECTIONS

Muscle tone is regulated by intrinsic circuits of the spinal cord and by several descending pathways such as the medial and lateral vestibulospinal tracts. The lateral vestibulospinal tract modulates muscle tone based on information about the body's equilibrium derived from the maculae of the otolith organs. The medial vestibulospinal tract, by comparison, ensures that movement of the neck and trunk is coordinated with eye movements triggered by stimulation of the semicircular canals.

The lateral vestibulospinal tract facilitates extensor motor neurons.

Lateral Vestibulospinal Tract. The lateral vestibulospinal tract originates in the lateral and inferior vestibular nuclei and terminates on both α- and γ-motor neurons in the anterior horn (see Chapter 3, Figure 3-23). Although the lateral vestibulospinal tract descends the full length of the spinal cord, most of its axons terminate at cervical and lumbar levels. Stimulation of the lateral vestibulospinal tract releases glutamate or acetylcholine, which facilitates extensors and inhibits flexors of the ipsilateral arm and leg.

The actions of the lateral vestibulospinal tract normally are modulated by descending inhibitory corticobulbar projections and opposed by the rubrospinal tract. Extensor posturing, more commonly referred to as *decerebrate rigidity*, is caused by the unopposed action of the lateral vestibulospinal and pontine reticulospinal tracts on the α- and γ-motor neurons of the ventral horn. Patients with upper brainstem lesions may show pathologic extension of the arms and legs in response to noxious stimulation. The clearest demonstrations of decerebrate rigidity are seen in experimental preparations following intercollicular section of the brainstem (Figure 8-14). Decerebrate rigidity is typically accompanied by hyperactive deep tendon reflexes. Decerebrate rigidity may be exacerbated by coincident damage to the flocculonodular lobe of the cerebellum whose GABAergic projections to the lateral vestibular nucleus normally provide additional restraint. The severity of decerebrate rigidity can be relieved if some of the excitatory input to the vestibular nuclei is removed by sectioning the vestibular nerves or the dorsal roots.

Medial Vestibulospinal Tract. Stimulation of the labyrinth, in addition to initiating the VOR, triggers the *vestibulo-collic reflex*, a series of compensatory head movements designed to stabilize the head in space during movement. The vestibulo-collic reflex is

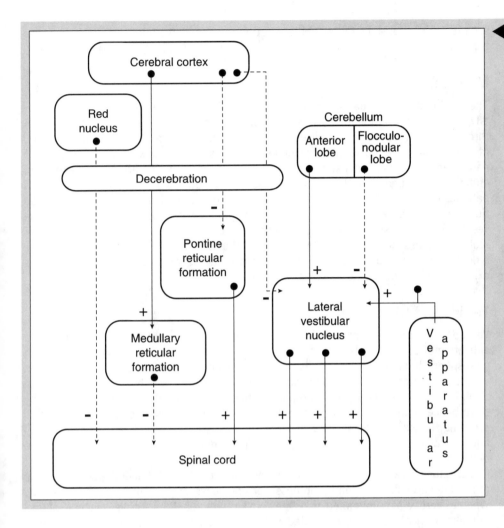

FIGURE 8-14
Neural Circuits Underlying Decerebrate Rigidity. Decerebrate rigidity occurs following isolation of the spinal cord and caudal brainstem from more rostral regions of the brain. This damage has three actions. First, the lateral vestibular nucleus and the pontine reticular formation are released from the inhibitory control of the cerebral cortex. This disinhibition facilitates extensor motor neurons of the arms and legs. Second, projections from the red nucleus to the spinal cord, which would normally inhibit extensor motor neurons, are severed. Third, the medullary reticular formation, which also inhibits extensor motor neurons and remains connected to the spinal cord, is inoperative because it has lost its excitatory input from the cerebral cortex. The net effect is a profound and unopposed facilitation of the extensor motor neurons of the arms and legs by the lateral vestibular nucleus and the pontine reticular formation.

mediated by the medial vestibulospinal tract, which consists of descending projections from the medial vestibular nucleus to cervical α- and γ-motor neurons that innervate the neck muscles. The medial vestibulospinal tract descends through the caudal brainstem and cervical cord within the medial longitudinal fasciculus (see Chapter 3, Figure 3-23; Chapter 4, Figure 4-10). The medial vestibulospinal tract also terminates bilaterally within the reticular formation of the caudal brainstem; its projections to the spinal cord are strictly ipsilateral.

Efferent Projections. Small groups of neurons located near the lateral border of the abducens nucleus project via the vestibular nerve to the hair cells of the maculae and cristae. These crossed and uncrossed cholinergic projections are believed to modulate the dynamic range of the vestibular hair cells.

CLINICAL SIGNS AND SYMPTOMS

Whereas other sensory systems thrive on change, the vestibular system works full-time to maintain the status quo. Under most circumstances, the vestibular system restores balance by adjusting muscle tone, posture, or the extraocular eye muscles. Extreme or unfamiliar movements that overwhelm the vestibular system cause sensory, motor, and autonomic symptoms. These symptoms also may be caused by an inability to reconcile information derived from different sensory systems, for example, vision and balance. Unilateral dysfunction of the vestibular end organ, nerve, or nuclei may produce a neurophysiologic imbalance, which has a similar effect. In short, vestibular signs and symptoms are caused by failure of the vestibular system to restore the status quo. These sensory, motor, and autonomic effects range from mildly unpleasant to totally disabling.

Motion Sickness

Motion sickness is caused by a mismatch of sensory signals.

The combination of visual, kinesthetic, somatosensory, and vestibular information usually presents an unambiguous assessment of how the body is oriented, moving, or both through the environment. When these sensory systems provide discordant information, motion sickness may occur. Motion sickness usually starts as malaise but may progress to nausea and vomiting. Other symptoms of motion sickness may include profuse sweating, chills, pallor, hyperventilation, and dizziness. Thus, motion sickness is not considered a pathologic response but rather a normal response to mismatched sensory stimuli. When riding in a car, for example, the stationary image of the dashboard may clash with the vestibular and kinesthetic sensations caused by motion of the car. Thus, the sensation of motion sickness may be relieved by looking out the car window or exacerbated by reading a book. People gradually adapt to the sickness-inducing stimulus, as suggested by the expression to "acquire one's sea legs."

Vertigo and Dizziness

Vertigo is the illusion of movement of either self or environment caused by asymmetric activation of the vestibular system. In addition to the perception of movement, which corresponds to activity in the cerebral cortex, the sufferer exhibits ocular, postural, and autonomic symptoms. Ocular signs may include nystagmus, which is a rhythmic oscillation of the eyes caused by a disturbance of the VOR. Postural imbalance is caused by disturbances in the descending vestibulospinal systems. Autonomic symptoms, such as sweating, nausea, vomiting, and hyperventilation, are due to activation of medullary autonomic areas, including the area postrema, the nucleus of the solitary tract, and the dorsal motor nucleus of the vagus.

Dizziness, unlike vertigo, has no localizing value.

Dizziness is a more diffuse phenomenon that includes lightheadedness, sensations of swimming or floating, and giddiness but not necessarily an illusion of movement. Whereas vertigo and its related signs are considered the hallmark of vestibular dysfunction, dizziness has no signs associated with it and usually originates outside the vestibular system. Dizziness has no localizing value.

Meniere's Disease

Tinnitus is a ringing, buzzing, or clicking sound that the patient localizes to the ear.

Meniere's disease is a disorder of the inner ear characterized by recurrent attacks of tinnitus, sensorineural hearing loss, and vertigo. Attacks range in duration from minutes to hours during which the symptoms of vertigo gradually dissipate. A permanent loss of hearing usually takes place on the affected side during the first few years; eventually, the disease becomes bilateral. The symptoms of Meniere's disease are caused by distortion of the membranous labyrinth by endolymphatic hydrops, the overaccumulation of endolymph. Hydrops is caused by impaired resorption rather than overproduction of endolymph. Spontaneous remission of Meniere's disease is common and is probably caused by fistulization between the endo- and perilymphatic compartments, which permits excess endolymph to drain. The etiology of Meniere's disease is unknown.

Nystagmus

The direction of nystagmus is defined by its quick phase because it is easier to observe.

Nystagmus is a pathologic oscillation of one or both eyes in one or more planes. Nystagmus involves a slow saccade in one direction followed by a quick excursion in the opposite direction. Despite the fact that the slow phase is the pathologic component of nystagmus and the quick phase is merely a compensatory adjustment, the quick phase is used to define the direction of nystagmus because it is more easily detected. Spontaneous nystagmus may signal damage to the vestibular apparatus or nerve, the brainstem, or the cerebellum. For patients with suspected lesions in these areas, induction of nystagmus is an important part of the clinical examination because it enables the physician to observe the operation of the vestibular system.

Nystagmus can be induced in healthy individuals by either caloric stimulation of the external auditory meatus or bodily rotation. Caloric stimulation creates convection currents in the semicircular canals, which induces endolymphatic flow. The easiest semicircular canal to stimulate is the horizontal canal because it lies closest to the external ear. The patient's head is typically elevated at a 60° angle to align the horizontal canal with the vertical plane. Irrigating the ear with cool (30°C) water creates convection currents in the endolymph, which then flows away from the ampulla. The resultant hyperpolarization of the hair cells causes the patient's eyes to turn slowly toward the stimulated ear; the rapid phase is in the opposite direction (**c**old, **o**pposite). The effect is reversed if warm water is used (**w**arm, **s**ame).

Under certain circumstances, rotation of the head is capable of inducing nystagmus. As described above, the VOR is a set of compensatory eye movements that oppose normal head rotation. Unusually large rotations of the head, which force the eyes beyond the limits imposed by the orbits, initially trigger a normal VOR. When the eyes reach the limit of their excursion, they quickly rebound to a central fixation point and then resume their slow movement opposite to the direction of head rotation. The initial, slow component opposes the rotation of the head while the fast component follows the rotation.

In the clinic, nystagmus can be invoked with the aid of a Bárány chair. The Bárány chair allows the patient to be rotated at a constant speed for 15–20 seconds in one direction before the rotation is suddenly stopped. Prior to stopping, the movement of the endolymph matches that of the labyrinth; after stopping, the inertia of the endolymph carries it through the ampulla, which stimulates the crista. The abrupt stop causes the patient's eyes to move slowly in the *same* direction as the prior rotation. These slow excursions are punctuated by quick movements in the direction opposite of the chair's rotation. For example, if the patient were rotated to the left, the slow phase of nystagmus would be to the left, and the quick phase would be to the right. This patient, if asked to point at a stationary target, would past-point, that is, point further to the left. If this patient were to stand up, there would be a tendency to fall in the direction of the prior rotation. The Bárány chair, unlike caloric stimulation, requires specialized equipment and does not permit separate testing of each ear.

The mnemonic COWS (**c**old, **o**pposite; **w**arm, **s**ame) summarizes the direction of rapid eye movement following caloric stimulation of the ear

Hot air (and hot endolymph) rise.

RESOLUTION OF CLINICAL CASE

M. L. was diagnosed with benign paroxysmal positional vertigo (BPPV), the most common type of vertigo. Idiopathic BPPV may strike at any age, but the highest prevalence is in the elderly, and women are more commonly afflicted than men. Postmortem studies have shown that patients with BPPV have utricular degeneration. It is believed that otoconia liberated from the diseased utricle migrate into the semicircular canals, typically the posterior one. Attacks of vertigo are triggered when angular rotation pushes these "floaters" into the ampulla and against the cupula. In most cases, BPPV resolves itself spontaneously within 1 month. Physicians often prescribe exercises designed to dislodge the debris from the cupula and disperse them into the endolymph of the utricle and saccule.

REVIEW QUESTIONS

Directions: For each of the following questions, choose the **one best** answer.

1. Which of the following statements best describes the lateral vestibulospinal tract?

   (A) It descends into the spinal cord as a caudal continuation of the medial longitudinal fasciculus (MLF)

   (B) It descends ipsilaterally from its origin in the medial vestibular nucleus

   (C) It facilitates the extensors of the arms and legs

   (D) It extends only as far as the cervical spinal cord and plays an important role in the postural control of the head

   (E) Together with the rubrospinal tract, it controls posture by facilitating the extensor muscles of the legs

2. An unconscious 23-year-old man is brought into the emergency room; he was found lying on the sidewalk outside a tavern, and his wallet was missing. Blood oozed from the deep scalp laceration at the mastoid protuberance and the external auditory meatus. After ruling out injury to the cervical spine, the attending physician performed the doll's eye maneuver. As a diagnostic test, the doll's eye maneuver usually does not pinpoint damage within the brain, but rather rules out damage to particular structures. Which of the following structures can be assessed by the doll's eye maneuver?

   (A) Medial vestibulospinal tract

   (B) Lateral vestibulospinal tract

   (C) Thalamic vestibular relay

   (D) Vestibular nerve

   (E) Cerebellum

3. Which of the following areas receives a direct projection from vestibular neurons located in Scarpa's ganglion?

   (A) Cerebellum

   (B) Nucleus abducens

   (C) Brainstem reticular formation

   (D) Medial longitudinal fasciculus (MLF)

   (E) Spinal cord

4. Which of the following statements about the vestibular nuclei is true?

   (A) Projections from the medial vestibular nucleus to the contralateral abducens nucleus are inhibitory

   (B) Commissural connections between vestibular nuclei are excitatory for linear acceleration and inhibitory for angular acceleration

   (C) Electrical stimulation of the fastigial nucleus decreases extensor muscle tone

   (D) The superior vestibular nucleus receives afferent projections from the semicircular canals and modulates muscle tone

   (E) Direct projections from the vestibular nuclei to the neostriatum help regulate voluntary motor control

5. Which of the following events would be caused by turning the head to the left?

(A) Neural activity in the vestibulocochlear nerve on the left side of the head increases

(B) The stereocilia of the horizontal semicircular canal on the left side of the head bend away from the utricle

(C) Endolymph flows toward the utricle on the right side of the head

(D) Descending lateral vestibulospinal projections execute compensatory adjustments of the head and neck

(E) Right nystagmus in the left eye

6. Which of the following procedures exacerbates the symptoms of decerebrate rigidity?

(A) Sectioning the dorsal roots in the cervical enlargement

(B) Lesioning the lateral vestibular nucleus

(C) Denervation of the labyrinths

(D) Sectioning the ventral roots in the cervical enlargement

(E) Electrical stimulation of the vestibular nerve

ANSWERS AND EXPLANATIONS

1. The answer is C. The ability of the lateral vestibulospinal tract to facilitate extensors is illustrated in cases of decerebrate rigidity. The lateral vestibulospinal tract descends the full length of the spinal cord within the anterior funiculus. The medial vestibulospinal tract, on the other hand, descends within the MLF only as far as the cervical cord and controls posture of the head. The rubrospinal tract facilitates flexors, which is why it normally counteracts the action of the lateral vestibulospinal tract.

2. The answer is D. The doll's eye maneuver tests the integrity of the vestibulo-ocular reflex (VOR) circuit, which includes the vestibular labyrinths, both vestibular nerves, the vestibular nuclei, and the motor nuclei and nerves of the extraocular eye muscles. The medial and lateral vestibulospinal tracts, which descend to the spinal cord, are not part of the VOR circuit. The doll's eye maneuver operates without participation from the forebrain areas such as the thalamus or cortex. The integrity of the cerebellum cannot be ascertained with the doll's eye maneuver.

3. The answer is C. Although most primary vestibular fibers project to the vestibular nuclei, some enter the juxtarestiform body and project directly to the cerebellar flocculus. The brainstem reticular formation, the abducens nucleus, and the spinal cord all receive secondary vestibular projections. The MLF contains secondary fibers that originate in the vestibular nuclei.

4. The answer is B. Turning the head to the left causes inertial flow of the endolymph to the right. This movement causes depolarization of the receptors of the left crista ampullaris and hyperpolarization of those on the right side. Inhibitory commissural projections reinforce the complementary output from the opposing semicircular canals. The situation is different during linear acceleration because all otolith organs move in concert. These commissural connections reinforce the output from the opposite side. Choice A is incorrect because the vestibulo-ocular reflex (VOR) requires that the abducens muscle on one side be stimulated by the vestibular nucleus on the contralateral side. Choice C is incorrect because the fastigial nucleus would activate the vestibular nuclei and increase extensor muscle tone. Choice D is incorrect because the superior vestibular nucleus plays a key role in the VOR, not muscle tone. Finally, choice E is incorrect because there are no direct projections from the vestibular nuclei to the basal ganglia.

5. The answer is A. Turning the head to the left causes endolymph in the left horizontal semicircular canal to flow from the ampulla into the utricle, which increases neural activity in the ipsilateral vestibulocochlear nerve. On the contralateral side, the endolymph pushes the stereocilia away from the utricle causing a decrease in neural activity on that side. Rotation of the head triggers compensatory movements of the head and neck, but these adjustments are made by the medial vestibulospinal tract. Nystagmus is a pathologic oscillation of the eyes, which is unlikely to be seen in a normal person during movement of the head.

6. The answer is E. One of the primary determinants of muscle tone in the extensor muscles is the level of neural activity in the lateral vestibular nuclei. Procedures that increase the activity of the lateral vestibular neurons such as electrical stimulation of the vestibular nerve increase extensor tone. Other procedures such as denervation of the labyrinths or lesioning the lateral vestibular nucleus have the opposite effect. Sectioning the dorsal roots eliminates sensory input from the annulospiral endings, another source of extensor facilitation. Sectioning the ventral roots denervates the muscles.

ADDITIONAL READING

Benson AJ: The vestibular sensory system. In *The Senses*. Edited by Barlow HB, Mollon JD. New York, NY: Cambridge University Press, 1989, pp 333–368.

Ryu JH: Anatomy of the vestibular end organ and neural pathways. In *Otolaryngology—Head and Neck Surgery*. Edited by Cummings CW, Fredrickson JM, Harker LA, et al. St. Louis, MO: Mosby, 1993, pp 2609–2631.

Wazen JJ: Dizziness and hearing loss. In *Merritt's Textbook of Neurology*. Edited by Rowland LP. Philadelphia, PA: Williams and Wilkins, 1995, pp 30–35.

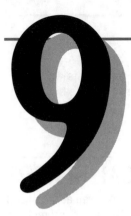

CHEMICAL SENSES

INTRODUCTION OF CLINICAL CASE

T. R., a 30-year-old female victim of an automobile accident, was brought to the emergency room with an assortment of cuts and bruises on her forehead probably caused when her head struck the windshield. T. R. regained consciousness shortly after arriving at the hospital but was mildly confused. The attending physician ordered frontal and lateral computed tomography (CT) scans of the head, which showed that T. R. had a broken nose but no skull fracture or evidence of intracranial bleeding. The patient showed no signs of hemiplegia, aphasia, or cranial nerve palsies but was dizzy and had a severe headache. By the time she was discharged from the emergency room, T. R. was no longer dizzy, and her headache had improved considerably. Her nose had stopped bleeding but was now slowly discharging a small amount of clear fluid. The physician diagnosed a mild concussion and instructed the patient to go home and rest. Her husband was instructed to awaken T. R. every 3 hours during the night. One week later during her follow-up examination, T. R. mentioned that food seemed tasteless since the accident. The physician tested her sense of taste with a sugar packet that he picked up at the emergency room coffee station. After T. R. correctly identified the sugar, the physician completed the neurologic examination; all other tests were unremarkable. To this day, T. R. steadfastly insists that she has no sense of taste but has not been re-examined.

OVERVIEW OF THE CHEMICAL SENSES

The chemical senses include the so-called *common chemical sense* as well as smell and taste. The common chemical sense, which is the most primitive of the three, protects us from noxious odors and fluids. Taste and smell guide a variety of motivated behaviors and, in humans, have an important bearing on the quality of life. Unlike other sensory systems, taste and smell often evoke strong hedonic reactions that range from delight to disgust.

Smell and taste stand at the threshold between the internal milieu and the outside world. From this vantage point, smell and taste monitor and control food selection to ensure that our diets are both safe and nutritious. The virtually seamless coordination of smell and taste belies the fact that each is a separate sense with its own receptors, pathways, and percepts. Smell results from chemical stimulation of receptors located in the nasal cavity. Taste sensation arises following chemical stimulation of receptors located throughout the oral cavity. Flavor is the fusion of gustatory, olfactory, and somatosensory (i.e., touch, pain, or hot or cold temperature) stimulation that takes place during eating.

Flavor is an amalgam of taste, smell, and somesthetic sensations.

THE COMMON CHEMICAL SENSE

The common chemical sense detects noxious chemical stimulation of mucous membranes such as the eyes, nose, mouth, respiratory tract, and anal and genital openings. The pain caused by chemical irritation triggers lacrimal and withdrawal reflexes, which protect the organism from prolonged, potentially damaging stimulation. The range of chemical stimuli is virtually limitless and may include substances such as pungent spices (e.g., onion, garlic, chili pepper), lacrimators (e.g., tear gas), sternutators (chemicals that cause sneezing such as black pepper), and skin irritants. High concentrations of some olfactory and gustatory stimuli (e.g., hydrochloric acid [HCl], sodium chloride [NaCl]) have irritant properties as well. The receptors for the common chemical sense are free nerve endings, which lack the specialization and sophistication of the olfactory and gustatory end organs. Because the common chemical sense is closely aligned with the sense of pain, the physiological responses it evokes are both reflexive and protective. For example, sneezing, closure of the nares and glottis, respiratory depression, and increased nasal secretion limit exposure to noxious stimulation of the nasal cavity.

OVERVIEW OF OLFACTION

Smell serves several important functions in humans, and its loss by either trauma or disease has serious consequences, especially on the quality of life. It is estimated that 1% of the population has a complete and permanent olfactory deficit. Olfactory dysfunction is particularly common in the elderly, the most rapidly expanding segment of the population.

Olfactory Epithelium

Olfactory transduction takes place within the *olfactory epithelium* located along the posterodorsal roof of the left and right nasal cavities, the medial nasal septum, and part of each superior nasal turbinate. The olfactory epithelium consists of olfactory receptors intermixed with *sustentacular, basal (stem) cells*, and *Bowman's glands* (Figure 9-1).

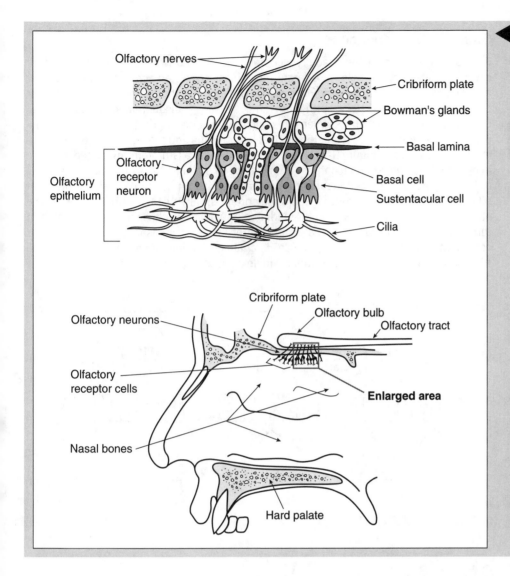

Diagram of the Olfactory Epithelium in Situ. *The enlarged area (top) illustrates the axons of olfactory receptor neurons entering the cranium through small foramina in the cribriform plate of the ethmoid bone.*

Unlike the common chemical sense, which relies on free nerve endings, the receptors in the olfactory system are bipolar neurons. The distal end of each *olfactory receptor neuron (ORN)* has a knob-like swelling capped with a tuft of cilia. The cilia are covered with receptor-binding sites and coated by mucus secreted by the Bowman's glands. The sustentacular cells are glial-like cells that provide structural and metabolic support for the receptors. Various immunoglobulins, antimicrobial proteins, and enzymes secreted by the sustentacular cells protect the ORNs from environmental toxins and viruses that invade the nasal cavity with each breath. Whether ORNs succumb to these external agents or are preprogrammed for death, they are replaced continuously over the lifetime of the organism. The life span of ORNs varies from 30 to 120 days in mammalian species. Replacement cells are derived by mitosis of basal cells. The relatively rapid turnover of ORNs may make them susceptible to radiation therapy and antineoplastic agents, which target rapidly dividing cells.

ORNs have a life span of 30–120 days.

The extremely fine unmyelinated axons of the ORNs form the olfactory nerve (cranial nerve I), which enters the cranial vault through small perforations in the *cribriform plate* of the ethmoid bone. Head trauma severe enough to shift the brain within the skull may stretch or sever the delicate olfactory axons during their passage through the cribriform plate. Although some regeneration of the olfactory filia is possible, local edema and scar formation usually limit it. In most cases, olfactory deficits caused by head trauma are permanent. Interestingly, patients who have lost their sense of smell are unaware of their olfactory impairment; instead, they report an inability to taste food.

Olfactory Transduction

For molecules to engage the olfactory receptors, they must traverse the mucous layer that covers the olfactory epithelium. Odorant molecules are carried across the mucous layer by proteins called *odorant-binding molecules*. Odorant-binding molecules also clear odorants from the olfactory epithelium after sensory transduction has taken place. Olfactory transduction starts when an odorant molecule binds to one of the trans-membrane receptor proteins located on the olfactory cilia and triggers one of two second-messenger pathways (Figure 9-2). The first pathway uses a G-protein–mediated increase in cyclic adenosine monophosphate (cAMP) to open sodium (Na^+) channels. The influx of Na^+ depolarizes the cell leading to the generation of an action potential at the axon hillock. Pleasant fruity and floral odors may preferentially use the cAMP pathway. The other pathway relies on a G-protein–mediated activation of phospholipase C, which in turn increases the intracellular concentration of inositol triphosphate (IP_3). Increased concentrations of IP_3 open calcium (Ca^{2+}) channels, which depolarize the ORNs. The IP_3 pathway has not been linked to any single class of odorants.

FIGURE 9-2 ▶
Pathways of Olfactory Transduction. Two separate pathways, one using cyclic adenosine monophosphate (cAMP) and the other inositol triphosphate (IP_3), mediate olfactory transduction. AC = adenyl cyclase; G = G protein; OBP = olfactory-binding protein; PLC = phospholipase C.

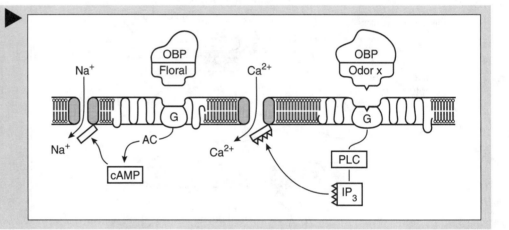

Olfactory Bulb

Axons of the olfactory nerve enter the anterior cranial fossa and terminate in the ipsilateral olfactory bulb. The *olfactory bulb* is a flattened sphere sandwiched between the cribriform plate and the ventral surface of the orbital cortex (Figure 9-3). The olfactory bulb consists of six distinct layers. Starting from the outer surface, these layers are: (1) *the olfactory nerve layer*, (2) *the glomerular layer*, (3) *the external plexiform layer*, (4) *the mitral cell layer*, (5) *the granule cell layer*, and (6) the *anterior olfactory nucleus*. The elaborate circuitry of the olfactory bulb (described below) converts the signals received from the olfactory cilia into highly processed codes before sending the message to the forebrain.

Olfactory nerve axons line the surface of the rostral olfactory bulb before piercing its surface and terminating in spherical acellular areas called *glomeruli*. The neurotransmitter used by ORNs is not known. The glomerulus is an elaborate plexus in which the axons of ORNs synapse with the axons and dendrites of *periglomerular cells* and the apical dendrites of mitral and tufted cells (Figure 9-4). The somas of the periglomerular cells form a calyx around each glomerulus. The axons and dendrites of one periglomerular cell may infiltrate as many as 10 neighboring glomeruli. Periglomerular cells, which use γ-aminobutyric acid (GABA), dopamine, substance P, and enkephalin as neurotransmitters, improve quality coding in the olfactory bulb by inhibiting neighboring glomeruli. Mitral and tufted cells are the efferent neurons of the olfactory bulb. The olfactory input from the ORNs undergoes tremendous convergence as it passes through the olfactory bulb. For every 1000 axons that enter a glomerulus, only 1 dendrite exits. The glomeruli also receive projections from the contralateral olfactory bulb, as well as noradrenergic,

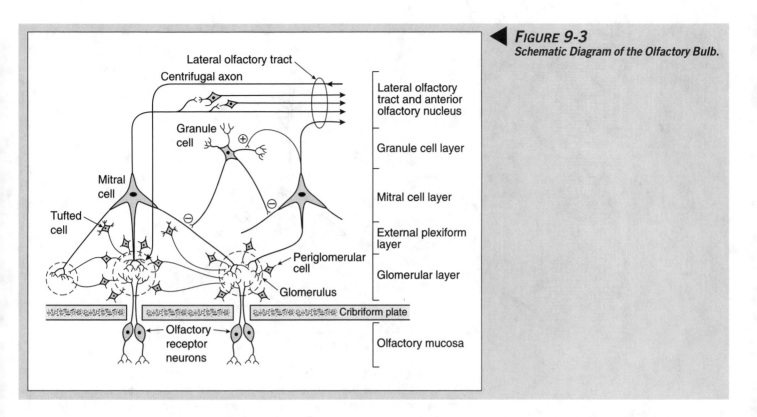

◀ FIGURE 9-3
Schematic Diagram of the Olfactory Bulb.

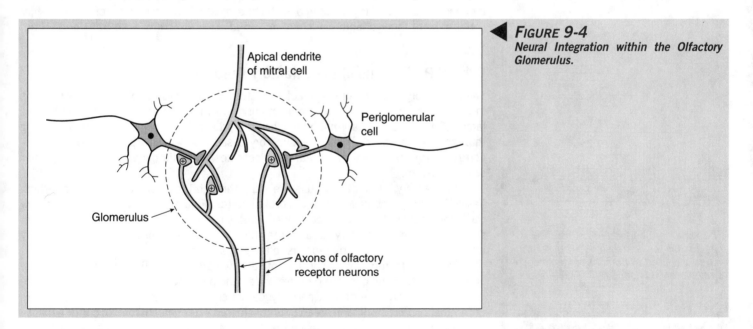

◀ FIGURE 9-4
Neural Integration within the Olfactory Glomerulus.

serotonergic, and cholinergic projections from the locus ceruleus, midline raphe, and basal forebrain, respectively.

As the apical dendrites of the mitral and tufted cells pass through the external plexiform layer, they are inhibited by GABAergic dendrodendritic synapses from *granule cells*. Because granule cell inhibition is initiated by excitatory axodendritic synapses from the mitral cells, the *mitral cells* are, in effect, terminating their own signal (Figure 9-5). This recurrent inhibitory circuit may improve the temporal resolution of the olfactory system by limiting the duration of mitral cell responsiveness. Granule cells, like the glomeruli, also receive projections from the anterior olfactory nucleus bilaterally, other parts of the olfactory cortex, and the limbic system.

Granule cells in the olfactory bulb have no axons.

FIGURE 9-5 ▶
Local Circuits of the Olfactory Bulb. Recurrent inhibition of mitral cells is mediated by granule cells.

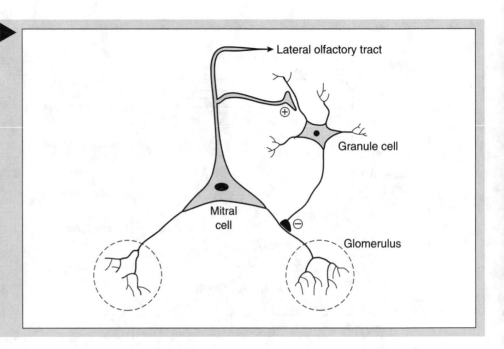

FIGURE 9-5 ▶
Local Circuits of the Olfactory Bulb. Recurrent inhibition of mitral cells is mediated by granule cells.

The core of the olfactory bulb is formed by axons of mitral and tufted cells, which exit the caudal end of the bulb and form the *lateral olfactory tract* (see Figure 9-3). Within this medullary core lie scattered clusters of cells, which collectively constitute the anterior olfactory nucleus. Although the anterior olfactory nucleus does not have a laminar structure, it is considered to be the most rostral extension of the olfactory cortex. The anterior olfactory nucleus may mediate interhemispheric transfer of olfactory memories.

Central Projections of the Olfactory Bulb

The central organization of the olfactory system differs from the other sensory systems in several important ways. First, projections from the olfactory bulb are entirely ipsilateral. Second, smell information reaches the primary olfactory cortex without passing through the thalamus. Third, the olfactory system projects to paleocortex and neocortex. Fourth, the olfactory system has closer ties to the limbic system than any other sensory system.

All olfactory information enters the brain through the *lateral olfactory tract*, which lies within the olfactory sulcus of the orbital cortex (Figure 9-6). As the lateral olfactory tract approaches the anterior perforated substance, it divides into lateral and medial striae. The lateral olfactory stria is the main conduit for cortically bound olfactory information; the medial stria projects to the septal area.

Primary olfactory cortex consists of four cytoarchitecturally distinct regions: the anterior olfactory nucleus, the *piriform cortex*, the periamygdaloid cortex, and the entorhinal cortex. The piriform and periamygdaloid cortices are three-layered *paleocortex*. Entorhinal cortex (Brodmann area 28) is considered a transitional form of cortex because it resembles paleocortex and neocortex. As in other cortical regions, pyramidal cells located in the deep layers constitute the efferent neurons of the primary olfactory cortex. Primary olfactory cortex projects to the insula and *orbitofrontal cortex*, as well as the cortical and medial amygdaloid nuclei, the hypothalamus, the lateral preoptic area, the *mediodorsal nucleus of the thalamus*, and the diagonal band of Broca. Olfactory projections into the limbic forebrain provide an avenue for odors to affect visceral and emotional responses. Projections from the entorhinal cortex to the hippocampus may form the anatomic link for the strong associations between smell and memory. The entorhinal cortex also projects to the mediodorsal nucleus, which serves as the thalamic relay for olfactory information bound for the orbitofrontal cortex.

The ascent of smell information to the primary olfactory cortex without synapsing in the thalamus reflects the antiquity of the olfactory system. The olfactory projection to its

There is a medial olfactory stria but no medial olfactory tract.

The anterior perforated substance is named for its pincushion appearance, which is caused by branches of the medial striate artery that penetrate the brain here.

In certain species, the piriform cortex is pear-shaped.

The mediodorsal nucleus is the thalamic relay for smell.

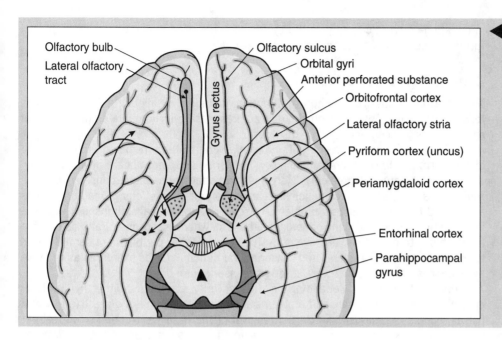

more recently evolved neocortical target, the orbitofrontal cortex, assumes a more conventional transthalamic route through the mediodorsal nucleus. Thus olfaction, like all other sensory systems, projects to *neocortex* via the thalamus.

Neural Coding of Odor Quality

The most persistent controversies in olfaction (and taste) concern the issue of quality coding. The problem in olfaction is particularly acute because we can identify thousands of different odors. Attempts to organize the olfactory world on the basis of chemical composition have been largely unsuccessful, but psychophysical studies have shown that most odors fall into one of several qualitative categories (Table 9-1). These qualitative categories typically refer to the substances or plant and animal sources that generate the odors such as orange, rose, or licorice. This insight, unfortunately, has done little to advance our understanding of quality coding in the olfactory system. Unlike primary colors, these qualitative categories cannot be used like building blocks to assemble new odors.

TABLE 9-1
Prototypical Stimuli of the Primary Odor Qualities

Odor Quality	Prototypical Stimuli
Flowery	Rose
Fruity	Fruit and wines
Ambrosial	Musk and sandalwood
Aromatic	Camphor and spices
Sweaty	Isovaleric acid
Rotten	Rotten eggs and feces
Stinging	Formic acid

The difficulty in determining how the nervous system codes for stimulus quality in the chemical senses has been attributed to our lack of understanding of basic transduction mechanisms. Recent breakthroughs in receptor transduction mechanisms should serve as a framework for future studies on quality coding within the central nervous system (CNS). Early speculation that individual smell (and taste) neurons would act as *labeled lines* responsive to only a single stimulus quality gave way as experimental data showed that most sensory neurons are *broadly tuned*, that is, they respond to a variety of stimuli. Broad tuning sacrifices specificity within individual neurons to increase the information-carrying capacity of the system. Coding of stimulus quality is discussed further in the section on taste.

Clinical Aspects of Olfaction

There are many causes of olfactory dysfunction, including nasal obstruction, toxic odors (e.g., formaldehyde, paint solvents), and fractures of the cribriform plate. Impairment of smell also may accompany certain diseases.

Olfactory deficits may be partial (*hyposmia*), complete (*anosmia*), or in rare cases, distorted (*dysosmia*) or even hallucinatory. Hyposmia and anosmia are *negative disturbances*, which vary in degree only. Dysosmias and olfactory hallucinations, by comparison, are *positive disturbances*, which have an entirely different etiology. Olfactory deficits are caused by either transport problems or sensorineural damage. Transport problems impede stimulus access to the olfactory epithelium, whereas sensorineural problems are associated with neurologic damage or dysfunction of either peripheral or central structures. Both transport problems and sensorineural deficits may be expressed as negative disturbances; positive deficits are strictly of sensorineural origin.

Transport problems, depending on their severity, can cause either hyposmia or anosmia. Because most transport problems are caused by paranasal disease (e.g., nasal polyps, neoplasms, sinusitis), surgical removal of the nasal obstruction often restores olfactory function. The range of causative factors for *sensorineural olfactory deficits*, on the other hand, is almost limitless. Viral infections, head trauma, radiation therapy, environmental toxins and pollutants, prescribed medication, and endocrine imbalances have been linked to sensorineural olfactory dysfunction. Olfactory deficits also accompany intracranial tumors (e.g., olfactory groove meningiomas, frontal lobe gliomas) that compress the lateral olfactory tract or the medial aspect of the temporal lobe. Hyposmia is an early presenting symptom of Alzheimer's disease and human immunodeficiency virus (HIV) infection and often accompanies idiopathic Parkinson's disease, Korsakoff's psychosis, and Huntington's disease.

Dysosmias and olfactory hallucinations are positive disturbances caused by abnormal patterns of neural activity. Patients with dysosmias report that normally pleasant smelling odors smell bad. Some dysosmias develop while the olfactory system is recovering from some insult, but most are idiopathic and the locus indeterminate. Olfactory hallucinations often accompany epileptiform activity within the medial temporal lobe and its limbic neighbors, the amygdala and hippocampus. Schizophrenic and psychotic patients often experience olfactory hallucinations. Almost all olfactory hallucinations are unpleasant.

Olfaction shows a gradual deterioration with age that accelerates rapidly after age 70. For patients in their 80s, anosmia is the rule rather than the exception. Although there may be multiple causative factors for the age-related decline of smell, erosion of the olfactory epithelium is one known cause. It also has been shown that few olfactory glomeruli persist beyond age 90. Age-related anosmia, through its deleterious effect on flavor perception, may have a significant impact on feeding and nutrition in the elderly.

> A positive disturbance does not reflect lost function but rather the expression of surviving structures.

> A negative disturbance is a function lost due to damage or pharmacologic blockade.

> Uncinate fits are seizures that involve the uncus of the temporal lobe; many are preceded by olfactory hallucinations or auras.

OVERVIEW OF TASTE

Taste receptors are not as primitive as those of either the common chemical sense or olfaction. Transduction of gustatory information takes place within specialized receptors rather than free nerve endings or bipolar neurons, and its central projections terminate in neocortex rather than paleocortex. Taste information mediates several ingestive reflexes as well as more complex behaviors such as foraging for food.

Taste Quality

> The four basic taste qualities are salty, sweet, sour, and bitter.

Taste stimuli often are grouped into four discrete qualitative categories: *salty, sweet, sour,* and *bitter* (Table 9-2). Some data suggest that the beef-like taste of monosodium glutamate may be a fifth primary taste quality, but there is no consensus on this point.

Each of these primary taste qualities is related to the safety and nutritional content of food. For example, sweet stimuli are eagerly ingested because most are sugars, carbohydrates, or other calorie-rich foods. Ingestion of salts replaces NaCl, a mineral that is continuously lost through sweating and urination. Sour and bitter stimuli are rejected because sourness and bitterness often are associated with food spoilage and poisons, respectively. There are exceptions to these rules, however. Saccharin, which tastes sweet, has no nutritional value, and lead acetate, a sweet-tasting salt, is poisonous. Lithium chloride, a toxic salt, tastes like sodium chloride.

Taste Quality	Prototypical Stimuli
Salty	Sodium chloride (NaCl)
Sweet	Sucrose
Sour	Hydrochloric (HCl) or citric acid
Bitter	Quinine hydrochloride (QHCl)

◀ **TABLE 9-2**
Prototypical Stimuli of the Primary Taste Qualities

Flavor is a synthesis of gustatory and somesthetic (touch, temperature, pain) input from the oral cavity, with odors released during mastication of food. Few people appreciate the contributions of odors to the flavor of food until a head cold blocks their nasal air flow. The overwhelming tendency to attribute olfactory stimulation to the palate accounts for the fact that most patients who report a loss of taste, in fact, are unable to detect odors.

Taste Buds

Taste buds are goblet-shaped clusters of specialized epithelium that communicate with the oral cavity through an apical *taste pore* (Figure 9-7). The apical taste pore enables fluids in the oral cavity to enter the papilla and bind with the taste receptors located inside. Each taste bud contains 50–150 *receptor, sustentacular,* and *basal cells* concentrically arranged like the segments of an orange. The receptor cells have an apical tuft of *microvilli* that protrudes into the taste pore, and numerous synapses along their basolateral surfaces. Taste buds have a life span of only 10–14 days. As taste cells degenerate, basal cells located at the perimeter of the bud migrate into the center of the bud and differentiate into receptor cells. Sustentacular cells provide support for the basal and receptor cells but do not play a direct role in taste transduction.

> Taste buds are microscopic structures embedded within taste papillae.

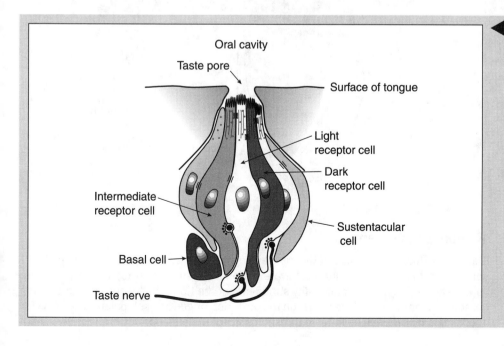

◀ **FIGURE 9-7**
Cross Section of an Individual Taste Bud.
Each taste bud has a concentric arrangement of basal, sustentacular, and receptor cells.

Taste receptor cells are divided into light, dark, and intermediate types based on the granularity of the cytoplasmic matrix. It is uncertain whether these cell types reflect different classes of receptor cell or different developmental stages of a single type. Synaptic vesicles are located along the basolateral surfaces of all three.

Distribution of Taste Buds

Taste buds are located on the tongue dorsum, soft palate, epiglottal folds, larynx, pharynx, and the upper one-third of the esophagus (Figure 9-8). Taste buds on the tongue are encased within papillae; those on the soft palate and epiglottis are embedded in the surface epithelium. There are no taste papillae on the ventral tongue surface and few, if any, along the midline of the dorsal surface. There are four different types of papillae within the oral cavity, but only three contain taste buds. *Fungiform papillae* line the lateral margin and the tip of the anterior tongue. *Foliate papillae*, which are buried within three or four vertically oriented trenches near the palatoglossal arches, have limited access to tastants except those released when food is crushed by the molars. *Circumvallate papillae*, numbering between seven and eleven, form a chevron near the base of the tongue. These bunker-like papillae have their taste buds in the walls of the trenches of the mucous-filled moats that surround these structures. *Filiform papillae*, which cover most of the tongue's dorsum, do not contain taste buds. These cone-shaped pillars of cornified epithelium give the tongue its rough texture.

Fungiform, from the Latin, means mushroom-like.

Foliate, from the Latin, means leaf-like.

FIGURE 9-8 ▶

Distribution of Taste Buds. *Inserts show cross sections of fungiform, foliate, and circumvallate papillae.*

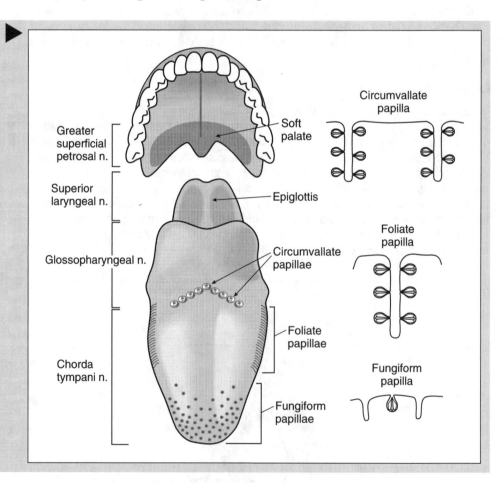

Regional Taste Sensitivity

Despite the fact that all parts of the oral cavity populated by taste papillae respond to all four of the basic taste stimuli, there are regional differences in taste threshold. The lowest thresholds for sweet and salty stimuli are at the tip of the tongue. The thresholds for sour and bitter stimuli are lowest on the posterior tongue and soft palate. The basis for these regional differences in taste thresholds is not understood.

Taste Transduction

Taste transduction begins when sapid stimuli bind to receptors located on the microvilli within the taste pore. Research within the last 5 years has shown that the mechanism for taste transduction is different for each of the primary taste qualities but probably similar across different classes of taste papillae (Figure 9-9). Salty taste depends on the dissociation of NaCl into Na^+ and chloride (Cl^-) ions. Transduction of salty taste is initiated by the voltage-independent diffusion of Na^+ ions through pores located along the surface of the microvilli. The influx of positively charged Na^+ ions depolarizes the receptor cell directly, which releases neurotransmitter from synapses at the base of the taste receptor cell. Although less certain, the initial step in sour transduction may depend on closure of potassium (K^+) channels by dissociated hydrogen (H^+) ions. The resultant increase in the intracellular K^+ concentration depolarizes the cell.

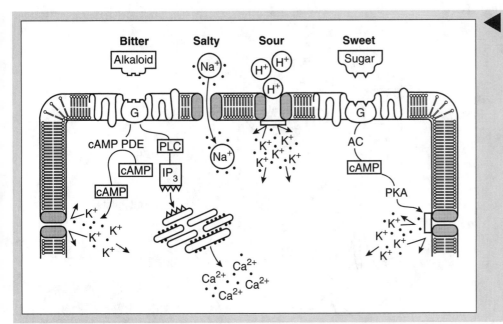

FIGURE 9-9
Taste Transduction Mechanisms for Bitter, Salty, Sour, and Sweet Stimuli. See text for details. AC = adenyl cyclase; cAMP = cyclic adenosine monophosphate; cAMP PDE = cyclic AMP phosphodiesterase; G = G protein; IP$_3$ = inositol triphosphate; PLC = phospholipase C; PKA = protein kinase A.

Sweet-tasting stimuli include carbohydrates (e.g., mono- and disaccharides), D-amino acids, dipeptides (e.g., aspartame), artificial sweeteners (e.g., saccharin, cyclamate), certain proteins (e.g., thaumatin, monellin), and some heavy metal salts (e.g., lead acetate). Although it is unclear how many different sweet receptors exist, once the receptors are activated, release of neurotransmitter is believed to depend on activation of a G-protein cascade ending in the release of the second messenger, cAMP. The transduction mechanism for sweet stimuli resembles that described above for pleasant smelling odors.

Bitterness, like sweetness, is associated with a wide range of chemically diverse agents. Bitter stimuli include many L-amino acids (e.g., L-phenylalanine, L-tryptophan), alkaloids (e.g., caffeine, quinine), glycosides (e.g., digitalis), divalent cations (e.g., Ca^{2+}, magnesium [Mg^{2+}]), and various peptides. Bitter stimuli are so widespread in the wild that bitterness could be described as the default taste quality. Several lines of evidence indicate that there are multiple bitter receptors and G-protein–activated transduction pathways. In some receptors, G proteins activate phospholipase C, which triggers an IP$_3$-mediated release of Ca^{2+} from intracellular stores and neurotransmitter release. The other bitter receptors use cAMP phosphodiesterase to decrease the intracellular concentration of cAMP, which in turn hyperpolarizes the cell by closing basolateral K^+ channels. Bitter transduction is similar in some respects to olfactory transduction.

> *Transduction of sweetness and bitterness resembles olfactory transduction.*

Taste Bud Innervation

The taste buds of the oral cavity are innervated by the trigeminal, facial, glossopharyngeal, and vagus nerves (Figure 9-10). Based on its embryology, the tongue is

> *The chorda tympani nerve (VII) innervates the taste buds on the anterior two-thirds of the tongue.*

The chorda tympani passes through the middle ear and is named after the tympanic membrane.

The glossopharyngeal nerve (IX) innervates the taste buds on the posterior one-third of the tongue.

Taste buds located within the foliate papillae are innervated by the chorda tympani nerve (anterior half) or the glossopharyngeal nerve (posterior half).

divided into anterior and posterior parts. Taste buds located on the *anterior two-thirds of the tongue* are innervated by the *chorda tympani* branch of the facial nerve and the lingual nerve, a branch of the trigeminal nerve. The chorda tympani nerve conveys gustatory information while the lingual nerve provides somatosensory innervation. Taste buds within the circumvallate papillae, as well as other stray taste buds on the *posterior one-third of the tongue*, are innervated by the *glossopharyngeal nerve*. The glossopharyngeal nerve contains gustatory and somatosensory fibers. The foliate papillae, which straddle the chorda tympani and glossopharyngeal fields, are innervated by both nerves. Taste buds on the soft palate are innervated by the *superior petrosal nerve*, a branch of the facial nerve, and the glossopharyngeal nerve; those within the esophagus and on the epiglottal surface are innervated by the *superior laryngeal nerve*, a branch of the vagus nerve. Although it has been established that taste buds synapse on these first-order taste nerves, the neurotransmitters have not been identified.

FIGURE 9-10 ▶
Peripheral and Central Taste Pathways. *Taste buds in the oral cavity are innervated by cranial nerves VII, IX, and X. Each of the first-order nerves terminates in the nucleus of the solitary tract (NST) of the medulla; second-order neurons ascend to the parvocellular division of the ventroposteromedial nucleus (VPMpc) of the thalamus. The primary taste cortex is located in the anterior insula. Gustatory information ascends from the oral cavity to cortex along ipsilateral pathways.*

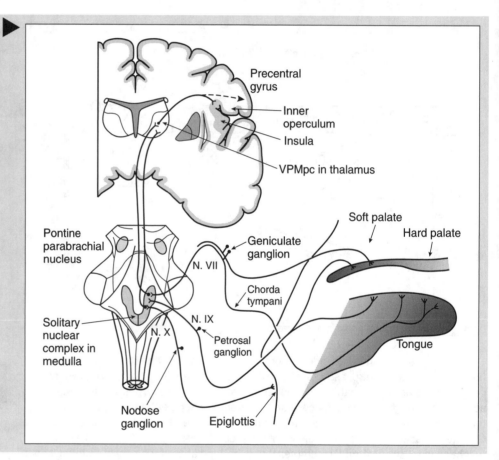

Central Gustatory Projections

The chorda tympani, glossopharyngeal, and vagus nerves are the distal processes of pseudounipolar neurons whose cell bodies are located within ganglia located near the brainstem (Table 9-3). Their central processes enter the rostral medulla and terminate in the *nucleus of the solitary tract (NST)* [see Chapter 4, Figure 4-10]. The NST contains a

TABLE 9-3 ▶
Location of Cell Bodies of Gustatory Nerves

Taste Nerves	Location of Cell Bodies
Chorda tympani nerve (VII)	Geniculate ganglion
Glossopharyngeal nerve (IX)	Petrosal ganglion
Superior laryngeal nerve (X)	Nodose ganglion

rough map of the tongue. Taste buds innervated by the chorda tympani nerve project to the rostral part of the NST while the glossopharyngeal and vagal nerves project to progressively more caudal regions of the nucleus. Axons of second-order neurons within the NST enter the *central tegmental tract* and ascend ipsilaterally to the *parvocellular division of the ventroposteromedial nucleus (VPMpc) of the thalamus* (see Figure 9-10; Chapter 5, Figure 5-10). Third-order neurons in the thalamus project to the *primary taste cortex* located at the junction of the anterior insula and the inner operculum. It has not been determined whether a minor projection to the foot of the precentral gyrus conveys gustatory information. Neurons in the primary taste cortex project to the caudolateral orbitofrontal cortex, which also receives convergent projections from the visual, somatosensory, and olfactory systems. The multimodal nature of the orbitofrontal cortex suggests that it may provide a neural substrate for flavor perception.

Taste Quality Coding

As in olfaction, supporters of the labeled line theory have had to explain why most taste neurons respond to more than one stimulus, that is, why they are broadly tuned. The ambiguity associated with broad tuning virtually demands that taste quality be represented by the pattern of activity across many neurons. This notion, referred to as pattern theory, has empirical support. Psychophysical and neurophysiologic experiments have shown that similar tasting chemicals evoke similar patterns of neural activity in the nervous system (Figure 9-11). The labeled line theory, on the other hand, emphasizes the activity of individual cells or groups of cells that respond similarly. The labeled line theory garners support from the fact that people typically use a limited vocabulary to describe taste quality. The mechanisms of taste transduction, although not fully understood, are consistent with the notion that only a limited number of stimulus qualities exists. Because the labeled line theory can be tested more easily than the across fiber pattern theory, it has received more criticism. At present, both theories have firm empirical support and a loyal following. Future studies are likely to show that the nervous system uses both to encode taste and smell quality.

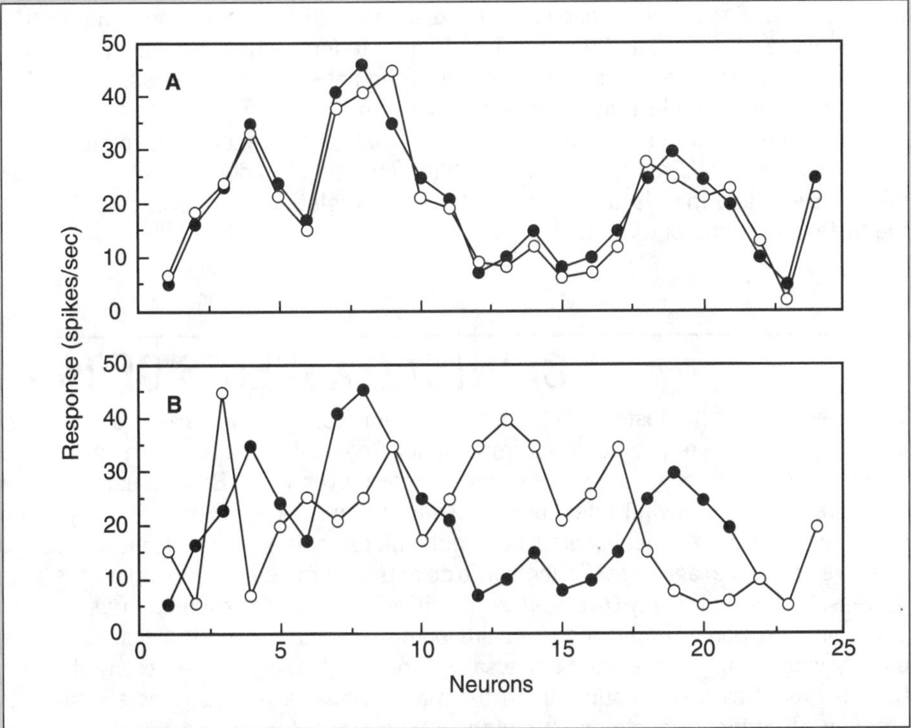

> The central ascending taste pathway is strictly ipsilateral.

FIGURE 9-11
Pattern of Neural Activity across Neurons.
(A) The pattern of neural activity across 24 neurons is very similar when two similar tasting chemicals are applied to the tongue. (B) When two dissimilar tasting chemicals are applied to the tongue, the pattern of activity across the same sample of 24 neurons is distinctly dissimilar.

Functions of the Gustatory System

Oral Reflexes. Foods with appetitive tastes initiate reflexive swallowing while aversive tastes (e.g., bitter or sour-tasting foods) trigger gapes and other oral motor reflexes that eject food from the mouth. These acceptance and rejection reflexes are executed by a circuit formed by the first-order taste neurons, interneurons within the NST and reticular formation, and output neurons within the facial and hypoglossal motor nuclei.

Stimulation of the epiglottal taste buds triggers the gag reflex, which prevents fluid aspiration into the upper airway. The superior laryngeal branch of the vagus nerve, which constitutes the afferent limb of this reflex, projects to the posterior NST whose cells act as interneurons for this reflex arc. The efferent limb of the gag reflex is executed by cholinergic neurons within the nucleus ambiguus.

The taste of food also triggers salivation, as well as other vagally mediated gastric and pancreatic secretions that aid digestion. Salivation is mediated by a four-neuron reflex involving the chorda tympani and glossopharyngeal nerves, neurons in the NST, preganglionic parasympathetic neurons in the superior and inferior salivatory nuclei, and the postganglionic parasympathetic neurons. The efferent projections of the superior salivatory nucleus are contained within the chorda tympani nerve; those of the inferior salivatory nucleus reside within the glossopharyngeal nerve. Food in the oral cavity also triggers gastric acid release, which prepares the stomach for the arrival of food. Oral administration of glucose releases pancreatic insulin. This preabsorptive release of insulin exceeds that following intravenous glucose administration. The efferent limb of these visceral reflexes is mediated by the subdiaphragmatic branch of the vagus nerve.

Taste and Learned Behaviors. Many animals, including humans, form strong associations between taste cues and the consequences of feeding. The clearest demonstration of this phenomenon is a *conditioned taste aversion (CTA),* the association between the taste of a novel food and subsequent gastrointestinal (GI) malaise. Ambient odors and the physical setting may interact with the learning and expression of CTAs but are of secondary importance. CTAs represent a form of classical conditioning in which the taste of the novel food serves as the *conditioned stimulus (CS).* The illness-inducing agent (e.g., *Salmonella,* radiation, or a toxic chemical) acts as the *unconditioned stimulus (UCS),* which evokes illness, the *unconditioned response (UCR).* Sometimes only a single pairing of the CS (taste) and the UCS is sufficient to form a CTA. Radiation and cancer chemotherapy are potent emetics, which, in some patients, may act as UCSs that link food consumed at the last meal before therapy with GI malaise.

The ability to associate taste with the beneficial consequences of feeding forms the basis for conditioned taste preferences. When an animal is depleted of an individual micronutrient and then is given an opportunity for repletion, a preference develops for the taste of that micronutrient.

CLINICAL ASPECTS OF TASTE

Bell's palsy is caused by damage to the facial nerve.

The innervation of the taste buds by three different cranial nerves makes a total loss of taste (*ageusia*) unlikely, though not impossible. Regional ageusias, however, are more common following local trauma to primary taste nerves (e.g., Bell's palsy) or central structures, as well as viral infections involving the middle ear. Because the gustatory system emphasizes the quality of taste stimulation rather than its locus, most people are unaware of regional ageusias. Patients who do notice a problem may report a generalized decrease in taste intensity (*hypogeusia*). Positive disturbances such as *dysgeusias* and *phantoms* are poorly understood but are potentially more serious because they are usually long-lasting and almost universally unpleasant. Dysgeusias are errant perceptions triggered by a sapid stimulus in the mouth while taste phantoms appear in the absence of verifiable gustatory stimulation. Some dysgeusias and phantoms have a metallic taste while others assume a bitter or fecal quality. Dysgeusias and phantoms triggered by trauma or disease may respond to sectioning of one or more of the remaining taste nerves; those that appear spontaneously are more resistant to treatment.

RESOLUTION OF CLINICAL CASE

Taste loss following traumatic closed-head injury is rare and not well understood. Careful testing of patients who report permanent taste loss shows that, in most cases, their sense of smell has been disrupted, and that taste perception is intact. Most people, and many physicians, appreciate the enormous contribution of olfactory information to the perception of flavor only when they have a head cold that prevents food-associated odors from reaching the olfactory epithelium. When T. R. hit her head on the windshield, her brain surged forward and struck the inner surface of the skull causing a concussion. Such severe brain movement may sever the delicate olfactory nerves where they pass through the cribriform plate. When the olfactory nerves are merely stretched, there may be some recovery of olfactory function. In this case, T. R. showed a permanent anosmia, which suggests that her olfactory nerves were severed in the accident. Another issue that should have been addressed in the emergency room was the leakage of clear fluid from the nose (rhinorrhea) of this patient. Rhinorrhea following head trauma may signal cerebrospinal fluid leakage into the nasal cavity through a fracture of the cribriform plate. Fractures of the cribriform plate provide opportunities for bacteria in the nasal cavity to infect the meninges, a serious, but preventable complication of head trauma.

REVIEW QUESTIONS

Directions: For each of the following questions, choose the **one best** answer.

1. Which of the following areas receives a direct projection from the olfactory bulb?
    - **(A)** Orbitofrontal cortex
    - **(B)** Piriform lobe
    - **(C)** Insula
    - **(D)** Nucleus of the solitary tract (NST)
    - **(E)** Mediodorsal thalamic nucleus

2. The taste transduction mechanism for NaCl involves
    - **(A)** reversible binding to receptors located on the microvilli of the taste bud, which triggers Ca^{2+} entry into taste cells
    - **(B)** direct entry of Na^+ ions into the cell through ion-sensitive gates, which causes direct depolarization of the taste cell
    - **(C)** reversible binding to receptors located on the apical surface of the taste bud, which triggers a G-protein–mediated release of cAMP
    - **(D)** A G-protein–initiated cascade that involves the second messenger inositol triphosphate (IP_3)

3. Receptors for the common chemical sense are located throughout the nasal and oral cavities, as well as the eyes, the anogenital openings, and the gastrointestinal tract. From the standpoint of perception, which of the following sensory modalities is most closely related to the common chemical sense?
    - **(A)** Taste
    - **(B)** Smell
    - **(C)** Flavor
    - **(D)** Touch
    - **(E)** Pain

4. What is the source and destination, respectively, of gustatory information carried by the central tegmental tract?
    - **(A)** The medulla and the ipsilateral mediodorsal (MD) nucleus of the thalamus
    - **(B)** The nucleus of the solitary tract (NST) and the ipsilateral primary gustatory cortex
    - **(C)** The parvocellular division of the ventroposteromedial nucleus (VPMpc) of the thalamus and the ipsilateral primary gustatory cortex
    - **(D)** The NST and the contralateral MD nucleus of the thalamus
    - **(E)** The medulla and the ipsilateral VPMpc of the thalamus

Directions: The group of questions below consists of lettered choices followed by several numbered items. For each numbered item, select the appropriate lettered option with which it is most closely associated. Each lettered option may be used once, more than once, or not at all.

Questions 5–9

Match the following.

  (A) Only smell
  (B) Only taste
  (C) Both taste and smell
  (D) Neither taste nor smell

5. Receptor cells regenerate

6. Transduction involves second messengers

7. Receptor cells are neurons

8. Apical end of receptors are capped by microvilli

9. Central projections are primarily contralateral

ANSWERS AND EXPLANATIONS

1. The answer is B. The piriform cortex, which is the largest division of the primary olfactory cortex, receives direct projections from the olfactory bulb via the lateral olfactory stria. The mediodorsal nucleus of the thalamus, which projects to the orbitofrontal cortex, receives olfactory projections from the entorhinal cortex. The olfactory system does not project to the insula or the NST.

2. The answer is B. Positively charged Na+ ions do not bind reversibly to receptors located on the membrane but rather pass into the cell through ion channels. Because these positive ions depolarize the cell directly, no second messengers are required to complete the transduction process.

3. The answer is E. Regardless of origin, the sensation mediated by the common chemical sense is pain, which is discussed in Chapter 6.

4. The answer is E. Ascending gustatory information ascends from the medulla to the ipsilateral VPMpc of the thalamus. The MD nucleus is a relay for olfactory information bound for the orbitofrontal cortex. The pontine parabrachial nucleus is an obligatory gustatory relay in nonprimate species only; in humans the central tegmental tract ascends to the thalamus without synapsing in the pons.

5–9. The answers are: 5-C, 6-C, 7-A, 8-B, 9-D. Gustatory and olfactory receptors cells regenerate, probably because of the harsh environments they inhabit. Second messengers are not used for all stimuli, but gustatory and olfactory receptors use them. Only olfactory receptors are neurons; the gustatory system uses specialized receptor cells. Only taste receptor cells are capped by microvilli; olfactory neurons have tufts of cilia at the apical end. The central projections of the olfactory and gustatory systems are primarily ipsilateral.

ADDITIONAL READING

Doty RL, Bartoshuk LM, Snow JB Jr: Causes of olfactory and gustatory disorders. In *Smell and Taste in Health and Disease*. Edited by Getchell TV, Doty RL, Bartoshuk LM, et al. New York, NY: Raven Press, 1991, pp 449–462.

Duncan HJ, Smith DV: Clinical disorders of olfaction. In *Handbook of Olfaction and Gustation*. Edited by Doty RL. New York, NY: Marcel Dekker, 1995, pp 345–365.

Kinnamon SC, Cummings TA: Chemosensory transduction mechanisms in taste. *Ann Rev Physiol* 54:715–731, 1992.

Kratskin IL: Functional anatomy, central connections, and neurochemistry of the mammalian olfactory bulb. In *Handbook of Olfaction and Gustation*. Edited by Doty RL. New York, NY: Marcel Dekker, 1995, pp 103–126.

Miller IJ: Anatomy of the peripheral taste system. In *Handbook of Olfaction and Gustation*. Edited by Doty RL. New York, NY: Marcel Dekker, 1995, pp 521–547.

Price JL: Olfactory system. In *The Human Nervous System*. Edited by Paxinos G. New York, NY: Academic Press, 1990, pp 979–998.

Pritchard TC: The primate gustatory system. In *Smell and Taste in Health and Disease*. Edited by Getchell TV, Doty RL, Bartoshuk LM, et al. New York, NY: Raven Press, 1991, pp 109–125.

Ronnett GV: The molecular mechanisms of olfactory signal transduction. In *Handbook of Olfaction and Gustation*. Edited by Doty RL. New York, NY: Marcel Dekker, 1995, pp 127–145.

10 VISUAL SYSTEM

INTRODUCTION OF CLINICAL CASE

A 37-year-old woman was seen by her family physician because of recurring headaches and blurred vision. She also reported difficulty reading from left to right because she could not see the next word. An ophthalmoscopic examination found no evidence of papilledema or retinopathy. In both eyes the optic cup had a well-defined margin, and there were no signs of vascular hemorrhage, aneurysm, or retinal exudates. Both the lens and vitreous were free of opacities. The eyes displayed direct and consensual pupillary light reflexes, and there was no indication of a relative afferent pupillary defect. The patient did not have double vision, and eye movements appeared normal. A test of visual acuity revealed bilateral loss of the temporal fields and complete loss of macular vision in the left eye. Although the patient did not exhibit any other physical symptoms, her blood was drawn for an endocrine evaluation, and she was taken to a nearby medical center for a magnetic resonance imaging (MRI).

OVERVIEW OF THE VISUAL SYSTEM

Most people rely on vision more than any other sensory system to acquire information about the external world. Our visual system creates a vivid spatial representation of the world, which allows us to determine the size, shape, color, and location of objects in three-dimensional space. When these objects move, our visual system informs us of their direction and relative speed. Furthermore, our motor system receives projections from the visual system to guide eye movements and enable skillful interactions with objects in our environment.

The visual system includes the eyes and all of the central pathways in the brain that receive information from the eyes. The central visual pathways extend from the front of the brain to the back of the cerebral cortex and project to several intermediate regions in the diencephalon and brainstem. Because of this widespread distribution, the visual system can be affected by many diseases or injuries. The central pathways of the visual system are precisely organized, and knowledge of this system is critical for determining the location of lesions that impair vision and other central nervous system (CNS) functions.

THE EYE

The eyes are highly specialized structures that allow light to be perceived by the CNS. In the posterior part of each eye lies the retina, a laminated neural structure that transduces light into neural signals. The neuronal circuits of the retina transform light information into a neural code that is used by the brain to construct a visual representation of the external world.

Development of the Eye

The eye is an outgrowth of the brain.

The eyes begin to develop from the prosencephalon during the third week of embryologic growth. On day 22, the optic vesicles extend from both sides of the ventral forebrain and remain connected to the diencephalon by hollow optic stalks (Figure 10-1). As the optic vesicles grow laterally, their distal ends enlarge and gradually displace the overlying mesenchyme until they appose the surface ectoderm. After the ectoderm thickens and forms the lens placode, the underlying optic vesicle induces the lens placode to invaginate and form the lens vesicle. Cells in the neck of the lens vesicle fuse together and cause the lens vesicle to separate from the surface ectoderm before it develops into the lens of the eye.

Formation of the lens vesicle is accompanied by invagination of the distal end of the optic vesicle into a two-layered structure called the optic cup. After the lens vesicle separates from the ectoderm, the distal rim of the optic cup bends inward and embraces the lens vesicle to form the iris. The inferior surface of the optic cup is indented by the optic fissure, a small cleft that contains mesenchyme and hyaloid blood vessels that supply the retina and the lens vesicle. The edges along the optic fissure eventually grow around the hyaloid vessels and fuse together. With further development, the distal tributaries of the hyaloid vessels degenerate, but the proximal branches remain intact to become the central retinal artery and vein.

The optic cup is composed of two distinct layers. The inner, thicker layer is called the nervous layer because it differentiates into the neuronal layers of the retina. The outer, thinner layer is called the pigment layer because it is the predecessor to the pigment epithelium. These layers are separated by the intraretinal space, a slender cavity that originates from the lumen of the optic vesicle and gradually disappears as the pigment and nervous layers grow closer together to form a fully developed retina. Sometimes the pigment and nervous layers become separated later in life, and this is known as a retinal detachment.

The lens vesicle induces cell proliferation in the nervous layer, causing it to form a thick neuroepithelium that differentiates into several layers of neurons. Axons from the

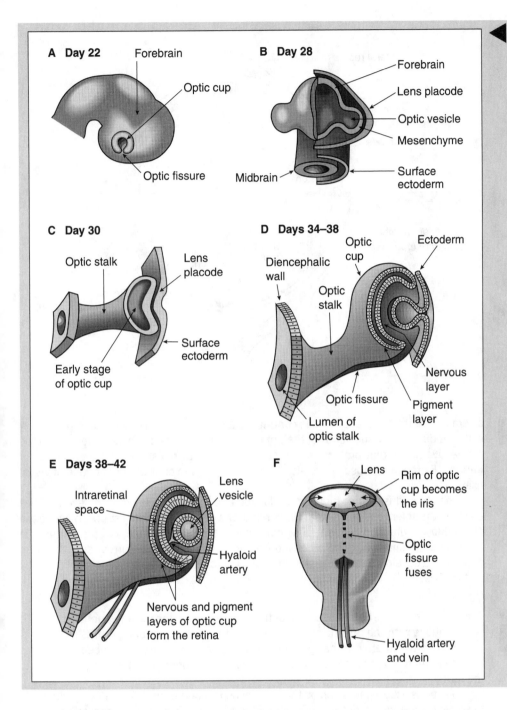

A Day 22
Forebrain
Optic cup
Optic fissure

B Day 28
Forebrain
Lens placode
Optic vesicle
Mesenchyme
Midbrain
Surface ectoderm

C Day 30
Optic stalk
Lens placode
Early stage of optic cup
Surface ectoderm

D Days 34–38
Optic cup
Ectoderm
Diencephalic wall
Optic stalk
Nervous layer
Pigment layer
Optic fissure
Lumen of optic stalk

E Days 38–42
Intraretinal space
Lens vesicle
Hyaloid artery
Nervous and pigment layers of optic cup form the retina

F
Lens
Rim of optic cup becomes the iris
Optic fissure fuses
Hyaloid artery and vein

FIGURE 10-1
Development of the Eye. (A) Surface view of the optic vesicle evaginating from the ventral surface of the forebrain. (B–E) Sectional views showing the development of the optic stalks and the induction of the lens from the surface ectoderm. (F) The optic fissure closes around the hyaloid artery and vein.

retinal ganglion cells eventually grow across the inner surface of the nervous layer and migrate into the lumen of the optic stalk, which they eventually fill as they form the optic nerve. Optic nerve fibers from both eyes proceed caudally until they meet at the optic chiasm located at the base of the brain. The optic nerve fibers originating from the nasal half of each retina (approximately 60% of the fibers) cross through the midline of the optic chiasm before entering the brain.

Anatomy of the Eye

The eye is a complex structure that contains many intricate components. The major components of the eye are shown in Figure 10-2.

SCLERA AND CHOROID

Most of the eye is covered by an extremely tough membrane called the sclera or, more commonly, the "white of the eye." Except for the region overlying the pupil and iris, the

FIGURE 10-2
Components of the Eye. Horizontal section through the right eye illustrates the visual axis and its relationship to the lens, the macula, and other structures in the eye.

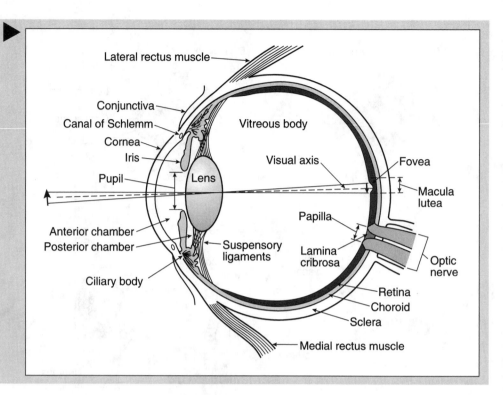

FIGURE 10-2
Components of the Eye. Horizontal section through the right eye illustrates the visual axis and its relationship to the lens, the macula, and other structures in the eye.

The sclera protects the eye.

sclera surrounds the eyeball and is continuous anteriorly with the cornea and posteriorly with the dura mater surrounding the optic nerve. The sclera consists of dense, fibrous connective tissue that protects the interior of the eye by resisting punctures and other injuries. Extraocular muscles are attached to the sclera to control the direction of visual fixation.

The choroid is a thin, highly vascularized and pigmented layer of the eye that lies between the sclera and the retina. Branches of the ophthalmic artery supply blood to the choroid layer, which in turn supplies nutrients to the photoreceptors of the retina. The sclera and the choroid are both derived from mesenchyme tissue surrounding the optic cup. During development, the distal rim of the choroid differentiates into the ciliary body and the iris.

CORNEA

The cornea refracts light more than any other part of the eye.

The cornea forms the anterior surface of the eye and covers the iris and pupil. Although it is continuous with the opaque sclera, the cornea is transparent and permits light transmission into the interior of the eye. The cornea has a highly curved surface that refracts light more than any other component in the eye and is essential for focusing images onto the retina.

Due to its exposed location on the anterior aspect of the eye, the cornea is vulnerable to abrasion by small particles. To detect minor irritants, the cornea is densely innervated by a plexus of free nerve endings that originate in the ophthalamic division of the trigeminal ganglion. The central projections of these neurons terminate in the facial nucleus to mediate the corneal blink reflex.

IRIS

The iris controls the amount of light entering the eye.

The iris is an adjustable, pigmented diaphragm that controls the size of the pupil and, hence, modulates the amount of light entering the eye. Pupil diameter can vary from 1 to 8 mm and is controlled by two sets of nonstriated muscles in the iris. Thus, the pupil constricts during contraction of the pupillary sphincter and dilates during contraction of the pupillary dilator. The sphincter is an annular muscle located around the inner rim of the iris and receives parasympathetic innervation from a small number of postganglionic neurons of the ciliary ganglion located in the posterior orbit. By comparison, the dilator muscle has a radial organization around the circumference of the pupil and is located along the posterior wall of the iris. The dilator muscle receives sympathetic innervation from postganglionic neurons of the superior cervical ganglion located in the trunk of the neck. Damage to these sympathetic neurons causes Horner's syndrome, which is characterized by a small pupil (miosis) and partial eyelid drooping (pseudoptosis).

CILIARY BODY

The ciliary body has a ring-like structure that follows the outer perimeter of the iris and consists mainly of muscle fibers that lie underneath the ciliary processes and the ciliary epithelium. The ciliary processes produce aqueous humor, a clear fluid similar to cerebrospinal fluid. Aqueous humor carries nutrients to the lens and the cornea. Suspensory ligaments (or zonal fibers) connect the ciliary body to the equator of the lens.

The ciliary muscle develops from mesenchyme tissue and differentiates into three layers of annular, oblique, and longitudinal fibers. Contraction of these fibers causes the ciliary body to move slightly towards the equator of the lens, and this small movement reduces tension along the suspensory ligaments to allow accommodation of the lens (Figure 10-3). The ciliary muscle is innervated by most of the postganglionic neurons in the ciliary ganglion.

> *Ciliary muscles control the shape of the lens.*

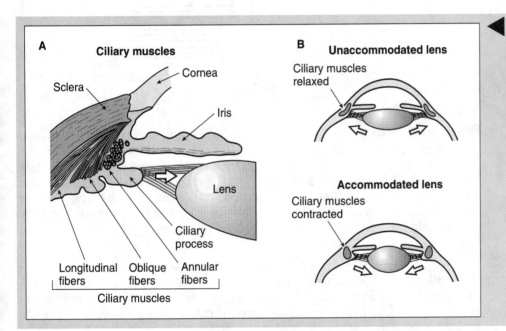

FIGURE 10-3
Ciliary Muscles. (A) This diagram shows the structure of the three sets of ciliary muscle fibers after removing the cornea and sclera. The arrow indicates the direction of movement of the ciliary body during contraction of the ciliary muscles. (B) The ciliary muscles control the shape of the lens. When distant objects are viewed, the ciliary muscles are relaxed, and this flattens the lens. When nearby objects are viewed, the ciliary muscles contract, and this allows the lens to bulge because of decreased tension along the suspensory ligaments.

LENS

The lens is a transparent, oval-shaped structure composed of interlocking crystalline fibers enclosed in a basement membrane called the lens capsule. The main function of the lens is to alter light refraction to focus on objects at different distances from the eye. Because the lens capsule and its enclosed fibers are highly elastic, the shape of the lens varies with changes in the amount of tension along the suspensory ligaments. The curvature of the lens surface determines the degree of light refraction; therefore, lens shape is controlled within narrow limits to bend light rays more or less as the eye focuses on near or distant objects, respectively. Thus, light refraction is greatest when the lens bulges during contraction of the ciliary muscles and is lowest when the lens flattens during relaxation of the ciliary muscles (see Figure 10-3).

The lens may become cloudy in older individuals and interfere with visual acuity. This condition, known as a cataract, is easily corrected by surgically removing the cloudy lens and implanting a plastic lens in the lens capsule.

> *The lens focuses light onto the retina.*

RETINA

During embryologic development, the nervous layer of the optic cup differentiates into several layers of neurons to form the retina. One layer in the retina is composed exclusively of photoreceptors, which transduce photons of light into neural signals that are

> *Photoreceptors transduce light into neural impulses.*

subsequently processed by neighboring layers of neurons. Ultimately, these signals are sent to ganglion cells whose axons converge at the optic disk and project to the brain as the optic nerve. The detailed structure of the photoreceptors and the other layers of the retina are discussed below.

The structure of the retina varies considerably across its surface. The macula lutea, which lies in the center of the retina, represents the central part of the visual field. A small depression in the macula lutea, called the fovea, has the highest density of photoreceptors and, consequently, has the highest spatial resolution of the visual field. The optic disk, which lies medial to the macula lutea, indicates the point at which the optic nerve emerges from the retina. There are no photoreceptors at the optic disk, and hence, it is often called the blind spot (Figure 10-4).

FIGURE 10-4 ▶

Blind Spot. To demonstrate the blind spot, close your left eye and view the plus sign with your right eye while holding the page 1 foot away. The filled circle "disappears" when its image is projected onto the optic disk. The blind spot is usually not noticed because the visual system "fills-in" the missing portion of the visual scene. This is demonstrated by viewing the lower portion of the figure as described above; all the lines appear continuous despite the presence of a gap.

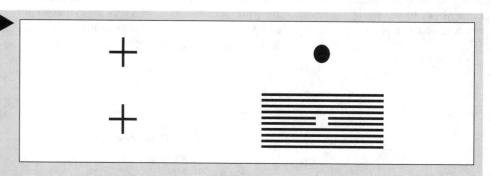

The pigment epithelium supports the cellular functions of the retina.

PIGMENT EPITHELIUM

The pigment epithelium develops from the pigment layer of the optic cup and lies between the choroid on its outer surface and the photoreceptors on its inner surface. The proximity of the pigment epithelium and the photoreceptors allows interactions that are vital to visual functions. The pigment epithelium also contains a high concentration of melanin, which absorbs light and reduces the reflection of light onto the photoreceptors.

OPTIC NERVE

The optic nerve is composed of myelinated axons that convey visual information from the retina to the brain. The central retinal artery and vein travel through the center of the optic nerve and supply blood to the inner layers of the retina. At the posterior surface of the optic disk, the optic nerve and retinal blood vessels perforate the sclera and choroid at the lamina cribrosa (Figure 10-5). The three meningeal layers (i.e., dura mater, arachnoid, pia

FIGURE 10-5 ▶

Optic Nerve. Horizontal section through the optic nerve shows the nerve fibers perforating the sclera to form the lamina cribrosa.

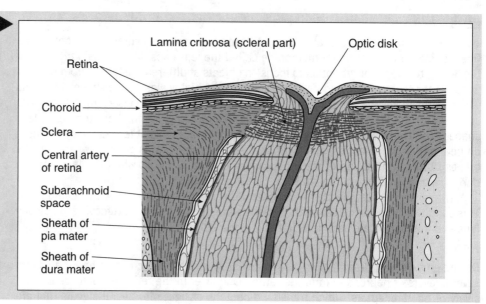

mater) lining the optic nerve are continuous with the meninges that surround the brain. As the optic nerve enters the eye, the dura mater merges with the sclera.

FLUID-FILLED CHAMBERS IN THE EYE

The chambers lying anterior and posterior to the lens are filled with two types of fluid. Aqueous humor is a clear, watery fluid that is secreted by the ciliary process into the posterior chamber between the iris and the lens (see Figure 10-2). Aqueous humor in the posterior chamber passes through the pupil and into the anterior chamber, which lies between the iris and the cornea. The aqueous humor supplies nutrients to the lens and cornea before it leaves the anterior chamber via the canal of Schlemm located near the junction of the iris and cornea. When the outflow of aqueous humor is impeded, the intraocular pressure increases and may lead to glaucoma.

The vitreous body, the large spherical chamber between the lens and the retina, is filled with a thick, gelatinous fluid called vitreous humor (see Figure 10-2). The vitreous humor maintains the shape of the eyeball and contains phagocytic cells that remove blood and other cellular debris that might interfere with light transmission.

Ophthalmoscopic Examination of the Eye

An ophthalmoscope is used to look through a patient's pupil to inspect the retina, the optic disk, and the blood vessels on the inner surface of the retina (Figure 10-6). The macula lutea ("yellow spot") is the general area in the center of the retina that lies between a ring of vascular arcades. The fovea appears as a small bright spot in the center of the macula, and it contains a small depression, the foveola, which is totally devoid of

Macula lutea is the region in the retina that represents the central part of the visual field.

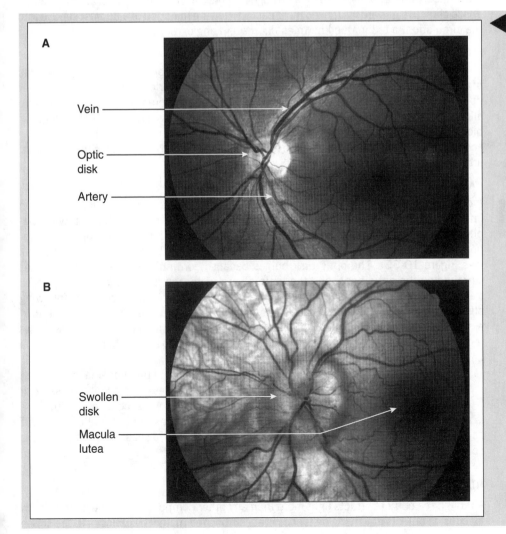

A

Vein

Optic disk

Artery

B

Swollen disk

Macula lutea

◀ **FIGURE 10-6**
Ophthalmoscopic Views of the Eye. *(A) Optic disk in a normal individual. The margins of the optic disk are well defined, and the central retinal artery and vein are seen emerging from the optic cup before bifurcating into branches that radiate along the surface of the retina. (B) Retina with papilledema. The margins of the optic cup are blurred because the optic disk is swollen. (Courtesy of Dr. Thomas Gardner and Mr. Timothy Bennett, Pennsylvania State University College of Medicine, Hershey, Pennsylvania.)*

retinal vessels. The foveola and the surrounding part of the macula lack surface blood vessels because this region is supplied by capillaries in the choroid layer. The macula has a darkly stained appearance because it contains the highest density of photoreceptors and, thus, has a high concentration of melanin and other pigments. The macular region, especially the fovea and foveola, consists mainly of cones, which subserve color vision and the perception of fine details. The optic disk, or papilla, is located approximately 3 mm medial to the macula lutea and appears as a bright pinkish disk. The central part of the disk is lighter in color and represents a depression or cup in the optic disk, which is close to the underlying sclera. The central retinal artery and vein pass through the optic disk and radiate into several branches across the surface of the retina.

Ophthalmoscopic (or funduscopic) examination is an important part of every neurology examination because the appearance of the retina might be altered by head trauma or by a variety of systemic diseases. Furthermore, the central retinal artery and vein lie on the surface of the retina, and inspection of their "nude" state provides an opportunity to detect signs of vascular disease produced by diabetes mellitus, hypertension, or arteriosclerosis.

DIABETIC RETINOPATHY

The most serious ocular complication of chronic diabetes mellitus is retinopathy. Although insulin administration may control blood sugar levels, vascular pathology may continue to progress in this disease. Diabetes mellitus produces morphologic changes in the endothelial cells and basement membranes of blood vessels throughout the body, including the eye where diabetes may lead to occlusion or leakage of the retinal capillaries. Thus, the ophthalmoscopic hallmarks of diabetic retinopathy are a scattering of microaneurysms and blot-like hemorrhages where the capillary walls are weakened. These clinical signs are visualized more easily following injection of a fluorescent dye into the circulation, a technique known as fluorescein angiography.

HYPERTENSIVE AND ARTERIOSCLEROTIC RETINOPATHY

The central retinal artery is really an arteriole, but in the sclerotic state, it may show signs of arteriosclerosis. In the sclerotic state, the normally red arteriole appears lighter in color due to thickening of its vessel wall. In hypertension, an increase in vascular pressure allows the arterioles to compress the veins wherever they cross each other in the retina. If blood pressure is not controlled, hemorrhages and hard exudates (cellular debris) may accumulate in the posterior part of the fundus. Chronic hypertension is the main cause of arteriosclerosis.

PAPILLEDEMA

Papilledema is a swollen or "choked" optic disk.

Increased intracranial pressure produced by a brain tumor, cerebral hemorrhage, or an infection of the CNS invariably causes a swelling of the optic disks. Although papilledema does not normally affect vision, it is recognized during a funduscopic examination because the swelling obliterates the optic cup and blurs the margins of the optic disk (see Figure 10-6B). The optic disk bulges because continuity between the meninges surrounding the optic nerve and the brain allows increased intracranial pressure to be transmitted through the subdural space. Alternatively, papilledema may appear following obstruction of venous outflow that occurs secondary to increased pressure in the cavernous sinus that, in turn, elevates the pressure of the ophthalmic vein. In either case, the optic disk is compliant where the sclera is perforated at the lamina cribrosa by the departing optic nerve fibers.

An increase in intracranial pressure is not the only cause of papilledema, but it is the most common. Papilledema can also be produced by decreases in intraocular pressure or by a marked elevation in blood pressure. As papilledema becomes more advanced, there is an increase in venous engorgement, vascular hemorrhages, and retinal exudates. If papilledema is not treated, vision may become impaired due to secondary atrophy of the optic nerve.

Image Formation on the Retina

Although the cornea refracts light more than any other component of the eye, the ability to focus on objects at varying distances is accomplished mainly by changes in the shape of the lens (Figure 10-7). When we focus on distant objects, the lens becomes thin and flat. For nearby objects, the lens becomes thicker in order to bend light rays to a greater degree.

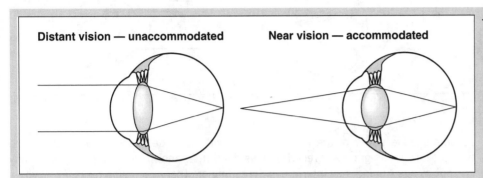

Distant vision — unaccommodated   Near vision — accommodated

◄ **FIGURE 10-7**
Accommodation. *When viewing nearby objects, the lens thickens to increase the angle of refraction.*

The shape of the lens is controlled by two opposing forces: the innate elasticity of the lens and tension along the suspensory ligaments. When the ciliary muscle relaxes, the ciliary body retracts, and the suspensory ligaments pull on the equator of the lens to flatten it. By contrast, contraction of the ciliary muscle causes the ciliary body to move toward the lens, and the decreased tension along the suspensory ligament allows the elastic lens to form a more convex shape.

The shape of the lens and the size of the pupil are adjustable to focus images on the retina.

The clarity of images on the retina is partly determined by the size of the pupil. As with microscopes and other optic instruments, light rays passing through the edge of the lens are subjected to chromatic and spherical aberrations. With a small pupil, most light entering the eye is transmitted through the center of the lens, and this reduces optical distortion. Photographers employ the same principle when they reduce the aperture of a camera to improve the depth of field so that objects located at varying distances from the camera are brought into focus. A small pupil, however, interferes with visual acuity by reducing the amount of light entering the eye. For this reason, the visual system adjusts the size of the pupil to limit optical distortion and maximize the depth of field according to the ambient illumination.

ACCOMMODATION–CONVERGENCE REACTION

The ability to focus on objects near the face is accomplished by coordinating the activities of several muscles in a response called the accommodation–convergence reaction. This ocular reflex is clinically important and can be demonstrated by having a patient fixate on the examiner's finger as it is moved toward the nose. As the patient watches the approaching finger, the eyes converge toward the midline. This convergence response is mediated by contraction of the medial recti muscles of both eyes. Also, as the eyes converge, the lens in each eye becomes more spherical, and both pupils constrict. This accommodation response is mediated by simultaneous contraction of the ciliary muscle and the pupillary sphincter, both of which receive parasympathetic innervation from postganglionic neurons in the ciliary ganglion.

MYOPIA AND HYPEROPIA

Myopia and hyperopia represent refractive errors in which light rays are not properly focused on the retina because the focal plane of the lens and the shape of the eye are mismatched (Figure 10-8). Myopia, or nearsightedness, results when distant objects are focused in front of the retina either because the cornea is too curved or the eyeball is too long. Hyperopia, or farsightedness, results when nearby objects are focused behind the retina either because the cornea is not curved enough or because the eyeball is too short. Both types of refractive errors can be corrected with an appropriate set of concave (for myopia) or convex (for hyperopia) lenses.

Myopic individuals are "nearsighted"; images from distant objects are focused in front of the retina.

Hyperopic individuals are "farsighted"; images from near objects are focused behind the retina.

PRESBYOPIA

In nearly all persons, aging causes the lens to lose elasticity and limits the degree of curvature that can be achieved by the lens when the ciliary muscle is fully relaxed. As the

FIGURE 10-8 ▶

Hyperopia and Myopia. *Hyperopic (far-sighted) individuals focus light behind the retina because the eyeball is too short. Myopic individuals focus light in front of the retina because the eyeball is too long. The* dashed lines *indicate how these refractive errors are corrected by the appropriate lenses.*

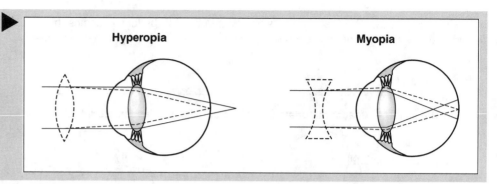

Presbyopia
With age the lens loses elasticity and is unable to accommodate to nearby objects.

accommodative power of the lens decreases with age, the closest point that can be brought into focus gradually recedes. This condition, known as presbyopia, is usually present by age 45 and may interfere with reading or other near-vision tasks. Presbyopia can be corrected by an appropriate set of convex lenses.

THE RETINA

The retina originates from the neural tube during embryologic development and is, therefore, considered part of the CNS. Consistent with its origin, the retina contains a variety of neurons that are organized into circuits for processing visual information.

Laminar Organization of the Retina

The retina contains five types of neurons: photoreceptors, bipolar cells, ganglion cells, horizontal cells, and amacrine cells. These neurons and their processes are organized into several layers that are identified with respect to the vitreous body (Figure 10-9). The outer nuclear layer, which is adjacent to the pigment epithelium and is most distant from

FIGURE 10-9 ▶

Organization of the Retina. *(A) Photomicrograph of the human retina. (Courtesy of Dr. Eric Lieth, Pennsylvania State University College of Medicine, Hershey, Pennsylvania.) (B) Diagram of the neuronal components in the retina. Vertical transfer of information from photoreceptors to bipolar cells and then to ganglion cells provides the most direct route into the brain. Horizontal cells and amacrine cells mediate lateral interactions between neighboring parts of the retina.*

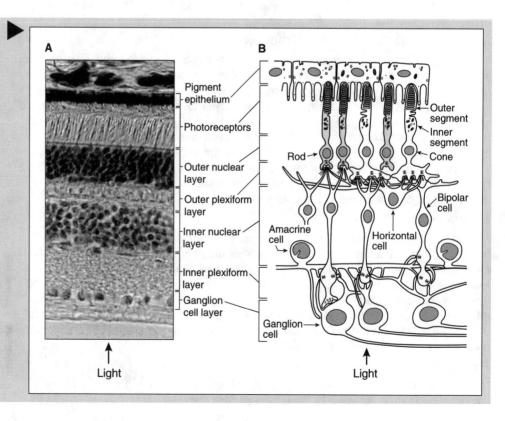

the vitreous body, contains two types of photoreceptor cells: rods and cones. The outer plexiform layer lies closer to the vitreous body and contains rod and cone presynaptic terminals as well as postsynaptic processes originating from bipolar and horizontal cells. The cell bodies of the bipolar and horizontal cells reside in the inner nuclear layer, which also contains the cell bodies of amacrine cells. Progressing toward the vitreous humor, the inner plexiform layer contains the synaptic connections between the bipolar, amacrine, and ganglion cells. Finally, the cell bodies of the ganglion cell layer give rise to a layer of nerve fibers that converge in the optic disk and exit the retina as the optic nerve.

The five types of retinal neurons are organized into simple circuits for conveying visual information to the brain. Photoreceptors, bipolar cells, and ganglion cells process visual information in a serial fashion and represent the most direct route for sending visual information to the brain. Horizontal cells and amacrine cells mediate lateral interactions between adjacent groups of photoreceptors, bipolar cells, and ganglion cells. These lateral connections enable neighboring parts of the retina to compare the intensity of light coming from contiguous regions of the visual field. Abrupt changes in illumination indicate important features of an object, and the lateral connections of horizontal and amacrine cells serve to enhance the detection of these features.

Photoreceptors

Rods and cones are the only cells in the visual system that are directly activated by light. Both types of photoreceptors have a similar structure and are composed of outer and inner segments that are connected by a cilium (Figure 10-10). The outer segments

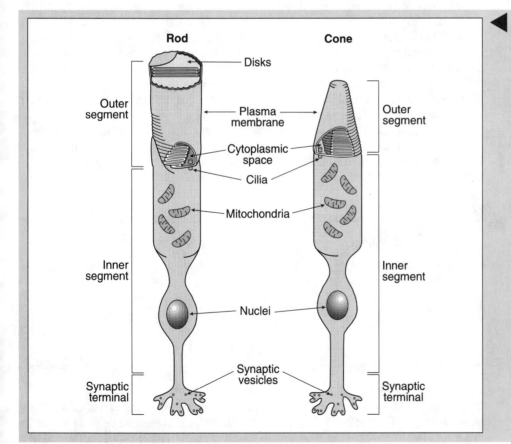

FIGURE 10-10

Photoreceptors. Although similar in structure, cones have short outer segments and contain fewer disks than rods. The outer segments contain photopigments and other proteins needed for transducing light into electrophysiologic signals; the inner segments contain organelles that synthesize the components of the outer segments. The synaptic terminals contain vesicles and neurotransmitter molecules.

contain stacks of membranous disks that are loaded with photopigments and other proteins needed to transduce light into neural signals. The inner segments contain a nucleus, mitochondria, and organelles needed for biosynthesis of disks and other molecules used in phototransduction. The inner segments also synthesize synaptic vesicles and maintain the synaptic terminals in the outer plexiform layer.

Most students are initially surprised to learn that photoreceptors are in the outermost layer of the retina because this means light must pass through several layers of cells and their processes before reaching the rods and cones. Fortunately, the inner layers of the retina absorb very little light and are essentially transparent. The location of photoreceptors in the outer layer of the retina reflects their physiologic dependence on the pigment epithelium. Thus, as new disks are formed at the base of the outer segment, the oldest disks at the tip of the outer segment are shed into the intraretinal space. The life span of a disk is only 12 days, and to accommodate this turnover rate, detached disk fragments are removed from the intraretinal space by the phagocytic activity of the pigment epithelium. The pigment epithelium also recycles bleached photopigment molecules after they participate in phototransduction. A retinal detachment interferes with these critical functions and causes the photoreceptors to degenerate.

PHOTOTRANSDUCTION

Phototransduction is the process by which photoreceptors convert light energy into neural signals. This process involves one light-sensitive step that is followed by a cascade of biochemical reactions, which alter the membrane potential of the photoreceptor. The only light-dependent step in the transduction process involves the absorption of a photon of light by a photopigment molecule. There are only a few types of photopigments, and all of them consist of a protein covalently linked to 11-*cis* retinal, an aldehyde derivative of the carotenoid alcohol known as vitamin A. Photopigments differ according to their ability to absorb certain wavelengths of visible light, and the protein component determines the spectral characteristics of each type of photopigment. In rods, the protein coupled to 11-*cis* retinal is opsin, and the combination of opsin and 11-*cis* retinal is called rhodopsin. Cones have one of three different proteins that combine with 11-*cis* retinal, and each is sensitive to a different range of wavelengths in the visible spectrum.

Photopigments *are the combination of a protein and 11-*cis *retinal.*

Opsin molecules are integrated into the disk membrane, and each molecule contains 348 amino acid residues, which span the disk membrane seven times. The hydrophobic transmembrane regions are connected by hydrophilic loops of amino acids that extend into the cytoplasm of the outer segment. Cross-links within the transmembrane regions form a tight pocket around a bound molecule of 11-*cis* retinal. Hence, the conformational structure of the opsin molecule resembles the structure of metabotropic neurotransmitter receptors as described in Chapter 1.

The absorption of light by a photoreceptor causes a cascade of biochemical events.

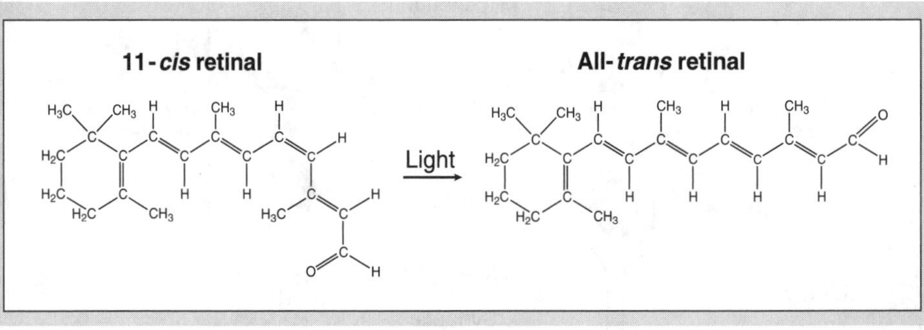

When a photon of light is captured by rhodopsin, the conformational structure of retinal is altered from the 11-*cis* form to the all-*trans* form (Figure 10-11). The all-*trans* isomer does not conform to the opsin binding site, however, and this causes a conformational change in opsin, which then activates a G protein called transducin. In response,

FIGURE 10-11 ▶
Photoactivation of Retinal. *Absorption of light alters the conformational structure of retinal from the 11-*cis *form to the all-*trans *configuration.*

transducin stimulates phosphodiesterase to hydrolyze a nucleotide called cyclic guanosine monophosphate (cGMP). Removal of cGMP from the cytoplasm causes the closure of sodium (Na^+) channels in the outer segment (Figure 10-12). Thus, activation of a single rhodopsin molecule stimulates hundreds of transducin molecules, each of which hydrolyzes hundreds of cGMP molecules. It has been estimated that a single photoactivated rhodopsin molecule may close 300 Na^+ channels or nearly 3% of the Na^+ channels that are normally open in a dark-adapted rod.

After all-*trans* retinal detaches from the protein component, it is reduced to all-*trans* retinol, which enters the pigment epithelium where it is recycled back into 11-*cis* retinal. Subsequently, 11-*cis* retinal is transported from the pigment epithelium to the photo-

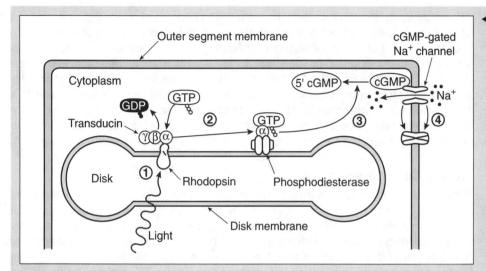

Phototransduction. *Phototransduction in rods involves four steps: (1) light stimulates rhodopsin to activate the G protein transducin; (2) transducin activates phosphodiesterase; (3) phosphodiesterase hydrolyzes cGMP to convert it to 5' cGMP; (4) the removal of cGMP from the cytoplasm closes the cGMP-gated Na+ channels. GTP = guanosine triphosphate; GDP = guanosine diphosphate.*

receptor outer segments where it combines with a protein to form a new photopigment molecule.

Photoreceptor Membrane Potentials. In darkness, cGMP maintains open Na+ channels and permits a passive flow of Na+ into the cytoplasm of the outer segment of the photoreceptor. The steady influx of Na+ in the dark depolarizes the photoreceptor and maintains the membrane potential at −40 mV. In this partially depolarized state, the photoreceptor's inner segments allow potassium (K+) to leak out of the cell through K+ channels. Thus, the steady influx of Na+ into the outer segment is balanced by an efflux of K+ from the inner segment, and together these ionic movements establish a circular flux of current known as dark current (Figure 10-13). The concentration gradients for K+ and Na+ are maintained at physiologic concentrations by ion pumps in the inner segment that use metabolic energy to pump Na+ out and K+ in (see Chapter 1).

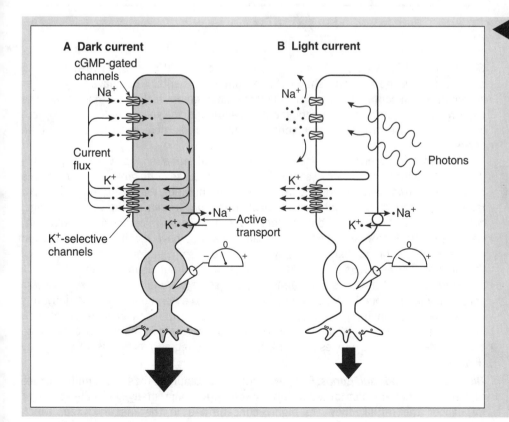

FIGURE 10-13

Photoreceptor Membrane Potentials. *(A) In the dark, cGMP-gated Na+ channels are open and allow a passive influx of Na+ current, which depolarizes the photoreceptor to −40 mV. Further depolarization is prevented by leakage of K+ current from the inner segment. Concentration gradients of Na+ and K+ are maintained by ion pumps in the inner segment. (B) During light stimulation, removal of cGMP causes Na+ channels to close, and the photoreceptor hyperpolarizes because K+ continues to leak out of the inner segment. Shading indicates depolarization, and arrow size indicates the magnitude of neurotransmitter release.*

Following illumination of the retina, the Na+ channels close, and the decrease in Na+ influx causes the membrane potential to become hyperpolarized because K+ continues to leak out of the inner segment. Although the membrane potential never shifts completely to the equilibrium potential for K+ (−80 mV), illumination may cause hyperpolarization to −65 mV. Like other neurons, the vesicular release of neurotransmitter from a photoreceptor requires depolarization of the membrane potential, and it is during darkness that photoreceptors release the most neurotransmitter. In moderate levels of illumination, the amount of neurotransmitter release fluctuates continuously in response to changes in brightness. Thus, transmitter release decreases with a gain in luminance and increases when luminance declines.

ROD AND CONE COMPARISONS

Although rods and cones are both sensitive to light, important distinctions between these cells allow them to serve different visual functions. Rods and cones differ in several respects, including size, shape, types of photopigment, retinal distribution, and their synaptic connections with other neurons (Table 10-1). The rod system is specialized to detect low levels of illumination and stimulus motion. By comparison, the cone system needs higher levels of illumination to operate and is specialized to resolve spatial detail with greater acuity than the rod system.

TABLE 10-1 ▶
Structural and Functional Differences between Rods and Cones

Properties of Rods	Properties of Cones

High sensitivity to light
    Large amounts of photopigment
    Scotopic (night) vision
	Low sensitivity to light
	    Smaller amounts of photopigment
	    Photopic (day) vision

Low spatial acuity
    Highly convergent retinal circuits
    Located outside fovea
	High spatial acuity
	    Retinal circuits less convergent
	    Concentrated in fovea

Achromatic
    One photopigment (rhodopsin)
	Chromatic
	    Three color-sensitive photopigments

Sensitivity to Illumination. The most striking structural difference between rods and cones concerns the size and shape of their outer segments. Rods have longer outer segments which contain more disks and more photopigment molecules than cones. The large number of disks and photopigment molecules in the rod, coupled with a more efficient rhodopsin transduction mechanism, makes rods more sensitive to light than cones.

Human vision occurs over a much wider range of illumination than would be possible if rods and cones had the same sensitivity to light. Because of its greater sensitivity, the rod system allows vision during the low levels of illumination that occur in the scotopic range (e.g., starlight). At higher levels of illumination, known as the mesopic range, colors can barely be detected because both rods and cones are responsive. In daylight, vision is determined mainly by cones because the rods have reached their saturation point and are unable to distinguish any further increase in illumination. This range of illumination, known as photopic vision, mediates most of our visual perceptions.

Scotopic: *Rod vision*
Photopic: *Cone vision*

Differences in the sensitivity and time course of the rod and cone systems are apparent whenever one leaves a brightly lighted area to enter a dark room. Initially, it is impossible to see anything because neither the cones nor the rods are sensitive at such low light levels. In a few minutes, however, rhodopsin levels in the rods become more concentrated, and this process of dark adaptation enables greater visual sensitivity (Figure 10-14).

Distribution of Rods and Cones. Each eye contains 100 million rods and 6 million cones that are differentially distributed within the retina. Although many cones are scattered throughout the retina, they are highly concentrated in the macula lutea, which

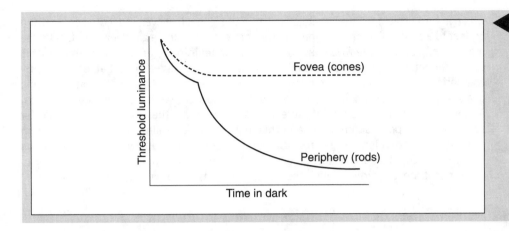

► **FIGURE 10-14**
Dark Adaptation. *This figure illustrates changes in threshold sensitivity as a function of elapsed time in the dark. The light intensity of a small target was constantly adjusted to a level that was barely detectable. The threshold sensitivity of the fovea depends mainly on cones, whereas peripheral sensitivity depends mainly on rods.*

represents the central 5° of the visual field. The fovea, which lies in the center of the macula, is totally devoid of rods and contains only cones. In contrast, rods are densest in the region surrounding the macula lutea.

These regional variations reflect the distinct functions of the macula lutea and the surrounding parts of the retina. Whereas the macula lutea has high spatial acuity, the surrounding regions are specialized for detecting visual motion. Thus, reading and other tasks that require high spatial resolution are dependent on visual signals received from the macula. The peripheral retina, by comparison, is responsible for initiating changes in visual attention that occur in response to objects moving in the peripheral part of the visual field.

There are several reasons why the fovea and the rest of the macula have better spatial resolution than surrounding parts of the retina. First, the fovea is devoid of any overlying blood vessels that might interfere with light transmission. Second, the inner layers of the retina are displaced laterally so that light can interact directly with photoreceptors in the fovea without having to pass through multiple layers of neurons (Figure 10-15). Finally, the fovea only contains cones, and these cones are much narrower than those in the rest of the retina; this permits the fovea to have a much higher density of photoreceptors than the surrounding retina.

Another factor contributing to the regional variation in visual acuity concerns the degree of synaptic convergence in the rod and cone systems. A tremendous amount of convergence exists in the retina, and this fact can be appreciated simply by comparing the relative number of cell bodies in the different layers of the retina as shown by Figure 10-9A. As this figure indicates, a large number of photoreceptors send information to a much smaller number of ganglion cells. Thus, many rods project to a few bipolar cells,

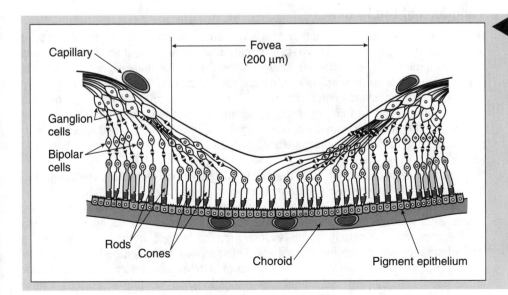

► **FIGURE 10-15**
Macula Lutea. *A cross section through the macula lutea shows how bipolar and ganglion cells are displaced from the central part of the fovea. Only cones are present in the center of the fovea, and each cone communicates with one bipolar and one ganglion cell.*

which in turn project to fewer ganglion cells. In the fovea, however, individual cones often project to a single bipolar cell, which in turn projects to a single ganglion cell. Unlike the rod system, cones in the fovea have a private channel into the brain, which enables this part of the retina to provide the visual system with a high degree of spatial resolution. By comparison, a ganglion cell activated by the rod system cannot signal the exact position of a stimulus in the visual field because it receives convergent inputs from multiple rods. Although convergent circuits interfere with spatial acuity, they provide a substrate for spatial and temporal summation, and this increases the likelihood that a rod ganglion cell will respond when several rods are sequentially activated by a moving stimulus (Figure 10-16). Because of these convergent circuits, our attention is often drawn to objects that move rapidly through the peripheral parts of our visual field.

FIGURE 10-16 ▶

Retinal Circuits. (A) In the fovea, cones have one-to-one communication with bipolar and ganglion cells, which allows the cone system to determine the exact location of a stimulus (x) in the visual field. Arrows indicate the flow of information in the retina. (B) In the periphery, many rods project to a few bipolar cells, which project to even fewer ganglion cells. Because of spatial and temporal summation, the convergent circuits of the rod system enhance sensitivity to moving stimuli but at the expense of spatial resolution.

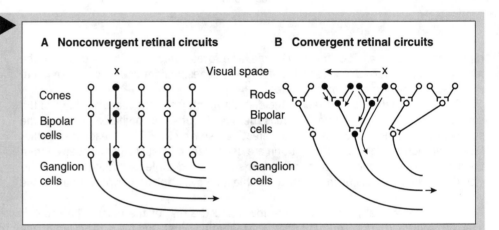

A **Nonconvergent retinal circuits**   B **Convergent retinal circuits**

Visual space

Cones   Rods

Bipolar cells   Bipolar cells

Ganglion cells   Ganglion cells

Macular degeneration is the leading cause of blindness in the elderly.

Macular Degeneration. The importance of the macula for resolving spatial detail is underscored by the degree of visual impairment that accompanies macular degeneration. In many adults, the choroid undergoes age-related degenerative changes that allow blood and other fluids to leak into the retina at the posterior fundus. As the intraretinal space becomes filled with fluid, the macula detaches from the pigment epithelium and eventually forms a scarred region. Patients with macular degeneration may have normal peripheral vision, but the loss of macular vision is disabling because the patient cannot drive a car, and reading becomes difficult. Although macular degeneration is the leading cause of blindness in persons older than 75, the cause of this disease is unknown, and there is no cure.

Functions of the Retina

One of the main tasks of the visual system is to identify objects in the external world. To accomplish this, the brain must extract information about form and shape from variations in light intensity. Abrupt changes in light intensity, or luminance contrast, provide important cues about the shape of an object. Thus, the amount of light reflected from an object is usually constant along its flat surfaces but varies significantly at its corners. In addition, light reflected from an object is significantly different in intensity and color from the light originating from the background. Thus, the contrast in light reflected from the corners and edges of an object are used by the visual system to recognize shape and form.

The process of using contrast to identify the edges and corners of an object begins in the retina. Unlike most sensory systems that transmit peripheral signals directly to the CNS with little modification, the retina performs a significant amount of processing before sending visual information to the brain. Neurons in the inner layers of the retina receive photoreceptor output, which is closely related to light intensity, and convert it into information about luminance contrast. Thus, signals conveyed by the optic nerve fibers do not simply represent the absolute amount of light coming from a particular point in the visual field but, instead, signal spatial locations that contain abrupt changes in light intensity. By transforming light intensity into information about contrast, the retina enhances our ability to perceive the edges of an object.

CENTER–SURROUND RECEPTIVE FIELDS

Much of our knowledge about the retina comes from physiology experiments in which the responses of individual neurons were recorded while stimulating their receptive fields with small spots of light. Experiments performed by Stephen Kuffler in the 1950s showed that ganglion cells have circular receptive fields, and that their responses to light depend on whether the light stimulates the center or the perimeter of their receptive fields. These studies led to the characterization of two classes of retinal neurons: "on-center" and "off-center" ganglion cells (Figure 10-17). Thus, an on-center ganglion cell is excited when light strikes the center of its receptive field but is inhibited when light stimulates the perimeter of its receptive field. In contrast, an off-center cell is inhibited by light in the center of its receptive field center but is excited by light in the perimeter.

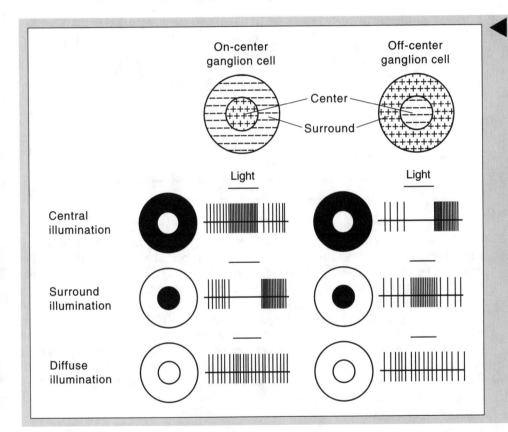

FIGURE 10-17
Center–Surround Receptive Fields. *On-center and off-center ganglion cells respond differentially to light stimulating the center or perimeter of their receptive fields.*

The total population of retinal ganglion cells is divided into equal numbers of on-center and off-center cells. Both types of cells are distributed uniformly across the retina to respond to changes in light intensity that might occur in any part of the visual field. Thus, light and dark edges in the visual field are detected by both types of ganglion cells. Bright light on one side of an edge is signaled by an increase in the firing rate of on-center cells, whereas the darker side of the edge is signaled by an increase in the firing rate of off-center cells. Off-center ganglion cells are necessary because the spontaneous activity of on-center cells is low, and a decrease in illumination would not be effectively signaled by a decline in their firing rate.

How do cells with circular receptive fields signal the presence of a linear edge of light and dark? The answer to this question is clear from an analysis of ganglion cell responses during different stimulus conditions. The best stimulus for exciting an on-center ganglion cell is a small spot of light that stimulates only the center of the receptive field, whereas the best stimulus for exciting an off-center ganglion cell is a ring of light that illuminates only the perimeter of the receptive field. In both types of cells, the optimal responses can be suppressed by shining light onto the antagonistic region of the receptive field. Thus, illumination of the receptive field perimeter effectively inhibits on-center cells, whereas illumination of the receptive field center suppresses the responses of off-center cells. Consequently, retinal ganglion cells respond poorly to diffuse illumination that stimulates both regions and respond best to stimuli that differentially illuminate the center and surrounding parts of the receptive field (see Figure 10-17). Few visual stimuli, however, consist of small circular lights that stimulate only the center or surround of a ganglion cell's receptive field. Most objects are defined by corners or linear edges in which there is a distinct change in the density of reflected light. Although ganglion cells have circular receptive fields, the configuration of antagonistic center–surround regions allows them to respond differentially to linear edges of light and dark that fall across their receptive fields (Figure 10-18).

Ganglion cells respond best when a light–dark edge falls on their receptive field.

FIGURE 10-18 ▶

Ganglion Cell Responses to Light–Dark Edges. *This figure illustrates the responses of matching sets of on-center and off-center ganglion cells to a light–dark edge. Both types of cells respond best when their receptive fields subtend the light–dark edge. The two sets of cells show different response patterns that distinguish the light and dark sides.*

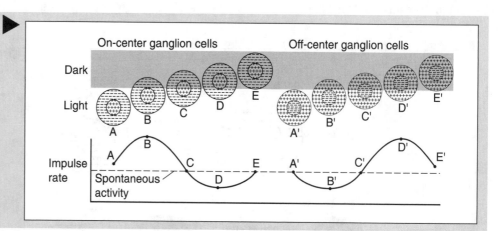

These observations suggest that the rate of activity in a ganglion cell is a code for the amount of contrast between the center and surrounding part of its receptive field. This is important because luminance contrast represents the basis for distinguishing an object from its background. The antagonistic center–surround properties of ganglion cells also explain why perception of brightness depends on the background luminance. When an object reflecting a uniform amount of light is presented against a background of varying illumination, our perception does not match the physical stimulus. As illustrated by Figure 10-19, perception of brightness is based on the activity of retinal ganglion cells that respond to the contrast in illumination across neighboring parts of the visual field. Because ganglion cells enhance contrast, a moderately bright region may appear brighter or darker depending on its background.

CIRCUIT MECHANISMS

The antagonistic center–surround properties of on-center and off-center ganglion cells are determined mainly by the afferent connections of the bipolar cells. Bipolar cells, like ganglion cells, have antagonistic center–surround receptive fields and are classified as

FIGURE 10-19 ▶

Perceptual Contrast. *The center panel reflects a constant amount of light throughout its extent but appears brighter or darker depending on the background illumination. The uniform shading of the center panel can be confirmed by covering the upper and lower panels.*

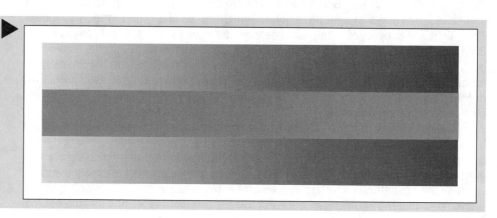

on-center or off-center cells. The primary difference is that bipolar cells, unlike ganglion cells, do not discharge action potentials because they do not contain voltage-gated Na+ channels. Since bipolar cells have relatively short processes, their graded potentials are able to spread passively to their synaptic terminals without a significant reduction in amplitude.

In response to small spots of light stimulating the center of their receptive fields, on-center bipolar cells depolarize and off-center bipolar cells hyperpolarize (Figure 10-20). To understand these responses, it is important to remember that light hyperpolarizes photoreceptors, and this reduces their release of neurotransmitter, which, for both rods and cones, is always glutamate. Although glutamate is an excitatory neurotransmitter in most brain regions, it produces opposite effects on off-center and on-center bipolar cells because these cells contain different types of glutamate receptors. Thus, glutamate opens Na+ channels in off-center bipolar cells, and the resulting influx of Na+ depolarizes these cells. In contrast, glutamate closes the Na+ channels of on-center bipolar cells but opens their K+ channels; consequently, these cells are hyperpolarized by the efflux of K+. Since light reduces glutamate release, on-center cells are excited by light in the center of their receptive fields, whereas off-center cells are inhibited when their receptive field centers are illuminated.

Glutamate has opposite effects on off-center (excitatory) and on-center (inhibitory) bipolar cells.

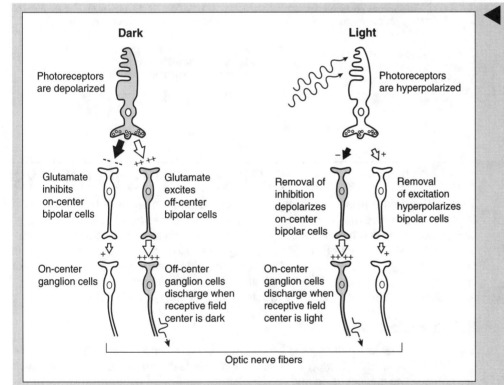

◀ **FIGURE 10-20**
On-Center and Off-Center Responses. *Photoreceptors in the dark or light are depolarized (shaded) or hyperpolarized (unshaded) and release more or less glutamate from their synaptic terminals. Glutamate is inhibitory (dark arrows) or excitatory (light arrows), depending on the postsynaptic receptors on the bipolar cells. Arrow size indicates the magnitude of neurotransmitter release.*

Light produces opposite effects on the rate of bipolar cell activity, depending on whether it stimulates the center or the surrounding part of the cell's receptive field. This antagonistic property is mediated by a lateral network of horizontal cells interconnecting neighboring groups of photoreceptors (Figure 10-21). Bipolar cells do not receive direct synaptic contacts from horizontal cells; instead, horizontal cells synapse directly on the terminals of photoreceptors. This configuration allows horizontal cells to regulate one group of photoreceptors in response to membrane potential changes in a neighboring group of photoreceptors. When a local group of photoreceptors is hyperpolarized by light, the horizontal cells within that group cause adjacent groups of photoreceptors to become depolarized. Thus, on-center bipolar cells are hyperpolarized by light in the peripheral part of their receptive field because the horizontal cells mediate an increase in glutamate

Horizontal cells cause neighboring photoreceptors to release more glutamate.

release from nearby photoreceptors. Hence, horizontal cells provide a mechanism for mediating opposite responses in adjacent groups of photoreceptors, and this mechanism is used to enhance luminance contrast.

FIGURE 10-21 ▶

Horizontal Interactions. This diagram shows how horizontal cells alter responses of an on-center bipolar cell. (1) Light hyperpolarizes photoreceptors in the surround region. (2) As the photoreceptors release less excitatory neurotransmitter, this hyperpolarizes postsynaptic horizontal cells. (3) As the horizontal cells release less inhibitory neurotransmitter, nearby photoreceptors are depolarized. (4) The depolarized photoreceptors release more inhibitory neurotransmitter onto the on-center bipolar cell.

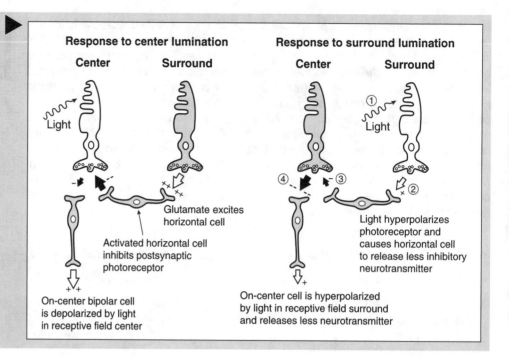

CENTRAL VISUAL PATHWAYS

The visual system consists of a diverse set of pathways and interconnected structures in the brain that analyze the information received from the retina. Visual perception of form, color, motion, and depth is mediated by multiple cortical areas in the occipital, temporal, and parietal lobes. Other brain regions, such as the superior colliculus and specific parts of the motor system, use visual information to guide eye movements and to direct changes in visual attention. Finally, retinal projections to the brainstem mediate pupillary reflexes while projections to the hypothalamus regulate circadian rhythms.

Retinal Projections

Each retina contains 1 million ganglion cells whose axons converge at the optic disk and exit the eye as the optic nerve. The optic nerve proceeds toward the optic chiasm, which lies between the diencephalon and the pituitary gland. At that point, nearly 60% of the optic nerve fibers cross the midline and continue centrally as the optic tract. The fibers of the optic tract enter the brain and terminate in the thalamus, the hypothalamus, or the midbrain.

PRIMARY VISUAL PATHWAY

Most retinal ganglion cells project to the lateral geniculate nucleus, which resides in the caudal part of the ventral thalamus (see Chapter 7, Figure 7-26). Lateral geniculate neurons send efferent projections into the optic radiation and terminate in the primary visual cortex, which occupies the superior and inferior banks of the calcarine sulcus in the occipital lobe (Figure 10-22). The primary visual cortex (Brodmann area 17) is often called the striate cortex because freshly cut sections of this area reveal prominent horizontal striations, which represent the myelinated fibers passing horizontally within certain cortical layers. The disynaptic retinogeniculostriate pathway forms the primary visual pathway in the brain and is responsible for conveying information essential for

Primary Visual Pathway
Retina → lateral geniculate nucleus → striate cortex

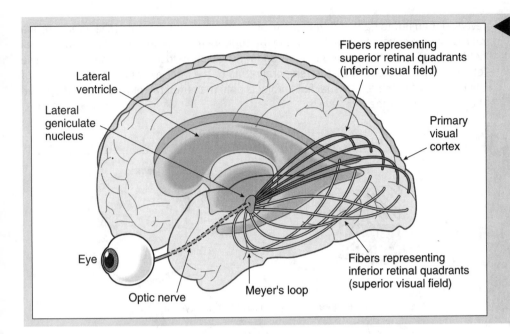

Lateral
ventricle

Lateral
geniculate
nucleus

Fibers representing
superior retinal quadrants
(inferior visual field)

Primary
visual
cortex

Eye

Optic nerve

Meyer's loop

Fibers representing
inferior retinal quadrants
(superior visual field)

◀ **FIGURE 10-22**
Primary Visual Pathways. *This is a lateral view of the brain showing the disynaptic retinogeniculostriate pathway. Geniculo-striate projections (or optic radiations) course along the lateral margin of the lateral ventricle; the fibers conveying information from the inferior retina course through the temporal lobe (Meyer's loop) before terminating in the inferior bank of the calcarine sulcus.*

most aspects of visual perception. A lesion in any part of this pathway causes partial or total blindness.

SECONDARY VISUAL PATHWAYS

Another set of projections from the retina terminates in the midbrain to mediate pupillary light reflexes (see Chapter 4). The afferent part of the pupillary light reflex consists of ganglion cell axons that project to the pretectal olivary nucleus, which lies rostral and lateral to the superior colliculus. Neurons in the pretectal olivary nucleus project bilaterally to preganglionic parasympathetic neurons in the Edinger-Westphal nucleus, which in turn innervate the ciliary ganglion (see Chapter 4, Figure 4-31). Postganglionic parasympathetic neurons in the ciliary ganglion innervate the ciliary muscle and the pupillary sphincter of the iris. Thus, in response to shining a light in either eye, the bilateral projections from the pretectal olivary nucleus mediate both direct and consensual pupillary constriction.

If a shadow is cast over either eye, both pupils dilate. Although the pathway mediating this sympathetic response remains uncertain, it is thought that retinal projections to the midbrain reticular formation serve the afferent part of this reflex. The midbrain reticular formation sends descending projections to the intermediolateral cell column of the thoracic spinal cord, which contains preganglionic cholinergic cells that project to the superior cervical ganglion. Postganglionic neurons in the superior cervical ganglion ascend in association with blood vessels and innervate the dilator muscle of the iris.

Other retinal ganglion cells project to the superior colliculus, which lies in the tectum of the midbrain. The superior colliculus uses visual, auditory, and somatosensory information to coordinate head and eye movements in response to stimulation in these sensory modalities (see Oculomotor Mechanisms later in this chapter).

Finally, a few retinal ganglion cells also project to the suprachiasmatic nucleus of the hypothalamus. This brain region uses variations in light intensity to control a broad range of physiologic processes that have circadian rhythms.

Visual Fields

The visual space seen by each eye is called the visual field for that eye (Figure 10-23). For descriptive reasons, each visual field is subdivided by vertical and horizontal lines that intersect the point in space fixated by the fovea. Each visual field is composed of left, right, superior, and inferior hemifields, which are represented by corresponding parts of the retina. Visual images are inverted by the lens, however, and the visual fields are reversed from left to right and from top to bottom on the retina. Hence, the inferior retina represents the superior visual field while the superior retina represents the inferior visual field. The retinal representation of left and right visual fields is more complicated. The left visual field projects onto the temporal retina of the right eye and the nasal retina of the left eye while the right visual field projects onto the temporal retina of the left eye and the nasal retina of the right eye.

FIGURE 10-23 ▶

Visual Fields. (A) Fixated images are projected onto the retina upside down and reversed from left to right. (B) Visual fields for each eye are asymmetric because the nasal retina (which views the temporal field) is larger than the temporal retina. (C) The brain fuses the information from each eye into a single image centered around the fixation point. The visual field can be subdivided into left, right, inferior, and superior hemifields.

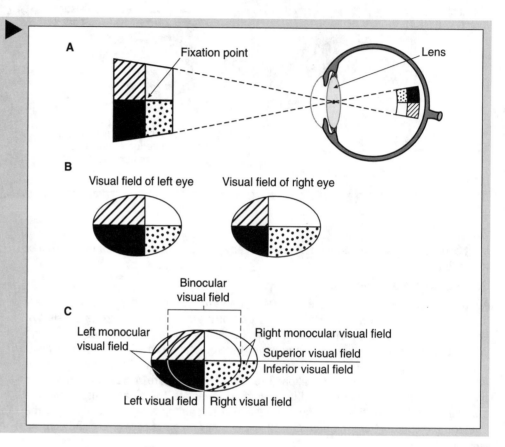

The nasal retina is more extensive than the temporal retina.

Both eyes are usually aimed at the same fixation point, and consequently, most of their visual fields have substantial overlap. The overlapping region is called the binocular visual field because every point in this area is seen by both eyes; the nonoverlapping regions are called monocular visual fields because they are seen only by one eye (Figure 10-24). The monocular visual fields are crescent-shaped areas that surround the peripheral edge of each side of the binocular visual field and are seen only by the extreme medial portion of the ipsilateral nasal retina. You can demonstrate to yourself the existence of monocular visual fields by rapidly closing and opening each eye in an alternating sequence. As your field of view switches from one eye to the other, you should notice that objects in the extreme lateral part of one eye's visual field (viewed by the nasal retina) are not seen by the other eye, in part, because the latter view is blocked by the nose. In fact, the temporal retina is less extensive than the nasal retina and contributes only 40% of the fibers that comprise the optic nerve; the other 60% of the fibers originate from the nasal retina.

Each cortical hemisphere receives visual information from the contralateral visual field only. While axons originating from the nasal half of each retina decussate in the optic chiasm, those fibers coming from the temporal half remain ipsilateral (see Figure 10-24B). Hence, the optic nerve contains fibers representing both sides of the visual field, but the optic tract and more posterior structures represent only the contralateral visual field. Thus, the purpose of the optic chiasm is analogous to the internal arcuate fibers (in the somatosensory system) or to the pyramidal decussation (in the motor

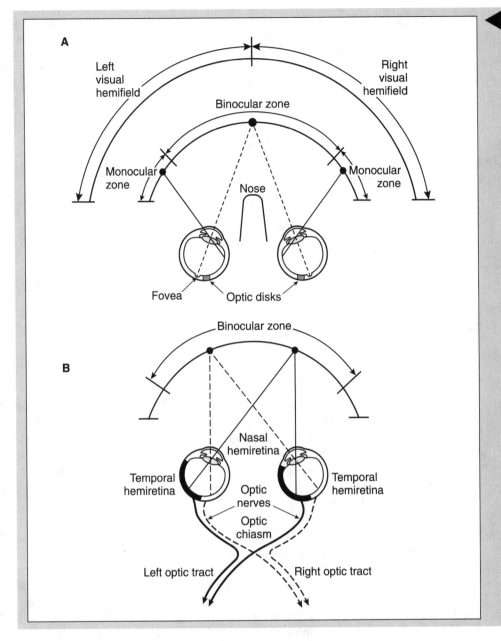

◀ **FIGURE 10-24**
Visual Field Projections onto the Retina.
(A) Different parts of the visual field are shown relative to the fixation point. The binocular visual field is seen by both eyes; monocular visual fields are seen only by the extreme medial portion of the nasal retina. (B) Each point in the binocular visual field projects onto a corresponding point in the temporal and nasal retina of both eyes. The partial decussation in the optic chiasm allows information from each side of the visual field to be sent only to the contralateral hemisphere.

system): all of these tracts allow information concerned with one side of the body to be processed by the opposite side of the brain.

Topography of the Visual Pathways

The visual system uses orderly retinotopic projections to construct precise maps of the visual world in the lateral geniculate nucleus and the primary visual cortex. Thus, neighboring ganglion cells in the retina project to neighboring neurons in the lateral geniculate nucleus, which in turn project to neighboring neurons in the striate cortex. These orderly projections indicate that the visual system relies on the spatial location of neural activity to code the position of objects in the visual field.

Visual field defects are highly correlated with the location of damage in the visual system, and for this reason, it is important for physicians to understand certain features of the retinotopic projection system. The macular part of the retina, which represents the central 5 degrees of the visual field, is represented in the posterior half of the lateral geniculate nucleus and in the posterior half of the striate cortex. The superior half of the retina projects to the medial half of the lateral geniculate nucleus, which in turn projects

The lateral geniculate nucleus and striate cortex contain retinotopic maps of the contralateral visual field.

through the optic radiations en route to the superior bank of the calcarine sulcus. By comparison, the inferior half of the retina projects to the lateral half of the lateral geniculate nucleus, which in turn projects anterolaterally into the temporal lobe to form Meyer's loop, before coursing posteriorly to terminate in the lower bank of the calcarine sulcus (see Figure 10-22). Due to these projection patterns, the superior visual field is represented in the lower bank of the calcarine sulcus, whereas the lower visual field is represented in the upper bank (Figure 10-25).

FIGURE 10-25 ▶

Primary Visual Cortex. This diagram shows how one-half of the visual field is mapped onto the primary visual cortex of the contralateral hemisphere.

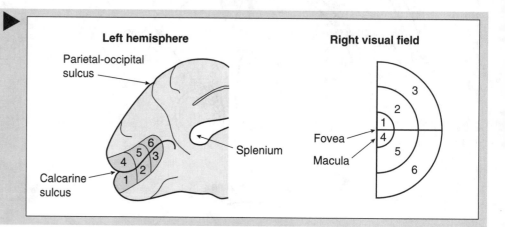

Although the visual system is retinotopically organized, the visual maps in the lateral geniculate nucleus and the striate cortex are highly distorted. Nearly half of the neurons in both regions respond to macular stimulation even though the macula represents only a small fraction of the total visual field. The distorted representation of the central visual area reflects the high density of ganglion cells in the macula and the fact that cones, which have a one-to-one synaptic relationship with the axons of the optic nerve, provide a disproportionate share of visual input to the brain.

Visual Field Deficits

It is not uncommon for patients suffering from a cerebral vascular accident (or stroke) to experience loss of vision, or anopsia, in part of the visual field. One consequence of the visual system's retinotopic organization is that limited damage in one part of this system produces a specific visual field deficit. After carefully mapping the visual field of each eye and noting where vision is impaired, knowledge of the retinotopic organization of the visual system should enable a physician to deduce the precise location of a CNS lesion.

Visual field defects provide important clues about the location of lesions in the CNS.

The relationship between lesions in the visual system and specific visual field deficits is illustrated in Figure 10-26. As indicated, damage to one retina or to one optic nerve only affects vision for the corresponding eye. Lesions affecting more posterior parts of the visual system, however, involve the visual fields of both eyes. When the crossing fibers of the optic chiasm are damaged, the visual field deficit is called heteronymous because the visual loss occurs in nonoverlapping parts of the visual fields of both eyes. Tumors of the pituitary gland that compress decussating fibers in the optic chiasm produce heteronymous bitemporal hemianopsia.

Damage to the visual system at sites posterior to the optic chiasm always affects the same part of the visual field in each eye, and such visual field deficits are said to be homonymous. A complete lesion of the right optic tract, for example, produces left homonymous hemianopsia. More caudal lesions are less likely to produce complete hemianopsia, however, because the optic radiations occupy an extensive region that is unlikely to be completely destroyed by a single lesion. Damage to Meyer's loop on the right side produces a quadrantic anopsia in the left superior visual field without affecting vision in the inferior quadrant. Finally, a stroke in the upper or lower cortical bank of the calcarine sulcus may produce a quadrantic anopsia with macular sparing. Although the basis for macular sparing is uncertain, anastomoses between the middle cerebral artery

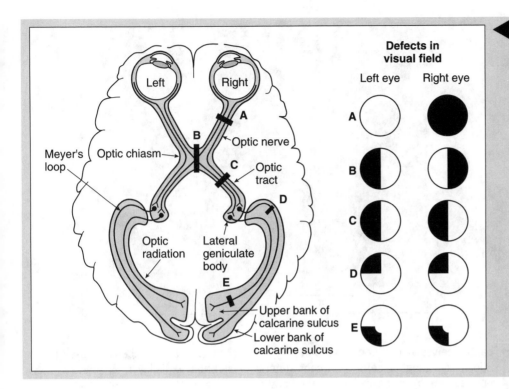

FIGURE 10-26
Visual Field Deficits. Lesions in the visual system are correlated with specific visual field deficits. *(A) Blindness in the right eye. (B) Bitemporal heteronymous hemianopsia. (C) Left homonymous hemianopsia. (D) Superior quadrantic anopia. (E) Inferior quadrantic anopsia with macular sparing.*

and the posterior cerebral artery may permit the flow of blood to the occipital pole following a stroke in the posterior cerebral artery.

RELATIVE AFFERENT PUPILLARY DEFECT

The results of testing a patient's visual fields should always be used in conjunction with other tests to determine the likely location of a lesion in the visual system. If a partial lesion of the optic nerve is suspected, the swinging light test can be used to compare pupillary light reflexes elicited from each eye. In this test, a bright flashlight is swung from one eye to the other while the patient stares ahead in a dimly lit room. Dysfunction in one optic nerve usually causes the affected eye to respond more slowly or less completely than the normal eye. In left optic neuritis, for example, both pupils constrict equally when the right eye is illuminated. When the light is moved to the left eye, however, the speed and amplitude of the left pupil response are decreased relative to the response of the right eye. A partial optic nerve lesion may also cause the affected eye to constrict only transiently during sustained illumination. The clinical value of the swinging light test relies on the fact that the speed and amplitude of the pupillary reflex are proportional to the number of intact fibers in the optic nerve.

A relative pupillary defect may also occur if the optic tract has a lesion or is compressed by a tumor. Even though the optic tract contains fibers from both eyes, a slower pupillary reflex is more likely to be elicited when light is shone into the eye with temporal hemianopsia because fibers from the nasal retina, which is more extensive than the temporal retina, have been damaged. The eye located ipsilateral to the optic tract lesion has nasal hemianopsia, but since at least 60% of its nerve fibers are intact, it can mediate a quicker pupillary light reflex.

Lateral Geniculate Nucleus

The lateral geniculate nucleus is a small, laminated structure in the caudal thalamus that relays information from the retina to the striate cortex. As shown in Figure 10-27, the lateral geniculate nucleus contains six layers that vary in neuronal composition. The most ventral layers are called magnocellular layers 1 and 2 because they are composed of large multipolar neurons with large dendritic fields. More dorsally, layers 3 through 6 are called parvocellular layers because they contain much smaller neurons.

Each layer of the lateral geniculate nucleus represents the contralateral visual field

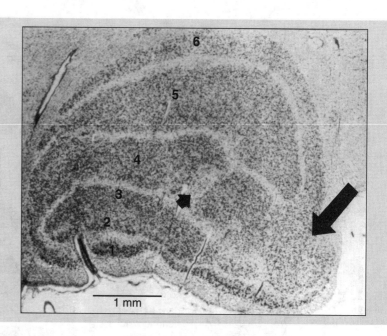

FIGURE 10-27 ▶

Lateral Geniculate Nucleus. A coronal section illustrates the six layers of the lateral geniculate nucleus. Layers 1 and 2 are the magnocellular layers; layers 3, 4, 5, and 6 are the parvocellular layers. The small arrow indicates the representation of the blind spot in layer 4; the large arrow indicates where layers 4 and 6 have merged together to represent the monocular segment. (Source: Reprinted with permission from Hickey TL, et al: Variability of laminar patterns in the human lateral geniculate nucleus. Comp Neurol 183:221–246, 1979.)

1 mm

Layers 2 and 3, which are the same as 5, receive inputs from the contralateral eye on the same (ipsilateral) side.

and receives visual input from only one eye. Layers 1, 4, and 6 receive crossed projections from ganglion cells in the contralateral nasal retina, while layers 2, 3, and 5 receive projections from the ipsilateral temporal retina. This pattern of retinal projections explains two morphologic features of the lateral geniculate nucleus (see Figure 10-27). First, the monocular visual field is represented within layers 1, 4, and 6 at the bilaminar segment; layers 2, 3, and 5 are absent because no part of the temporal retina views this part of the visual field. Second, a cell-sparse region appears in layers 4 and 6, but not in layers 3 and 5, because this area corresponds to the blind spot located in the nasal retina. Lateral geniculate neurons in the blind spot representation disappear during embryologic development because they never receive functional inputs from the contralateral retina.

Each layer of the lateral geniculate nucleus receives retinotopic projections so that the contralateral visual field is represented six times along its dorsal–ventral extent. Neurons located directly above or below each other in different layers of the lateral geniculate nucleus represent the same point in the visual field even though they receive projections from different eyes. The receptive fields of neurons in the lateral geniculate nucleus, like those of the retinal ganglion cells, have concentric center–surround receptive fields with "on" and "off" antagonistic regions.

MAGNOCELLULAR AND PARVOCELLULAR COMPARISONS

Although their receptive field organizations are similar, neurons in the parvocellular and magnocellular layers differ in several important respects. Parvocellular neurons tend to have smaller receptive fields and are color sensitive, whereas magnocellular neurons have larger receptive fields and respond equally to all colors. Magnocellular neurons display transient responses to a flash of light; parvocellular neurons, by comparison, exhibit sustained responses. These functional differences are directly related to the types of retinal ganglion cells that project to the magnocellular and parvocellular layers.

Structural and functional criteria have been used to classify retinal ganglion cells into two different subtypes (Table 10-2). Retinal ganglion cells that project to the magnocellular layers of the lateral geniculate nucleus are called M cells; those that project to the parvocellular layers are called P cells. The M cells have large cell bodies and large dendritic fields that integrate visual information from a wider expanse of the retina; P cells are smaller and respond only to a tiny part of the retina. The P ganglion cells tend to be concentrated near the fovea, whereas the M ganglion cells are scattered throughout the retina. Finally, the terminal arborizations of the P ganglion cells are smaller and more densely packed than those of the M ganglion cells.

The functions of the M and P cell types have been studied by analyzing the effects of focal lesions in the lateral geniculate nucleus. Lesions restricted to the parvocellular layers impair color vision and reduce visual acuity. Removal of the magnocellular layers,

M Ganglion Cells	P Ganglion Cells
Large receptive fields	Small receptive fields
Large dendritic arbors	Small dendritic arbors
Large soma	Small soma
Magnocellular projections	Parvocellular projections
Broad terminal arbors	Narrow terminal arbors
Layers 1 and 2 of the lateral geniculate	Layers 3, 4, 5, and 6 of the lateral geniculate
Involved in motion processing	Involved in visual acuity
Scattered throughout the retina	Concentrated in the fovea
Brief, transient responses	Sustained responses
Insensitive to color	Color sensitive

however, does not affect color vision or visual acuity but interferes with motion perception. These results suggest that the parvocellular layers are critical for detailed visual discrimination, whereas the magnocellular layers detect and analyze moving objects.

Visual Cortex

One of the most striking aspects of the brain is the enormous amount of cortex that is devoted to visual functions. The visual cortex includes all of the occipital lobe and a substantial portion of the temporal and parietal lobes (Figure 10-28). The cerebral cortex contains at least 25 distinct regions that are concerned exclusively with visual function and another six areas that play a limited role in visual processing.

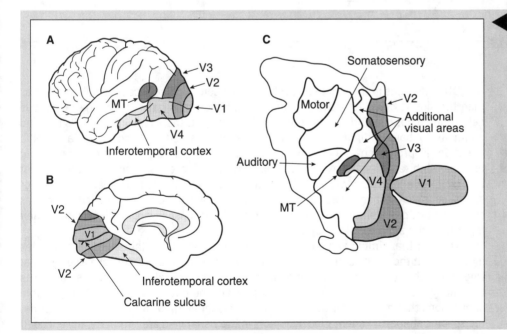

FIGURE 10-28
Visual Cortex. (A) Lateral view of cerebral hemisphere showing the location of the striate cortex (V1) and other major visual areas including V2, V3, and V4. (B) Medial view. (C) A flattened view of the cortex, which reveals the area devoted to motor and sensory functions. More than 25 distinct regions in the visual cortex occupy approximately 40% of the total cortical area. MT = medial temporal area.

STRIATE CORTEX

The striate cortex is called the primary visual cortex (V1) because it is the primary target of the lateral geniculate nucleus. The striate cortex occupies both banks of the calcarine sulcus and contains a complete topographical map of the contralateral visual field.

Unlike neurons in the retina or the lateral geniculate nucleus, neurons in the striate cortex do not respond to circular spots of light. In the 1960s, David Hubel and Torsten Wiesel showed that striate cortical neurons respond to rectangular stimuli that have a light–dark edge. Responses of striate neurons vary as a function of the orientation of

Neurons in the striate cortex detect specific features in the visual world.

the stimulus so that each neuron has a preferred orientation (Figure 10-29). Striate cortical neurons that respond to stationary bars of light at a preferred orientation are called simple cells. Simple cell response properties are a product of convergent inputs from lateral geniculate neurons whose circular receptive fields occupy adjacent, linear parts of the visual field. The dependence of simple cells on convergent inputs from the lateral geniculate nucleus is evident from the fact that simple cells tend to reside near layer IV, which receives the geniculocortical projections.

Simple cells detect specific orientations.

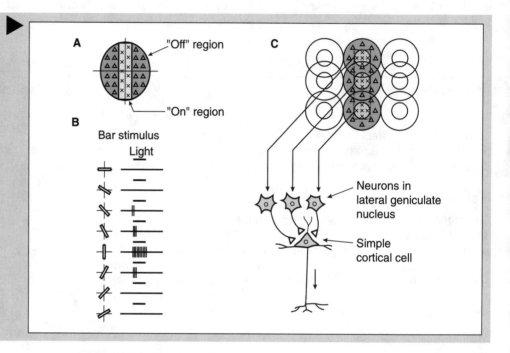

FIGURE 10-29
Simple Cell Receptive Fields. *(A) Simple cells in the striate cortex have rectangular receptive fields with excitatory (on) and inhibitory (off) regions. (B) Simple cells are orientation sensitive. (C) The rectangular receptive field of a simple cell results from convergent inputs from lateral geniculate neurons with aligned receptive fields.*

Other neurons in the striate cortex have more complicated receptive field properties than the simple cells. Neurons classified as complex cells have much larger receptive fields and do not respond well to stationary bars of light. Instead, complex cells respond optimally to bars of light that are appropriately oriented and moving in a specific direction. Neurons known as hypercomplex cells also have a preferred orientation but become inhibited if the bar exceeds a specific length. These response properties suggest that complex and hypercomplex cells receive convergent inputs from specific classes of simple cells that respond to adjacent parts of the visual field. Complex and hypercomplex cells are most prevalent in layers II, III, V, and VI, and these layers receive much of their input from the simple cells located near layer IV.

Complex cells are orientation and direction selective.

The fact that simple and complex cells respond only to certain stimulus attributes indicates that the striate cortex is organized to detect particular aspects of a visual scene. One reason the striate cortex is several times larger than the lateral geniculate nucleus is that many more neurons are required to construct the circuits that detect all possible orientations that may appear in any part of the visual field. With these built-in circuits, the specific shape and orientation of objects in the visual field are automatically encoded by the activity in specific populations of striate neurons.

Columnar Organization of the Striate Cortex. The striate cortex is organized into repeating modules or columns of cells that respond to particular stimulus features in one part of the visual field. The columnar organization of the striate cortex was discovered by comparing the response properties of neurons that were successively encountered during electrode penetrations in this region (Figure 10-30). If the electrode traveled orthogonal to the cortical surface, the electrode encountered neurons with similar receptive fields and orientation preferences. If the electrode traveled parallel to the cortical surface, the orientation preferences gradually shifted until, after approximately 800 μm, a complete range of orientations was encountered.

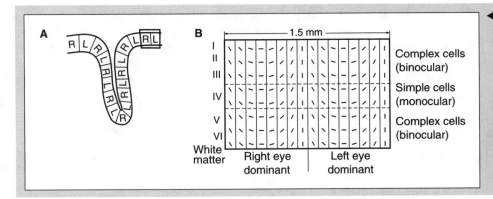

► **FIGURE 10-30**
Columnar Organization. *(A) Diagram of the striate cortex with an inset of two adjacent ocular dominance columns. (B) Each ocular dominance column contains a series of smaller orientation columns arranged systematically to represent orientations spanning 180 degrees. Simple cells respond to one eye and reside near layer IV. Complex cells may respond to both eyes and usually reside above and below layer IV. R = right; L = left.*

Each neuron in layer IV of the striate cortex responds entirely to photic stimulation of one eye or the other but not to both eyes (see Figure 10-30). Left and right eye dominance occurs in alternating bands of neurons 800 μm wide called ocular dominance columns. Neurons located above and below layer IV may respond to both eyes but tend to be more responsive to the eye that activates the neurons in layer IV. Hence, the ocular dominance of these neurons indicates the presence of a columnar organization in the striate cortex. The basis for ocular dominance columns is determined exclusively by the projection pattern from the lateral geniculate nucleus. Each 800 μm–wide band in layer IV receives its visual information either from layers 2, 3, and 5 (representing the ipsilateral eye) or from layers 1, 4, and 6 (representing the contralateral eye) of the lateral geniculate nucleus.

Electrophysiologic studies have shown that orientation and ocular dominance columns are superimposed on one another in the striate cortex. Each ocular dominance column (800 μm) contains an orderly representation of all possible orientation preferences. Thus, within two adjacent ocular dominance columns, all possible orientations are represented twice, once for each eye. Other stimulus attributes such as color sensitivity, motion sensitivity, and spatial frequency are also organized into columns or modules that repeat at regular intervals throughout the striate cortex. Neurons sensitive to color, for example, are clustered into segregated regions called "blobs" that contain high concentrations of cytochrome oxidase.

Stereopsis. Neurons located above or below layer IV of the striate cortex may respond to visual inputs from both eyes. For some of these neurons, the information received from each eye represents adjacent parts of the visual field, and the binocular responses of these neurons are used for coding depth perception. Stereopsis, or vision with two eyes, is critical for depth perception because objects outside the plane of fixation evoke images with some degree of retinal disparity (Figure 10-31). To understand how retinal disparity contributes to depth perception, use only one eye to look at the tip of your finger as you position it in front of an object located a few yards away. As you continue to fixate on your fingertip, open the other eye and you will notice that you perceive two images of the distant object. Fortunately, your visual system interprets the doubled image as an indication of depth and does not conclude that the object magically replicated itself!

Although the neuronal circuits that mediate stereopsis are not entirely understood, it is well established that binocular responses in the striate cortex depend on normal inputs from both eyes during early postnatal development. Binocular responses do not develop if the cortex is deprived of images from one eye because of uncorrected refractive errors, if the lens is cloudy (congenital cataract), or if images from both eyes cannot be fused because the extraocular muscles fail to align the eyes properly (amblyopia or "lazy eye"). If binocular responses do not develop, retinal disparity is an ineffective cue for depth perception, and this may impair performance in certain visual-motor tasks. Therefore, children should be screened for visual problems at an early age so that corrective actions can be taken as soon as possible.

EXTRASTRIATE CORTEX

Anatomic, physiologic, and behavioral studies have identified numerous cortical areas around the striate cortex that process visual information. Those areas located close to V1

> *Binocular vision leads to retinal disparity, an important cue for depth perception.*

are named according to their functional proximity to the striate cortex (i.e., V2, V3, or V4); other extrastriate visual areas are named according to their anatomic location (e.g., middle temporal cortex). Extrastriate cortex includes all of the occipital lobe that lies outside of Brodmann area 17 as well the posterior part of the parietal lobe and the ventral part of the temporal lobe. The striate cortex communicates with these regions by means of short corticocortical association fibers.

FIGURE 10-31 ▶

Retinal Disparity. Binocular vision results in retinal disparity for objects that lie outside the plane of fixation. In this illustration, two objects are aligned so that their images fall on the fovea of the right eye. The images fall on different parts of the left retina because the background object is located further away.

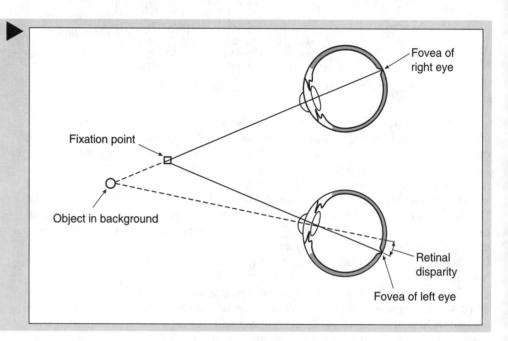

Processing Streams. Stimulus features such as form, color, and motion are analyzed by separate areas within the extrastriate cortex. These areas are organized into processing streams in which information is passed sequentially from one cortical area to the next by a series of corticocortical connections. There are at least two major processing streams in the extrastriate cortex and both originate in the magnocellular and parvocellular layers of the lateral geniculate nucleus (Figure 10-32). The parvocellular and magnocellular layers of the lateral geniculate nucleus project to distinct subdivisions of layer IV in the striate cortex, which in turn project to separate parts of the V2 cortex. The magnocellular and parvocellular regions of V2 form the origin of two separate and divergent processing streams that extend across the remaining extrastriate cortical areas.

FIGURE 10-32 ▶

Visual Processing Streams. (A) Lateral view of the brain showing the location of visual processing streams for object recognition and motion perception. (B) Information from the parvocellular and magnocellular layers of the lateral geniculate nucleus is sent through a hierarchical network of cortical areas. Although separate pathways may process specific attributes of a stimulus, lateral connections (reciprocal arrows) may unify different stimulus features into a single percept. MT = medial temporal area.

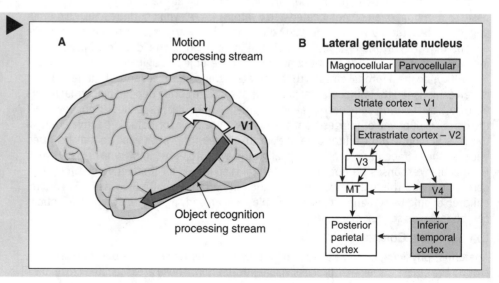

The processing stream derived from the parvocellular layers of the lateral geniculate nucleus receives high-resolution information from the macula and is concerned with form perception and object recognition. Regions in V1 and V2 that analyze form and pattern information project to parts of the extrastriate cortex such as area V4 and the inferior part of the temporal lobe. By comparison, the processing stream derived from the magnocellular pathway analyzes the motion and spatial relationships of objects in the visual field. The magnocellular pathway receives most of its visual input from the retina surrounding the macula. The parts of V1 and V2 that analyze motion and spatial position project to medial parts of the extrastriate cortex, including V3, the medial temporal (MT) area, and the posterior part of the parietal lobe. Some evidence suggests the presence of another processing stream for analyzing color information, but this pathway is largely a subset of the parvocellular processing stream.

Parvocellular Stream
Form and pattern perception

Magnocellular Stream
Analysis of moving stimuli

The segregation of visual functions into distinct anatomic pathways is reflected by the specificity of symptoms resulting from focal lesions in the extrastriate cortex. Patients that sustain damage to area MT, for example, cannot interpret moving objects in a meaningful way. Patients having this disorder, called akinetopsia, recognize objects at rest but report that rapidly moving objects seem to appear suddenly at one position and then at another. Other patients with selective damage to the extrastriate cortex are unable to perceive color even though their cones function normally. These achromatopsic individuals recognize objects and perceive motion, but their visual world is composed entirely of shades of gray.

There is strong evidence for divergent processing streams in the extrastriate cortex, but it is not clear how segregated pathways might bind different parts of a visual stimulus into a single percept. For example, when we see a red car moving along the highway, our visual system automatically links the separate features of this stimulus (i.e., "movement," "red," "car") to form a unified perception. Lateral connections between regions at the same level (e.g., V4, MT) of the processing streams might provide an anatomic substrate for unifying the various stimulus attributes into a single perception (see Figure 10-32). Recent evidence suggests that these lateral connections are responsible for synchronizing neuronal discharges in the connected regions. Thus, when separate visual features of the same object are analyzed independently by separate cortical areas, synchronous discharges in both regions may provide a perceptual mechanism for binding these stimulus features together.

Lateral connections between the processing streams unify separate features into the perception of a single stimulus.

OCULOMOTOR MECHANISMS

To acquire a vivid spatial representation of the world, the visual system constantly directs the motor system to move the eyes so that points of visual interest are fixated by the fovea. Thus, signals received from the visual system are used by different structures in the motor system to control the direction and amplitude of eye movements precisely.

Saccadic Eye Movements

We acquire most visual information by making a series of brief, ballistic eye movements that are known as saccades. We emit high rates of saccadic eye movements but are unaware of these movements because the visual system uses only information acquired during the fixation periods to create a stable representation of the world. Otherwise, the external world would appear to be moving around us because the visual fields are constantly changing with each successive eye movement.

Saccadic eye movements have two motor components: an initial pulse phase followed by a tonic step phase. The pulse phase, which represents the actual ballistic movement of the eyes, is initiated by a burst of activity in the extraocular motor nuclei. The velocity and amplitude of the pulse phase are determined by the number of active motor neurons and their firing rates. Once the pulse phase has been completed, the eyes remain fixated on a target during the step phase because the extraocular muscles are tonically active. The exact position of the eyes during the step phase is determined by the rate of activity in the neurons innervating each pair of extraocular muscles.

Neural Control of Saccadic Eye Movements

The frontal eye fields and the superior colliculus are responsible for issuing the motor commands that initiate saccadic eye movements. Both of these brain regions receive afferent signals from the visual system and send descending projections to the brainstem nuclei that control horizontal and vertical eye movements (Figure 10-33).

FIGURE 10-33 ▶

Oculomotor Pathways. Lateral and medial views of the brain depicting the location of the oculomotor structures and their interconnections that mediate saccadic eye movements. RiMLF = rostral interstitial nucleus of the medial longitudinal fasciculus; INC = interstitial nucleus of Cajal; SC = superior colliculus; PPRF = paramedian pontine reticular formation. III, IV, and VI = cranial nerve nuclei.

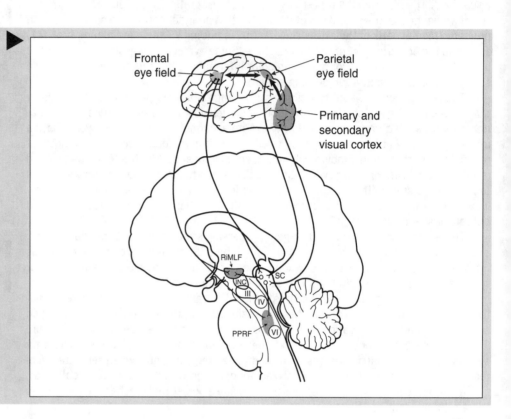

HORIZONTAL AND VERTICAL GAZE CENTERS

A saccadic eye movement in any direction is composed of a movement vector in the horizontal direction and a movement vector in the vertical direction. Rather than relying on a single brain region to calculate the muscle contractions needed for a particular saccade, the brainstem contains two separate nuclear regions, known as gaze centers, that independently calculate the motor output needed to produce movement vectors in the vertical or horizontal directions. Thus, all saccadic eye movements represent the combined output of activity from the horizontal and vertical gaze centers.

Horizontal gaze movements are controlled by the paramedian pontine reticular formation (PPRF). The PPRF is an elongated region within the rostral and caudal pontine reticular formation, which lies adjacent to the midline. The PPRF sends excitatory projections to the ipsilateral abducens nucleus and inhibitory projections to the contralateral abducens nucleus. The abducens nuclei innervate the lateral rectus muscle of the ipsilateral eye and send crossed projections to the part of the oculomotor complex that controls the medial rectus muscle of the contralateral eye. Hence, the PPRF on each side coordinates the contractions of the lateral rectus and medial rectus muscles of both eyes to execute conjugate horizontal eye movements.

Vertical saccades are controlled by two regions located in the rostral part of the midbrain. The rostral interstitial nucleus of the medial longitudinal fasciculus (RiMLF) controls the pulse phase of vertical saccades, while a nearby region, the interstitial nucleus of Cajal, controls the step phase. Both of these midbrain nuclei project bilaterally to the oculomotor complex, which executes vertical eye movements by activating the superior and inferior rectus muscles.

SUPERIOR COLLICULUS

The superior colliculus is a laminated structure that receives direct projections from certain types of retinal ganglion cells, especially M cells, which respond to stimuli moving in the peripheral part of the visual field. Thus, one function of the superior colliculus is to re-orient visual attention by sending commands to the motor system so that the eyes track specific targets moving through the visual field.

The upper layer of the superior colliculus receives topographical projections from both the retina and the ipsilateral striate cortex. These afferent projections form a detailed map of the contralateral visual field, and each site in this map represents a potential target for visual fixation. Thus, electrical stimulation of one point in the superior colliculus elicits saccadic eye movements to the corresponding part of the contralateral visual field. Physiologic recordings have also shown that saccadic eye movements to a visual target are preceded by increased neuronal activity at the corresponding site in the superior colliculus.

The deeper layers of the superior colliculus receive visual inputs from the upper layers of the superior colliculus, as well as auditory inputs from the inferior colliculus and somatosensory inputs from the nucleus gracilis and nucleus cuneatus. Hence, the superior colliculus plays a key role in visual fixation by using a variety of sensory modalities to guide eye and head movements to external stimuli.

Projections from the deep layers of the superior colliculus are used to initiate saccadic eye movements and maintain tracking movements of the eyes and head on a moving stimulus. The ventral part of the superior colliculus contains a precise motor map that specifies the direction of eye movements to any point in the contralateral visual field. The ocular motor responses are mediated by ipsilateral tectofugal projections to the nucleus RiMLF, the interstitial nucleus of Cajal, and the PPRF. In addition, the superior colliculus sends descending projections to the spinal cord (tectospinal tract) to control head and neck movements.

Reflexive eye movements to objects moving in the peripheral part of the visual field are mediated by the superior colliculus.

FRONTAL EYE FIELDS

Each frontal lobe contains a small area that mediates voluntary and memory-guided eye movements to sites in the ipsilateral visual field. Known as Brodmann area 8, the frontal eye fields are located in the posterior part of the middle frontal gyrus and, like other parts of the motor system, receive functional projections from the cerebellum and basal ganglia. The frontal eye fields also receive massive projections from the extrastriate cortex via the superior longitudinal fasciculus. This visual information is used by the frontal eye fields to direct the eyes toward those parts of the visual field that have visual interest.

Voluntary eye movements are mediated by the frontal eye fields.

Efferent projections from the frontal eye fields descend through the internal capsule and crus cerebri to terminate in the ipsilateral superior colliculus, RiMLF, and interstitial nucleus of Cajal. Additional fibers proceed further caudally and decussate in the rostral pons to terminate in the PPRF. Consistent with these projections, unilateral activation of the frontal eye field produces saccadic eye movements to the contralateral visual field. A unilateral lesion of the frontal eye fields may briefly impair saccadic eye movements in the ipsilateral direction, but it does not produce permanent deficits because the superior colliculus and frontal eye fields provide redundant control of the extraocular eye muscles.

RESOLUTION OF CLINICAL CASE

The clinical case in this chapter illustrates signs of pituitary adenoma. Most tumors of the pituitary gland are benign, and pituitary adenomas may go undetected if they are asymptomatic. Pituitary adenomas are classified as secretory or nonsecretory. Secretory tumors, which are less common, release anterior pituitary hormones such as prolactin, growth hormone, adrenocorticotropic hormone, follicle-stimulating hormone, or luteinizing hormone. Nonsecretory tumors may cause headaches or produce visual field deficits if the tumor extends superiorly and compresses the fibers of the optic chiasm. Due to the retinotopic arrangement of the optic chiasm, visual loss initially occurs in the superior temporal quadrants and then spreads into the inferior temporal quadrants. Although bitemporal hemianopsia is a classic sign of pituitary adenoma, any pattern of visual loss can occur, including unilateral or homonymous hemianopsia, because the tumor may grow asymmetrically and affect one side of the optic chiasm. Pituitary tumors may also invade the cavernous sinus and compromise the third, fourth, or sixth cranial nerves to produce diplopia. The best diagnostic procedure for evaluating pituitary adenoma is a MRI scan because it provides an image of soft tissue without interference from the surrounding bone. Pituitary adenomas can be surgically excised, and the mortality rate for this procedure is less than 1%. This patient's vision was restored after successful transsphenoidal pituitary surgery.

REVIEW QUESTIONS

Directions: For each of the following questions, choose the **one best** answer.

1. Which of the following structures participates in the accommodation–convergence reflex?
   - **(A)** Edinger-Westphal nucleus
   - **(B)** Pigment epithelium
   - **(C)** Pupillary dilator
   - **(D)** Superior colliculus
   - **(E)** Lateral rectus muscles

2. Which condition is least likely to be detected by ophthalmoscopic examination?
   - **(A)** Diabetic retinopathy
   - **(B)** Bitemporal hemianopsia
   - **(C)** Papilledema
   - **(D)** Hypertension
   - **(E)** An increase in intracranial pressure

3. Which of the following conditions would produce a bitemporal visual field deficit?
   - **(A)** Occlusion of the posterior cerebral artery
   - **(B)** An increase in intracranial pressure
   - **(C)** Compression of the optic chiasm by a pituitary adenoma
   - **(D)** Compression of the oculomotor nerve by an aneurysm of the superior cerebellar artery
   - **(E)** Transection of one optic nerve

4. Retinal disparity is important for which of the following visual functions?
   - **(A)** Color vision
   - **(B)** Visual acuity
   - **(C)** Motion detection
   - **(D)** Depth perception
   - **(E)** Saccadic eye movements

5. What ocular function would be impaired by a retinal detachment?
   - **(A)** Phototransduction
   - **(B)** Pupillary constriction
   - **(C)** Accommodation of the lens
   - **(D)** Conjugate eye movements
   - **(E)** Blood flow through the central retinal artery

6. A patient has a left homonymous superior quadrantic anopsia without macular sparing. Which of the following structures is most likely to be damaged?
   - **(A)** Right lateral geniculate nucleus
   - **(B)** Left optic tract
   - **(C)** Optic radiations in Meyer's loop on the right side
   - **(D)** Optic radiations in Meyer's loop on the left side
   - **(E)** Striate cortex in the lower bank of the right calcarine sulcus

ANSWERS AND EXPLANATIONS

1. The answer is A. Accommodation of the lens is mediated by projections from the Edinger-Westphal nucleus to the ciliary ganglion, which in turn innervates the ciliary body and the pupillary sphincter muscle. Convergence is mediated by contraction of the medial rectus muscles, not the lateral rectus muscles.

2. The answer is B. Bitemporal hemianopsia is a visual field deficit that is caused by a lesion in the optic chiasm, and it is not evident from an ophthalmoscopic examination. Papilledema, or swelling of the optic disk, can be determined by a funduscopic examination and is almost always produced by an increase in intracranial pressure. Diabetic retinopathy and hypertension produce noticeable changes in the appearance of blood vessels of the retina.

3. The answer is C. A bitemporal visual field deficit is a classic finding with a pituitary adenoma. Compression of the nerve fibers coursing through the optic chiasm is likely to affect noncorresponding (heteronymous) parts of the visual fields of both eyes. When more posterior structures in the visual system are affected, such as the striate cortex, the visual field deficit is always homonymous. Transection of one optic nerve would affect the visual field of only one eye. Increased intracranial pressure or altered function of the oculomotor nerve do not cause visual field deficits.

4. The answer is D. Retinal disparity is an inherent property of binocular vision that provides cues for depth perception. Color vision, visual acuity, motion detection, and saccadic eye movements do not depend on binocular vision.

5. The answer is A. A retinal detachment widens the distance between the photoreceptors and the pigment epithelium and, consequently, interferes with phagocytosis of membranes sloughed off from the photoreceptor's outer segments. The photoreceptors would begin to deteriorate, and phototransduction would soon be impaired. The remaining ocular functions would not be affected by a retinal detachment.

6. The answer is C. Loss of the left visual field in both eyes indicates a lesion in the right hemisphere posterior to the optic chiasm. Quadrantic anopsias usually result from partial damage to the optic radiations or their terminals in the striate cortex. Loss of the superior visual field indicates an injury to Meyer's loop or to the lower bank of the calcarine sulcus, but since the macula was not spared, damage to Meyer's loop is more likely.

ADDITIONAL READING

Behrens MM: Impaired vision. In *Merritt's Textbook of Neurology*, 9th ed. Edited by Rowland LP. Baltimore, MD: Williams & Wilkins, 1995, pp 35–42.

Felleman DJ, Van Essen DC: Distributed hierarchical processing in primate cerebral cortex. *Cerebral Cortex* 1:1–47, 1991.

Hart WMJ: *Adler's Physiology of the Eye: Clinical Application*, 9th ed. St. Louis, MO: Mosby Year Book, 1992.

Hubel DH: *Eye, Brain and Vision*. New York, NY: W. H. Freeman, 1988.

Koretz JF, Handelman GH: How the human eye focuses. *Sci Am* 259:92–99, 1988.

Sterling P: Retina. In *The Synaptic Organization of the Brain*. Edited by Shepard GM. New York, NY: Oxford University Press, 1990, pp 170–213.

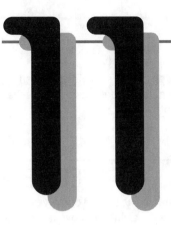

MOTOR SYSTEM

CHAPTER OUTLINE

INTRODUCTION OF CLINICAL CASE

B. T., a 40-year-old man with a litany of seemingly unrelated symptoms, scheduled an appointment with his physician at the behest of his wife. B. T. and his wife both agreed that he had not been himself lately. Nervous and jittery most of the time, B. T. had developed multiple tics and jerky involuntary movements of the arms. He also noted that his piano playing had deteriorated recently. Perhaps coincidentally, B. T.'s father had developed similar motor problems when he was about 50 years old, but he died in an automobile accident before seeing a physician. B. T. dismissed his wife's concerns that business woes were pushing him toward a nervous breakdown, but it was true that he had been depressed recently. Although he tried, B. T. was unable to provide a rational explanation for why he had been polishing the tines of an old pitchfork in the garage last week. There were two noteworthy observations during the neurological examination. Muscle tone and strength appeared normal, but the patient was unable to sustain a tight handgrip. In addition, it was difficult for B. T. to track the physician's moving pen visually unless it moved very slowly. The physician prescribed a mild antidepressant and asked that B. T. undergo genetic testing before his next appointment.

OVERVIEW

Movement is a fundamental activity. The motor system enables us to feed ourselves, fight and flee our adversaries, reproduce, work, and play. When the ability to move is lost, the effect can be catastrophic. Paralysis in the advanced stages of amyotrophic lateral sclerosis (ALS or Lou Gehrig's disease) is so profound that patients are described as "locked-in" because the only voluntary movement they retain is the ability to move their eyes.

The central organization of the motor system is deceptively complex. Motor control is distributed across the spinal, brainstem, cerebellar, subcortical, and cortical levels of the nervous system. The spinal cord and brainstem contain the motor neurons that constitute the final common pathway for motor execution. Subcortical and cerebellar areas initiate movement as well as refine the temporal and spatial precision. Volitional control of movement is vested in the cerebral cortex. This multitiered system is tightly interwoven with the visual, auditory, and somatosensory systems, which provide the spatial and temporal contexts within which movement takes place.

Previous chapters have discussed control of the extraocular eye muscles as well as the roles of the spinal cord and brainstem in movement and visceromotor and somatomotor reflexes. This chapter discusses cortical, subcortical, and cerebellar motor areas and how movement is generated by their coordinated actions.

CORTICAL CONTROL OF MOVEMENT

The motor cortex consists of three contiguous areas located in the posterior part of the frontal lobe: *primary motor cortex*, *premotor cortex*, and *supplementary motor area*. The division of the motor cortex into three areas is based on their histologic and connectional differences as well as functional differences that have been illustrated by clinical and experimental studies. The cooperative action of these three areas is essential for voluntary execution of skilled movements.

Primary Motor Cortex

Movement can be evoked by electrical stimulation of many areas of the cerebral cortex, but the excitation thresholds vary considerably. Sir Charles Sherrington, after noting that the precentral gyrus had the lowest threshold, designated this area as the primary motor (MI) cortex. The MI cortex or Brodmann area 4 covers the precentral gyrus from the depths of the midsagittal sulcus to the lateral sulcus (see Chapter 5, Figure 5-10). Histologically, the MI cortex consists almost exclusively of pyramidal cells with a prominent layer V and an almost nonexistent layer IV. Because the MI cortex lacks granule cells, it is referred to as agranular cortex. Betz cells, the largest of the pyramidal cells (70–90 µm), are the histologic hallmark of Brodmann area 4, but other than their size, they have no special significance.

Electrical stimulation of the MI cortex contracts individual muscles.

Studies conducted on neurosurgical patients and animals have shown that electrical stimulation of the MI cortex evokes contractions of individual muscles of the body on the contralateral side and the upper face, tongue, jaw, larynx, and pharynx bilaterally. Studies in which widespread areas of the MI cortex were tested have shown that the entire body is represented along the precentral gyrus in a fashion similar to that of the primary somatosensory cortex on the postcentral gyrus (Figure 11-1). The organization of the *motor homunculus* is related to the degree of fine motor control, not to the size of the peripheral muscle or limb. Thus, a larger part of the MI cortex is devoted to control of the hands and face than to the torso and legs. Focal stimulation of the MI cortex has shown

Homunculus means "small person" in Latin.

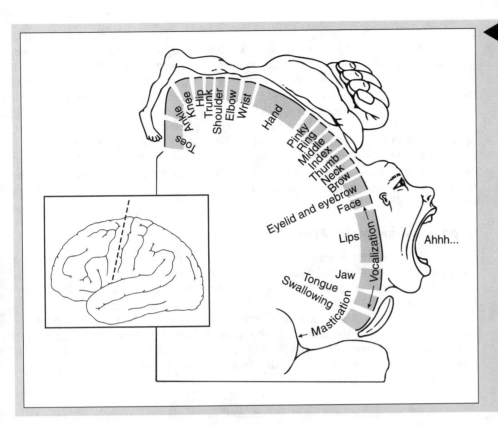

Somatotopic Map of Primary Motor Cortex. *The disproportionate sizing of the body reflects differences in fine motor control.*

that neurons related to particular muscles or muscle groups have a columnar organization, an obvious analogy to the primary somatosensory, auditory, and visual cortices described previously. Individual muscles, especially those related to the digits, are represented at multiple loci across cortex. It is believed that muscles with a multiple representation have a wider movement repertoire than muscles represented only at a single site.

Electrophysiologic recordings from animals trained to aim a joystick at a target have shown that the activity of individual neurons in the MI cortex is correlated with the direction and force of arm movement. The activity of individual neurons, though consistent, is too variable to account for the high degree of motor precision shown by the animals. Apparently, precise movements are not controlled by any one cortical neuron but rather by the combined output from a large pool of neurons. Motor precision produced by the composite output of a neuron pool is analogous to coding of sensory quality by a pool of sensory neurons, as proposed by the across fiber pattern theory (see Chapter 9).

Because the MI cortex executes movement by controlling individual muscles, movements that require coordination of different parts of the body (e.g., bending over to pick up an object) must be orchestrated by some part of the brain that projects to the MI cortex. The premotor and supplementary motor areas plan and coordinate movements through their projections to the MI cortex. The MI cortex, in addition to the projections it receives from the premotor and supplementary motor areas, also receives direct projections from sensory areas within the parietal lobe and the thalamus, as well as indirect projections from the basal ganglia and cerebellum. Collectively, these projections provide the MI cortex with the set of instructions required for the execution of skilled movements.

The responsibility for coordination of complex movements lies in the premotor and supplementary motor cortices.

Premotor Cortex

The premotor motor cortex or Brodmann area 6 is located immediately anterior to the MI cortex and contains several motor homunculi; none are as well-defined as the motor map in the MI cortex (see Chapter 5, Figure 5-10). Compared to the MI cortex, movements evoked by electrical stimulation of the premotor cortex are more complex (e.g., simultaneous turning of the torso and head) and require stronger electrical currents. The premotor cortex creates complex movements through its descending and corticocortical

Electrical stimulation of the premotor cortex produces complex movements.

projections. Some descending projections of the premotor cortex terminate on reticulospinal neurons in the brainstem, which control the axial and proximal musculature. Other corticospinal projections from the premotor cortex terminate in the ventral horn of the spinal cord. Corticocortical projections from the premotor cortex to the MI cortex control the distal musculature. These corticocortical and corticoreticular projections enable the premotor cortex to create a motor template for complex and coordinated movements of the torso, arms, and fingers. These motor templates are based, in part, upon visual and tactile information received from the posterior parietal cortex.

Neurons in the premotor cortex increase their firing rate prior to the onset of movement and neural activity in the MI cortex. These data, as well as the clinical literature (see below), suggest that the premotor cortex functions as a form of higher-order motor cortex.

Supplementary Motor Area

The supplementary motor area (MII) forms the medial part of Brodmann area 6 that is buried within the longitudinal fissure (see Chapter 5, Figure 5-10). Like the premotor cortex, the MII cortex influences voluntary movement primarily though its efferent projections to the MI cortex. The MII cortex has a homunculus, but it is not as well defined as the map in the MI cortex. Electrical stimulation of the MII cortex produces complex movements of the axial muscles contralaterally or the proximal muscles bilaterally. Because neuronal activity in the MII cortex increases prior to the onset of movement, it has been suggested that the MII cortex rehearses complex, internally generated movements (Figure 11-2).

FIGURE 11-2 ▶

Areas of Cortex Activated during Three Different Movement-related Behaviors. Subjects were given an injection of radioactive xenon to visualize the active cortical areas during each task. (A) Simple task: Repeated apposition of the index finger and the thumb. This simple movement activates the finger areas of the primary motor and sensory cortices along the central sulcus. (B) Complex task: Apposition of several fingers to the thumb, one at a time in a specified order. This more complex task activates the same motor and sensory areas as the first task as well as circumscribed areas in the premotor and MII cortices. (C) Mental rehearsal: The subjects remain motionless but rehearse the complex task. Only the MII cortex is active during mental rehearsal. From these results Roland et al. (1980) concluded that the premotor cortex creates the template for executing the complex movement while the MII cortex is involved in cognitive preparation prior to movement.

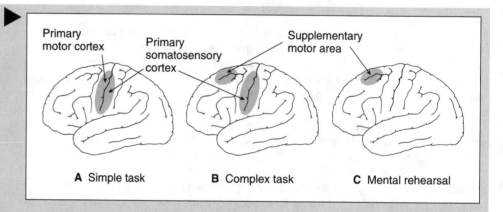

Primary motor cortex
Primary somatosensory cortex
Supplementary motor area

A Simple task   **B** Complex task   **C** Mental rehearsal

Posterior Parietal Cortex

Brodmann areas 5 and 7 are sensory association areas that are indispensable to the motor system (see Chapter 5, Figure 5-10). To operate properly, the motor system must have a spatial context in which to operate. The *posterior parietal lobe* uses visual, auditory, somatosensory, vestibular, and proprioceptive information to construct a map of the immediate extrapersonal space. Projections from the posterior parietal cortex to the premotor and supplemental motor areas of the frontal lobe are important for reaching, grasping, and tracking nearby objects. Patients with damage to the posterior parietal cortex neglect the contralateral visual and tactile fields (see Chapter 5). Although sensory neglect is not a motor deficit per se, sensory assessment of the extrapersonal space by the posterior parietal cortex is essential for movement to take place.

Descending Projections from Motor Cortex

The seven major descending pathways that exit the motor cortex terminate in the spinal cord, red nucleus, reticular formation, brainstem, thalamus, striatum, and pons. The corticobulbar projections that control movement of the mouth and face were discussed in Chapter 4. The corticothalamic, corticostriatal, and corticopontine projections contribute to the elaborate neural loops through the basal ganglia and cerebellum that modulate motor performance; each is discussed later in this chapter. The corticospinal, corticorubral, and corticoreticular pathways have direct control of body movements.

The *corticospinal tract* is the pathway responsible for fine motor control of the digits (see Chapter 3, Figures 3-27 and 3-28). Naturally, more than half of its axons terminate in the anterior horn of the cervical enlargement. Despite its close association with precision movements, only 30% of the corticospinal tract originates in the MI cortex; the remaining axons derive from Brodmann area 6 (20%) and the parietal lobe (40%). The descending projections from the postcentral gyrus terminate in the posterior horn and modulate sensory information derived from the dorsal roots.

The *corticorubral tract* originates in both the MI and premotor cortices. Neurons in the MI cortex terminate in a somatotopic fashion within the red nucleus. Neurons in the MI cortex that control the fingers terminate on neurons in the red nucleus that, in turn, project to the lateral half of the anterior horn and primarily affect the distal musculature. The *corticoreticular/reticulospinal pathway* and the *corticorubral/rubrospinal pathway* originate in the MII and premotor cortices, project to the medial half of the anterior horn, and control the axial and proximal muscles (see Chapter 3, Figure 3-23). The rubrospinal and reticulospinal tracts coordinate complex, cooperative movements of the axial and proximal muscles such as turning the head and torso while moving the arms and hands.

The reticulospinal pathways originate in the pons and medulla.

Lesions of Motor Cortex

Motor deficits caused by cortical lesions vary according to the size and location of the damage. Unlike lower motor neuron damage, which usually causes paralysis, lesions of the motor areas in the frontal lobe produce severe weakness, known as paresis. In addition, patients with cortical lesions rarely show the degree of spastic paralysis that accompanies damage to lower levels of the corticospinal system.

Patients with damage to the motor cortex demonstrate a flaccid paralysis with slow recovery that begins in the axial and proximal musculature and gradually moves toward the digits. Movement of the trunk and arms survives damage restricted to the MI cortex because most descending projections to the axial and proximal musculature originate in the premotor cortex. Patients with damage to the MI cortex may show some recovery in the digits but are unlikely to recover independent control of their fingers. The inability to fractionate motor control of the fingers interferes with manual dexterity. Thus, damage to the MI cortex interferes with motor proficiency rather than the ability to comprehend, learn, or remember a motor sequence.

Fine control of the digits is controlled by the primary motor cortex.

Paresis or motor weakness is more common than paralysis.

Patients with cortical damage rarely show extensor rigidity but will show a positive Babinski sign.

Lesions in the premotor cortex cause paresis of the axial and proximal muscles and interfere with the choreography of complex movements. Complex motor sequences are still possible following damage to the premotor cortex, but execution is slow. Because movements generated by the premotor cortex are heavily dependent on the map of the extrapersonal space generated by the posterior parietal cortex, visually guided movements are severely affected by damage to the premotor cortex.

Whereas lesions in the premotor cortex interfere with visually guided movements, damage to the MII cortex interferes with internally generated movement sequences. Damage to the MII cortex interferes with goal-directed behaviors that require planning and execution of complex motor sequences. For example, monkeys with lesions in the MII and premotor cortices attempt to obtain treats by reaching through a transparent screen rather than reaching around it. Lesions in the MII cortex also may produce motor apraxia, an inability to perform certain acts that cannot be attributed to paralysis per se.

These patients may be able to use each hand independently but not cooperatively (e.g., holding a lid open with one hand while removing an object with the other).

Modulation of the Motor System

The MI cortex is responsible for executing voluntary movement but is very dependent on input from other areas of the brain. As discussed above, the visual, auditory, and somatosensory systems provide the motor system with information about the environment within which the next movement will take place. Two other parts of the brain, the basal ganglia and the cerebellum, support volitional movement in other ways. The basal ganglia initiate and terminate movements while the cerebellum improves the precision of skilled or complex movements. Whereas damage to the motor cortex, its descending pathways, or the lower-order neurons that innervate muscles produces either paresis or paralysis, lesions within the basal ganglia or cerebellum only degrade motor performance. Nevertheless, both the basal ganglia and cerebellum are vital components of the motor system.

> *The basal ganglia initiate and terminate movements.*

> *The cerebellum improves motor precision.*

BASAL GANGLIA

The *basal ganglia* consist of several subcortical nuclei of telencephalic and diencephalic origin located within the ventral forebrain (Table 11-1). Other midbrain nuclei, such as the *substantia nigra* and *ventral tegmental area (VTA)*, have close anatomic and functional ties with the basal ganglia. Although best known for their motor functions, the basal ganglia also contribute to cognition. This section emphasizes the relationship between the basal ganglia and movement.

TABLE 11-1 ▶

Components of the Basal Ganglia

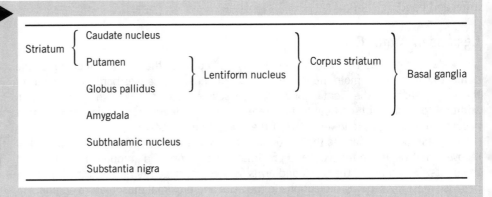

The basal ganglia are divided on functional grounds into *input nuclei*, *output nuclei*, and *intrinsic nuclei* whose interconnections form two types of intrinsic circuits (Figure 11-3). The *direct circuits* initiate movement while the *indirect circuits* suppress them. These direct and indirect circuits are the keys to understanding the operation of the basal ganglia and its contributions to normal and pathologic movement. The basal ganglia contain at least four separate sets of direct and indirect circuits: somatomotor, association, limbic, and oculomotor.

Gross Anatomy

The basal ganglia include the *caudate nucleus*, the *putamen*, the *nucleus accumbens*, the *globus pallidus*, and the *amygdala*. Several other nuclei (*subthalamic nucleus*, VTA, substantia nigra) with close ties to the basal ganglia also are discussed in this section. Despite spreading from the telencephalon to the mesencephalon, the basal ganglia and related nuclei form a coherent and integrated system.

The caudate nucleus and the putamen have the same cytoarchitecture and many of the same afferent and efferent connections and, for these reasons, often are referred to as

> *The basal ganglia include the caudate nucleus, the putamen, the nucleus accumbens, the globus pallidus, and the amygdala.*

> *The caudate nucleus and putamen form the striatum or* **neostriatum**.

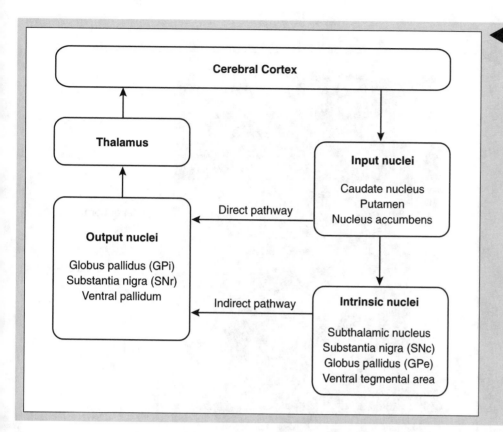

◄ **FIGURE 11-3**
Flow Diagram Showing the Input, Output, and Intrinsic Nuclei of the Basal Ganglia.
GPi = internal globus pallidus; GPe = external globus pallidus; SNr = substantia nigra pars reticulata; SNc = substantia nigra pars compacta.

a single entity, the *neostriatum*. Both parts of the neostriatum are embryologic derivatives of the same cells but during development become almost completely separated from one another by the ingrowing fibers of the internal capsule. Rostrally, the putamen is continuous with the head of the caudate nucleus in two places, along the medial edge of the internal capsule and through perforations in the internal capsule called *striatal bridges* (Figures 11-4 and 11-5).

The caudate nucleus consists of three parts: a large head, a body that tapers posteriorly, and a long, cycle-shaped tail, all closely associated with the ventricular system. The head of the caudate nucleus forms the lateral wall of the anterior horn of the lateral ventricle and for this reason is an important radiologic landmark (Figure 11-5; see Figure 11-4). From the foramen of Monro posteriorly, the body of the caudate nucleus lies on the dorsolateral surface of the thalamus. The tail of the caudate nucleus descends into the inferior horn of the lateral ventricle and ends immediately posterior to the amygdala.

The putamen is the largest component of the basal ganglia and lies lateral to the internal capsule and the globus pallidus. The putamen and its medial neighbor, the globus pallidus, form a wedge-shaped region called the *lenticular nucleus* (see Chapter 5, Figure 5-1A). A thin layer of myelinated fibers separates the putamen from the globus pallidus; another layer of fibers divides the globus pallidus into *internal (GPi)* and *external (GPe) pallidal segments*. The last part of the basal ganglia, the amygdala, is discussed with the rest of the limbic system in Chapter 13.

The globus pallidus is closely associated with the subthalamic nucleus, a lens-shaped nucleus sandwiched between the zona incerta and the internal capsule in the caudal diencephalon (see Chapter 5, Figures 5-1C and 5-1D). Immediately caudal to the subthalamic nucleus lie the substantia nigra (see Chapter 4, Figure 4-25) and the VTA (see Chapter 5, Figure 5-1E), which have close ties to the basal ganglia. The substantia nigra was introduced in Chapter 4; the VTA lies medial to the nigra. The substantia nigra consists of two functionally distinct layers. The dorsally located *pars compacta (SNc)* region contains large pigmented, dopaminergic neurons while the ventrally located *pars reticulata (SNr)* region contains small GABAergic neurons. Like the separate pallidal segments, the two parts of the substantia nigra have different connections and functions.

The putamen and globus pallidus form the ***lenticular*** *nucleus.*

The globus pallidus also is known as the ***pallidum***.

FIGURE 11-4 ▶
Photomicrograph of the Rostral Striatum in the Coronal Plane (Weigert Stain). (Source: Reprinted with permission from Dr. Malcolm B. Carpenter, Professor and Chairman Emeritus, Uniformed Services University of the Health Sciences, Bethesda, Maryland.)

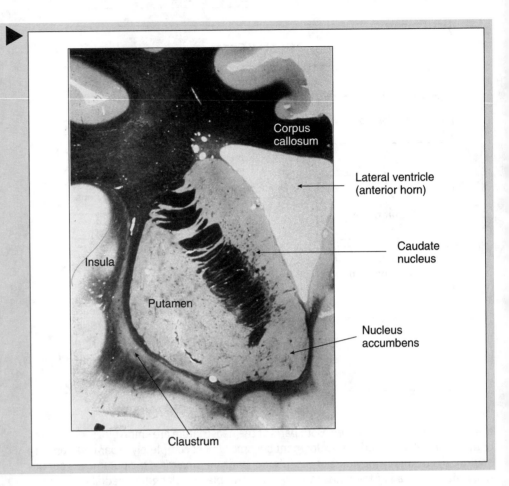

FIGURE 11-5 ▶
Lateral View of the Caudate and Putamen. This drawing emphasizes the continuity of the putamen with the head and body of the caudate nucleus. Rostrally, the head of the caudate nucleus and the putamen are continuous with one another through the nucleus accumbens. Further caudally, the caudate nucleus and putamen are partially separated by the developing fibers of the internal capsule; thin webs of tissue that connect the putamen with the body of the caudate nucleus are called striatal bridges.

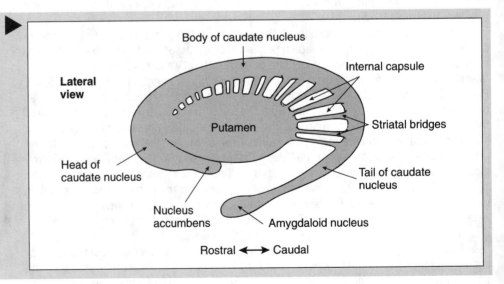

Input Nuclei

Almost all afferent projections to the basal ganglia enter through the neostriatum and most of those originate in the cerebral cortex (see Figure 11-3). Cortical association areas in the frontal, parietal, and temporal lobes project primarily to the caudate nucleus; the putamen receives most of its input from the primary sensory and motor cortices. Clusters of neurons within the putamen receive motor and sensory projections from the same part of the body (e.g., the same joint or the same limb). In general, these glutamatergic, corticostriatal projections overlap the dopaminergic projections from the substantia nigra, SNc. Cortical projections to the nucleus accumbens and the ventral neostriatum come from the insula, the amygdala, the olfactory cortices, and the hippocampal formation. Evidence that the sensorimotor and limbic areas of the cerebral cortex project to segregated parts of the neostriatum and nucleus accumbens suggests that the basal ganglia consist of separate functional channels or processing streams.

Corticostriatal projections use glutamate and are excitatory.

The striatum consists of several different cell types, but the complexity of the striatum derives primarily from its chemical diversity. More than 90% of the neurons in the striatum are *medium spiny neurons*, which project to the globus pallidus and substantia nigra. All of the medium spiny neurons are GABAergic, but most contain a neuropeptide that serves as a second neurotransmitter. Those that project to the GPi and the SNr contain substance P and dynorphin; others that project to the GPe have GABA co-localized with enkephalin. These co-localized peptides enable the GABAergic medium spiny neurons to activate different populations of neurons selectively. Intrinsic connections within the striatum are mediated by aspiny neurons, which contain either GABA, acetylcholine, neuropeptide Y, or somatostatin.

Medium spiny cells are projection neurons.

Output Nuclei and Pathways

Basal ganglia output arises from the internal segment of the GPi, the SNr, and the ventral pallidum. The inhibitory GABAergic neurons of the GPi and SNr project to the ventral anterior (VA) and ventral lateral (VL) nuclei of the thalamus, which in turn project to the premotor and supplementary motor cortices (see Chapter 5, Figures 5-1A and 5-1B). These pathways are critical for initiation of movement.

The GPi, SNr, and ventral pallidum are the output nuclei of the basal ganglia.

The efferent projections from the GPi to the thalamus follow two separate pathways, the ansa lenticularis and the lenticular fasciculus (Figure 11-6; see Chapter 5, Figures 5-1A and 5-1B). Axons forming the lenticular fasciculus exit the dorsal surface of the GPi, perforate the internal capsule and subthalamic nucleus, and run medially along the ventral border of the zona incerta until they merge with the thalamic fasciculus, which enters the thalamus from the ventrolateral side (see Chapter 5, Figure 5-1B). The thalamic fasciculus also contains crossed cerebellothalamic fibers. Axons forming the ansa lenticularis exit the GPi from its ventral surface, wrap around the medial tip of the internal capsule, and join the thalamic fasciculus.

*The two efferent pathways of the globus pallidus are the **ansa lenticularis** and the **lenticular fasciculus**.*

Intrinsic Nuclei

The afferent and efferent projections of the intrinsic nuclei remain within the basal ganglia. The intrinsic nuclei of the basal ganglia include the GPe, the subthalamic nucleus, the VTA, and the SNc. Some of the intrinsic nuclei modulate activity in other parts of the basal ganglia; others act as logical switches, which enable the output nuclei to either increase or decrease the likelihood that movement will occur.

The intrinsic nuclei of the basal ganglia include the GPe, the subthalamic nucleus, the VTA, and the SNc.

Dopaminergic projections from the SNc terminate throughout the caudate nucleus and putamen. A smaller mesolimbic dopaminergic pathway originates in the VTA and terminates in the limbic areas of the striatum (nucleus accumbens, ventral striatum). These ascending dopaminergic projections modulate the effects of the excitatory projections from the cerebral cortex.

The dopaminergic projection to the striatum is referred to as the nigrostriatal dopaminergic system.

The subthalamic nucleus is a critical component of the disinhibitory circuit that determines the output of the basal ganglia (see Neural Models of Basal Ganglia Function below). Most afferent projections to the subthalamic nucleus originate in the GPe whose activity may increase or decrease as a function of its input from the striatum. When neural activity in the subthalamic nucleus increases, its excitatory projections increase the inhibitory output of its target nuclei, the GPi and the SNr, on the thalamus. As thalamic activity decreases, it becomes more difficult to initiate movement. Conversely, damage to the subthalamic nucleus increases the incidence of spontaneous movements.

The dopaminergic projections to the nucleus accumbens, ventral striatum, and medial frontal cortex is referred to as the mesolimbic dopaminergic system.

***Disinhibition:** Turning off the fire extinguisher that was dousing the fire, allowed the fire to spread (see Chapter 1).*

Clinical Aspects

Disorders of the basal ganglia do not cause paralysis or paresis but rather unwanted movements or a general poverty of movement. Symptoms associated with the basal

FIGURE 11-6 ▶
Photomicrograph of the Lenticular Fasciculus and Thalamic Fasciculus (Weigert Stain).

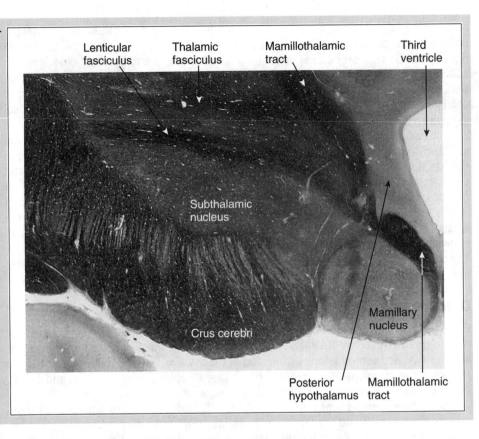

Lenticular fasciculus

Thalamic fasciculus

Mamillothalamic tract

Third ventricle

Subthalamic nucleus

Mamillary nucleus

Crus cerebri

Posterior hypothalamus

Mamillothalamic tract

---

ganglia are classified as negative and positive signs. *Negative symptoms* (or signs) are deficiencies in the patient's motor repertoire. In Parkinson's disease, a *hypokinetic disorder*, patients exhibit muscle rigidity and bradykinesia. *Positive symptoms* are movements over which the patient has no control such as tics (twitches) and tremors. Because patients with Huntington's disease, hemiballism, and athetosis display positive symptoms, these are *hyperkinetic disorders*.

Parkinson's Disease. Parkinson's disease is a chronic, progressive disorder of unknown origin that affects both motor and cognitive skills. The cardinal symptoms of Parkinson's disease include *resting tremor*, muscle rigidity, and slowness of movement. The onset of Parkinson's disease is typically signaled by the resting tremor in one hand (pill-rolling) that disappears during volitional movement and increases during stress or emotional turmoil. Over time, tremor may appear in the lips, tongue, ipsilateral foot or the other hand; eventually the tremor spreads to the axial musculature of the body (Figure 11-7). Increased muscle tone in both extensors and flexors produces a plastic or *"lead pipe" rigidity*. Movements also may have a *cogwheel* appearance. Parkinson's patients also have difficulty initiating movements *(akinesia)*; when movements do occur, they are slow *(bradykinesia)* and lack normal amplitude *(hypokinesia)*. Spontaneous, automatic movements of the face and eyes are replaced by a *mask-like expression* and an unblinking (reptilian) stare. As the akinesia progresses, speech becomes more difficult, and the patient speaks less often and more softly until mutism ensues. Loss of postural reflexes causes bowing of the head and trunk forward along with flexed elbows, hips, and knees. Walking consists of short steps and a shuffling gait with the hands positioned in front of the body. Like the motor system, thinking slows appreciably; approximately 30% of Parkinson's disease patients develop dementia.

Although the etiology of Parkinson's disease is not known, Parkinson-like symptoms may accompany other diseases or be evoked by drugs (e.g., dopamine antagonists) or toxins (e.g., carbon monoxide, manganese, cyanide), hypoxia, trauma, and tumors. Parkinson-like symptoms and Parkinson's disease are caused by depletion of striatal dopamine secondary to degeneration of dopaminergic neurons within the SNc. The first symptoms of Parkinsonism appear after approximately 70%–80% of the SNc cells die; as cell death within the SNc continues, the number of symptoms and their severity increase.

Pill-rolling is a rhythmic movement of the thumb across the other fingers performed in combination with rotation of the wrist.

Patients with *cogwheel rigidity* move their limbs in a choppy, ratchet-like fashion.

Akinesia is difficulty starting movements.

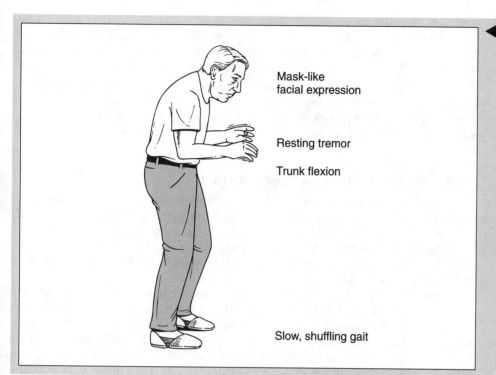

Mask-like facial expression

Resting tremor

Trunk flexion

Slow, shuffling gait

Treatment of Parkinson's disease emphasizes dopamine repletion; surgical intervention is the treatment of last resort. Replacement therapy is designed to increase dopamine levels in the brain either by administering a dopamine precursor (e.g., L-dopa) or a dopamine agonist (e.g., bromocriptine). To limit peripheral conversion of L-dopa into dopamine, a decarboxylase inhibitor such as carbidopa usually is administered. Surgical intervention may be attempted in long-term Parkinson patients who no longer respond to pharmacologic treatment. Coagulation of the GPi reduces tremor and rigidity and improves akinesia. Due to the proximity of the internal capsule and optic tract to the GPi, pallidotomy patients risk hemiparesis and homonymous hemianopsia. The effectiveness of surgical implantation of dopaminergic neurons from the patient's adrenal cortex or from the substantia nigra of fetal donors remains controversial.

Dopamine does not cross the blood–brain barrier, but its precursor, L-dopa, does.

Huntington's Chorea. Huntington's chorea is a hereditary disease of adult onset characterized by motor, cognitive, and behavioral deterioration. The hallmark of Huntington's disease is the involuntary, dance-like or *choreiform movements* of the limbs. Early in the disease, these choreic movements and small tics may be incorporated into ongoing voluntary movements of the arms and legs. As these movements increase in magnitude, they begin to overshadow normal motor behavior. In advanced cases, the choreiform movements abate as rigidity and bradykinesia ensue. Even more debilitating are the cognitive impairments that eventually develop into global dementia.

Huntington's disease was first described by George Huntington in 1872.

Huntington's chorea is characterized by degeneration of the medium spiny projection neurons, first in the caudate nucleus and eventually in the putamen and globus pallidus. Shrinkage of the caudate nucleus caused by cellular degeneration is visible with magnetic resonance imaging (MRI). The cause of Huntington's disease is a mutation of chromosome 4 that produces a proliferation of a normal trinucleotide pattern. The probability of Huntington's disease rises dramatically if the length of this trinucleotide pattern exceeds a critical length. Recently developed genetic tests that measure the length of this trinucleotide repeat are used to confirm Huntington's chorea in symptomatic patients and diagnose family members who are still asymptomatic.

Neuronal degeneration observed in Huntington's and Parkinson's disease may be caused by amino acid excitotoxicity.

Huntington's disease is marked by a loss of striatal neurons.

Hemiballismus. Hemiballismus is a hyperkinetic disorder of the basal ganglia marked by a series of involuntary ballistic movements of one arm or leg. The most common cause of hemiballismus is a focal stroke involving the subthalamic nucleus; the symptoms are expressed by the contralateral extremities. Destruction of the subthalamic nucleus decreases the inhibitory output from the GPi, which allows activity in the ventral anterior (VA)

*Patients with **hemiballismus** have ballistic movements of the limbs.*

and ventral lateral (VL) nuclei of the thalamus to increase above normal levels. Dopamine-blocking (e.g., haloperidol) or dopamine-depleting (e.g., reserpine) drugs alleviate the symptoms of hemiballismus by increasing neural activity in the subthalamic nucleus.

Athetosis. Athetosis is an involuntary, slow, writhing movement of the hands and fingers. In general, the movements in athetosis are slower than those observed in chorea, but all gradations are possible making the distinction between the two disorders impossible in some instances. Postmortem studies have implicated damage to the globus pallidus and thalamus.

Neural Models of Basal Ganglia Function

The basal ganglia, working in concert with the thalamus, form parts of several loops that begin and end in the cerebral cortex. The somatomotor and oculomotor circuits modulate body and extraocular eye movement. The limbic and association circuits are not as well understood, but appear to involve cognition, emotion, and behavior. These four circuits share common features; the somatomotor circuit, which is the best understood of the four, is described below.

Recent clinical and experimental studies have provided fresh insights into the functional organization of the basal ganglia. The most useful model, which views the output of the basal ganglia as a balance between so-called direct and indirect pathways, has been well articulated by Graybiel, Alexander, DeLong and Strick among others. In this model, the direct pathway promotes movement through its excitatory projections while the indirect pathway suppresses movement. The direct and indirect somatomotor circuits include the input, output, and intrinsic nuclei described above (see Figure 11-3). In normal individuals, the output of the direct and indirect circuits is balanced, in part, by the opposing actions of dopaminergic nigrostriatal projections on the D_1 and D_2 receptor subtypes within the putamen (Figure 11-8A). Neurons with D_2 receptors are inhibited by dopamine and project to the GPe while neurons with D_1 receptors are excited by dopamine and project to the GPi and SNr. In Parkinson's disease, the loss of dopamine's inhibitory action on the D_2 receptors leads to an increase in subthalamic nucleus activity, which ultimately leads to hypokinesia (Figure 11-8B). In hemiballismus, the

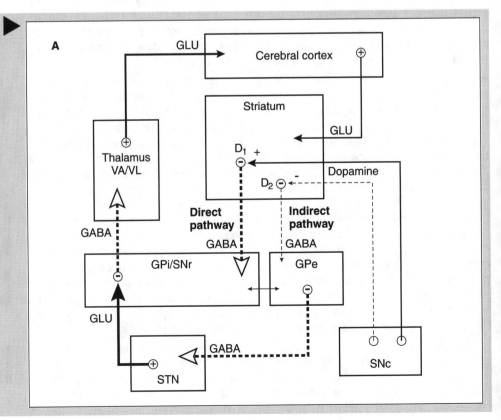

FIGURE 11-8A

Basal Ganglia Circuits. Both the direct and indirect circuits begin with activation of the striatum by a glutamatergic corticostriatal projection. In the normal individual, the activation of striatal GABAergic neurons inhibits GABAergic neurons within the internal globus pallidus (GPi) and the pars reticulata (SNr). Reduced activity in the GABAergic neurons of the GPi and SNr allows the ventral anterior (VA) and ventral lateral (VL) nuclei to increase their activity, which in turn activates the supplementary motor cortex. GABA = γ-aminobutyric acid; STN = subthalamic nucleus.

dopaminergic projections are intact, but damage to the subthalamic nucleus disinhibits the thalamus, which through its projections to the supplementary and premotor cortices, triggers involuntary movements (Figure 11-8C).

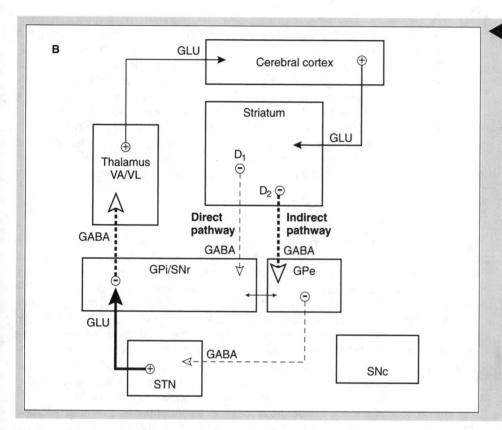

FIGURE 11-8B

In Parkinson's disease, the hypokinetic symptoms are caused by a diminution of cortical activation by the thalamic motor nuclei. Nigral degeneration affects both the direct and indirect circuits of the basal ganglia. The GABAergic neurons in the direct circuit decrease their firing rate, which, by releasing GPi and SNr, suppresses the motor thalamus. The GABAergic striatal neurons of the indirect circuit respond to the loss of dopamine by increasing their activity, which reduces the inhibitory effect of the external globus pallidus (GPe) on the subthalamic nucleus. Increased activity in the subthalamic nucleus further enhances the inhibitory effect of the GPi and SNr on the motor thalamus. Inhibition of the motor nuclei of the thalamus ultimately produces less activation of the motor cortex.

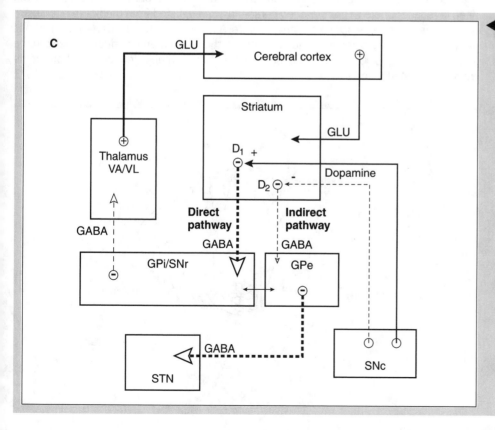

FIGURE 11-8C

In hemiballismus, the hyperkinetic symptoms are caused by focal damage to the subthalamic nucleus. Normally, the glutamatergic projections from the subthalamic nucleus to the GPi and SNr suppress the motor nuclei of the thalamus (see Figure 11-8A). After damage to the subthalamic nucleus, the thalamic motor nuclei are disinhibited and provide excessive activation of the motor cortices.

CEREBELLUM

Overview

The *cerebellum* does not initiate movement or directly control the musculature but nevertheless plays a vital role in voluntary movement, posture, muscle tone, and balance. The cerebellum guides volitional movement in two ways. Ballistic movements too fast to benefit from sensory guidance (e.g., swatting a mosquito) are orchestrated by the cerebellum based on previous experience. More deliberate actions (e.g., threading a needle) are guided in real time by tactile, proprioceptive, and visual feedback to the cerebellum. Although this sensory information does not enter the conscious sphere, its loss has serious clinical implications. Following cerebellar damage, gait, balance, and delicate movements are severely impaired. Other data suggest that the cerebellum contributes to motor learning and language; for clinicians, however, these functions are of secondary importance.

Gross Anatomy

The cerebellum, the largest resident of the posterior cranial fossa, is connected to the brainstem by three stout fiber bundles that contain all of its afferent and efferent projections: the *inferior*, *middle*, and *superior cerebellar peduncles*. The tentorium covers the dorsal surface of the cerebellum and secures it to the inner surface of the skull. The cerebellar cortex consists of small gyri called *folia*, but unlike the cerebral cortex, its much finer gyral pattern buries 85% of the cortical surface. Although none of the cerebellar gyri have names, several of the larger fissures have been named, and they separate the three cerebellar lobes. The *primary* and *posterolateral fissures* divide the cerebellum into the *anterior*, *posterior*, and *flocculonodular lobes*, respectively (Figure 11-9; see Chapter 2, Figure 2-10). The cerebellar cortex consists of two hemispheres, a vermal region that straddles the midline, and an intermediate paravermal region (Figure 11-10).

The cortical mantle rests upon the *arbor vitae*, a dense bundle of myelinated fibers that reciprocally connect the cerebellar cortex with various brainstem nuclei and the deep cerebellar nuclei. The *four deep cerebellar nuclei*, listed from medial to lateral, are the *fastigial*, *globose*, *emboliform*, and *dentate*. Almost all cerebellar efferent projections originate in the deep cerebellar nuclei. Although the deep cerebellar nuclei receive some afferent projections from extracerebellar sources, most of their afferent projections come from the cerebellar cortex.

> *The primary fissure is the deepest of the cerebellar sulci.*

> **Arbor vitae** means "tree of life" in Latin.

> *The subcortical nuclei of the cerebellum usually are referred to as the deep cerebellar nuclei.*

FIGURE 11-9 ▶
Midsagittal Section of the Cerebellum.

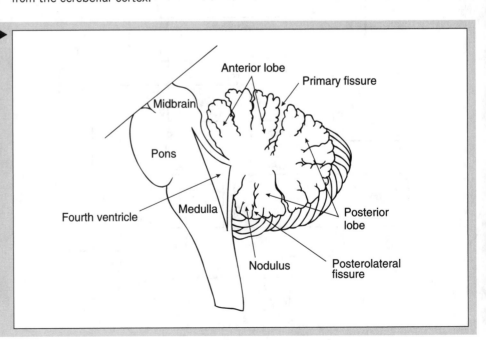

Anterior lobe
Primary fissure
Midbrain
Pons
Fourth ventricle
Medulla
Nodulus
Posterior lobe
Posterolateral fissure

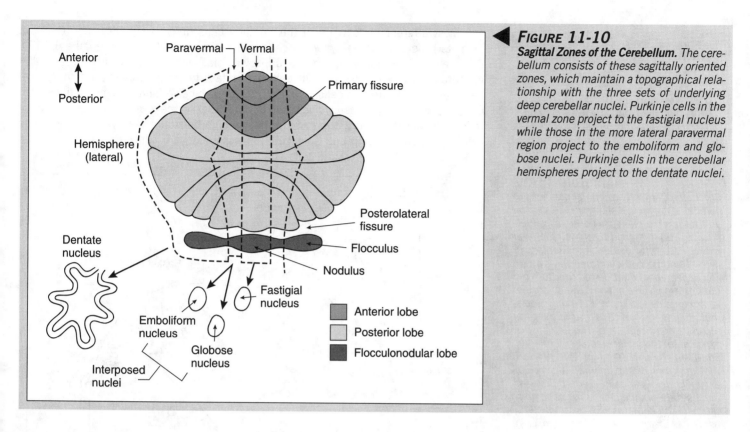

FIGURE 11-10
Sagittal Zones of the Cerebellum. The cerebellum consists of these sagittally oriented zones, which maintain a topographical relationship with the three sets of underlying deep cerebellar nuclei. Purkinje cells in the vermal zone project to the fastigial nucleus while those in the more lateral paravermal region project to the emboliform and globose nuclei. Purkinje cells in the cerebellar hemispheres project to the dentate nuclei.

Cortical Cytoarchitecture

The most important neural elements of the cerebellar cortex are the large (40–75 μm diameter), flask-shaped, *Purkinje neurons* (Table 11-2; see Chapter 1, Figure 1-1). The Purkinje cells have a distinctive fan-like dendritic tree whose flat surface is oriented perpendicularly to the long axis of the folia (see Figure 11-11). Purkinje cells use GABA as an inhibitory neurotransmitter and are the sole efferent neurons of the cerebellar cortex.

TABLE 11-2
Cerebellar Cortical Neurons

Cell Type	Location	Afferent Source	Efferent Targets	Neurotransmitters	Action
Purkinje	Purkinje layer	Granule cell Basket cells Stellate cells Climbing fibers	Deep cerebellar nuclei Lateral vestibular nuclei	GABA	Inhibition
Granule	Granule layer	Mossy fibers Golgi cells	Purkinje cell dendrites Basket cells Stellate cells Golgi cells	Glutamate	Excitation
Basket	Molecular layer	Granule cells	Purkinje cell bodies	GABA	Inhibition
Stellate	Molecular layer	Granule cells		Taurine (?)	Inhibition
Golgi	Granule	Mossy fibers	Purkinje cell dendrites Glomerulus	GABA	Inhibition

Note. GABA = γ-aminobutyric acid.

The Purkinje cells speak for the cerebellar cortex.

Granule cells are the only excitatory neuron of the cerebellar cortex.

Most afferent projections to the Purkinje cells derive from the small (5-8 μm diameter), densely packed *granule cells* located in cerebellar cortex (Figure 11-11). Granule cells have multiple, short dendrites with claw-like endings within the cerebellar glomeruli described below. Granule cells use glutamate or aspartate to excite the apical dendrites of the Purkinje cells. Purkinje cells also receive inhibitory projections from Golgi neurons, *basket cells*, and stellate cells. Basket cells are the most effective inhibitory neuron of this group because their axon arborizations encircle each Purkinje cell's soma. Stellate cells and Golgi cells are less effective because they synapse on the distal dendrites of the Purkinje cells.

FIGURE 11-11 ▶

Cerebellar Cortex. *The cellular elements of cerebellar cortex are shown in the sagittal and transverse planes. The large, goblet-shaped Purkinje cells form a single layer along the ventral border of the molecular layer. Purkinje cell dendrites have a fan-like appearance when viewed sagittally but not the transverse plane. The molecular layer contains few cells, but many fibers, including the apical dendrites of the granule cells and Golgi cells. The granule cell axons enter the molecular layer, bifurcate, and form the parallel fibers that run with the long axis of the folium. Basket cell axons form a pericellular nest that embraces the Purkinje cell somas. The granule cell layer contains cerebellar glomeruli as well as their cellular constituents, granule cells and Golgi cells. Input to the cerebellar cortex is provided by mossy fibers and climbing fibers.*

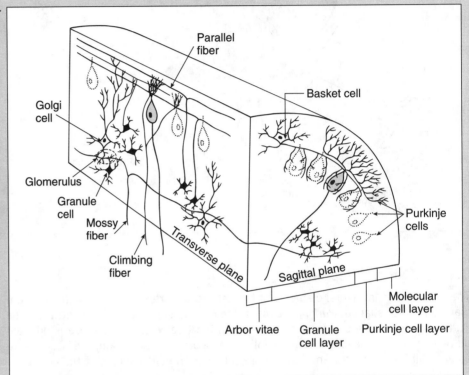

The cerebellar cortex consists of three layers that, unlike the cerebral cortex, show no regional variation (Figure 11-12). The *molecular layer*, which lies closest to the pia mater, consists primarily of granule and Golgi cell axons and the expansive dendritic trees of the underlying Purkinje cells. The Purkinje cells form a one-cell thick layer located along the ventral margin of the molecular layer. The deepest layer of the cerebellar cortex is the *granule cell layer*, whose constituent neurons are packed so tightly that adjacent neurons seem to touch one another.

Cortical Circuitry

*Most cerebellar afferent projections end as **mossy fibers**.*

Glomerulus (pl. glomeruli) means "ball" in Latin.

Afferent projections to cerebellar cortex terminate as either *mossy fibers* or *climbing fibers*. Mossy fiber projections originate in the spinal cord, medulla, and pons and terminate within glial encapsulated structures called *glomeruli* that are scattered throughout the granule cell layer of the cerebellar cortex (Figure 11-13). The mossy fiber designation derives from the moss-like appearance of the lobulated enlargements of the afferent terminals that provide for high-fidelity transmission of afferent information. The *mossy fiber rosette* forms the centerpiece of the glomerulus, which also includes granule cell dendrites and Golgi cell axons and dendrites. The only excitatory input to the glomerulus is provided by the mossy fiber. Glomerular output is conveyed by the granule cells whose axons ascend to the superficial part of the molecular layer, bifurcate, and run the length of the folia parallel to the cortical surface and perpendicular to the dendritic fans of the Purkinje cells. The *parallel fibers* pass through the outstretched dendrites of the Purkinje cells like electrical wires passing through the upper limbs of trees. The lengthy course of each parallel fiber enables individual granule cells to influence a widespread area of the cerebellar cortex.

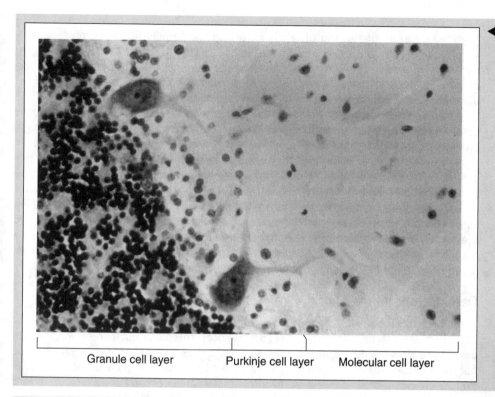

FIGURE 11-12
Photomicrograph of Cerebellar Cortex. *This section, stained for both cell bodies and myelin, shows the molecular, Purkinje, and granule cell layers. (Source: Reprinted with permission from Dr. Malcolm B. Carpenter, Professor and Chairman Emeritus, Uniformed Services University of the Health Sciences, Bethesda, Maryland.)*

Granule cell layer   Purkinje cell layer   Molecular cell layer

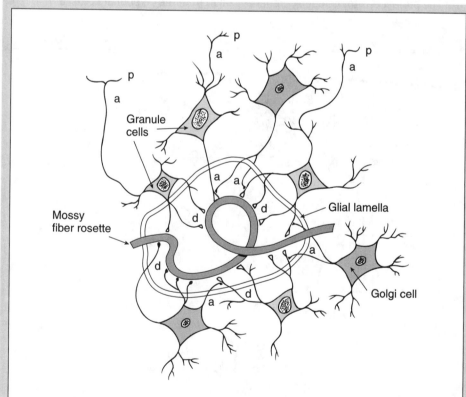

FIGURE 11-13
Cerebellar Glomerulus. *Mossy fibers terminate in a series of convoluted and lobulated processes called mossy fiber rosettes. The mossy fiber rosette forms the core of the cerebellar glomerulus, a glial encapsulated synaptic ensemble that also contains dendrites of several local granule cells and axons from local Golgi cells. The inhibitory Golgi cells terminate presynaptically on granule cell dendrites. The mossy fiber provides the excitatory input to the glomerulus while the granule cells serve as the efferent components. p = parallel fiber; a = axon; d = dendrite.*

Projections from the inferior olivary nuclei enter the molecular layer and terminate as climbing fibers on the dendritic trees of the Purkinje cells (Figure 11-14). Climbing fibers are so named because they climb the dendritic tree of Purkinje cells like vines on a trellis. Although one climbing fiber may target several Purkinje cells, each Purkinje cell receives only one climbing fiber. Through its multiple excitatory synapses, the climbing fiber exerts a powerful excitatory effect on each Purkinje cell.

The action potentials of a Purkinje cell vary as a function of the type of excitatory input it receives. Simple spikes, similar to those seen throughout the nervous system, are

Climbing fibers originate in the inferior olivary nucleus.

If Purkinje cells and climbing fibers were married to one another, the Purkinje cells would be monogamous and the climbing fibers would be polygamous.

triggered by excitation of the distal dendrites by the parallel fibers. Complex spikes, which have a prolonged and elaborate multiphasic waveform, are evoked by the multiple, excitatory synapses of the climbing fibers on the Purkinje cell. It is possible that the changes in calcium conductance produced by complex spikes may trigger a cascade of intracellular second messenger–mediated events related to motor learning.

The cerebellar cortex also receives noradrenergic projections from the locus ceruleus, dopaminergic projections from the substantia nigra and VTA, and serotonergic projections from the raphe nuclei. These projections are distributed throughout all layers of the cerebellar cortex and, to a lesser degree, the deep cerebellar nuclei. Like similar projections to the cerebral cortex, these neurotransmitters modulate ongoing activity at their target.

The cerebellar cortex contains several topographical maps of the body, but none are as well organized as those of the primary somatosensory cortex. In the cerebellar cortex, the orderly representation of one body part (e.g., one arm) may be juxtaposed to a detailed map of a leg. This so-called fractured somatotopy may be the basis for coordinating multiple parts of the body during complex movements.

Deep Cerebellar Nuclei

The fastigial, globose, emboliform, and dentate nuclei contain the primary efferent neurons of the cerebellum (Figure 11-15). The deep cerebellar nuclei receive collateral projections from brainstem and spinal cord neurons that project to the cerebellar cortex, but most of their afferent projections derive from the cerebellar cortex. Their output is exclusively excitatory and mediated by either glutamate or aspartate.

The projections to the deep cerebellar nuclei from the cerebellar cortex define three

The dentate nucleus is referred to as the "cerebellar olive" because its crumpled appearance resembles the inferior olivary nucleus.

FIGURE 11-14 ▶

Purkinje Cell Circuitry. A transverse section through a folia shows the fan-like profile of the cerebellar Purkinje cell. Climbing fibers, which originate from neurons of the inferior olivary nucleus, climb the dendritic tree of the Purkinje cell–like vines on a trellis. The Purkinje cell axon shown leaving the ventral surface of the soma terminates in one of the deep cerebellar nuclei. The basket cell is named for its basket-like termination around Purkinje cell soma.

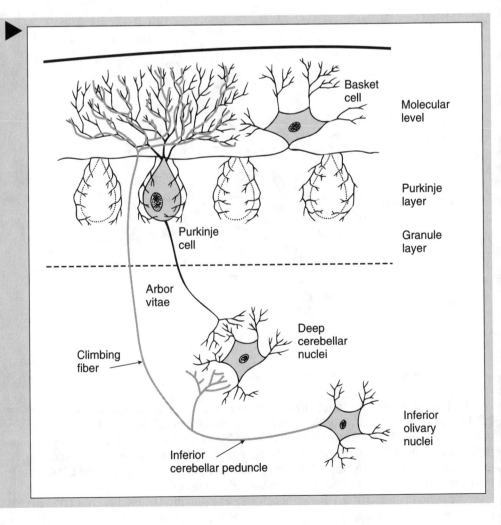

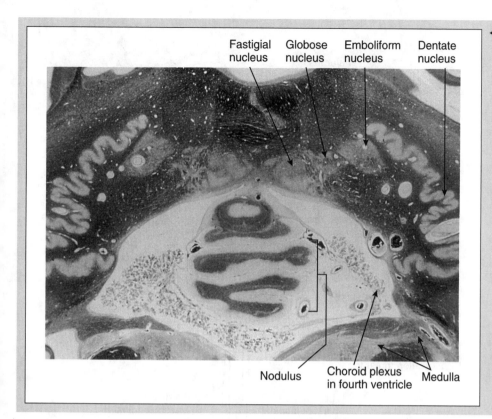

Fastigial nucleus   Globose nucleus   Emboliform nucleus   Dentate nucleus

Nodulus   Choroid plexus in fourth ventricle   Medulla

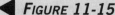

FIGURE 11-15
Photomicrograph of the Deep Cerebellar Nuclei. *Coronal section of the base of the cerebellum showing the four deep cerebellar nuclei. (Source: Reprinted with permission from Dr. Malcolm B. Carpenter, Professor and Chairman Emeritus, Uniformed Services University of the Health Sciences, Bethesda, Maryland.)*

sagittally oriented zones (see Figure 11-10). The fastigial nuclei receive most of their projections from the *vermal zone* of the cerebellar cortex. The more laterally located interposed (emboliform, globose) and dentate nuclei receive most of their projections from the *paravermal* and *lateral zones* of the cerebellar cortex, respectively. These sagittally oriented zones are related to the functional organization of the cerebellum.

The afferent and efferent projections of the cerebellum form three sagittal planes: vermal, paravermal, and lateral.

Together, the globose and emboliform nuclei comprise the interposed nuclei.

Functional Organization of the Cerebellum

The cerebellum provides the sensory interface with the environment that the motor system requires for precise operation. As an embryologic derivative of the alar plate, the cerebellum receives significant projections from the somatosensory, vestibular, visual, and auditory systems. The pattern of cerebellar afferent projections forms three functional modules: the *vestibulocerebellum*, the *cerebrocerebellum*, and the *spinocerebellum*.

Vestibulocerebellum. The vestibulocerebellum consists of the flocculonodular lobe as well as parts of the vermis and fastigial nuclei. As its name implies, the vestibulocerebellum contributes to balance, posture, and visual fixation through its close relationship to the vestibular system. Secondary projections from the vestibular nuclei and primary projections from Scarpa's ganglion enter the cerebellum through the juxtarestiform body located along the medial aspect of the inferior cerebellar peduncle (Figure 11-16). The vestibulocerebellum also receives significant visual and somatosensory projections from the contralateral inferior olivary nuclei.

The vestibulocerebellum adjusts posture and maintains balance through its efferent projections to the vestibular nuclei and the reticular formation (see Figure 11-16). Purkinje cells of the flocculonodular lobe have direct, inhibitory projections to the ipsilateral lateral vestibular nuclei. Excitatory projections to the vestibular nuclei and the ipsilateral reticular formation originate in the fastigial nucleus and exit the cerebellum through the juxtarestiform body (see Chapter 8, Figure 8-9). Fastigial projections to the contralateral reticular formation form the uncinate fasciculus, a small myelinated tract that exits the cerebellum along the dorsal surface of the superior cerebellar peduncle. These excitatory fastigiobulbar projections use glutamate or aspartate as their neurotransmitter.

*The oldest division, the **vestibulocerebellum**, also is known as the archicerebellum.*

Most of fibers of the inferior cerebellar peduncle are olivocerebellar projections.

The juxtarestiform body, a component of the inferior cerebellar peduncle, contains reciprocal connections between the cerebellum and the brainstem as well as first-order vestibulocerebellar fibers.

FIGURE 11-16 ▶

Projections of the Vestibulocerebellum. The efferent projections of the vestibulo-cerebellum originate in the vermis and the fastigial nuclei.

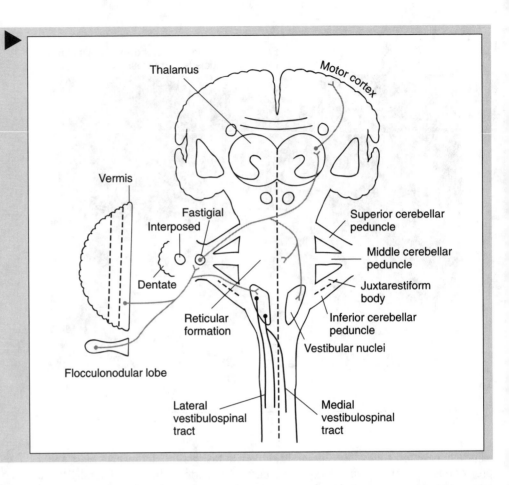

Stimulation of the flocculonodular lobe reduces extensor muscle tone.

*The newest division, the **cerebrocerebellum**, also is known as the neocerebellum.*

In feedback mode, the cerebellum uses sensory information to make contemporaneous adjustments in a motor sequence.

Clinical signs related to damage of the vestibulocerebellum include disorders of balance, gait, posture, and eye movement (e.g., nystagmus). These patients often assume a *broad-based gait* to compensate for their poor balance and may not show a normal vestibulo-ocular reflex (VOR).

Cerebrocerebellum. The lateral zones of the anterior and posterior lobes constitute the cerebrocerebellum. In addition to improving motor precision, the cerebrocerebellum plans and initiates complex movements.

The cerebrocerebellum is part of a multisynaptic pathway that begins and ends in the cerebral cortex (Figure 11-17). This loop starts in the sensory and motor areas adjacent to the central sulcus, descends through the posterior limb of the internal capsule, and terminates in the pontine nuclei. Efferent projections from the pontine nuclei cross the pons and enter the cerebellum through the middle cerebellar peduncle. The deep cerebellar nuclei receive some collateral projections, but most terminate as mossy fibers. Other olivocerebellar projections conveying visual and somatosensory information terminate as climbing fibers on Purkinje cells in the lateral zone. As the recipient of both motor output and sensory feedback, the cerebrocerebellum is positioned to compare intended movements with actual movements. Purkinje cell axons in the cerebrocerebellum terminate in a topographical manner within the dentate nuclei. Efferent projections of the dentate nucleus form the superior cerebellar peduncle, which exits the cerebellum rostrally and decussates in the caudal mesencephalon. Most projections from the dentate nucleus terminate in the VL nucleus of the thalamus, which in turn projects to Brodmann areas 4 and 6. The *feedback* provided by this cerebro-cerebello-thalamo-cortical pathway improves motor precision by matching intended and actual movements.

The cerebrocerebellum also guides movement in a *feedforward* manner. In feedforward mode, the cerebrocerebellum predicts the speed, force, and direction of a movement prior to its first occurrence. For example, we know before we pick up a bowling ball that it will be heavy and should be cradled from the bottom. A different strategy is used to pick up fragile items like a wedge of cake. Our past experience with bowling balls and

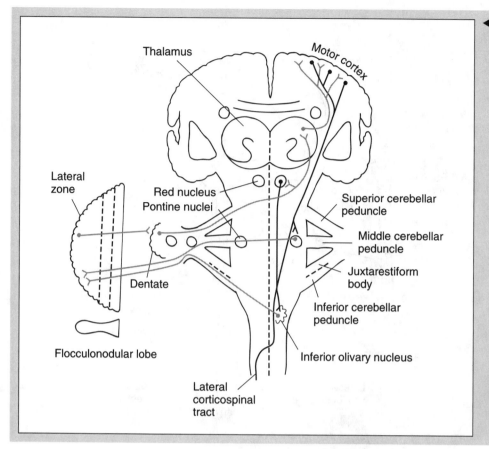

FIGURE 11-17
Cerebrocerebellar Circuitry. *The ascending projections from the cerebellum cross to the contralateral side of the brain. Because descending corticospinal projections cross back, cerebellar damage causes ipsilateral motor deficits.*

cakes is sufficient to create a motor template appropriate for each item. When we encounter an item that is heavier than expected, we usually abort the grasp and reposition our grip or stance to address the item again with better results.

In feedforward mode, the cerebrocerebellum also guides movements that are too quick to benefit from feedback (e.g., a golf swing). Swinging a golf club takes only a fraction of a second to complete, which is too brief a period to benefit from sensory feedback; proper execution depends on past experience. For an experienced golfer, the golf swing is an automatic movement orchestrated by the cerebellum; conscious (i.e., originating in the cerebral cortex) manipulation of the swing is usually counterproductive. After adopting a new golf swing, it is necessary to practice until the cerebellum assumes control of it and executes it automatically.

> *In feedforward mode, the cerebellum uses previous experience to generate a motor sequence.*

Spinocerebellum. The spinocerebellum consists of the vermal and paravermal zones of the anterior and posterior lobes and the fastigial and interposed nuclei, respectively. The vermal and paravermal zones adjust torso and limb position based on feedback from muscle spindles (Ia) and Golgi tendon organs (Ib). Kinesthetic information from the upper limbs is conveyed by the cuneocerebellar tract while the lower limbs are innervated by the dorsal and ventral spinocerebellar tracts. The courses of these ascending pathways differ substantially, but all three convey information from the periphery to the ipsilateral side of the cerebellum (see Chapter 3).

> *The **spinocerebellum** is known as the paleocerebellum.*

Projections from the vermal and paravermal zones of the cerebellum originate from the fastigial and interposed nuclei (Figure 11-18). Projections from the fastigial nuclei to the vestibular nuclei and reticular formation, like those of the vestibulocerebellum described above, enable the vermal zone to adjust the axial musculature of the body. The projections from the paravermal zone to the interposed nuclei, by comparison, control the distal musculature and modulate muscle tone. Axons originating in the interposed nuclei exit the cerebellum through the superior cerebellar peduncle, decussate in the lower mesencephalon, and ascend to the red nucleus and the VL nucleus of the thalamus, which projects to the MI cortex (see Chapter 4, Figure 4-24). The projections to the red nucleus terminate in the caudal, magnocellular region from which the rubro-

> *Cerebellar lesions affect the ipsilateral side of the body.*

FIGURE 11-18 ▶
Projections of the Spinocerebellum. *Efferent projections of the spinocerebellum resemble those of the vestibulocerebellum and the cerebrocerebellum.*

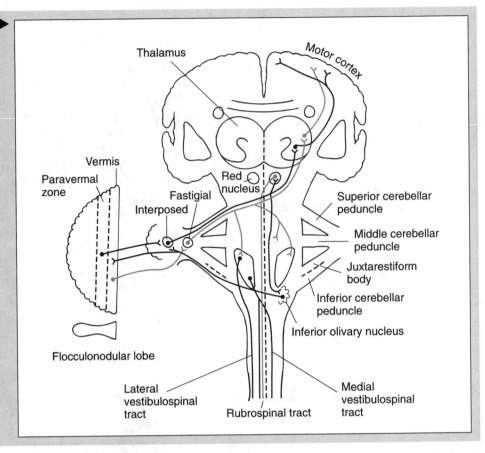

FIGURE 11-18 ▶
Projections of the Spinocerebellum. *Efferent projections of the spinocerebellum resemble those of the vestibulocerebellum and the cerebrocerebellum.*

spinal tract originates. The rubrospinal tract works in concert with the corticospinal tract to facilitate the flexors of the distal musculature.

As would be predicted from the efferent projections of the spinocerebellum, damage to the vermal and paravermal areas upsets balance and control of the proximal musculature. Spinocerebellar damage also disrupts velocity and force of individual movements as well as the timing of complex movements. It is unusual, however, for patients to have damage restricted to the spinocerebellum.

Clinical Aspects

Despite the importance of the cerebellum to movement, its removal does not cause paralysis or paresis. Indeed, patients with cerebellar damage can do everything that a healthy person can, but the quality of performance is poor. The core deficit underlying all cerebellar symptomology appears to be poor temporal coordination because cerebellar damage disrupts the timing sequences that coordinate complex, multijoint/multimuscle movements related to balance, posture, walking, reaching, speaking, and visual fixation.

Ataxia. Damage to the lateral zone, by affecting the coordination of the extremities, results in an unsteady gait. Ataxic patients may compensate by assuming a broad-based stance, but falls are common, usually after staggering toward the side of the lesion. The staggering of ataxic patients resembles that of drunkenness; similarly, one diagnostic test for cerebellar ataxia is heel–toe walking. Ataxia may be accompanied by *myoclonic movements.*

The *Romberg test* is used to determine whether an ataxic gait is of spinal or cerebellar origin. Standing is a postural reflex that depends on visual, vestibular, and kinesthetic projections to the cerebellum. Visual feedback, which the physician can manipulate easily by asking patients to close their eyes, is a critical component. When patients with cerebellar damage stand and close their eyes, they often lose their balance and fall if left unsupported. This is a positive Romberg sign. Although some patients with spinal cord damage may have difficulty standing, closing their eyes does not exacerbate their condition.

Cerebellar ataxia resembles drunkenness.

Myoclonic movements are abrupt, almost shock-like movements of a muscle group or limb.

When patients with cerebellar ataxia close their eyes, they risk falling (Romberg sign).

Dysmetria. Patients with dysmetria are unable to gauge the distance to a target accurately. Reaching motions overshoot the target and may be accompanied by tremor and oscillating movements until the patient eventually homes in on the target. Patients with saccadic dysmetria show a similar pattern of overshoot and oscillation during visual fixation.

Hypotonia. Cerebellar damage produces hypotonia through reduced activation of the α- and γ-motor systems. Loss of muscle tone can be observed by direct inspection or by testing for motor rebound. Testing for rebound involves pulling against the patient's flexed arm and then suddenly letting go. Normal patients will prevent the arm from striking them in the face.

Dysdiadochokinesia. One of the hallmark symptoms of cerebellar damage is dysdiadochokinesia, an inability to perform rapid, alternating movements. Patients with cerebellar damage are unable to pronate and supinate their hands while patting their thighs rapidly.

Decomposition of Movement. Patients with cerebellar damage often have trouble initiating movements, especially those that involve either multiple muscle groups or coordination of the axial and distal musculature. To compensate, patients may decompose complex movements into their component parts. For example, swinging a tennis racket, which normally involves a sweeping arm motion combined with rotation of the torso would be performed as serial rather than simultaneous motions. Decomposition of movement is caused by a breakdown in timing between agonist and antagonist muscle groups and gives movement a robotic appearance.

> *Dysmetria* describes arm movements that overshoot or undershoot their target.

> *Dysdiadochokinesia* describes an inability to perform rapidly alternating movements.

RESOLUTION OF CLINICAL CASE

B. T. was showing early signs of Huntington's chorea. At this time, B. T.'s symptoms are mild. He shows minor choreiform movements of the arms and minor impairment of manual dexterity. These problems will progress until the diagnosis of Huntington's chorea is unmistakable. Although it is too soon to tell if his business problems reflect cognitive impairment, eventually B. T. will not be able to manage either his business or his family affairs. Odd and inexplicable behaviors like polishing the pitchfork may increase over time. B. T. would likely respond to antidepressants. The physician may be able to make a more certain diagnosis after receiving the results from the genetic testing.

REVIEW QUESTIONS

Directions: For each of the following questions, choose the **one best** answer.

1. One positive symptom of Parkinson's disease is
   (A) bradykinesia
   (B) tremor
   (C) facial akinesia
   (D) lead pipe rigidity
   (E) mutism

2. The only excitatory neuron in the cerebellar cortex is the
   (A) basket cell
   (B) Purkinje cell
   (C) granule cell
   (D) Golgi cell
   (E) stellate cell

3. Efferent projections from the globus pallidus to the thalamus
   (A) project to nuclei, which in turn project to Brodmann area 6
   (B) overlap those originating from the contralateral deep cerebellar nuclei
   (C) project to nuclei, which in turn project to the primary motor cortex
   (D) overlap those originating in the substantia nigra
   (E) originate from cells in the lateral pallidal segment

4. If a patient experienced a seizure in the shoulder and the epileptiform activity spread laterally across cortex, how would the seizure spread across the body?
   (A) Shoulder, elbow, wrist, fingers, face, and mouth
   (B) Shoulder, face, mouth, fingers, and wrist
   (C) Shoulder, trunk, leg, and foot
   (D) Shoulder, elbow, wrist, fingers, maxillary face, and ophthalmic face
   (E) None of the above

5. Which of the following nuclei of the basal ganglia is the key excitatory relay in the indirect pathway?
   (A) Striatum
   (B) Subthalamic nucleus
   (C) Substantia nigra, pars compacta (SNc)
   (D) Internal segment of the globus pallidus (GPi)
   (E) External segment of the globus pallidus (GPe)

6. A 62-year-old woman presented with an 8-month history of gradually progressive incoordination of the right arm and leg. Examination revealed hypotonia and ataxia of the limbs on the right side. The most likely diagnosis is

- **(A)** a stroke involving the anterior spinal artery on the left side above the pyramidal decussation
- **(B)** a tumor within the right cerebellar hemisphere
- **(C)** a tumor within the left subthalamic nucleus
- **(D)** a stroke involving the crus cerebri on the right side
- **(E)** a tumor at the C5 level of the spinal cord affecting most of the lateral funiculus on the right side

ANSWERS AND EXPLANATIONS

1. The answer is B. Tremor is an involuntary shaking that appears most often in the hands, lips, and tongue, but in advanced cases, may involve the trunk. Because these tremors are involuntary, they are positive signs that the basal ganglia are unable to suppress. Bradykinesia, facial akinesia, lead pipe rigidity, and mutism are negative signs, caused by pathologic retardation of normal movement by ineffective basal ganglia.

2. The answer is C. Granule cells are the only excitatory neurons in the cerebellar cortex. Granule cells and climbing fibers, which originate in the inferior olivary nuclei, excite Purkinje cells. Basket cells, Purkinje cells, Golgi cells, and stellate cells are inhibitory.

3. The answer is A. The efferent projections of the internal pallidal segment (GPi) terminate in the ventral anterior and ventral lateral nuclei of the thalamus, which in turn project to Brodmann area 6. These pallidothalamic projections do not overlap other ascending projections from the substantia nigra or the cerebellum.

4. The answer is A. Seizures that spread across the motor cortex follow a pattern known as the Jacksonian march, named after the 19th century neurologist who first reported the phenomenon. As epileptiform activity spreads across the motor cortex, the seizure progresses across the body following the pattern of the motor homunculus, that is, shoulder, elbow, wrist, fingers, face, and mouth.

5. The answer is B. The subthalamic nucleus is the key relay in the indirect pathway because it modulates the suppressive effect of the basal ganglia on the motor nuclei of the thalamus. The striatum, SNc, GPi, and GPe contribute to both the direct and indirect pathways.

6. The answer is B. A tumor in the right cerebellum produces limb incoordination on the ipsilateral side. An infarct of the anterior spinal artery on the left side above the pyramidal decussation would produce a spastic paralysis on the right side. Left-side damage to the subthalamic nucleus would produce ballistic movements of the right limbs, but not incoordination, per se. An infarct of the right crus cerebri would produce a left-sided spastic paralysis. Damage to the lateral funiculus at C5 most likely would affect the α-motor neurons of the anterior horn and cause a flaccid paralysis.

ADDITIONAL READING

Alexander GE, DeLong MR, Strick PL: Parallel organization of functionally segregated circuits linking basal ganglia and cortex. *Ann Rev Neurosci* 9:357–381, 1986.

Bastien JJ, Thach WT: Cerebellar outflow lesions: a comparison of movement deficits resulting from lesions at the levels of the cerebellum and thalamus. *Ann Neurol* 38:881–892, 1995.

DeLong MR: Primate models of movement disorders of basal ganglia origin. *Trends Neurosci* 13:281–285, 1990.

DeLong MR, Wichman T: Basal ganglia—thalamocortical circuits in Parkinsonian signs. *Clin Neurosci* 1:18–26, 1993.

Georgopoulos AP, Kalaska JF, Caminiti R, Massey JT: On the relations between the direction of two-dimensional arm movements and cell discharge in primate motor cortex. *J Neurosci* 2:1527–1537, 1982.

Goetz CG, DeLong MR, Penn RD, Bakay RAE: Neurosurgical horizons in Parkinson's disease. *Neurology* 43:1–7, 1993.

Roland PE, Larsen B, Lassen NA, Skinhof E: Supplementary motor area and other cortical areas in organization of voluntary movements in man. *J Neurophysiol* 43:118–136, 1980.

Tanji J: The supplementary motor area in the cerebral cortex. *Neurosci Res* 19:251–268, 1994.

Tanji J, Shima K: Role for supplementary motor area cells in planning several movements ahead. *Nature* 371:413–416, 1994.

Thach WT, Goodkin HP, Keating JG: The cerebellum and the adaptive coordination of movement. *Ann Rev Neurosci* 15:403–442, 1992.

12

NEURAL AND NEUROENDOCRINE CONTROL OF AUTONOMIC FUNCTION

INTRODUCTION OF CLINICAL CASE

After months of gradually deteriorating health, L. J., a 47-year-old man, finally scheduled an appointment with his physician following a recent bout of unrelenting headaches. L. J. reported unusual fatigue and an almost unquenchable thirst. For L. J., the thirst was not as much of a problem as the frequent urination, which interfered with sleep, work, shopping, and travel. During this visit, L. J. also asked for a new eyeglass prescription.

Testing of L. J. was performed over a 3-day period. Reflexes were normal, and there was no evidence of papilledema. His urine had a low specific gravity (1.003), but glucose was within the normal range. A subcutaneous injection of vasopressin reduced the volume of urinary output and increased its osmolarity. L. J.'s vision, which had been corrected to 20/20 with his current eyeglasses, was only 20/40 now. A magnetic resonance imaging (MRI) scan of the head was scheduled, and additional blood was taken. After reviewing the results of the MRI, the physician requested that L. J. have his visual fields measured in the ophthalmology clinic; a bitemporal hemianopsia was detected.

OVERVIEW

The autonomic nervous system (ANS) regulates the cardiovascular, pulmonary, gastrointestinal, renal, hepatic, excretory, and reproductive systems of the body to meet the body's changing needs for oxygen, nutrients, and electrolytes and maintain proper serum osmolarity and core body temperature. During stressful situations or exercise, the ANS releases glycogen from the liver and increases cardiopulmonary output while diverting energy from the skin and digestive tract. At rest, the process is reversed as energy stores are increased. In short, the ANS adjusts visceral activity to meet the ever changing demands placed on the body, a process called *homeostasis*.

Autonomic function is under both neural and hormonal control. Neural control ensures quick and timely activation, but the effects are often short-lived. Hormonal effects are more persistent but develop more slowly. Homeostasis requires the coordinated action of both systems. Neural control of autonomic function originates from multiple areas in the brain and spinal cord while hormonal control comes from both central (e.g., hypothalamus, hypophysis) and peripheral (e.g., adrenal gland, gonads) sites.

*In the somatomotor system, a single neuron constitutes the **final common pathway**.*

In the visceromotor system, the final common pathway involves two neurons.

Although the ANS is predominantly a motor system, it differs significantly from the somatic motor system. The most obvious difference between the somatic and visceral motor systems is the relative lack of volitional control over autonomic function. In addition, their degree of reliance on central innervation differs. Denervation of somatic muscles causes paralysis, but denervated viscera and glands continue functioning, although they are unable to respond to a physiologic challenge such as exertion. Activation of the ANS often affects multiple systems in the body, unlike the somatic motor system, which is capable of more discrete actions. Not surprisingly, there are a host of anatomic differences between the somatic and visceral motor systems.

AUTONOMIC NERVOUS SYSTEM

The ANS consists of the SNS, the PNS, and the ENS.

The ANS consists of three divisions: the *sympathetic nervous system (SNS)*, the *parasympathetic nervous system (PNS)*, and the *enteric nervous system (ENS)*. The SNS and PNS control smooth muscle, cardiac muscle, and glandular secretory cells. Although most smooth muscle lines the viscera of the thoracic and abdominal cavities, other sites under autonomic control include the iris, the vasculature of the skin and muscles, sweat glands, and muscles of piloerection. Many, but not all, receive complementary innervation from both the SNS and PNS. The ENS is a semiautonomous neural network that controls intestinal motility and digestive secretions. Mechanical and chemosensory feedback from receptors in the walls of the thoracic, abdominal, and pelvic viscera as well as the upper gastrointestinal tract reach the central nervous system (CNS) along multiple pathways (see below).

The PNS saves energy; the SNS spends energy.

Sympathetic Nervous System

The SNS is responsible for flight or fight behaviors.

The SNS mobilizes the body's resources for fight or flight behaviors. Sympathetic effects include widespread changes in cardiac, pulmonary, hepatic, and gastrointestinal activity, all of which are intended to ready the body for some type of emergency. Sympathetic activation takes place quickly, but its effects are relatively short-lived. The organization of the SNS is ideally suited for these purposes.

SNS postganglionic sympathetic neurons are located in ganglia adjacent to the thoracolumbar segments of the spinal cord.

Sympathetic *preganglionic neurons* are located in the lateral horn (Rexed lamina VII) of the spinal cord between segments T1 and L2–L3 (Figure 12-1; see Chapter 3,

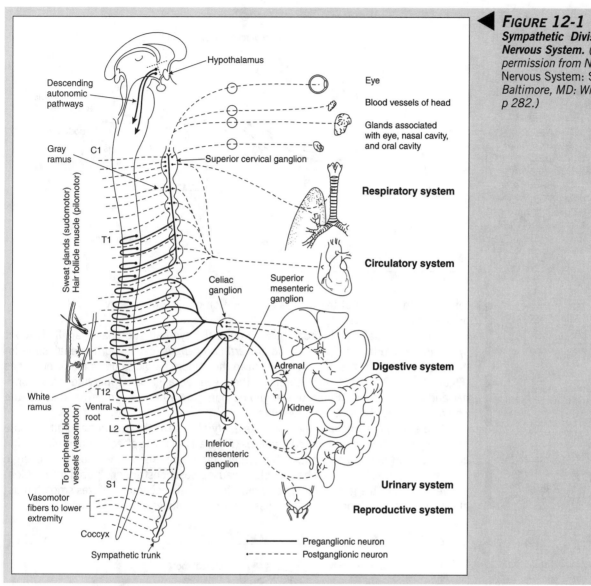

FIGURE 12-1
Sympathetic Division of the Autonomic Nervous System. (Source: *Reprinted with permission from Noback CR, et al:* Human Nervous System: Structure and Function. *Baltimore, MD: Williams & Wilkins, 1996, p 282.)*

Figure 3-8D). Most preganglionic axons exit the spinal cord and travel with the ventral root a short distance before forming the *white communicating ramus* that enters the *paravertebral ganglia* (Figure 12-2). The paravertebral ganglia form a continuous column called the *sympathetic chain* that stretches along the lateral margin of the vertebral column from the base of the skull to the coccyx. Within the ganglia, there is substantial synaptic convergence between the preganglionic and postganglionic neurons. The axons of *postganglionic neurons* exit the paravertebral ganglia as the *gray communicating ramus*; these axons rejoin their respective spinal nerves and distribute to a variety of peripheral structures including blood vessels, sweat glands, and hair follicles. None of these structures, however, receive complementary innervation from the PNS.

At thoracic, lumbar, and sacral levels, the sympathetic chain ganglia have a one-to-one relationship with their corresponding spinal nerves (see Figure 12-1). In the cervical spinal cord, however, sympathetic preganglionic fibers from the eight segments coalesce into three ganglia, the most important of which is the superior cervical ganglion. Postganglionic neurons in the *superior cervical ganglion* innervate visceral targets within the head such as the sweat and lacrimal glands, the pupillary dilator muscle, and the levator palpebrae muscle. The superior cervical ganglion also innervates the vasculature of the skin, whose somatosensory innervation derives from the first four cervical nerves. Damage to the superior cervical ganglion or its afferent projections from the brainstem produces pupillary constriction (miosis), loss of sweating (anhidrosis), drooping of the eyelid

A ganglion (pl. ganglia) is a collection of neurons located outside the CNS.

The **white communicating rami** consist of thinly myelinated, preganglionic fibers.

The sympathetic chain ganglia run from the base of the skull to the coccyx.

The **gray communicating rami** consist of unmyelinated, postganglionic fibers.

FIGURE 12-2 ▶
Sympathetic Efferent Pathways. *Sympathetic preganglionic neurons exit the spinal cord through the ventral roots and join the spinal nerves briefly before entering the sympathetic chain ganglia as the white rami and synapsing on the postganglionic neurons. Postganglionic neurons exit the chain ganglia within the gray rami, rejoin the spinal nerves, and synapse on sebaceous glands and piloerector muscles of the skin and blood vessels of the limbs.* (Source: *Reprinted with permission from Hardy SGP, et al: Viscerosensory pathways. In* Fundamental Neuroscience. *Edited by Haines DE. New York, NY: Churchill Livingstone, 1997, p 422.*)

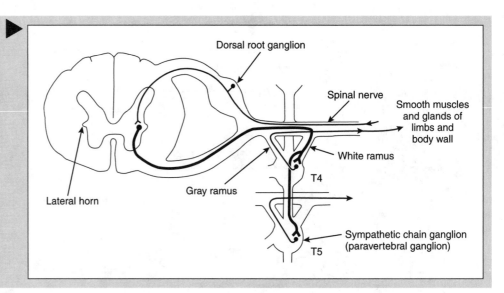

> The preganglionic axons that project to the prevertebral ganglia are called splanchnic nerves.

> The neurosecretory cells of the adrenal cortex develop from chromaffin cells of the neural crest.

> Functionally, the chromaffin cells of the adrenal medulla are analogous to the postganglionic neurons of the sympathetic ganglion.

(ptosis), and flushing of the face, a constellation of symptoms known as Horner's syndrome (see Chapter 4).

Some preganglionic neurons pass through the sympathetic chain ganglia without synapsing and terminate in one of the *prevertebral ganglia* (celiac, aorticorenal, superior mesenteric, inferior mesenteric) adjacent to the abdominal aorta or its major branches (Figure 12-3). Postganglionic neurons in the prevertebral ganglia innervate the abdominal and pelvic viscera. Some preganglionic parasympathetic neurons synapse on the *chromaffin cells* of the *adrenal medulla*.

In the SNS preganglionic neurons use *acetylcholine* as their neurotransmitter while postganglionic neurons use *norepinephrine* (Figure 12-4). The effects of norepinephrine administration depend on whether the target organ contains alpha- or beta-adrenergic receptors. Stimulation of alpha-receptors causes vasoconstriction, pupillary dilation, and relaxation of the gut. Adrenergic stimulation of beta-receptors relaxes smooth muscle, which causes bronchodilation, vasodilation in skeletal muscles, and decreased

FIGURE 12-3 ▶
Pathways of the Cardiac and Splanchnic Nerves. *The cardiac and splanchnic nerves are preganglionic axons that pass through the sympathetic chain ganglia without synapsing and terminate in the prevertebral ganglia.* (Source: *Reprinted with permission from Hardy SGP, et al: Viscerosensory pathways. In* Fundamental Neuroscience. *Edited by Haines DE. New York, NY: Churchill Livingstone, 1997, p 257.*)

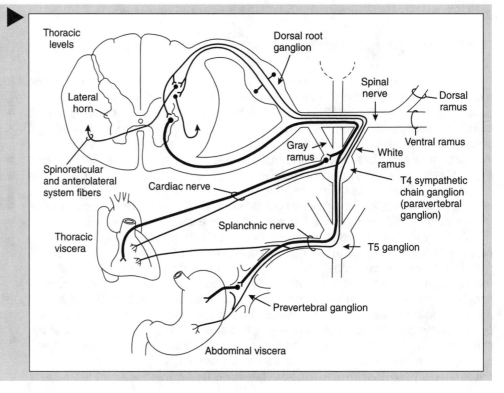

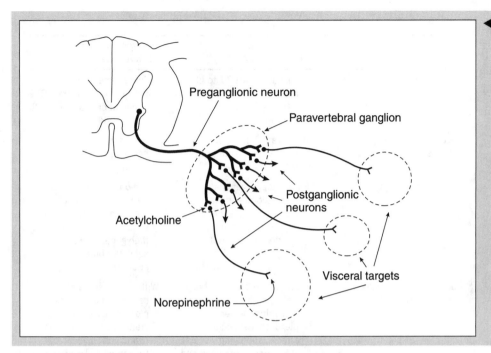

◀ **FIGURE 12-4**
***Efferent Limb of the Sympathetic Nervous
System.*** *The widespread effects of the
sympathetic nervous system are due, in
part, to the fact that individual preganglionic neurons which synapse on many
postganglionic neurons.*

intestinal peristalsis as well as increased heart rate and contractility. Epinephrine, a more
effective agonist than norepinephrine at both alpha- and beta-adrenergic receptors, is
used as a bronchodilator for asthma attacks and a cardiac stimulant following arrest of
the heart.

Preganglionic projections to the adrenal gland coordinate the widespread actions of
the SNS. In most of the SNS, preganglionic neurons project to postganglionic neurons,
which in turn release norepinephrine at terminals within the target organ. In the adrenal
medulla, the chromaffin cells act as the postganglionic neurons of the sympathetic chain
ganglion but release epinephrine into the systemic circulation to achieve the widest
possible distribution. By activating the adrenal medulla, the SNS prepares both the
visceral and somatic musculature for emergency mobilization.

Most fibers conveying pain from the abdominal and pelvic viscera enter the CNS
through the sympathetic nerves. The cell bodies of these visceral afferent neurons are
located in the dorsal root ganglia. Although the central projections of these *visceral
afferent neurons* cells have not been completely elucidated, some ascend with the
anterolateral system to the ventral posterior nucleus of the thalamus. Other nociceptive
sensations are relayed by the reticular formation to the hypothalamus. Unlike the somatosensory system, visceral afferent sensations are poorly localized; indeed, sensations
from the viscera often refer to skin, muscles, or limbs (see Chapter 6).

> *Exception: postganglionic neurons that in-
> nervate sweat glands are cholinergic.*

Parasympathetic Nervous System

The PNS is most active when the time for flight or fight has passed and the body is ready
to rest and digest. The PNS conserves energy by slowing cardiopulmonary function and
attending to digestion (salivation, gastrointestinal peristalsis, secretion), urination, defecation, and reproduction. The differences between the SNS and the PNS are listed in
Table 12-1.

Parasympathetic preganglionic neurons, like their sympathetic counterparts, have
their embryologic origin in the general visceral efferent (GVE) cell column (see Chapter 4,
Figure 4-1). Unlike the sympathetic preganglionic neurons which are distributed
throughout the thoracolumbar spinal cord, however, parasympathetic preganglionic neurons are located in the brainstem and in sacral segments S2, S3, and S4 (Figure 12-5).
The parasympathetic preganglionic neurons in the sacral spinal cord are located along
the lateral edge of the central gray, despite the fact that there is no lateral horn per se at
sacral levels.

Like the SNS, the efferent pathway of the PNS consists of preganglionic neurons

> *The PNS takes over when it is time to rest
> and digest.*

> *Preganglionic parasympathetic neurons
> are located in the brainstem and at sacral
> cord levels.*

TABLE 12-1 ▶

Comparison of the Sympathetic and Parasympathetic Divisions of Autonomic Outflow

Feature	Sympathetic (Thoracolumbar)	Parasympathetic (Craniosacral)
Location of preganglionic cell bodies	Spinal segments T1 to L2 mainly within the intermediolateral cell column	Spinal segments S2–S4 in the intermediate gray; GVE nuclei of cranial nerves III, VII, IX, and X
Location of preganglionic fibers	White rami T1 to L2, sympathetic trunks, and splanchnic nerves	Pelvic nerves and cranial nerves III, VII, IX, and X
Location of postganglionic cell bodies	Paravertebral ganglia and prevertebral ganglia (celiac, aorticorenal, superior mesenteric, inferior mesenteric)	Ganglion cell clusters in walls of viscera and cranial nerve autonomic ganglia (ciliary—III; pterygopalatine and submandibular—VII; otic—IX)
Location of postganglionic nerve fibers	Fibers to structures of body wall and limbs in gray rami and spinal nerves; plexuses associated with arteries supplying visceral structures of the head and body cavities	Within the viscera of body cavities; short nerves or plexuses extending from cranial ganglia to target organs; often accompany trigeminal nerve branches in head
Target effectors	Smooth muscle, cardiac muscle, and secretory cells throughout body	Mostly viscera of the head thoracic, abdominal, and pelvic cavities
Primary neurotransmitter of preganglionic neurons	Acetylcholine	Acetylcholine
Primary neurotransmitters of postganglionic neurons	Norepinephrine	Acetylcholine
General physiologic effects	Mobilization of resources for intensive activity	Promotion of restorative processes

NOTE. GVE = general visceral efferent.
Source: Reprinted with permission from Hardy SGP, et al: Viscerosensory pathways. In *Fundamental Neuroscience*. Edited by Haines DE. New York, NY: Churchill Livingstone, 1997, p 257.

The organ specificity of the PNS derives, in part, from the use of a long preganglionic axon and a short postganglionic axon.

and postganglionic neurons. In contrast to the chain ganglia of the SNS, the parasympathetic postganglionic neurons are located in discrete ganglia close to their visceral targets. For example, the postganglionic neurons that innervate the iris are located in the ciliary ganglion within the eye itself. Because the parasympathetic postganglionic neurons are adjacent to their visceral targets, the preganglionic axon is much longer than the postganglionic axon. This contrasts with the SNS in which preganglionic axons are shorter than the postganglionic fibers.

The proximity of the autonomic ganglia to their respective target organs reflects the specificity of parasympathetic action compared to the more diffuse action of the SNS. The specificity of the PNS also is reflected in the synaptic organization of the parasympathetic ganglia where preganglionic axons typically synapse on relatively few postganglionic neurons (Figure 12-6). Both pre- and postganglionic neurons in the PNS use acetylcholine as their neurotransmitter.

Afferent projections from non-nociceptive receptors in the pharynx, larynx, trachea, lungs, esophagus, heart, stomach, and liver form the afferent limbs of visceromotor, vasomotor, and secretory reflexes. Afferent projections from these visceral areas enter the CNS through the glossopharyngeal and vagus nerves and terminate in the caudal half of the nucleus of the solitary tract (NST). Local projections from the NST contribute to a number of vital reflexes (see below and Chapter 4). Ascending projections to the hypothalamus and pontine parabrachial nuclei enable afferent information from the viscera to reach the limbic forebrain (see Chapter 13).

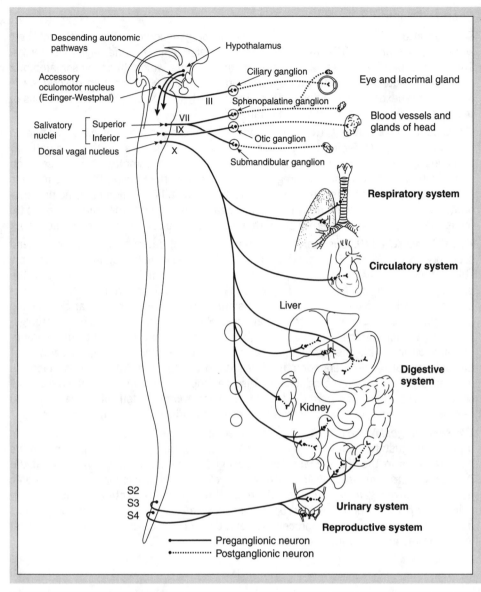

Parasympathetic Division of the Auto-nomic Nervous System. (Source: *Re-printed with permission from Noback CR, et al:* Human Nervous System: Structure and Function. *Baltimore, MD: Williams & Wilkins, 1996, p 284.*)

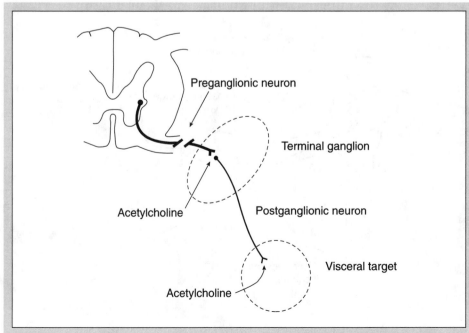

Efferent Limb of the Parasympathetic Nervous System. *The relatively discrete actions of the parasympathetic nervous system are due to the fact that individual preganglionic neurons synapse on only a few postganglionic neurons.*

CRANIAL DIVISION

The cranial division of the PNS consists of the preganglionic parasympathetic fibers within the oculomotor (III), facial (VII), glossopharyngeal (IX), and vagus (X) nerves. These nerves participate in a variety of autonomic reflexes, which, like their somatomotor counterparts, consist of both afferent and efferent limbs. This section describes the autonomic reflexes associated with cranial nerves III, VII, IX, and X; other functions of these cranial nerves are described in Chapter 4.

Oculomotor Nerve (CN III). The accommodation reflex is triggered by visual fixation on nearby objects. The afferent limb of the accommodation reflex is a multineuron pathway that ends in the Edinger-Westphal nucleus of the oculomotor complex. The efferent limb begins with the parasympathetic preganglionic neurons in the Edinger-Westphal nucleus that synapse with postganglionic neurons located in the ciliary ganglion of the posterior orbit. The postganglionic neurons in the ciliary ganglion innervate the ciliary muscles (to focus the lens) and sphincter muscles (to constrict the pupil) during accommodation.

Facial Nerve (CN VII). Gustatory stimulation of the oral cavity triggers salivatory and secretory reflexes that aid digestion. The facial nerve, which responds to gustatory stimulation of the anterior tongue, projects to the NST, which in turn projects to the *superior salivatory nucleus.* Preganglionic parasympathetic neurons in the superior salivatory nucleus project to the pterygopalatine and submandibular ganglia via the intermediate nerve, a branch of the facial nerve. Postganglionic neurons in the pterygopalatine ganglion innervate the lacrimal glands (tears) while those in the submandibular ganglion innervate the submandibular and sublingual glands (saliva). Regrowth of damaged facial nerve fibers sometimes results in crossed innervation of the lacrimal and salivary glands, which produces the disorder popularly known as "crocodile tears." Other efferent projections from the NST to the dorsal motor nucleus of the vagus (DMX) release gastric acid from the stomach and insulin from islet cells in the pancreas.

Glossopharyngeal Nerve (CN IX). Salivation mediated by the inferior salivatory nucleus is triggered by gustatory stimulation of the glossopharyngeal nerve, which projects to the NST. Neurons in the NST synapse on preganglionic parasympathetic neurons in the *inferior salivatory nucleus,* which in turn project to the *otic ganglion.* Postganglionic neurons in the otic ganglion complete the reflex through their projections to the secretory cells of the parotid gland. The glossopharyngeal nerve also contains afferent projections from baroreceptors and chemoreceptors (oxygen and carbon dioxide concentrations) located in the carotid sinus and carotid body, respectively (Figure 12-7).

> The superior salivatory nucleus is located near the medial edge of the NST.

> Patients with "crocodile tears" report that foods or beverages that normally produce salivation induce tearing instead.

> Baroreceptors detect changes in blood pressure.

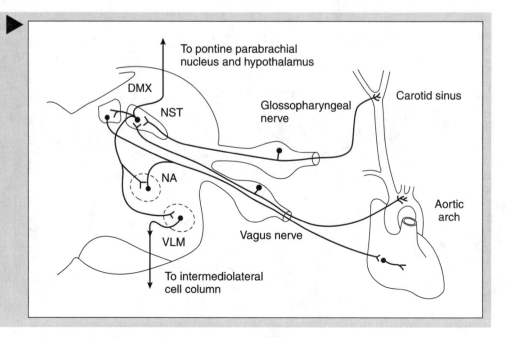

FIGURE 12-7

Carotid Sinus Reflex. Afferent projections from receptors located in the carotid sinus and aortic arch terminate in the caudal part of the nucleus of the solitary tract (NST). Ascending projections enter the limbic system through the pontine parabrachial nucleus. Efferent projections from the dorsal motor nucleus of the vagus (DMX) and the nucleus ambiguus make compensatory adjustments to the heart. NAS = nucleus ambiguus; VLM = ventral lateral medulla.

To pontine parabrachial nucleus and hypothalamus

DMX

NST

Glossopharyngeal nerve

Carotid sinus

NA

Aortic arch

Vagus nerve

VLM

To intermediolateral cell column

Vagus Nerve (CN X). The vagus nerve is a mixed nerve of branchiomeric origin that contains both special visceral afferent (SVA) fibers and general visceral afferent (GVA) fibers. The SVA fibers innervate taste buds around the epiglottis (see Chapter 9). The GVA fibers from the pharynx, larynx, trachea, lungs, esophagus, heart, liver, pancreas, stomach, and liver mediate a number of autonomic reflexes. The afferent limb of these reflexes is carried by the vagus nerve to the NST.

Fluid or mechanical stimulation of the larynx and pharynx initiates coughing, gagging, and vomiting reflexes designed to preserve airway patency. These reflexes are executed by projections from the DMX to the nucleus ambiguus, the phrenic nucleus, and the motor neurons in the thoracic spinal cord.

Other GVA fibers that innervate *baroreceptors* and *chemoreceptors* along the aortic arch and right atrium are vagal analogs to the pressure and chemical sensors in the *carotid sinus* and *carotid body* described above (see Figure 12-7). Feedback from the baroreceptors decrease heart rate and blood pressure by simultaneously increasing parasympathetic control of the heart while decreasing sympathetic activation. The parasympathetic effects are mediated by excitatory projections from the NST to the DMX and the nucleus ambiguus. Decreases in sympathetic tone are mediated by inhibitory projections from the NST to the rostral ventrolateral medulla.

Afferent projections from the thoracic and abdominal viscera to the NST ascend to the *paraventricular nucleus (PVN)* of the hypothalamus and the pontine parabrachial nucleus. The PVN affects cardiovascular function directly via descending sympathetic projections to the thoracic spinal cord and indirectly through vasopressin release by the neurohypophysis. Visceral afferent information that reaches the pontine parabrachial nucleus is relayed to the amygdala, the hypothalamus, and the bed nucleus of the stria terminalis, which are involved with emotion, motivation, and learning.

SACRAL DIVISION

The sacral division of the PNS consists of preganglionic neurons located in the lateral part of the central gray of sacral segments S2, S3, and S4. Preganglionic axons exit the spinal cord with the ventral roots and course directly to the target organs where they synapse with the postganglionic neurons. The short postganglionic axons innervate the bladder, descending colon, rectum, and reproductive organs.

Enteric Nervous System

The ENS controls the motility of the gastrointestinal tract as well as secretions of the pancreas and gallbladder. The ENS consists of sensory receptors located throughout the gut that are linked with motor neurons by interneurons of the myenteric and submucosal plexuses. Food in the lumen of the gastrointestinal tract initiates secretion of gastric acid and bile into the stomach and small intestine as well as peristaltic movements, which propel food through the gastrointestinal tract. Although the ENS usually operates independently of the CNS, during emergencies the SNS may interrupt peristalsis and secretion.

AUTONOMIC FUNCTIONS

Micturition

In healthy individuals, urinary retention and evacuation depend on the cooperation among the SNS, PNS, and the somatic motor system. In general, urination is controlled by parasympathetic pathways, while urinary retention is maintained by sympathetic and somatomotor circuits (Figure 12-8).

Urination depends upon the cooperation of the SNS, the PNS, and the somatic motor system.

Micturition involves volitional control as well as an elaborate hierarchy of segmental and suprasegmental reflexes organized across spinal, brainstem, and cortical levels. The reflexes associated with micturition allow urination and some aspects of urinary retention to be controlled by the ANS.

Most of the neural circuitry that prevents urinary incontinence is located in the

FIGURE 12-8 ▶

Urinary Retention and Evacuation. *Control over micturition is exerted by the cerebral cortex, the pons, and the spinal cord. Urinary retention* (left) *is initiated by neurons in the cerebral cortex and pons, which facilitate sympathetic preganglionic neurons in spinal segments T12–S2 and somatic motor neurons at sacral levels. Urinary evacuation is initiated by cortical and pontine neurons, which (1) relax the internal and external sphincter muscles by inhibiting the retentive circuits described above and (2) contract the detrusor muscle of the bladder.*

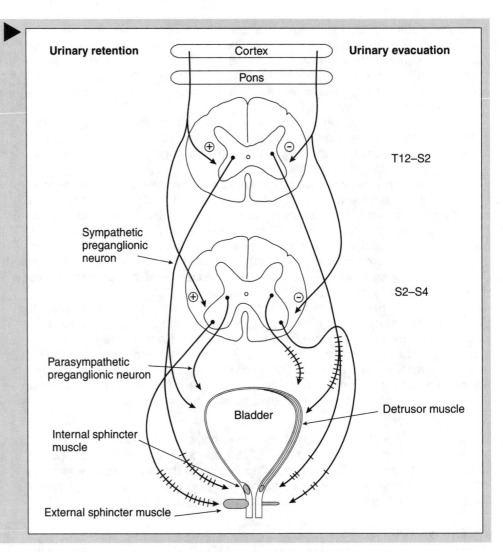

FIGURE 12-8 ▶

Urinary Retention and Evacuation. *Control over micturition is exerted by the cerebral cortex, the pons, and the spinal cord. Urinary retention* (left) *is initiated by neurons in the cerebral cortex and pons, which facilitate sympathetic preganglionic neurons in spinal segments T12–S2 and somatic motor neurons at sacral levels. Urinary evacuation is initiated by cortical and pontine neurons, which (1) relax the internal and external sphincter muscles by inhibiting the retentive circuits described above and (2) contract the detrusor muscle of the bladder.*

spinal cord. Bladder distention, detected by stretch receptors and nociceptors in the bladder walls, is transmitted to the spinal cord through the dorsal roots. When bladder distention is low, somatomotor neurons in the anterior horn of the S2–S4 segments (Onuf nucleus) reflexively tighten the striated muscles of the external urinary sphincter. Additional security is provided by sympathetic preganglionic neurons in the T12–S2 segments that contract the smooth muscles of the internal urinary sphincter and relax the detrusor muscles that line the walls of the bladder. These retentive mechanisms are facilitated by direct and indirect projections from the pons and cerebral cortex which activate the somatomotor neurons in the Onuf nucleus.

For urination to take place, the retentive reflexes are inhibited by micturition centers in the pons and cerebral cortex. Information regarding bladder distention ascends within the anterolateral, dorsal column, and medial lemniscal pathways to the ventral posterolateral nucleus of the thalamus; tertiary neurons in the thalamus may project to the parietal operculum of the postcentral sulcus. When bladder distention reaches a threshold level, we become conscious of the need to urinate. After retreating to a private area, voluntary urination is initiated by the cortical micturition center located along the medial wall of the superior frontal gyrus.

To urinate, the pons must release the internal and external sphincters that retain urine. Other descending projections from the pons to the S2–S4 segments engage preganglionic parasympathetic axons that contract the detrusor muscles of the bladder. Once the *micturition reflex* has begun, it continues until the bladder is virtually empty.

The widely distributed circuitry for micturition makes the system vulnerable to injury. Damage to the medial frontal lobes produces involuntary micturition, also known as an *uninhibited bladder*. Lesions that interrupt supraspinal micturition pathways produce an *automatic bladder*, which, as the name implies, voids automatically after filling to capacity. Damage to the sacral cord or the root fibers within the cauda equina produces an *atonic bladder*, which fills to capacity but, lacking parasympathetic control, cannot be emptied voluntarily. Some patients with an atonic bladder can void by compressing their abdominal muscles; most must be catheterized.

Erection and Ejaculation

The physiologic mechanisms that operate the male and female sex organs are remarkably similar and, like micturition, reflect the coordinated actions of the SNS, PNS, and the somatic motor system. Penile erection and clitoral erection are initiated by peripheral or psychogenic stimulation and executed by parasympathetic preganglionic neurons located in the S2–S4 segments of the spinal cord. Production of the ejaculate by the seminal vesicles and prostate gland and secretions from the vaginal walls are controlled by sympathetic and parasympathetic neurons in the thoracic, lumbar, and sacral spinal cord. Following seminal emission into the posterior urethra by the SNS, somatic motor reflexes initiate ejaculation.

Defecation

The stimulus for defecation is distention of the sigmoid colon by feces. Fecal matter is retained by an internal smooth muscle sphincter and an external striated muscle sphincter. The internal sphincter is innervated by sympathetic and parasympathetic fibers derived from the lower lumbar and sacral segments of the spinal cord, respectively. The external sphincter, unlike other striated muscles, is under both reflexive and voluntary control. Reflexive control preserves continence during sleep. Distention of the sigmoid colon produces simultaneous parasympathetic relaxation of the internal sphincter accompanied by tightening of the external sphincter. Defecation takes place following voluntary relaxation of the external sphincter.

Damage to the descending pathways leading to the parasympathetic preganglionic neurons of the sacral cord produces fecal retention, but lesions in the sacral cord or the cauda equina paralyze the external sphincter muscle, which causes fecal incontinence.

Denervation Hypersensitivity

Denervation of voluntary muscles causes paralysis and atrophy. Muscles and glands under autonomic control remain functional following denervation but develop a hypersensitivity to their normal neurotransmitters and agonists. For example, patients with Horner's syndrome demonstrate miosis due to interruption of the autonomic pathway that innervates the ciliary muscles of the eye. When the patient is aroused, circulating levels of epinephrine increase and activate the denervated, but hypersensitive, ciliary muscles. In patients with Horner's syndrome denervation hypersensitivity can be tested by dripping a 0.1% epinephrine solution into the conjunctival sac of the eye. Epinephrine at this dilution has no effect on healthy individuals but produces pupillary dilation in patients with sympathetic denervation.

GENERAL ORGANIZATION OF THE NEUROENDOCRINE SYSTEM

The combined and coordinated actions of the hypothalamus and hypophysis regulate a host of vital behavioral and endocrine processes. The hypothalamus is capable of targeting specific viscera or glands through autonomic and somatic motor pathways. More sweeping effects are mediated by hormones secreted either by the hypothalamus or by other endocrine sites controlled directly or indirectly by the hypothalamus (e.g., pituitary, gonads, adrenal medulla). Hormones released by the pituitary, which serves as the master gland of the endocrine system, influence growth, metabolism, parturition, lactation, reproduction, and water retention.

Medial frontal lobe damage produces an **uninhibited bladder**.

An **automatic bladder** fills to capacity and then voids automatically.

Lower motor neuron damage at the sacral level produces an **atonic bladder**.

Erection is driven by the PNS.

Lower motor neuron damage at the sacral level produces fecal incontinence.

Pituitary Gland

The pituitary gland or *hypophysis* resembles a small sack suspended from the ventral surface of the diencephalon into its bony case, the sella turcica (Figure 12-9). The stalk-like *infundibulum* provides a structural and functional link between the pituitary and the overlying hypothalamus. The pituitary consists of anterior (*adenohypophysis*) and posterior (*neurohypophysis*) lobes, which differ dramatically in terms of their development, anatomy, and function. The adenohypophysis develops as an outpouch from the underlying ectoderm of *Rathke's pouch*, originally part of the roof of the palate. As the immature adenohypophysis migrates dorsally, it fuses with the cells of the neurohypophysis, which forms as an evagination of the hypothalamic floor.

The **adenohypophysis** *is a derivative of non-neural ectoderm; the* **neurohypophysis** *develops from neuroepithelium.*

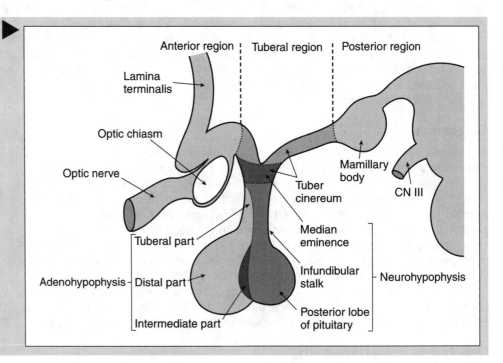

FIGURE 12-9 ▶
Diagram of the Hypothalamus and Hypophysis. *(Source: Reprinted with permission from Nolte J:* The Human Brain: An Introduction to Functional Anatomy. *Baltimore, MD: Mosby–Year Book, 1993, p 265.)*

The pituitary gland releases hormones that act on the body, the viscera, or other endocrine glands such as the gonads, the adrenals, and thyroid (Table 12-2). Hormone release from the adenohypophysis is triggered by regulatory hormones synthesized in the hypothalamus and transported vascularly to the anterior hypophysis through the *hypothalamic-hypophyseal portal system.* Two other hormones, vasopressin and oxytocin, are synthesized in the hypothalamus and transported axoplasmically by the *tuberoinfundibular tract* to the posterior hypophysis where they are released directly into the systemic circulation. The hypothalamic-hypophyseal portal system and the tuberoinfundibular tract are discussed below.

The hypothalamus is connected to the pituitary gland by the hypothalamico-hypophyseal tract and the tuberoinfundibular tract.

TABLE 12-2 ▶
Adenohypophyseal Hormones and Their Hypothalamic-Releasing Factors

Hypothalamic-Releasing Hormone	Adenohypophyseal Hormone
Thyrotropin-releasing hormone	Thyrotropin
Gonadotropin-releasing hormone Luteinizing hormone–releasing hormone	Luteinizing hormone; follicle-stimulating hormone
Corticotropin-releasing hormone	Adrenocorticotropin
Prolactin inhibitory factor, dopamine	Prolactin
Growth hormone–releasing hormone	Growth hormone (somatocrinin)
Growth hormone–inhibiting hormone	Growth hormone (somatostatin)

Hypothalamus

The hypothalamus constitutes only 4 g or 0.5% of the brain but is a critically important part of the brain. With the exception of the cerebral cortex, whose large size easily dwarfs the hypothalamus, no other area of the brain is involved in as many diverse functions. The pervasive effects of the hypothalamus derive from its widespread connections with other parts of the CNS and its neurohormonal control of the hypophysis.

The hypothalamus is a complex structure that consists of approximately 12 nuclei; most are small and poorly differentiated and are named according to their positions relative to the floor of the diencephalon or the third ventricle. For clarity of exposition as well as functional reasons, the hypothalamus typically is divided into coronal and sagittal zones.

When viewed in the coronal plane, the hypothalamus contains periventricular, middle, and lateral segments. The *periventricular segment* is a thin shell of neurons along the third ventricle whose *neurosecretory cells* regulate hormone release from the adenohypophysis. The *medial zone*, whose lateral boundary is marked by the fibers of the fornix, contains several distinct magnocellular nuclei that are closely related to the neurohypophysis. The *lateral segment* is a poorly differentiated region whose connections to the cerebral cortex, the extended amygdala, and other hypothalamic and brainstem nuclei enable it to link autonomic expression with behavior.

> In the coronal plane, the hypothalamus consists of periventricular, middle, and lateral segments.

In the sagittal plane the hypothalamus is divided into anterior (supraoptic), middle (tuberal), and posterior (mamillary) regions (Figure 12-10; see Figure 12-9). The *anterior hypothalamus* lies between the lamina terminalis and the caudal border of the optic chiasm (Figure 12-11; see Figure 12-10A; see Chapter 13, Figure 13-4). The *middle hypothalamus* surrounds the infundibular recess of the third ventricle, which lies between the optic chiasm and the mamillary bodies (see Figure 12-10B). The mamillary bodies, which form two prominent lumps on the basal surface of the diencephalon, mark the *posterior hypothalamus* (see Figures 12-10C and 12-11).

> In the sagittal plane, the hypothalamus consists of anterior, middle, and posterior zones.

ANTERIOR OR SUPRAOPTIC HYPOTHALAMUS

The narrow periventricular zone of the anterior and middle hypothalamus contains parvocellular neurons, which synthesize a host of hormones that modulate the activity of the anterior hypophysis (see below). The medial zone of the anterior hypothalamus

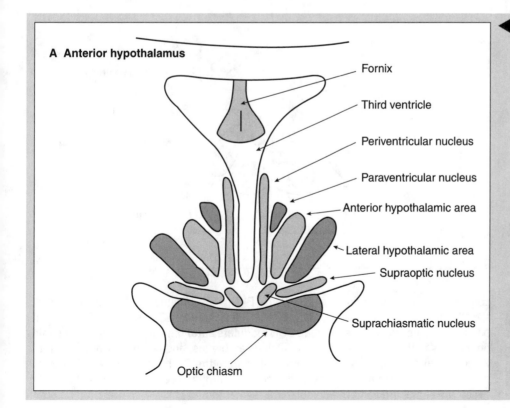

A Anterior hypothalamus

Fornix

Third ventricle

Periventricular nucleus

Paraventricular nucleus

Anterior hypothalamic area

Lateral hypothalamic area

Supraoptic nucleus

Suprachiasmatic nucleus

Optic chiasm

◀ *FIGURE 12-10A*
Diagram of the Hypothalamus in the Coronal Plane. *Anterior hypothalamus.* (Source: *Adapted from Freeman M: The hypothalamus. In* Neuroscience in Medicine. *Edited by Conn PM. Philadelphia, PA: J. B. Lippincott, 1995, p 266.)*

FIGURE 12-10B ▶
Diagram of the Hypothalamus in the Coronal Plane. *Middle hypothalamus.*

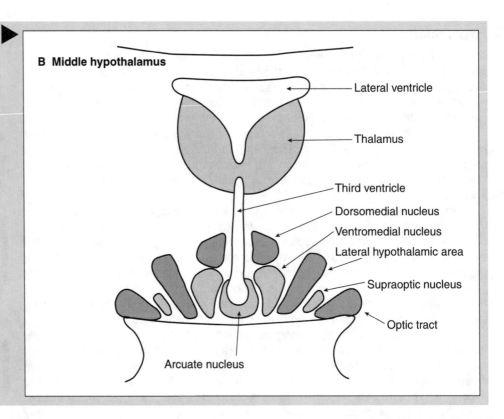

B Middle hypothalamus

Lateral ventricle

Thalamus

Third ventricle

Dorsomedial nucleus

Ventromedial nucleus

Lateral hypothalamic area

Supraoptic nucleus

Optic tract

Arcuate nucleus

FIGURE 12-10C ▶
Diagram of the Hypothalamus in the Coronal Plane. *Posterior hypothalamus.*

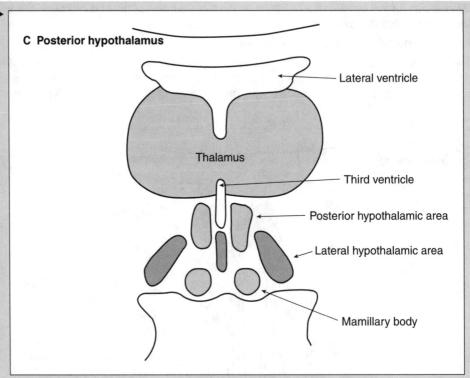

C Posterior hypothalamus

Lateral ventricle

Thalamus

Third ventricle

Posterior hypothalamic area

Lateral hypothalamic area

Mamillary body

The parvocellular neurons secrete hypophyseal-releasing hormones.

Magnocellular neurons in the SON and PVN synthesize and release vasopressin and oxytocin.

contains the *supraoptic nucleus (SON)* and PVN whose magnocellular neurons synthesize the hormones vasopressin and oxytocin (see Figures 12-10A and 12-11). Other parvocellular neurons in the PVN and SON modulate autonomic tone through descending projections to the DMX, the NST, the nucleus ambiguus, and respiratory neurons in the ventrolateral medulla. Descending projections from the PVN enter the medial forebrain bundle, a loose ensemble of fibers that courses through the lateral hypothalamus between the septal area and the dorsolateral tegmentum.

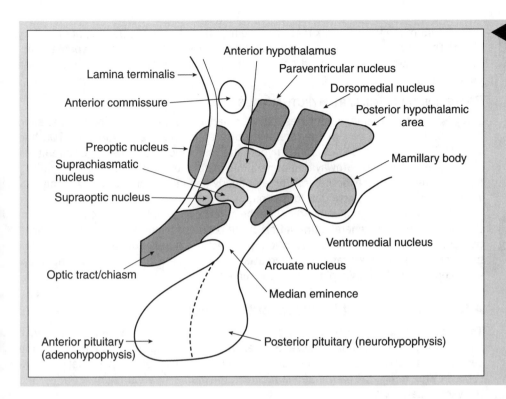

FIGURE 12-11
Diagram of the Hypothalamus and Hypophysis in the Sagittal Plane.

The nondescript *preoptic area*, which lies between the third ventricle and the basal nucleus of Meynert, is telencephalic in origin but for connectional and functional reasons is typically considered part of the anterior hypothalamus (see Figure 12-11). The preoptic area participates in temperature regulation as well as endocrine control of sexual behavior. In general, stimulation of the preoptic area and the anterior hypothalamus produces parasympathetic effects such as vasodilation, sweating, pupillary constriction, decreases in blood pressure and heart rate, and increased intestinal peristalsis and gastrointestinal secretion. The neighboring lamina terminalis contains two important circumventricular organs, the *organum vasculosum of the lamina terminalis (OVLT)* and the *subfornical organ (SFO)*. The OVLT and the SFO contribute to endocrine, autonomic, and behavioral control of water regulation.

> *The preoptic area participates in temperature regulation.*

> *The OVLT and SFO are located near the rostral tip of the third ventricle.*

The small, densely staining *suprachiasmatic nucleus*, perched on the superior surface of the optic chiasm, works in concert with the pineal gland to synchronize the body's circadian clock to the ambient day–night light cycle (see Figures 12-10A and 12-11). Information regarding the day–night cycle is relayed from the retina to the suprachiasmatic nucleus and, through an elaborate and not fully understood pathway, to the pineal gland. Circadian rhythms are discussed in more detail in Chapter 14.

> *The suprachiasmatic nucleus helps synchronize the body's circadian rhythm.*

MIDDLE OR TUBERAL HYPOTHALAMUS

The middle hypothalamic area contains the *arcuate nucleus* in the periventricular zone and the dorsomedial and ventromedial nuclei in the medial zone (see Figures 12-10B and 12-11).

The arcuate nucleus is located at the base of the third ventricle along the dorsal margin of the *median eminence* and infundibular stalk (see Figure 12-10). Like other parvocellular secretory hypothalamic nuclei, the arcuate nucleus modulates hormone secretion by the anterior pituitary. The ventromedial and paraventricular nuclei and the lateral hypothalamic area are part of the complex system that regulates food and water intake.

The lateral zone contains the *lateral hypothalamic area*, an important but indistinct region that stretches from the mid-hypothalamic level to the rostral border of the mid-brain tegmentum (see Figure 2-9). A variety of autonomic and behavioral functions are mediated by the widespread and often reciprocal connections between the lateral hypothalamus and the cerebral cortex, basal forebrain, and brainstem.

The base of the middle hypothalamus lies above the median eminence and the

The infundibulum is attached to the tuberal region of the hypothalamus.

infundibulum, the tubular stalk that links the hypothalamus to the peduncular pituitary gland. The infundibulum contains the tuberohypophyseal tract and the hypothalamic-hypophyseal portal system, which connect the hypothalamus and the hypophysis (see below).

POSTERIOR OR MAMILLARY HYPOTHALAMUS

The posterior hypothalamus includes the mamillary bodies, the posterior hypothalamic area, and the caudal part of the lateral hypothalamic area (see Figures 12-10C and 12-11). The *mamillary bodies* are the hypothalamic component of the Papez circuit, an elaborate multinuclear pathway that plays a role in emotion. Surrounding the mamillary bodies is the posterior hypothalamic area, a poorly defined region that merges caudally with the mesencephalic reticular formation.

Stimulation of the posterior hypothalamus produces sympathetic effects.

The posterior hypothalamic area, like the anterior hypothalamic area, is involved in thermoregulation. In general, stimulation of the posterior hypothalamus produces sympathetic effects such as vasoconstriction, piloerection, pupillary dilation, increases in blood pressure and heart rate, and decreased intestinal peristalsis and gastrointestinal secretion, all of which take place during emergencies.

Afferent and Efferent Pathways of the Hypothalamus

The hypothalamus has extensive and often reciprocal connections with a variety of forebrain structures including the septum, amygdala, hippocampus, thalamus, and the cerebral cortex. The major afferent and efferent projections of the hypothalamus are carried by the *fornix*, the *mamillothalamic tract*, the *medial forebrain bundle (MFB)*, and the ventral pathways.

The fornix is the primary efferent pathway of the hippocampal formation.

The massive C-shaped fornix is the largest and most easily recognized fiber tract within the diencephalon (see Chapter 2, Figure 2-21; see Chapter 13, Figure 13-2). The fornix consists primarily of axons from pyramidal cells of the hippocampal formation and subiculum. The fornix exits the posterior hippocampus and ascends toward the splenium of the corpus callosum before turning rostrally and coursing beneath the body of the corpus callosum. At the level of the interventricular foramen the fornix sweeps ventrally toward the anterior commissure and divides into two parts, a small precommissural limb that terminates in the septal area and a large postcommissural limb that projects to the medial hypothalamus before ending in the mamillary bodies. The efferent projections of the mamillary bodies form the mamillothalamic and *mamillotegmental tracts*. The

The mamillothalamic tract projects to the anterior nucleus of the thalamus.

mamillothalamic tract projects to the anterior nucleus of the thalamus, the first leg of the circuitous, multisynaptic pathway that eventually returns to the hippocampal formation (see Chapter 13, Figures 13-1 and 13-2). This circuit may contribute to memory retrieval and emotion. The mamillotegmental tract links the mamillary bodies with the locus ceruleus, the pontine parabrachial nucleus, the central gray, the DMX, the NST, and the spinal cord.

The hypothalamus and amygdala are reciprocally connected by the stria terminalis and the ventral pathways.

The hypothalamus and the amygdala are reciprocally connected by the *stria terminalis* and the ventral amygdalofugal pathway (VAFP). The stria terminalis originates in the corticomedial amygdaloid nuclei and runs dorsally and rostrally with the thalamostriate vein in the groove between the thalamus and the caudate nucleus. Most fibers of the stria terminalis terminate in the bed nucleus of the stria terminalis, but others continue caudally and terminate in the preoptic area and the anterior and ventromedial hypothalamus (see Chapter 13, Figure 13-2). Projections from the basolateral amygdala to the lateral hypothalamus form the VAFP (see Chapter 13, Figure 13-6). Some of the more anterior fibers of the VAFP destined for the preoptic area form the diagonal band of Broca.

The MFB is a loose ensemble of afferent and efferent projections that connect the hypothalamus with the forebrain and brainstem. Forebrain areas connected to the hypothalamus by the MFB include the septal area, the amygdala, the basal nucleus of Meynert, and the subiculum. As the MFB courses through the lateral hypothalamic area, some axons depart and other axons join until the composite tract exits the hypothalamus caudally and terminates in the brainstem tegmentum and central gray. Serotonergic, dopaminergic, and noradrenergic projections from the brainstem enter the hypothalamus through the MFB.

Other ascending and descending autonomic pathways between the hypothalamus and the brainstem are too diffuse for visual identification but are important nonetheless. Ascending projections from the NST to the hypothalamus relay afferent information from carotid baroreceptors and chemoreceptors as well as numerous thoracic and abdominal viscera. Brainstem and spinal autonomic reflexes are modulated by descending projections from a variety of central structures, but most notably the hypothalamus. Various brainstem nuclei (e.g., DNX, NST) and the brainstem tegmentum receive direct projections from the cerebral cortex, the lateral and paraventricular nuclei of the hypothalamus, and the mamillary nuclei, as well as indirect projections from the amygdala, hippocampus, and the limbic lobe. Descending projections to the spinal cord also originate in the hypothalamus and brainstem reticular formation. These descending autonomic pathways often are destroyed by tumors and strokes within the periaqueductal gray or lateral tegmentum. Interruption of the descending autonomic pathways within the brainstem or spinal cord produces Horner's syndrome (see above and Chapter 4).

Damage to descending autonomic pathways produces Horner's syndrome.

Hypothalamic-Hypophyseal Portal System and the Tuberoinfundibular Tract

Release of hormones synthesized and stored within the adenohypophysis is controlled by regulatory hormones secreted by the hypothalamus. These regulatory hormones are transported from the hypothalamus to the adenohypophysis by an elaborate vascular pathway called the hypothalamic-hypophyseal portal system (Figure 12-12). The so-called portal system consists of two capillary beds, one in the median eminence at the base of the hypothalamus and the other in the anterior lobe of the pituitary. The two capillary beds are connected by the *long portal veins* that run the length of the infundibulum.

The portal system consists of two capillary beds connected by long portal veins.

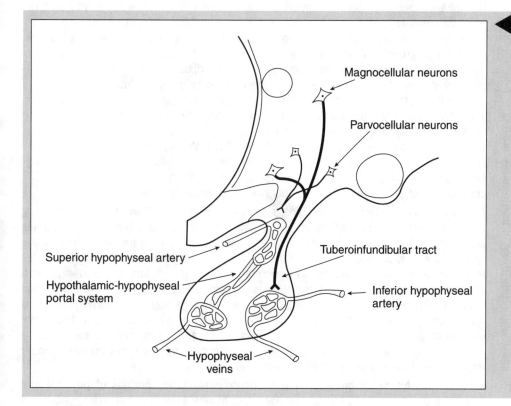

◀ **FIGURE 12-12**

Diagram of the Hypothalamic-Hypophyseal Portal System and Tuberoinfundibular Tract. *Oxytocin and vasopressin synthesized in the magnocellular neurons of the supraoptic and periventricular nuclei are transported axoplasmically along the tuberoinfundibular tract to the neurohypophysis. Oxytocin and vasopressin enter the systemic circulation through fenestrated capillaries of the hypophyseal veins. Regulatory hormones synthesized in the parvocellular neurons of the hypothalamus are released at axon terminals that line the capillary bed within the median eminence. After transport through the long portal veins to the adenohypophysis, these hypothalamic hormones regulate release of pituitary hormones into the systemic circulation.*

The regulatory hormones synthesized within hypothalamic neurons are axoplasmically transported to their terminals, which line the fenestrated capillaries of the venous plexus in the median eminence. The regulatory hormones flow through the long portal veins to the capillary bed within the adenohypophysis. The hypophyseal capillary bed provides the vascular link between the blood-borne hypothalamic hormones and the secretory cells of the adenohypophysis that release the appropriate pituitary hormones into the systemic circulation.

The tuberoinfundibular tract transports vasopressin and oxytocin, the hormones synthesized by the SON and PVN of the hypothalamus, to the posterior hypophysis (see Figure 12-12). Axons of the tuberoinfundibular tract, unlike normal axons, terminate on fenestrated capillaries within the posterior hypophysis. The fenestrated capillaries enable vasopressin and oxytocin to enter the systemic circulation. The terminals of the tuberoinfundibular tract on the capillary bed of the posterior hypophysis resemble the neurovascular link in the median eminence described above. No regulatory hormones are required for release of vasopressin and oxytocin from the posterior hypophysis.

The tuberoinfundibular tract transports vasopressin and oxytocin from the hypothalamus to the neurohypophysis.

Adenohypophyseal Hormones

Thyroid-Stimulating Hormone (TSH). Release of TSH from the anterior hypophysis increases secretion of thyroxin and diiodothyroxine from the thyroid gland, which controls the body's metabolic rate, temperature, and the level of general activity. TSH release is controlled by production of *thyroid-stimulating hormone–releasing hormone (THRH)* by parvocellular neurons in the PVN. *Hypothyroidism* caused by a deficiency of TSH is characterized by sluggishness and obesity. *Hyperthyroidism* caused by excessive production of thyroxin and diiodothyroxine promotes weight loss and nervousness.

THRH releases TSH from the anterior lobe of the pituitary gland.

Hypothyroidism is characterized by sluggishness and obesity.

Hyperthyroidism is characterized by nervousness and weight loss.

Two different releasing hormones (somatocrinin, somatostatin) control secretion of somatotropin.

Growth Hormones. The two growth hormones, *somatotropin* and *prolactin*, are essential for development of the bones, connective tissue, the viscera, and the reproductive organs. Growth hormone (*somatotropin*) release by the adenohypophysis is governed by two hypothalamic hormones, *growth hormone–releasing hormone (GHRH or somatocrinin)* and *growth hormone–inhibitory hormone (GHIH or somatostatin)*. Periods of growth occur when somatocrinin increases or somatostatin decreases in the blood. During childhood, somatotropin promotes bone and tissue growth; in adults, growth hormone enhances protein formation and maintains cellular integrity throughout the body. Whereas overproduction of growth hormone in children produces *gigantism*, underproduction results in *dwarfism*. Children with low levels of growth hormone may be given recombinant growth hormone at an early age to promote growth. In adults, overproduction of growth hormone causes *acromegaly*, a gross distortion and enlargement of the bones that is most noticeable in the face (protruding jaw), hands, and feet.

Prolactin, the hormone that promotes development of the mamillary glands, ovaries, and testes as well as milk synthesis, is released by the adenohypophysis at the command of the hypothalamus. Release of prolactin is restricted by dopamine and the hypothalamic hormone *prolactin inhibitory factor (PIF)*. Without PIF, prolactin would be secreted freely by the anterior hypophysis. Postpartum production of prolactin is triggered by suckling and has been shown to promote maternal behavior in rodents. The contribution of prolactin to maternal behavior in humans is uncertain.

Release of prolactin is modulated by dopamine and PIF.

Stress or other strong emotional stimuli interfere with nursing by preventing suckling-induced suppression of PIF secretion.

Gonadotropins. The two gonadotropins, *luteinizing hormone (LH)* and *follicle-stimulating hormone (FSH)*, have similar effects in the male and female. In the female, LH promotes corpora lutea formation and ovulation whereas in the male, LH stimulates testosterone synthesis and expression of secondary male sexual characteristics. FSH stimulates follicular growth in the ovaries and spermatogenesis in the testes. Release of both gonadotropins from the anterior hypophysis is governed by *gonadotropin-releasing hormone (GnRH*; also called *luteinizing hormone–releasing hormone [LHRH])*, which is synthesized in the preoptic areas and arcuate nucleus and released into the portal circulation. *Hypogonadotropic hypogonadism (Kallmann's syndrome)* is caused by a failure to secrete gonadotropic hormones due to a gene deletion that prevents proper migration and maturation of GnRH neurons.

Gonadotropin-releasing hormone (GnRH) also is called luteinizing hormone–releasing hormone (LHRH).

Patients with Kallmann's syndrome are anosmic because they lack olfactory receptor neurons.

Adrenocorticotropin Hormone (ACTH; Corticotropin). During periods of physical and psychological stress (e.g., trauma, hemorrhage, hyperthermia), the anterior hypophysis releases ACTH into the systemic circulation, which increases steroidal hormone production by the *adrenal cortex*. Two glucocorticoids, *cortisol* and *corticosterone*, protect the body from the adverse effects of stress by adjusting carbohydrate, fat, and protein metabolism. Release of ACTH by the anterior hypophysis is regulated by secretion of *corticotropin-releasing hormone (CRH)* from the parvocellular neurons in the PVN. Normally, release of the steroid hormones by the thyroid gland inhibits further secretion of ACTH by the pituitary.

Release of ACTH is controlled by CRH, which is secreted by the parvocellular neurons of the PVN.

Pituitary tumors that cause an oversecretion of ACTH result in elevated blood levels of cortisol and produce *Cushing's disease* which is characterized by hypertension, truncal obesity, and diabetes mellitus. Patients with *Addison's disease* have a diminished production of ACTH and demonstrate weakness, weight loss, increased skin pigmentation, hypotension, and hypoglycemia.

Neurohypophyseal Hormones

The neurohypophysis, unlike the adenohypophysis, does not synthesize hormones and thus does not rely on the hypothalamus for either release or inhibitory hormones. There are, however, two hormones that are synthesized in the hypothalamus and released by the neurohypophysis into the systemic circulation: *vasopressin* (also called *antidiuretic hormone [ADH]*) and *oxytocin*. Vasopressin and oxytocin are synthesized in separate populations of magnocellular neurons in the PVN and SON and transported by the tuberoinfundibular tract to the neurohypophysis. Once in the neurohypophysis, oxytocin and vasopressin are released into the blood through fenestrated capillaries. Although structurally similar nonapeptides, vasopressin and oxytocin have vastly different functions.

Vasopressin. Vasopressin acts as an antidiuretic hormone by decreasing water secretion by the kidneys. Vasopressin secretion is initiated in response to changes in blood pressure, blood volume, and serum osmolarity. Blood pressure and blood volume are measured by baroreceptors and mechanoreceptors in the carotid sinus, aortic arch, and right atrium. Serum osmolarity is measured directly by neurons in the SON and PVN. Water retention restores serum osmolarity and increases blood pressure and blood volume.

Damage to the hypothalamico-hypophyseal axis may disrupt vasopressin synthesis and release and cause diabetes insipidus. Patients with diabetes insipidus pass large volumes of urine (*polyuria*), have low urine osmolarity, reduced blood volume, increased thirst, and excessive water consumption (*polydipsia*). *Diabetes insipidus* is treated by vasopressin replacement.

Oxytocin. Oxytocin does not initiate labor but rather gradually intensifies uterine contractions until birth. Pitocin, a synthetic form of oxytocin, is used to induce labor in women who are past term and have not begun labor spontaneously. In postpartum women, oxytocin is released by stimulation of the nipple during suckling. Oxytocin initiates milk release (let-down), expression of milk from the mammary ducts, and restoration of the uterus. Oxytocin also may promote maternal behavior.

Functions of the Hypothalamic-Hypophyseal System

The coordinated actions of the hypothalamus and hypophysis influence body temperature, water and food regulation, growth, metabolism, cardiovascular function, and maternal and reproductive behavior.

Regulation of Temperature. Autonomic, endocrine, and behavioral responses that regulate body temperature are mediated by the anterior and posterior regions of the hypothalamus. Neurons in the preoptic area respond to changes in blood and skin temperature. Increases in core body temperature trigger parasympathetic responses such as decreased metabolism, increased sweating, and peripheral vasodilation. Sympathetic responses to decreases in core temperature include vasoconstriction, piloerection, and generation of heat generation through shivering; all are mediated by projections from the preoptic area to the posterior hypothalamus. These sympathetic and parasympathetic responses may be supplemented by appropriate changes in TSH production by the anterior pituitary and epinephrine secretion by the adrenal medulla. These physiologic responses usually are supported by appropriate behavioral responses such as closing a window, adjusting the room thermostat, or putting on a sweater. Damage to the preoptic area prevents vasodilation and sweating and ultimately produces hyperthermia.

Ingestive Behavior. Initial studies on feeding behavior demonstrated that rats with lesions of the lateral hypothalamus fail to eat (*aphagia*) and drink (*adipsia*) and must be fed intragastrically to prevent their starvation and death. Lesions of the ventromedial

Vasopressin is sometimes referred to as arginine vasopressin (AVP).

Vasopressin increases water retention by the kidney.

Oxytocin contracts the smooth muscle of the uterus during childbirth and releases milk from the mammary glands following parturition.

Psychogenic stimuli such as the sound of a crying child may trigger oxytocin release and milk let-down.

The anterior and posterior regions of the hypothalamus regulate body temperature.

Electrical stimulation of the lateral hypothalamus initiates feeding.

Electrical stimulation of the ventromedial hypothalamus stops feeding.

Adipsia *is an inability to drink.*

Aphagia *is an inability to eat.*

Sales of the serotonin agonist fenflura-mine, which decreases food intake, were stopped after concerns about its safety were raised.

Deprivation-induced drinking may be triggered by low blood pressure or low blood volume.

hypothalamus have the opposite effect: uncontrolled eating (*hyperphagia*) and drinking (*polydipsia*) lead to obesity. Division of the hypothalamus into a lateral feeding nucleus and a ventromedial satiety nucleus received further support from electrical stimulation experiments. More recent experiments, however, have shown that some of the initial results were due to inadvertent damage to fibers of passage. Although the field has abandoned the simplistic view of feeding and satiety centers, there is little doubt that the hypothalamus is intimately involved in the regulation of feeding and drinking.

Regulation of Food Intake. Recent studies examining the role of the hypothalamus in feeding have implicated the lateral nucleus, ventromedial nucleus, and PVN. Microinjections of norepinephrine and neuropeptide Y into the PVN increase feeding, particularly of carbohydrates. Consumption of fat increases following central injections of the peptide galanin; opioids increase consumption of protein. Feeding decreases following microinjections of dopamine and serotonin, but increases following injections of serotonin antagonists. These hypothalamic nuclei also may play a role in long-term weight regulation by monitoring systemic levels of *cholecystokinin (CCK)* and *leptin*. CCK is a peptide hormone secreted by the duodenum and upper intestine that terminates feeding and thus may act as a satiety signal. Interestingly, central administration of CCK also interrupts feeding. Leptin, a protein secreted by adipocytes, may be the sensory signal used by the hypothalamus for long-term weight regulation.

The sensory, autonomic, and endocrine connections of the PVN enable it to participate in a host of feeding-related activities. Projections from the NST to the PVN convey visceral information from the gastrointestinal tract, liver, and pancreas. The PVN also receives projections from other hypothalamic nuclei, various nuclei of the limbic system (amygdala, bed nucleus of the stria terminalis), and noradrenergic and dopaminergic areas in the brainstem. Release of TSH and CRH by the parvocellular neurons of the PVN affects the body's metabolism while secretion of vasopressin by the magnocellular neurons of the PVN affects water retention. Efferent projections from parvocellular neurons in the PVN to the brainstem and spinal cord modulate hormone release from the pancreas (insulin, glucagon) and catecholamine release from the adrenal medulla.

Regulation of Water Balance. Deprivation-induced drinking is triggered by significant blood loss or increased serum osmolarity (Figure 12-13). Decreases in blood volume (*hypovolemia*) caused by hemorrhage or excessive vomiting or diarrhea stimulate baroreceptors in the right atrium, carotid sinus, and aortic arch. Hypovolemic activation of the baroreceptor reflex, as discussed in the previous section, is mediated in part through afferent projections to the NST, some of which are relayed to the PVN. Hypovolemia also prompts the kidney to secrete renin, which initiates an enzymatic cascade that increases

FIGURE 12-13
Neural Circuitry Associated with Hypovolemic and Osmotic Regulation of Thirst. *PVN = paraventricular nucleus; SON = supraoptic nucleus; NST = nucleus of the solitary tract; OVLT = organum vasculosum of the lamina terminalis. PVN = paraventricular nucleus of the hypothalamus. (Source: Reprinted with permission from Carlson NR: Physiology of Behavior. Boston, MA: Allyn & Bacon, 1994, p 386.)*

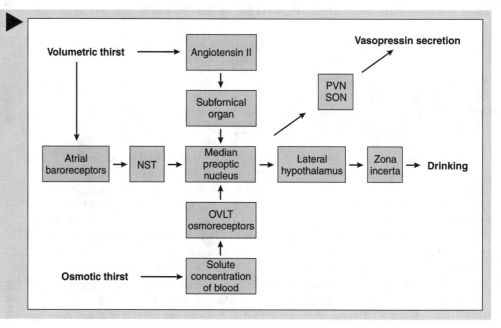

serum levels of *angiotensin II*. Angiotensin II not only increases blood pressure through vasoconstriction but also regulates water balance through endocrine, autonomic, and behavioral mechanisms. Angiotensin II triggers the release of aldosterone from the adrenal cortex and vasopressin from the neurohypophysis. The first step in vasopressin release is detection of circulating angiotensin II by neurons in the SFO. Efferent projections from the SFO to the magnocellular neurons of the SON and PVN release vasopressin from the neurohypophysis. Other SFO projections to the parvocellular neurons of the PVN increase blood pressure through autonomic areas of the brainstem and spinal cord.

Changes in serum osmolarity are detected by osmoreceptors located in the medial preoptic area and the adjacent OVLT. Projections from the medial preoptic area, the NST, and the DMX to the PVN trigger vasopressin release by the neurohypophysis.

Water depletion and increased serum osmolarity produce the sensation of thirst, an unpleasant sensation that is initiated and terminated by drinking. Lesion experiments have demonstrated that the *median* preoptic area is critical for initiation of drinking. The median preoptic area receives direct projections from osmoreceptors located in the OVLT and medial preoptic area and angiotensin II receptors located in the SFO.

Aldosterone improves conservation of sodium by the kidneys.

RESOLUTION OF CLINICAL CASE

All of the L. J.'s symptoms are consistent with mass effects caused by a pituitary adenoma. Polyuria and polydipsia were caused by inadequate production of ADH. Diabetes mellitus, which also causes polyuria and polydipsia, was ruled out because the urine had a low specific gravity and only a nominal amount of glucose. The second set of blood tests suggested that L. J.'s fatigue was caused by an abnormally low level of thyroxin, presumably due to a lack of TSH. The visual field defect and headache were caused by the tumor pressing against the crossing fibers of the optic chiasm. The MRI scan revealed a tumor around the infundibular stalk. L. J. was given hormone replacement therapy and scheduled for surgery to remove as much of the tumor as possible. Following radiation therapy, L. J. may have near normal ADH and TSH production and improved eyesight.

REVIEW QUESTIONS

Directions: For each of the following questions, choose the **one best** answer.

1. The neurotransmitters used by the preganglionic and postganglionic neurons of the parasympathetic nervous system (PNS) are
   - **(A)** acetylcholine and norepinephrine
   - **(B)** epinephrine and norepinephrine
   - **(C)** norepinephrine and acetylcholine
   - **(D)** acetylcholine and acetylcholine
   - **(E)** acetylcholine and glutamate

2. Receptors for the baroreceptor reflex are located in the
   - **(A)** organum vasculosum of the lamina terminalis
   - **(B)** subfornical organ
   - **(C)** left ventricle of the heart
   - **(D)** lungs
   - **(E)** carotid sinus

3. Diabetes insipidus is caused by a deficiency of
   - **(A)** thyroid-stimulating hormone (TSH)
   - **(B)** corticotropin-releasing hormone (CRH)
   - **(C)** insulin
   - **(D)** vasopressin
   - **(E)** thyroxin

4. A complete transection of the sacral spinal cord would produce an
   - **(A)** automatic bladder that fills to capacity before emptying automatically
   - **(B)** atonic bladder that is difficult, if not impossible, to empty voluntarily
   - **(C)** uninhibited bladder that empties when full but is under the patient's control
   - **(D)** empty bladder that drains urine as it fills
   - **(E)** inhibited bladder that empties only when it is filled to capacity

5. The vagus nerve, which contains afferent projections from the thoracic and abdominal viscera, terminates in the
   - **(A)** dorsal motor nucleus of the vagus (DMX)
   - **(B)** nucleus ambiguus
   - **(C)** Edinger-Westphal nucleus
   - **(D)** lateral hypothalamus
   - **(E)** nucleus of the solitary tract (NST)

Directions: The group of questions below consists of lettered choices followed by several numbered items. For each numbered item, select the appropriate lettered option with which it is most closely associated. Each lettered option may be used once, more than once, or not at all.

Questions 6–12

Match the following:

    (A) Only sympathetic nervous system (SNS)
    (B) Only parasympathetic nervous system (PNS)
    (C) Both SNS and PNS
    (D) Neither SNS nor PNS

6. Sweat glands

7. Rectal sphincters

8. Sex organs

9. Heart

10. Adrenal medulla

11. Muscles of the arms and legs

12. Blood vessels in the arms and legs

ANSWERS AND EXPLANATIONS

1. The answer is D. Both sympathetic and parasympathetic preganglionic neurons use acetylcholine. The postganglionic neurons in the PNS use acetylcholine while sympathetic postganglionic neurons use norepinephrine.

2. The answer is E. Baroreceptors are in the carotid sinus, the aortic arch, and the right atrium. The organum vasculosum of the lamina terminalis contains osmoreceptors that detect changes in serum osmolarity. Receptors in the subfornical organ detect elevated levels of serum angiotensin II associated with hypovolemia. There are no baroreceptors in the heart or the lungs.

3. The answer is D. Low levels of vasopressin or antidiuretic hormone cause diabetes insipidus, the main symptoms of which are polyuria and polydipsia. A deficiency of TSH would reduce thyroxin release by the thyroid gland. Hypothyroidism is characterized by sluggishness and obesity. Low levels of CRH would lower production of adrenocorticotropin hormone from the adenohypophysis and cause Addison's disease. Reduced production of insulin by the pancreas causes diabetes mellitus, whose hallmark symptoms are hyperglycemia and polyuria.

4. The answer is B. Complete transection of the sacral spinal cord produces an atonic bladder. Patients with an atonic bladder usually are unable to empty their bladders voluntarily and must be catheterized. Unless catheterized, their bladders are seldom empty. Filling to capacity is not sufficient to induce urination. An automatic bladder, which is caused by a lesion of the spinal cord above the sacral level, empties automatically when it reaches capacity. Patients with an uninhibited bladder have frontal lobe damage and are usually unaware that they are urinating.

5. The answer is E. Visceral afferent projections from the thoracic and abdominal viscera project to the caudal part of the NST. The DMX and the nucleus ambiguus contain parasympathetic preganglionic neurons that provide efferent control of the viscera. Neither the Edinger-Westphal nucleus nor the lateral hypothalamus receive visceral afferent projections.

6–12. The answers are: 6-A, 7-C, 8-C, 9-C, 10-A, 11-D, 12-A. Sweat glands have unopposed innervation of the SNS. The rectal sphincters, the sex organs, and the heart are innervated by the SNS and PNS. The adrenal medulla, which releases epinephrine into the systemic circulation during fight or flight situations, is innervated only by the SNS. The muscles of the arms and legs are innervated by the somatomotor rather than the autonomic nervous system, but the blood vessels of the arms and legs are under sympathetic control.

ADDITIONAL READING

De Groat WC, Steers WD: Neural control of the urinary bladder and sexual organs. In *Autonomic Failure*. Edited by Bannister R. New York, NY: Oxford University Press, 1988, pp 196–222.

Parent A: *Carpenter's Human Neuroanatomy*. Baltimore, MD: Williams & Wilkins, 1996.

Pick J: *The Autonomic Nervous System*. Philadelphia, PA: J. B. Lippincott, 1970.

13

LIMBIC SYSTEM

INTRODUCTION OF CLINICAL CASE

During the past 6 months, T. S., an 18-year-old woman, experienced recurring seizures. For several months the seizures occurred only once every 2 or 3 weeks, but more recently they have occurred at least once a week. The onset of each seizure was marked by unpleasant visceral sensations and a feeling of fear or dread. Initially, the behavioral manifestations of the seizures only included repetitive movements of the lips and tongue, but more recently they have expanded to include clonic, bilateral twitching of the face. The patient was not conscious of these motor events, and witnesses reported that she appeared confused for 30–60 minutes following these seizures. An electroencephalogram (EEG) revealed focal slowing and the presence of sharp waves or spikes in the midtemporal region of the cortex.

INTRODUCTION TO THE LIMBIC SYSTEM

The exact functional role of many forebrain structures is unclear because they form part of the neural substrate involved in mediating complex behaviors such as cognition or emotion. Such is the case with the amygdaloid complex, a multinuclear structure in the temporal lobe that is involved in regulating emotional behavior. Similarly, the hippocampal formation is another temporal lobe structure whose role in memory and related cognitive processes is poorly understood. Together, the amygdaloid complex and the hippocampal formation are the key structures in the so-called limbic system.

No single neural structure, however, is capable of mediating a complex process such as motivation, emotional behavior, or memory. The autonomic, cognitive, and behavioral responses associated with emotions, for example, are mediated by a distributed system of interacting neural structures that include the amygdaloid complex, the hypothalamus, the basal forebrain (i.e., septal nucleus, substantia innominata, nucleus basalis of Meynert), the nucleus accumbens and ventral striatum, the prefrontal and cingulate cortical areas, and a collection of somatic and autonomic motor nuclei in the brainstem. Thus, the amygdaloid complex and other parts of the limbic system act as an interface between the cerebral cortex and autonomic structures such as the hypothalamus and parts of the brainstem.

HISTORICAL VIEWS OF THE LIMBIC SYSTEM

In contrast to other cortical lobes, the limbic lobe is not demarcated by distinct fissures but is a synthesis of the medial cortical structures lying around the limbus, or rim, of the corpus callosum (Figure 13-1). As defined by Paul Broca in 1878, the limbic lobe includes the subcallosal area, the cingulate gyrus, the parahippocampal gyrus, and the underlying hippocampal formation. A specific function for the limbic lobe was proposed in the 1930s by James Papez after he observed emotional disturbances in some of his patients who had sustained damage in this area. Based on these observations and his knowledge of the gross morphology of the brain, Papez proposed a closed neural circuit that linked the hippocampus and cingulate gyrus for the purpose of expressing emotional behaviors. According to Papez, the hippocampus organized emotional "programs" that were communicated to the hypothalamus via the fibers of the fornix. The hypothalamus, particularly the mamillary body, executed these emotional programs via descending pathways to the brainstem while sending related information to other parts of the limbic lobe. Thus, the mamillothalamic tract conveyed emotional information to the anterior nucleus of the thalamus, which projects to the cingulate cortex via the thalamocortical radiations. Papez believed that the cingulate cortex represented the site for the conscious experience of emotions just as certain cortical areas represent the neural substrate for sensory perception. Since the cingulate cortex projects to the parahippocampal gyrus and the underlying hippocampus via the fibers of the cingulum, the major processing centers of the Papez circuit form a closed neural loop in which information may reverberate.

In the 1950s, Paul MacLean recognized that the limbic lobe was connected to many subcortical structures whose primary function was to regulate visceral functions. To make sense of these anatomic relationships, he developed the concept of a "limbic system" to

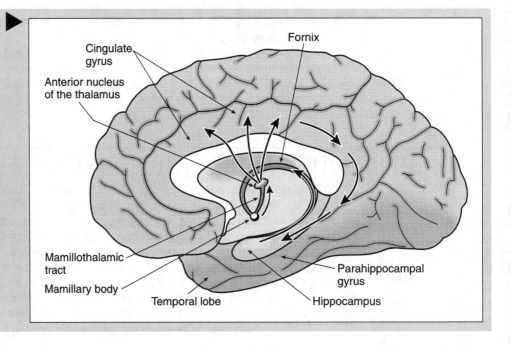

FIGURE 13-1 ▶

Papez Circuit. According to James Papez, information was sequentially processed in the limbic lobe as shown by the arrows in this diagram.

Cingulate gyrus

Fornix

Anterior nucleus of the thalamus

Mamillothalamic tract

Mamillary body

Temporal lobe

Parahippocampal gyrus

Hippocampus

explain how emotional affect influences autonomic responses. According to MacLean, the hypothalamus uses information received from a variety of limbic areas to coordinate the autonomic responses associated with different emotional states. In his view, the major subcortical nuclei in the limbic system included the amygdala, the septal nucleus, the nucleus accumbens, the substantia innominata, the hypothalamus, and the anterior and dorsomedial nuclei of the thalamus (Figure 13-2).

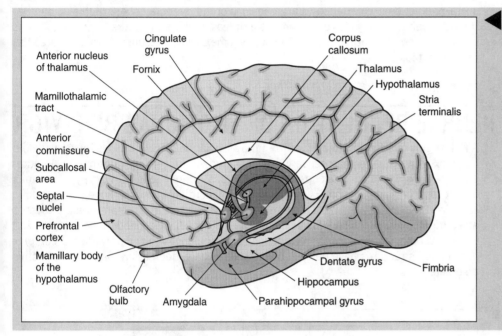

◀ **FIGURE 13-2**
Major Structures in the Limbic System. *The limbic system is composed of several cortical and subcortical structures located along the medial aspect of the brain. The amygdaloid complex and its connections regulate emotional behavior. The hippocampus and its connections consolidate information into long-term memory.*

Klüver-Bucy Syndrome

In the late 1930s, Paul Bucy and Heinrich Klüver showed that temporal lobe removal, which disrupts the Papez circuit, has profound effects on the social and emotional behaviors of rhesus monkeys. In contrast to wild monkeys, the monkeys that had their temporal lobes removed seemed less aggressive as indicated by their willingness to approach humans without attempting to bite or claw them. These monkeys also failed to vocalize or show other fearful reactions to snakes, which are strongly aversive to normal monkeys. Other observations, however, indicated that this behavioral tameness was a manifestation of a more general deficit in visual recognition. This view arose because monkeys with temporal lobe lesions are unable to recognize a wide range of behaviorally relevant stimuli, a phenomenon referred to as visual agnosia or "psychic blindness." These monkeys indiscriminately place a wide range of inanimate objects into their mouth and readily ingest fish, meat, feces, and other substances that normal monkeys avoid. Temporal lobectomy also disturbs their sexual behavior as indicated by repeated attempts to copulate with members of their own sex, with other species, or even inanimate objects. This constellation of behaviors subsequently became known as the Klüver-Bucy syndrome.

Klüver and Bucy thought that these behavioral changes were due to the loss of the hippocampus because it is the most salient structure in the temporal lobe. Additional studies, however, have shown that the Klüver-Bucy syndrome can be produced following removal of the amygdala alone. These findings suggest that amygdalectomy interferes with the ability to link past experiences to stimuli that have important behavioral consequences. The amygdala receives sensory information from many cortical areas and, thus, may provide the anatomic substrate for associating behaviorally significant stimuli with their positive or negative consequences. In this context, the behavioral disruptions that define the Klüver-Bucy syndrome may represent an inability to make appropriate sensory-affective associations.

Klüver-Bucy Syndrome
Placid behavior
Visual agnosia
Oral tendencies
Hypersexuality

Human patients with amygdaloid lesions exhibit behavioral changes that are remarkably similar to those seen in nonhuman primates. Amygdalectomy causes humans to become complacent and, for this reason, was often used in the past to treat individuals with a history of violent behaviors. Human patients with amygdaloid lesions also exhibit visual, auditory, or tactile agnosia and have an increased tendency to sniff objects and place them in their mouth. Damage to the amygdala also increases inappropriate sexual behavior, which takes the form of suggestive remarks and ill-conceived attempts to make sexual contact. Thus, the evidence from clinical and experimental data suggests that damage to the amygdala may interfere with the ability to link sensory stimuli to past social or emotional experiences. Larger lesions of the temporal lobe, which also damage the hippocampus, may also cause amnesia. In cases where the entire temporal lobe has been damaged, the patient is also likely to become aphasic because Wernicke's area has been affected.

NEURAL REGULATION OF EMOTIONAL BEHAVIOR

A rich supply of afferent projections from the association cortex provides the amygdaloid complex with visual, somatosensory, auditory, and viscerosensory information. In addition, the amygdaloid complex has dense, reciprocal connections with the hypothalamus and several brainstem nuclei, which allow it to coordinate a wide range of autonomic responses (Figure 13-3). These anatomic pathways suggest that the amygdala is located at a critical junction, which allows it to play a role in mediating emotion, personality, and other psychological processes. Neurochemical imbalances in the amygdaloid complex and related structures have been implicated in anxiety, depression, and other affective disorders.

FIGURE 13-3 ▶
Afferent and Efferent Connections with the Amygdala. *The amygdala uses sensory information received from the association cortex and other areas to coordinate the autonomic responses associated with emotional behavior.*

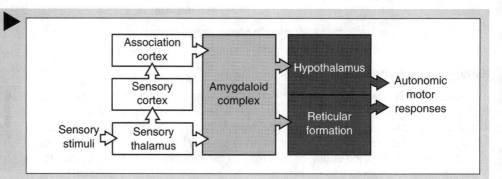

Anatomy of the Amygdaloid Complex

The amygdaloid complex is composed of several distinct nuclei that lie underneath the uncus, which is located in the rostromedial part of the temporal lobe (Figure 13-4). The amygdala is located just rostral to the hippocampal formation, and because of this proximity, temporal lobe damage may affect both of these structures. Although the amygdaloid complex is technically a part of the basal ganglia, its functional role and anatomic connections differ markedly from those structures.

NUCLEAR ORGANIZATION

The amygdaloid complex contains many nuclei that vary in neurochemical composition and differ according to their afferent and efferent connections. Since the nomenclature describing individual amygdaloid nuclei is inconsistent, many neuroanatomists prefer to organize them into basolateral and corticomedial groups.

Basolateral Nuclei. In humans, the basolateral nuclei are located in the lateral and ventral two-thirds of the amygdaloid complex. The basolateral part of the amygdaloid complex is considered a quasi-cortical structure because its anatomic features resemble the neocortex. Like the frontal cortex, the basolateral nuclei have reciprocal connections

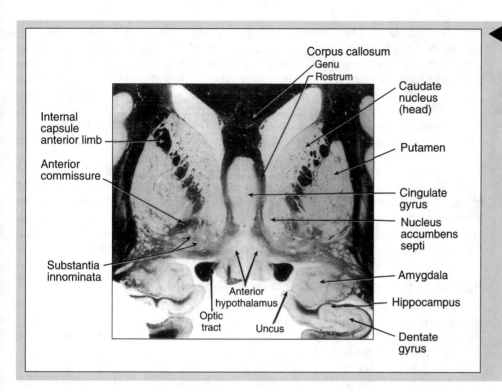

FIGURE 13-4
The Amygdala. This photomicrograph shows a cross section of the amygdaloid complex with respect to the nucleus accumbens, the basal forebrain, and the nuclei of the basal ganglia. (Source: Reprinted with permission from Carpenter M: Core Text of Neuroanatomy. Baltimore, MD: Williams & Wilkins, 1991, p 382.)

with the mediodorsal nucleus of the thalamus. The basolateral nuclei also have direct, sometimes reciprocal, connections with the prefrontal cortex, the cingulate gyrus, the insula, the parahippocampal gyrus, the subiculum, and adjacent gyri in the temporal lobe. Similar to the neocortex, the basolateral nuclei also receive diffuse cholinergic projections from the nucleus basalis of Meynert, which is located ventral to the anterior commissure. Finally, the basolateral nuclei project to motor areas in the frontal lobe and, like limbic cortical areas, send dense projections to the nucleus accumbens and ventral neostriatum.

Corticofugal projections from the temporal lobe, cingulate gyrus, and insula provide the basolateral nuclei with highly processed visual, auditory, somatosensory, and olfactory information (Figure 13-5). In addition to receiving projections from the dorsomedial thalamus, the basolateral nuclei receive projections from modality-specific thalamic nuclei such as the medial geniculate nucleus. These diverse connections provide a rich source of sensory information to the amygdala so that it may evaluate the social and emotional significance of a wide range of stimuli.

Basolateral nuclei receive visual, auditory, and somatosensory inputs.

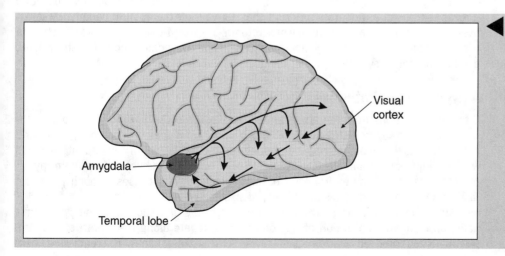

FIGURE 13-5
Visual Projections to the Amygdala. This diagram shows how visual information is transmitted through successive regions of the occipital and temporal lobes before it reaches the amygdaloid complex. The amygdala also projects to higher order visual processing regions in the temporal and occipital lobes.

Corticomedial nuclei receive olfactory and viscerosensory inputs.

Corticomedial Nuclei. The corticomedial nuclei, which includes the central nucleus, are located dorsomedially and only comprise one-third of the amygdaloid complex. Most afferent projections to the corticomedial nuclei originate from brain regions concerned with autonomic or viscerosensory functions. Thus, the corticomedial nuclei receive olfactory inputs directly from the olfactory bulb and indirectly from the adjacent pyriform cortex. The parabrachial nucleus of the pons, which receives viscerosensory information from the caudal nucleus of the solitary tract, sends a dense projection to the central amygdaloid nucleus. The ventromedial and lateral hypothalamic nuclei also project to the centromedial nuclei and, to a lesser degree, to the basolateral nuclei.

From an evolutionary perspective, the afferent connections of the corticomedial nuclei enable this part of the amygdaloid complex to evaluate the sensory properties of stimuli that are linked to survival and reproduction. Thus, olfactory information associated with food, predators, potential mates, and other stimuli are sent to the corticomedial nuclei. Ascending autonomic projections from the solitario-parabrachial pathway provide the amygdala with information needed to regulate visceral, cardiovascular, and respiratory functions.

ROLE OF THE AMYGDALA IN ANXIETY AND DEPRESSION

The neurochemical composition of the amygdaloid complex has drawn the attention of neuropharmacologists that develop drugs for treating mood disorders such as anxiety and depression. In this regard, the amygdala contains a high concentration of the amino acid γ-aminobutyric acid (GABA), which acts as an inhibitory neurotransmitter in most parts of the central nervous system (CNS). Although GABAergic neurons are found in all amygdaloid nuclei, the basolateral nuclei are noteworthy because they contain a high density of GABA receptors that specifically bind benzodiazepines (e.g., diazepam [Valium]) and other anxiolytic drugs. The benzodiazepines are not direct GABA agonists, but they act synergistically to enhance GABA binding, thereby promoting the inhibitory effects of this neurotransmitter. In animals, direct infusion of benzodiazepine into the amygdala reduces conditioned fear and other behavioral signs of anxiety. Hence, the therapeutic benefit of the benzodiazepines is derived, in part, from their ability to enhance GABA-mediated inhibition in the amygdala. This mechanism suggests that the placid behavior observed in the Klüver-Bucy syndrome may, to some extent, represent a reduction in fear and anxiety.

The amygdaloid complex receives dense, serotonergic projections from the dorsal and median raphe nuclei in the brainstem. Ascending dopaminergic projections from the ventral tegmental area and noradrenergic projections from the locus ceruleus also terminate in the amygdala, especially in the central nucleus. These neurochemical pathways are involved in modulating the degree of neuronal excitability in a number of forebrain regions. Given the amygdala's role in controlling emotions, it is not surprising that these monoaminergic systems have a strong influence on mood and other emotional behaviors. An imbalance in neurotransmitter release within the amygdaloid complex may lead to depression or other affective disorders. The clinical importance of the ascending serotonergic pathways is apparent from the large number of prescriptions for fluoxetine (Prozac) and other antidepressant drugs that derive their therapeutic benefits by selectively blocking the synaptic reuptake of serotonin. These antidepressants are effective, in part, because of their pharmacologic actions in the amygdaloid complex and related parts of the limbic system.

Amygdalofugal Pathways

Efferent projections from the amygdaloid complex are organized into two major pathways. One pathway, the stria terminalis, originates from the corticomedial nuclei and proceeds with the thalamostriate vein along the medial border of the caudate nucleus where it adjoins the thalamus (see Figure 13-2). The ventral amygdalofugal pathway, on the other hand, originates from the basolateral nuclei and passes through the basal forebrain before it terminates in a variety of structures.

Most fibers in the stria terminalis terminate in the bed nucleus of the stria terminalis, an elongated collection of neurons that aggregate along the length of the stria terminalis as it proceeds rostromedially towards the septal nucleus. The remaining fibers of the stria terminalis project to the septal nucleus and to parts of the hypothalamus including the medial preoptic area, the anterior hypothalamic nucleus, the ventromedial hypothalamus, and the lateral hypothalamus. The central amygdaloid nucleus and the bed nucleus of the stria terminalis also send descending projections to an assortment of brainstem nuclei including the parabrachial nucleus, the nucleus of the solitary tract, the dorsal motor nucleus of the vagus, the periaqueductal gray region, the ventral tegmental area, the substantia nigra, and parts of the reticular formation. Descending projections from these nuclei regulate the cardiovascular, respiratory, and gastric responses that occur during the expression of fear and other stress-related behaviors.

Fibers in the ventral amygdalofugal pathway proceed rostrally and medially as they pass through the substantia innominata. Many of these fibers make en passant synapses on acetylcholine-containing neurons in the basal forebrain (i.e., nucleus basalis of Meynert) before spreading to more diverse regions such as the septal nucleus, hypothalamus, cingulate cortex, and olfactory areas. Cholinergic fibers from the basal forebrain terminate diffusely throughout the cerebral cortex to enhance neuronal excitability, thereby enabling these cells to be more responsive to incoming sensory inputs. Other fibers of the ventral amygdalofugal pathway ascend to the medial prefrontal cortex either directly or indirectly via the mediodorsal nucleus of the thalamus. Thus, direct amygdalofugal projections to the prefrontal and cingulate cortical areas, as well as indirect projections through the basal forebrain and mediodorsal thalamus, provide parallel routes by which the amygdala may influence cognitive aspects of emotional behavior (Figure 13-6). Finally, the amygdaloid complex sends projections to the adjacent parts of the hippocampal formation, especially the subiculum and entorhinal cortex. These latter projections allow emotional states to influence learning and memory processes.

The **cortocomedial nuclei** give rise to the stria terminalis.

The **basolateral nuclei** give rise to the ventral amygdalofugal pathways.

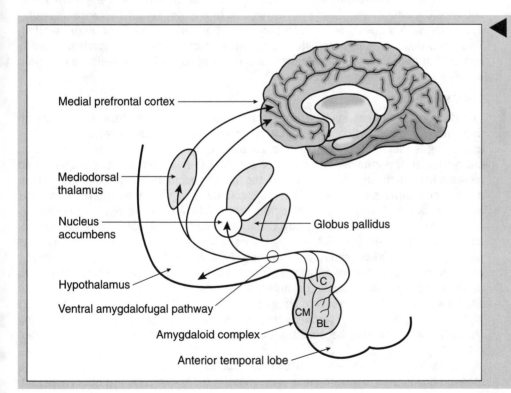

FIGURE 13-6
Amygdalofugal Projections. This diagram shows the basolateral (BL), corticomedial (CM), and central (C) amygdaloid nuclei and their efferent connections with structures in the thalamus, hypothalamus, and cortex. The amygdala projects directly to the prefrontal cortex and indirectly via the mediodorsal thalamus.

Nucleus Accumbens and Ventral Striatum

The nucleus accumbens lies lateral to the septal nucleus in the ventromedial part of the forebrain. Although it is considered part of the basal ganglia, functional studies suggest that the nucleus accumbens and ventromedial part of the neostriatum have an important role in motivation. Consistent with this functional view, these regions receive

Mesolimbic Dopamine System
This system is comprised of dopaminergic pathways to nucleus accumbens, ventral striatum, and medial prefrontal cortex.

substantial projections from the basolateral nuclei of the amygdaloid complex via the ventral amygdalofugal pathway. The nucleus accumbens also receives prominent projections from other limbic regions in the forebrain, especially the medial prefrontal cortex and the hippocampal formation.

The nucleus accumbens, ventral striatum, and the medial prefrontal cortex are major targets of ascending dopaminergic fibers that originate from the ventral tegmental area. Dopaminergic neurons in the ventral tegmental area and their forebrain targets comprise a medial subset of limbic structures that are known as the mesolimbic system. Projections from the central amygdaloid nucleus to the ventral tegmental area enable the amygdaloid complex to simultaneously engage the dopaminergic pathways as well as their forebrain targets.

MESOLIMBIC DOPAMINE AND THE NEURAL BASIS OF REWARD

The mesolimbic dopamine system and its projections to the nucleus accumbens play a critical role in the subjective experience of pleasure and rewarding. The search for a neural substrate for pleasure began in earnest after the discovery of intracranial self-stimulation by James Olds and Peter Milner in 1954. They found that rats implanted with stimulating electrodes would press a bar to deliver brief pulses of electrical current to specific brain regions. Electrical stimulation of the mesolimbic dopamine system was so rewarding that rats would self-stimulate this region for extended periods of time without eating or sleeping. Lesions of the mesolimbic dopamine system or infusions of dopamine antagonists into the nucleus accumbens greatly attenuate the rate of intracranial self-stimulation.

There is considerable debate regarding the exact function of the mesolimbic dopamine system. The synaptic release of dopamine increases significantly when animals are presented with rewarding stimuli such as food or the opportunity to engage in sexual behavior. Dopamine release can also be triggered by arbitrary stimuli that were previously associated with a reward or by novel stimuli that are encountered during exploration. Therefore, dopamine may mediate the pleasurable or reinforcing properties of many stimuli, but may also maintain alertness and increase psychological vigilance in certain situations.

DRUGS OF ABUSE

Drugs of abuse *increase mesolimbic dopamine transmission.*

Psychomotor stimulants such as amphetamine and cocaine produce an increase in dopaminergic transmission in the nucleus accumbens and other targets of dopamine-containing terminals. The motivation to use these drugs and the potential for addiction are related to the immediate feelings of pleasure that accompany the drug-induced increase in dopaminergic transmission in the nucleus accumbens. This view is based on a behavioral paradigm in which animals are trained to regulate their intake of amphetamine or cocaine. Animals will even administer amphetamine directly into the nucleus accumbens, a fact that strongly suggests that dopamine release in the nucleus accumbens is sufficient to maintain drug-taking behavior. Consistent with this view, the reinforcing effects of systemic administration of amphetamine or cocaine are blocked by direct infusions of dopamine antagonists into the nucleus accumbens. Thus, if low doses of dopamine antagonists are administered, animals work harder to self-administer more amphetamine or cocaine to overcome the partial block of dopamine transmission. When higher doses of dopamine antagonists are given, however, the animals stop administering amphetamine or cocaine because the postsynaptic dopamine receptors are saturated with antagonists.

Other classes of commonly abused drugs, such as alcohol, nicotine, and heroin, also increase dopaminergic transmission in the mesolimbic system, and this effect may form the basis for their reinforcing properties. These drugs act at multiple brain regions, however, and have additional pharmacologic properties that make it difficult to pinpoint the precise mechanisms that mediate their rewarding properties.

Despite the physiologic and social costs of drug abuse, the mesolimbic system serves an important function in normal behavior. In essence, the mesolimbic system rewards an organism for engaging in behaviors that lead to its success and survival. Sensory information is funneled into the amygdaloid complex so that an individual may recognize stimuli that have behavioral significance. Efferent projections from the amygdala coordinate a variety of autonomic responses; those which activate the mesolimbic dopaminergic system produce feelings of elation when a tangible reward has been obtained. Rewards increase the probability that the preceding behavior will recur, and natural rewards, such as food, fluid, and sex, promote behaviors that lead to the survival of an organism and its species. In humans, rewarding experiences are also produced by the attainment of abstract goals, which involve the expenditure of considerable energy over long periods of time. In the case of drug abuse, the natural mechanisms of the limbic system are circumvented by psychoactive drugs that directly activate dopaminergic transmission within the mesolimbic forebrain.

HIPPOCAMPUS

The hippocampus was originally thought to play a major role in the expression of emotional behavior because patients with severe damage to the hippocampus and surrounding temporal lobe structures showed clear signs of emotional disturbance. Subsequently, it became evident that most of the emotional changes produced by temporal lobe lesions were a consequence of damage to the amygdaloid complex alone. Although the hippocampal formation may have a role in emotional expression, selective damage to the hippocampus indicates that it has a specific role in learning and memory processing.

Anatomy of the Hippocampal Formation

The hippocampal formation is a collection of laminated structures that lie below the parahippocampal gyrus on the ventral aspect of the temporal lobe (Figure 13-7). Located immediately caudal to the amygdaloid complex, the hippocampal formation extends along the temporal horn of the lateral ventricle until it reaches the splenium of the corpus callosum. The hippocampal formation includes the dentate gyrus, the hippocampus proper, the subiculum, and the entorhinal cortex. The sigmoid configuration of these structures resembles the shape of a seahorse which, in Greek, is called a hippocampus.

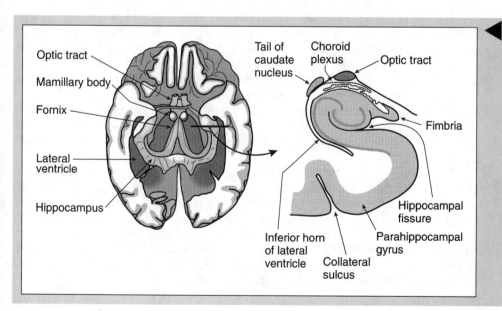

FIGURE 13-7
Hippocampal Formation. A ventral view of the hippocampus after removing the bottom half of the temporal lobe. A transverse section through the rostral part of the hippocampus is shown on the right.

DENTATE GYRUS AND HIPPOCAMPUS PROPER

The dentate gyrus and hippocampus form interlocking C-shaped structures when viewed in transverse section (Figure 13-8). Both structures contain three cortical layers, which define them as archicortex.

FIGURE 13-8 ▶

Hippocampus Proper and Dentate Gyrus.
This photomicrograph illustrates the laminar structure of the dentate gyrus and the cornu Ammonis (CA) subfields of the hippocampus. (Source: Courtesy of Dr. Malcolm Carpenter, Professor Emeritus, Uniform Armed Services University, Bethesda, Maryland.)

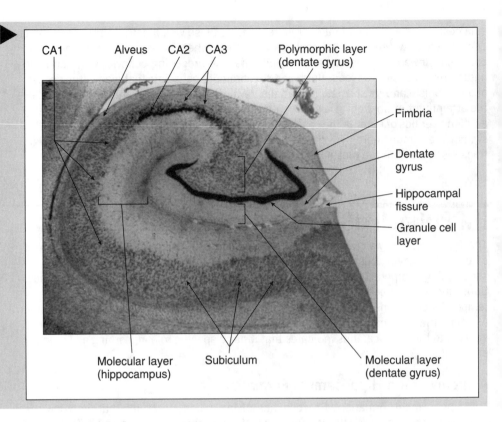

Cornu Ammonis *is Ammon's horn.*

The dentate gyrus contains a densely packed layer of granule cells that is easily seen in most histologic preparations of the hippocampal formation. The external side of the granule cell layer is encircled by the molecular layer, which contains a dense plexus of incoming axons, their terminals, and the dendrites extending from the granule cells. The polymorphic layer of the dentate gyrus, which lies within the hilus of the granule cell layer, contains interneurons, glia, and axons arising from the granule cells.

The hippocampus proper, which lies between the dentate gyrus and the subiculum, consists of a thick layer of pyramidal cells sandwiched between the more superficial polymorphic layer and a deeper molecular layer. As shown by Figure 13-8, the molecular layers of the hippocampus and dentate gyrus are continuous with each other. Apical dendrites from the pyramidal cells extend into the molecular layer of the hippocampus to receive synaptic inputs from the dentate gyrus. The polymorphic layer contains the axons and basal dendrites extending from the pyramidal neurons. The polymorphic layer is separated from the inferior horn of the lateral ventricle by a thin sheath of myelinated axons called the alveus, which contains the projection fibers originating from the hippocampus and subiculum.

The hippocampus is divided into subfields that vary in their cytologic appearance: CA1, CA2, and CA3. According to this nomenclature, in which CA stands for cornu Ammonis (Ammon's horn), the CA3 subfield begins at the polymorphic layer of the dentate gyrus and extends for several millimeters. The largest pyramidal cells in the hippocampus are located in the CA3 subfield where they are packed into a relatively thick layer. The CA2 subfield is a short transitional region between the more extensive CA3 and CA1 subfields. The CA1 subfield varies throughout its transverse axis, and its pyramidal cell layer gradually becomes thicker as it approaches the subiculum.

SUBICULUM

The subiculum is located in the superior part of the parahippocampal gyrus, partially buried within the ventral bank of the hippocampal fissure. The subiculum forms the transition between the trilaminar hippocampus and the six layers of the entorhinal cortex. Like the dentate gyrus and the hippocampus proper, however, the subiculum contains three layers and has a distinct layer of pyramidal neurons located between a superficial molecular layer and a deeper polymorphic layer. Pyramidal neurons in the subiculum provide the major subcortical projections of the hippocampal formation to the septal nucleus, the mamillary body, the nucleus accumbens, and the anterior nucleus of the thalamus.

ENTORHINAL CORTEX

The entorhinal cortex occupies the inferior part of the parahippocampal gyrus and extends laterally almost to the collateral sulcus. Although the entorhinal cortex contains six layers, it differs from traditional neocortex in several respects. Layer II, for example, contains distinct aggregates of large pyramidal neurons that form visible bumps on the surface of the parahippocampal gyrus. Layer IV is virtually absent in the entorhinal cortex and the pyramidal cells of layers III and V are closely apposed to one another. The pyramidal neurons in layers II and III of the entorhinal cortex are important because they provide the major route for transmitting information from the association cortex into the hippocampus.

INTRINSIC CIRCUITS IN THE HIPPOCAMPAL FORMATION

One of the prominent features in the neural circuitry of the hippocampal formation is the serial flow of information through each of its components (Figure 13-9). The entorhinal cortex begins this multisynaptic loop by projecting to the granule cells of the dentate gyrus. These entorhinal projections are called the perforant pathway because their fibers perforate the hippocampal fissure before terminating on granule cell dendrites in the molecular layer. The granule cells send a dense projection of axons, or mossy fibers, to the molecular layer of the CA3 subfield where they synapse on the apical dendrites of the pyramidal neurons. Axons from the CA3 pyramidal neurons bifurcate into two branches, one of which enters the alveus to exit the hippocampus in the fibers of the fornix. The collateral axons from the CA3 pyramidal neurons, called Schaffer collaterals, project to pyramidal neurons in the CA1 subfield which, in turn, project to the subiculum. Finally, pyramidal neurons in the subiculum complete the multisynaptic loop through the hippocampal formation by sending their axons to the entorhinal cortex.

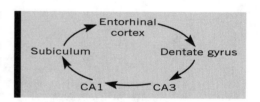

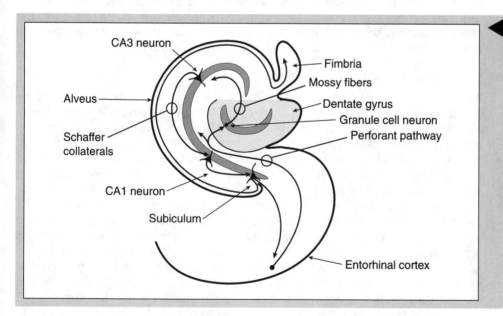

FIGURE 13-9

Intrinsic Hippocampal Circuits. The hippocampal formation contains a unidirectional circuit in which information is transmitted from the entorhinal cortex, to the dentate gyrus, to CA3, to CA1, and finally to the subiculum.

As the perforant pathway proceeds to the dentate gyrus, its axons form some en passant synapses with the distal dendrites of pyramidal neurons in CA1 and CA3, but there is no other opportunity for feedback processing within the hippocampal formation. The serial progression of information throughout the hippocampal formation is emphasized by the total absence of feedback projections from CA3 to the dentate gyrus and by a similar lack of projections from CA1 to CA3. All information processed by the dentate gyrus is transmitted to the CA subfield of the hippocampus; the dentate gyrus does not project to any other region of the brain.

This unidirectional flow of information through the hippocampal formation is conveyed entirely by excitatory connections. The perforant pathway, the mossy fibers, the
Schaffer collaterals, and the efferent projections from CA1 and the subiculum all use
glutamate as an excitatory neurotransmitter. Although GABAergic inhibitory interneurons
are present in the deeper parts of the granule cell layer of the dentate gyrus and the
polymorphic layers of the hippocampal CA fields, glutamate is the major neurotransmitter in each part of the hippocampal formation. The predominance of excitatory glutaminergic fibers in the hippocampal formation has, in part, made it vulnerable to seizure
activity, which quickly spreads to neighboring parts of the temporal lobe.

Neural Plasticity in the Hippocampus

To learn new information or to remember events of the past, the nervous system must
have the capacity for plasticity. In other words, the nervous system must be capable of
structural changes, or plasticity, to represent new memories. One possible mechanism
for plasticity involves the selective strengthening and weakening of synaptic connections. In 1949, Donald Hebb hypothesized that connections between a presynaptic and
postsynaptic neuron would become stronger if both neurons discharged at the same time.
This view, known as Hebb's postulate, is widely regarded as one of the mechanisms that
mediate learning. The ability to make these kinds of synaptic changes is a normal
function of the brain that occurs continuously throughout each person's life. Consistent
with its role in memory, numerous experiments have demonstrated the phenomenon of
synaptic plasticity in the hippocampus.

Most of our knowledge about hippocampal plasticity has been obtained from studies
conducted on rodents. When the rodent hippocampal formation is sectioned transversely, the multisynaptic pathways interconnecting the dentate gyrus with the hippocampus proper remain intact and neuronal responses can be recorded at each level of
this pathway. Thus, when thin slices of the hippocampal formation are placed in a warm
and oxygenated solution of artificial cerebrospinal fluid, pyramidal neurons in CA3 and
CA1 have normal membrane potentials that respond to electrical stimulation of the
perforant pathway or the Schaffer collaterals. This experimental technique has been
valuable for examining the cellular events that underlie neural plasticity.

LONG-TERM POTENTIATION

When a small population of Schaffer collaterals are electrically stimulated in a hippocampal slice, the orthodromic impulses excite the CA1 pyramidal neurons (Figure
13-10). If the same electrical test stimulus is delivered infrequently (e.g., once or twice
per minute), the amplitude of the CA1 excitatory postsynaptic potential (EPSP) remains
constant. If the Schaffer collaterals are repetitively stimulated by a train of electrical
pulses, known as tetanic stimulation, a subsequent test stimulus produces a much larger
EPSP in CA1. This potentiation in the size of the postsynaptic response may persist for
several hours and, therefore, this phenomenon is called long-term potentiation (LTP).
Synaptic potentiation is limited to those synapses that are activated repeatedly by tetanic
stimulation. For example, if two stimulating electrodes were used to activate separate
populations of Schaffer collaterals with a test stimulus, but tetanic stimulation was
administered by only one of these electrodes, LTP would appear only in the pathway that
received high-frequency stimulation (see Figure 13-10). It is thought that selective
potentiation of certain synapses, but not others, may mediate normal learning.

Synaptic responses in the hippocampus can be potentiated without using tetanic
stimulation, but only if the presynaptic and postsynaptic neurons are excited simultaneously. To demonstrate this effect, an intracellular electrode is used to briefly depolarize a CA1 neuron while a single electrical pulse is applied to the Schaffer collaterals.
After several trials of pairing postsynaptic depolarization with activation of the Schaffer
collaterals, the synaptic connections become potentiated. In this paradigm, however,
synaptic potentiation appears only when the presynaptic and postsynaptic neurons are
coactivated at precisely the same time, usually within an interval of 100 milliseconds
(ms) or less. This form of plasticity is thought to play a role in behavioral conditioning or
other types of associative learning.

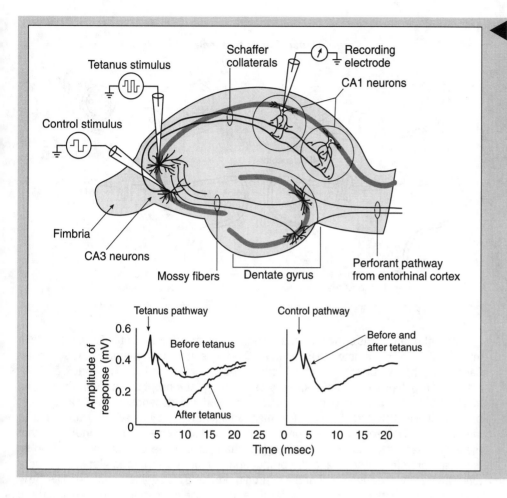

► **FIGURE 13-10**
Long-Term Potentiation. This diagram shows a slice of the rodent hippocampus in which a pair of stimulating electrodes is positioned at different sites in the CA3 subfield and an extracellular recording electrode is positioned in the CA1 subfield. When either part of the CA3 subfield is stimulated with a brief electrical pulse, CA1 neurons show a well-defined response. Following tetanic stimulation of one CA3 region, however, the CA1 response is potentiated when a brief pulse is applied to the same pathway. The CA1 response to pulse stimulation of the other CA3 subfield does not change.

LONG-TERM DEPRESSION

It is unlikely that learning and memory are mediated exclusively by increases in synaptic efficacy. If neural plasticity manifested itself only as an increase in synaptic strength, eventually all synapses would attain a maximum level of efficacy, and it would be difficult to encode new information. Experimentally it has been shown that certain patterns of electrical stimulation cause a decrease in synaptic efficacy. Thus, if Schaffer collaterals are stimulated at low frequencies (~1 hertz) for an extended period, a subsequent test stimulus elicits a weaker or depressed postsynaptic response in the CA1 subfield. This change may persist for several hours and can reverse the effects of LTP. Although the relationship between synaptic depression and learning is not understood, it is clear that synaptic strength can be attenuated in the hippocampus under certain circumstances.

CELLULAR BASIS FOR HIPPOCAMPAL PLASTICITY

The discovery of synaptic plasticity in the hippocampus has prompted considerable research to determine its cellular basis. Blockade of glutaminergic transmission prevents the development of LTP, and further analysis has shown that synaptic potentiation depends on the activation of a specific glutamate receptor, the *N*-methyl-D-aspartate (NMDA) receptor (see Chapter 1).

The postsynaptic effects of glutamate vary according to the types of glutamate receptors that are activated. If the neuron is at its resting membrane potential, glutamate binding to non-NMDA receptors allows an influx of sodium ions (Na^+). Glutamate is unable to activate NMDA receptors because NMDA-gated channels are blocked by magnesium ions (Mg^{2+}) whenever the membrane potential is negative (Figure 13-11). When the membrane potential becomes depolarized, the Mg^{2+} are expelled so that glutamate molecules may activate the NMDA receptors to allow an influx of both Na^+ and calcium ions (Ca^{2+}).

LTP depends on activation of glutamate NMDA receptors.

FIGURE 13-11 ▶

N-Methyl-D-Aspartate (NMDA) Receptors.
Magnesium ions (Mg²⁺) block NMDA receptors when the postsynaptic membrane is in its resting potential. Depolarization of the postsynaptic membrane removes the Mg²⁺ block and allows glutamate to activate NMDA receptors which allow an influx of sodium (Na⁺) and calcium (Ca²⁺) ions.

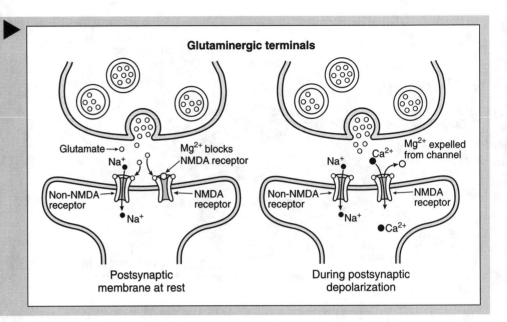

An influx of Ca²⁺ is critical for the induction and maintenance of LTP. An increase in intracellular Ca²⁺ promotes LTP, whereas Ca²⁺ chelators (compounds that sequester Ca²⁺ from the cytoplasm) effectively block the induction of LTP. The influx of Ca²⁺ activates two types of protein kinases (enzymes that phosphorylate certain protein molecules) that have been identified as Ca²⁺-calmodulin–dependent protein kinase and protein kinase C (Figure 13-12). The mechanisms of these kinases and their role in maintaining LTP have not been completely elucidated. Some evidence indicates that these Ca²⁺-activated proteins may trigger changes in gene expression that lead to increased protein synthesis and the production of more postsynaptic glutamate receptors. Other evidence suggests that the neuron produces a retrograde signal, such as nitric oxide, which directs the presynaptic terminal to release more glutamate in response to incoming action potentials.

FIGURE 13-12 ▶

Molecular Basis of Long-term Potentiation (LTP). *LTP depends on glutaminergic activation of N-methyl-D-aspartate (NMDA) receptors and the subsequent increase in calcium ion (Ca²⁺) influx. Increased levels of Ca²⁺ activate protein kinase C and Ca²⁺-calmodulin kinase II. These Ca²⁺-dependent enzymes may cause the metabolic machinery of the neuron to synthesize more glutamate receptors or release a retrograde signal which acts on the presynaptic terminal. Na⁺ = sodium ion.*

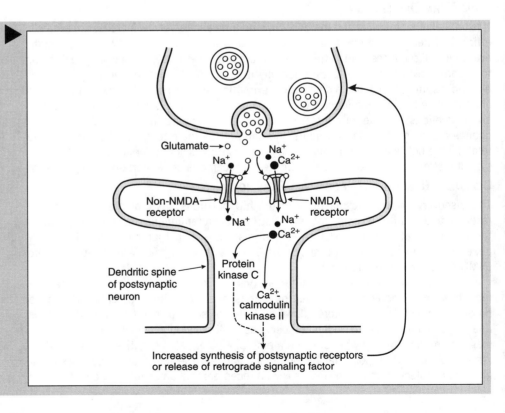

Regardless of the exact mechanisms by which Ca^{2+} induces LTP, the properties of LTP are reflected in the dynamics of the NMDA receptor. Thus, LTP is induced by high-frequency stimulation because the tremendous increase in the synaptic release of glutamate depolarizes the postsynaptic neuron enough to remove the Mg^{2+} block. Alternatively, LTP is induced by pairing weak presynaptic stimulation with direct depolarization of the postsynaptic cell because this also removes the Mg^{2+} block.

TEMPORAL LOBE EPILEPSY

Epilepsy is a neurologic disorder that is mediated by dysfunctional, synchronous, and rhythmic activity of large populations of neurons. Although epileptic seizures may occur throughout the cerebral cortex, most seizures are initiated in the hippocampus or in the adjacent temporal lobe. The propensity of the hippocampus for initiating seizures is directly related to the ease with which synaptic excitation can be potentiated in this brain region. Thus, the same mechanisms that mediate LTP may, under certain conditions, lead to excessive and uncontrollable neuronal activity.

The relationship between synaptic potentiation and seizure initiation is illustrated by kindling studies in which a weak electrical stimulus is delivered to the amygdaloid complex once a day. Initially, this stimulation does not elicit seizure activity or behavioral convulsions. After several daily sessions of stimulation, however, the same electrical stimulus evokes a full-blown seizure that is accompanied by convulsions. The pattern of hippocampal seizures elicited by kindling in animals is remarkably similar to the seizure activity seen in human epilepsy.

Kindling is the repetitive electrical stimulation of the amygdala, which leads to seizures.

Epileptic seizures in humans can be caused by trauma, tumors, infections, ischemia, and vascular malformations. Although no consensus has developed regarding how these factors alter the cellular and metabolic functions of hippocampal neurons, substantial evidence indicates that an increase in the extracellular concentration of potassiuim (K^+) [10–12 mM compared to a normal concentration of 3–5 mM] makes hippocampal neurons more excitable. The role of increased extracellular K^+ has received attention because certain forms of epilepsy are associated with low levels of adenosine triphosphate (ATP) and Na^+–K^+-adenosine triphosphatase (ATPase), both of which are needed to maintain the differential concentrations of Na^+ and K^+ across neuronal membranes. An increase in extracellular K^+ effectively shifts the K^+ reversal potential (E_K) more positive and, by causing a decrease in K^+ efflux, leads to partial depolarization of the resting membrane potential (see Chapter 1). Any diminishment in K^+ efflux also reduces the amplitude of long-latency inhibitory potentials, which are mediated by certain types of GABA receptors, namely the $GABA_B$ receptors, which promote K^+ efflux. Furthermore, in hippocampal neurons a brief burst of action potentials is immediately followed by a large hyperpolarization, or afterhyperpolarization, to prevent sustained repetitive firing. Since the afterhyperpolarization is mediated by a Ca^{2+}-dependent K^+ efflux, any reduction in K^+ outflow also interferes with the inhibition provided by the afterhyperpolarization. The net effect of all of these changes is to increase the excitability of hippocampal neurons.

Given its capacity for potentiating excitatory responses and its unidirectional circuit of excitatory connections, excessive activity in any part of the hippocampus may spread to the entorhinal cortex, which has access to widespread regions of the cerebral cortex. The behavioral manifestations of seizure activity in the cerebral cortex depend on the specific location and size of the affected area. Focal seizures that affect a small region of the motor cortex, for example, may produce mild twitching in a limb; more generalized seizures across a larger expanse of the cortex may lead to sensory hallucinations, uncontrollable convulsions, and loss of consciousness.

Epilepsy occurs in the hippocampus because it potentiates reverberating excitatory activity.

ROLE OF THE HIPPOCAMPUS IN MEMORY

Memory is a specific cognitive function that underlies our ability to learn new information. Although neural plasticity is necessary for learning and memory, there are different forms of neural plasticity that appear in various structures including the hippocampus and cerebral cortex. The hippocampus and surrounding structures play a special role in learning and memory, which we are just beginning to understand. Much of our knowledge comes from clinical studies correlating psychological performance with the findings of neuropathology.

Memory Classifications

Neuropsychologists classify memory into two broad categories: declarative memory and procedural memory. Declarative memory is concerned with the storage and retrieval of semantic information such as the meaning of words, famous dates in history, names of acquaintances, and other information that is encoded by language or other conscious methods (e.g., visual images). Procedural memory is concerned with the acquisition of motor skills that are performed without conscious awareness. Thus, keyboard typing or serving a tennis ball are examples of motor skills that are learned and perfected with practice. Once learned, these skills can still be performed after long intervals because the brain has "memorized" the motor programs that specify the timed sequence of muscle activity needed to perform these tasks.

The division of memory into procedural and declarative categories is appropriate from a neuroanatomical perspective because different brain regions are involved in storing these types of memory. The cerebellum, basal ganglia, and premotor cortex are critical for the long-term storage of procedural memories, whereas declarative memories depend on interactions between the hippocampus and widespread regions of the cerebral cortex.

Memory is also classified according to the time frame over which it persists (Figure 13-13). Immediate memory is the ability to hold an experience in mind for a brief instant and provides us with our sense of the present. Short-term memory describes the ability to remember information for short periods of time, usually for several seconds or minutes. Short-term memory is used to retain information until a task has been performed, at which time the information is rapidly forgotten. Memorizing a phone number and then forgetting it after completing the call is an example of short-term memory that is called working memory. Finally, information that can be retrieved after an interval of several days, weeks, months, or years is stored in long-term memory.

Declarative memories are encoded by language or visual images.

Procedural memories are encoded by motor performance.

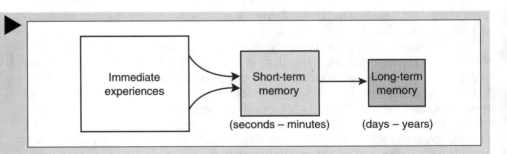

FIGURE 13-13 ▶
Time Course of Memory. How memory is stored depends on how long the information is needed. Only a fraction of our perceptual experiences are stored in short-term memory for a period of several seconds or minutes. Only a fraction of the information in short-term memory is consolidated into long-term memory for days, weeks, or years.

Consolidation is the transfer of short-term memory into long-term memory.

Retrieval is the process that brings memory into consciousness.

The ability to form and retrieve a memory involves several distinct processes. The process by which information is transferred from short-term memory into long-term memory is called consolidation. Some evidence indicates that consolidation depends on physical changes in synaptic connections, involving either the construction of new synapses or a change in the strength of existing synapses. The act of remembering refers to the process by which information is retrieved from long-term storage and is brought into consciousness (declarative memory) or is expressed as a motor skill (procedural memory). Thus, consolidation, long-term storage, and subsequent retrieval refer to distinct aspects of memory that may involve separate mechanisms and brain regions. The anatomic and physiologic basis for long-term memory is poorly understood, and considerable research is aimed at elucidating the mechanisms that mediate these processes.

Amnesia

Forgetting is a normal process that occurs over time in all individuals. For most of us, unimportant information is soon forgotten to facilitate our ability to remember significant information or to recall facts that we actively memorize for testing purposes. In some individuals, however, forgetting is a pathologic process that interferes with the ability to recall highly important information. In these cases, the pathologic loss of memory is classified as anterograde or retrograde amnesia. Anterograde amnesia is an inability to establish new memories (i.e., consolidation has been impaired) after some precipitating event or illness; retrograde amnesia is characterized by difficulty in retrieving information that had been consolidated into long-term memory.

Anterograde amnesia is the inability to establish new memory because of a defect in consolidation.

Retrograde amnesia is the inability to retrieve information from long-term memory.

ANTEROGRADE AMNESIA

The classic example of anterograde amnesia is represented by the case of H. M., a 27-year-old man who received a bilateral medial temporal lobectomy to alleviate seizures produced by a debilitating form of epilepsy. Since the age of 16, H. M. had suffered major seizures characterized by generalized convulsions, tongue-biting, urinary incontinence, and a loss of consciousness. Despite receiving heavy doses of different anticonvulsants, these attacks gradually increased in frequency and severity to the point where H. M. was unable to maintain a normal life.

When anticonvulsants are unsuccessful in managing temporal lobe seizures, the hippocampus and surrounding structures can be removed to reduce seizure activity. On this basis, H. M. underwent surgery in which the amygdala, uncus, parahippocampal gyrus, and the anterior two-thirds of the hippocampus were bilaterally removed. This surgery was performed in 1953, before it was known that the hippocampus was necessary for establishing memories. On recovering from his operation, however, it was clear that H. M. suffered from severe anterograde amnesia.

Approximately 19 months after his surgery, H. M. was examined by a psychologist to determine the precise nature of his amnesia. The severity of his memory defect was immediately apparent because H. M. was unable to recall any details of his life since the operation and was not even aware that he had received an operation. Despite this memory impairment, H. M. achieved an intelligence quotient (IQ) score of 112 on the Wechsler-Bellevue Intelligence Scale, a result that was similar to his preoperative score of 104. The examination also failed to reveal any deficits in perception, abstract thinking, reasoning ability, or motor learning.

On tests that measured declarative memory, H. M. was unable to demonstrate any memory for new stories or memorize word pairs that were presented to him a few minutes earlier. Whenever his attention was turned to a new task, H. M. was unable to recall the preceding task in which he had been engaged. These deficits indicate a profound loss of short-term and long-term memory. It is important to note, however, that H. M. was able to recall events that occurred prior to his operation. Indeed, when presented with pictures of celebrities, H. M. was able to name those people that became famous prior to his surgery. His ability to retrieve memories established before bilateral removal of the temporal lobes indicates that the hippocampus does not store information nor does it participate in the retrieval process. Instead, the inability to establish new declarative memories suggests that the main function of the hippocampus is to consolidate semantic information into long-term memory.

Causes of Anterograde Amnesia
Temporal lobe damage
Head trauma

RETROGRADE AMNESIA

By definition, retrograde amnesia means that a patient is unable to recall events that occurred prior to some precipitating event. In contrast to anterograde amnesia, which is produced by focal damage in the temporal lobe, retrograde amnesia is typically produced by pathologic processes that have more global effects on the cerebral cortex. Since long-term memories are stored in a distributed fashion throughout the cortex and related

Causes of Retrograde Amnesia
Alzheimer's disease
Head trauma
Electroconvulsive shocks

areas, any event that causes widespread neural dysfunction may interfere with the retrieval of long-term memories. Thus, retrograde amnesia can be precipitated by head trauma, electroconvulsive therapy, or generalized lesions such as those produced by Alzheimer's disease.

Head Trauma. It has long been known that patients may exhibit varying degrees of amnesia while recovering from the loss of consciousness associated with a severe head injury. Patients with head trauma are unable to remember events that immediately preceded the injury (retrograde amnesia) and may have difficulty recalling events that transpired after consciousness was regained (anterograde amnesia). In either case, the severity and duration of amnesia are directly related to the amount of brain damage. With a minor concussion, amnesia is rare, but following a severe contusion (i.e., bruise) of the brain, anterograde and retrograde amnesia may persist for several days or weeks. As these patients recover, their memory for events occurring before and after the injury is gradually restored until, eventually, no further recovery is apparent. The last memories to recover are those closest in time to the trauma, but events immediately preceding severe head trauma are never recalled because this information was not consolidated into long-term memory.

Electroconvulsive Therapy. Many patients suffering from epilepsy become depressed. In some of these individuals, the occurrence of an epileptic seizure alleviates their depression. This discovery prompted psychiatrists to treat depression by administering electrical shocks to the head to produce a full-blown seizure. Electroconvulsive therapy (ECT) is effective in the treatment of severe depression, but produces anterograde and retrograde amnesia.

Controlled studies of the effects of ECT on memory indicate that recent memories are more easily disrupted than older memories (Figure 13-14). In one study depressed patients were asked to identify the names of television programs that were shown for only 1 year between 1957 and 1972. Different sets of programs were presented to each patient before and after receiving ECT, and the portion of identified shows was plotted as a function of the time since each program was on the air. Results from this study indicated that memory for the programs declined over time, and this followed the same pattern of forgetting that is present in all individuals. Administration of ECT disrupted the ability to name the most recent programs but had little effect on the memory for programs seen several years earlier. These results suggest that the formation of a stable memory is a prolonged process. Administration of ECT interferes with the ability to retrieve memories that are still in a labile form but does not affect the retrieval of memories that had been consolidated for more than 2 years. With further passage of time, however, even stable memories are gradually degraded or become more difficult to retrieve.

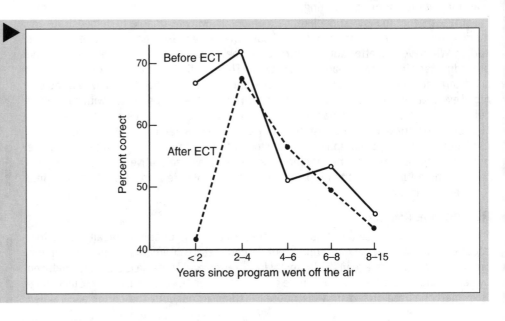

FIGURE 13-14 ▶

Amnesia Produced by Electroconvulsive Therapy (ECT). Patients with depression were asked to identify discontinued television programs that were aired for 1 year. Electroconvulsive shocks affected their memory for recent programs significantly more than their memory for older programs. (Source: Reprinted with permission from Squire LR, et al: Retrograde amnesia: temporal gradient in very long-term memory following electroconvulsive therapy. Science 187:77–79, 1975.)

Neural Substrate of Memory

The case of H. M. indicates that the hippocampus is necessary for memory consolidation but does not reveal the site of long-term memory storage. Accumulating evidence suggests that memories related to a particular sensory modality are stored in the corresponding cortical association area. Visual memory, for example, appears to be distributed throughout the inferior temporal gyrus. Neither the mechanisms by which the hippocampus consolidates information in the cerebral cortex nor the anatomic pathways employed in this process have been fully established. The prevailing presumption is that perceptual information is conveyed to the hippocampus from the association cortex and that this information is transformed by the hippocampus before it is returned to those association areas via the cortical projections of the subiculum and entorhinal cortex (Figure 13-15).

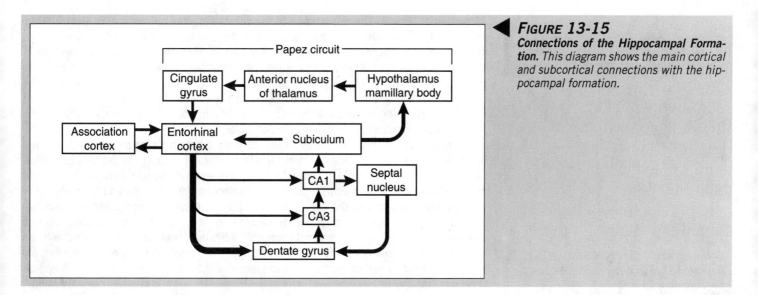

FIGURE 13-15
Connections of the Hippocampal Formation. *This diagram shows the main cortical and subcortical connections with the hippocampal formation.*

The hippocampal formation is also interconnected with a variety of subcortical structures within the diencephalon and basal forebrain (see Figure 13-15). The importance of these structures in memory has been demonstrated by several clinical cases, but their precise role in learning and memory has not been elucidated.

CORTICAL HIPPOCAMPAL CONNECTIONS

Extensive regions of the cerebral cortex project directly to the subiculum and entorhinal cortex or to adjacent parts of the parahippocampal gyrus (Figure 13-16). The cingulate gyrus sends a major projection to the entorhinal cortex via the cingulum, a thick bundle of fibers buried below the cingulate gyrus. Additional projections to the entorhinal cortex and subiculum originate from the dorsolateral prefrontal cortex (Brodmann areas 9, 10, and 46), the medial frontal cortex (Brodmann areas 25 and 32), and the orbitofrontal cortex. In the temporal lobe, the superior temporal gyrus, the perirhinal cortex, and the temporal pole all project to the entorhinal cortex. Finally, olfactory information reaches the hippocampal formation via projections from the piriform cortex and the periamygdaloid cortical area.

With the exception of the perforant pathway, efferent connections of the subiculum and entorhinal cortex have not been studied in detail. It is known that the entorhinal cortex and subiculum project to the perirhinal cortex, the cingulate gyrus, and the orbitofrontal cortex, but other long-range cortical projections are likely to exist as well. In addition, the entorhinal cortex has dense reciprocal connections with the parahippocampal gyrus, which projects to widespread regions in the temporal, parietal, and frontal lobes. Hence, the parahippocampal gyrus provides a major route by which the hippocampus influences diverse parts of the cerebral cortex.

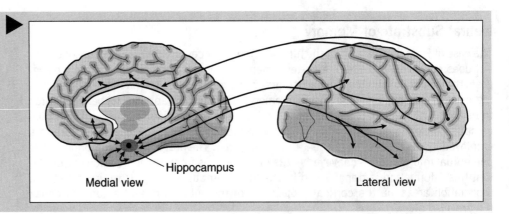

FIGURE 13-16
Long-term Memory Storage in the Cerebral Cortex. *Widespread regions of the cerebral cortex have reciprocal connections with the hippocampus, which may mediate the consolidation of short-term memory into long-term memory.*

Hippocampus

Medial view   Lateral view

Alzheimer's disease is characterized by an age-related pathologic decline in attention, reasoning, and memory.

Damaged Sites in Alzheimer's Disease
Basal forebrain
Hippocampal fields CA3, CA1
Subiculum
Entorhinal cortex
Association cortex

Alzheimer's Disease. The importance of the cerebral cortex for memory is illustrated by patients with Alzheimer's disease. Alzheimer's disease is a progressive neurologic disorder that is characterized by severe memory impairment and a progressive decline in attention, orientation, abstract reasoning, and language skills. In contrast to patients with medial temporal lobe damage, patients with Alzheimer's disease also experience difficulty retrieving distant memories. Although all individuals show some degree of mental deterioration with advancing age, the mental impairment associated with Alzheimer's disease is much more severe and debilitating.

A definitive diagnosis of Alzheimer's disease requires histologic examination of the brain. In Alzheimer's disease, there is significant loss of neurons in the hippocampus, subiculum, entorhinal cortex, and association cortex that may account for the severe memory impairment. Alzheimer's disease is also accompanied by a significant reduction in cholinergic neurons in the basal forebrain (i.e., substantia innominata, nucleus basalis of Meynert) and a concomitant decline in cholinergic markers (i.e., choline O-acetyltransferase) in the cerebral cortex. Finally, neuronal loss is correlated with an increase in the density of neurofibrillary tangles and amyloid plaques. Neurofibrillary tangles represent a pathologic form of intraneuronal cytoskeletal filaments, which appear to be produced by large pyramidal cells in the hippocampus and cerebral cortex. Amyloid plaques are extracellular deposits of proteinaceous material. It is not clear whether tangles and plaques cause the death of neurons or represent a by-product of neuronal death. Interestingly, the pathologic increase in plaques and tangles is more prevalent in association cortex than in primary sensory or motor cortices.

Although some forms of Alzheimer's disease have a genetic basis, the cause of this disease in most individuals is unknown. Because the incidence of Alzheimer's disease is age-related, familial patterns are more likely to be observed as more people live longer. Currently there is no cure or effective treatment for Alzheimer's disease.

SUBCORTICAL HIPPOCAMPAL PROJECTIONS

The septal nucleus is one of the few subcortical regions that sends a dense projection to the hippocampal formation (see Figure 13-15). Neurons in the medial septal nucleus project directly to the hippocampus via the fornix. Although some septohippocampal projections are GABAergic, most are cholinergic and, thus, comprise a portion of the basal forebrain cholinergic system. The septohippocampal projections terminate most densely in the dentate gyrus, subfield CA3, the subiculum, and the entorhinal cortex.

It has long been known that information having emotional significance is more likely to be consolidated into long-term memory. Consistent with this fact, the basolateral nuclei of the amygdaloid complex send a modest set of projections to the entorhinal cortex and the subiculum. Connections between the amygdala and hippocampus are reciprocal, but the amygdala exerts considerably more influence on the hippocampus than vice versa.

Monoaminergic influences on hippocampal processing are mediated by ascending projections from the brainstem. Thus, the hippocampus receives dopaminergic innervation from the ventral tegmental area, serotonergic innervation from the mesencephalic raphe nuclei, and noradrenergic innervation from the locus ceruleus. These modulatory pathways innervate widespread regions of the hippocampal formation but terminate most densely in the dentate gyrus.

Nearly all of the subcortical projections from the hippocampal formation are conveyed through the fornix. These projections originate from pyramidal neurons in subfields CA3 and CA1, as well as from the subiculum. The axons from these neurons proceed towards the inferior horn of the lateral ventricle to form a thin sheath, the alveus, that spreads along the ventricular surface of the hippocampus before emerging as the fimbria on the dorsomedial surface of the dentate gyrus. The fimbria proceeds caudally and medially with the hippocampus and lateral ventricle until it thickens to form the fornix, which arches under the splenium of the corpus callosum. At this point, some fibers in the fornix cross the midline within the hippocampal commissure, which interconnects the CA3 subfields of both hemispheres. The remaining fibers in the fornix proceed rostrally under the corpus callosum until they form the columns of the fornix, which enter the diencephalon between the interventricular foramen and the anterior commissure. At this point, the columns of the fornix divide into precommissural and postcommissural pathways. The smaller, precommissural fornix contains fibers arising from subfields CA3 and CA1, which terminate in the septal nucleus, the nucleus accumbens, and the medial frontal cortex. The more numerous fibers of the postcommissural fornix originate from the subiculum and terminate either in the mamillary body of the hypothalamus or in the anterior nucleus of the thalamus.

Korsakoff's Syndrome. Korsakoff's syndrome is a form of amnesia that is correlated with bilateral lesions in the mamillary bodies and mediodorsal nucleus of the thalamus. The cause of Korsakoff's syndrome is attributed to prolonged thiamine deficiency, which develops during chronic alcoholism (thiamine absorption is impaired in alcoholics). Patients with Korsakoff's syndrome are unable to remember recent events and tend to fabricate information to fill in the missing memory. Korsakoff's syndrome often appears with Wernicke's syndrome, another form of dementia induced by chronic alcoholism, which is associated with an ataxic gait and dysfunctional eye movements. Many neurologic problems occur in chronic alcoholics, and for this reason, Korsakoff's syndrome does not provide a clear picture of the relationship between amnesia and the underlying neuropathology. Nonetheless, autopsy findings from patients that had only the amnestic syndrome of Korsakoff's suggest that specific nuclei within the diencephalon play an important role in memory.

RESOLUTION OF CLINICAL CASE

This clinical case describes symptoms that are typical of temporal lobe epilepsy. This form of epilepsy, which is the most common type in adults, involves paroxysmal events in the amygdala, hippocampus, or parahippocampal gyrus. Temporal lobe epilepsy often begins in late childhood or adolescence, and though its cause is usually unknown, a history of febrile (fever-induced) seizures is not uncommon. A number of different criteria are used to classify seizures according to their severity. Thus, a partial seizure denotes epileptiform activity within a focal region of cortex, whereas a general seizure involves widespread cortical regions in both hemispheres. Consciousness is always preserved during a simple seizure but is impaired during a complex seizure. An aura usually precedes a complex-partial seizure, and the patient's description of the aura can be helpful in determining the focus of the epileptiform activity. An aura may have well-defined sensory characteristics such as visual, auditory, or olfactory hallucinations or may consist of general feelings of fear, detachment, or a sense of déjà vu. Complex-partial seizures are often marked by repetitive motor activity or automatisms, which affect the oral musculature (e.g., lip-smacking, tongue-biting, jaw movements). A loss of consciousness during a complex seizure is typically followed by a variable and prolonged period of confusion.

In most forms of epilepsy, seizures eventually recur and invariably increase in frequency and severity if left untreated. Successive seizures may cause brain damage and atrophy of the affected cortical sites, presumably due to the excitotoxic effects associated with excessive discharge of glutaminergic neurons (see Chapter 1). For this reason, it is imperative that patients diagnosed with epilepsy are treated to prevent further seizures. EEG uses scalp electrodes to display the spontaneous electrical activity that develops among populations of cortical neurons; thus, a routine EEG may characterize a specific epileptic syndrome even in the absence of behavioral symptoms.

No cure exists for epilepsy, but a variety of drugs are available to eliminate seizures or reduce their frequency. Since the propagation of seizure activity depends on excitatory neurotransmission, most drugs used in the treatment of epilepsy are anticonvulsants that act by attenuating neuronal excitability. Many anticonvulsant drugs inhibit neurons directly because they are GABAergic agonists (e.g., phenobarbital, valproic acid), while others reduce excitability by stabilizing the membrane conductance of Na^+ (e.g., carbamazepine, phenytoin). Patients who continue to have debilitating seizures after trying different classes of anticonvulsant drugs usually undergo surgical resection of the epileptic focus to control their seizures.

REVIEW QUESTIONS

Directions: For each of the following questions, choose the **one best** answer.

1. A focal lesion of the amygdaloid complex in a human is most likely to produce which of the following symptoms?

    (A) Agnosia

    (B) Amnesia

    (C) Anxiety

    (D) Aphasia

    (E) Automatism

2. Which of the following nuclei and neurotransmitters are associated with subjective feelings of pleasure?

    (A) Acetylcholine—nucleus basalis of Meynert

    (B) Dopamine—nucleus accumbens

    (C) γ-Aminobutyric acid (GABA)—amygdala

    (D) Glutamate—hippocampus

    (E) Serotonin—hypothalamus

3. Which of the following drugs produces its therapeutic benefit by increasing serotonergic transmission in the amygdala?

    (A) Amphetamine (Adderall)

    (B) Phenytoin (Dilantin)

    (C) Phenobarbital (Donnatal)

    (D) Fluoxetine (Prozac)

    (E) Diazepam (Valium)

4. Which of the following neural structures is most likely to be damaged in a chronic alcoholic?

    (A) Entorhinal cortex

    (B) Mediodorsal thalamus

    (C) Nucleus accumbens

    (D) Prefrontal cortex

    (E) Septal nucleus

5. Which of the following sequences correctly describes the flow of activity through a major loop in the limbic system?

    (A) Amygdala → mediodorsal thalamus → cingulate gyrus → entorhinal cortex → amygdala

    (B) Amygdala → mediodorsal thalamus → prefrontal cortex → hypothalamus → amygdala

    (C) Entorhinal cortex → dentate gyrus → CA3 → CA1 → subiculum → entorhinal cortex

    (D) Subiculum → CA1 → CA3 → dentate gyrus → entorhinal cortex → subiculum

    (E) Subiculum → cingulate gyrus → anterior thalamus → mamillary bodies → subiculum

6. Which cognitive process is impaired following damage to the hippocampus?

(A) Attention

(B) Consolidation

(C) Memory retrieval

(D) Motor learning

(E) Visual recognition

ANSWERS AND EXPLANATIONS

1. The answer is A. Agnosia is the most likely symptom of a focal lesion of the amygdaloid complex. This type of lesion produces a constellation of symptoms that resembles the Klüver-Bucy syndrome. Thus, human patients often have difficulty with stimulus recognition and may have visual, auditory, tactile, or olfactory agnosia. Amnesia may develop only if the lesion affects the hippocampal formation. Amygdaloid lesions produce a decrease, not an increase, in fear and anxiety. Aphasia is symptomatic of lesions in Broca's or Wernicke's area. An automatism is a repetitive motor activity that frequently occurs in the midst of an epileptic seizure.

2. The answer is B. Subjective feelings of pleasure, which can be caused by drugs such as cocaine and amphetamine, are increased by the synaptic release of dopamine in the nucleus accumbens. Direct infusions of dopamine antagonists into the nucleus accumbens cause animals to cease self-administration of amphetamine and cocaine. Cholinergic projections from the basal nucleus of Meynert are necessary for attention and other cognitive functions of the cerebral cortex. Diazepam (Valium) and other anxiolytics cause enhanced GABAergic transmission in the amygdala. Long-term potentiation is mediated by glutaminergic transmission in the hippocampus. Fluoxetine (Prozac) and other antidepressants increase serotonin release in the amygdala.

3. The answer is D. Fluoxetine (Prozac) inhibits the reuptake of serotonin at serotonergic terminals throughout the brain, including the amygdaloid complex. Amphetamine (Adderall) and cocaine act by different mechanisms to increase dopaminergic transmission in the basal ganglia and prefrontal cortex. Phenobarbital (Donnatal) and diazepam (Valium) enhance GABAergic inhibition at a number of sites in the brain.

4. The answer is B. The mediodorsal thalamus and the mamillary bodies are bilaterally damaged in chronic alcoholics who develop Korsakoff's syndrome. Loss of neurons in these areas is associated with amnesia for recent memories. The entorhinal cortex shows degenerative changes in Alzheimer's disease that account, in part, for memory impairment. The nucleus accumbens, the prefrontal cortex, and the septal nucleus are not damaged by disorders that affect memory processing.

5. The answer is C. Choice A is incorrect because the mediodorsal nucleus projects to the prefrontal cortex not to the cingulate gyrus. Choice B is incorrect because the prefrontal cortex projects mainly to the basal ganglia or to other parts of the motor system not to the hypothalamus. The pathway shown in D is the reverse of the correct answer. Choice E is incorrect because the subiculum projects directly to the mamillary bodies or the anterior thalamus but not to the cingulate gyrus.

6. The answer is B. Consolidation, the process of converting short-term memory into long-term memory, depends on hippocampal processing. Following damage to the hippocampus, it is still possible to learn a motor task, recognize visual patterns, or retrieve memories acquired previously. Attention is impaired in Alzheimer's disease or following damage to the anterior cingulate gyrus.

ADDITIONAL READING

Aggleton JP: The contribution of the amygdala to normal and abnormal emotional states. *Trends Neurosci* 16:328–333, 1993.

Davis M: The role of the amygdala in fear and anxiety. *Ann Rev Neurosci* 15:353–375, 1992.

MacLean PD: Some psychiatric implications of physiological studies on the frontaltemporal portion of the limbic system. *Electroencephal Clin Neurophysiol* 4:407–418, 1952.

McNamara JO: Cellular and molecular basis of epilepsy. *J Neurosci* 14:3413–3425, 1994.

Papez JW: A proposed mechanism of emotion. *Arch Neurol Psychiat* 38:725–743, 1937.

Pedley TA, Scheuer ML, Walczak TS: Epilepsy. In *Merritt's Textbook of Neurology*. Edited by Rowland LP. Baltimore, MD: Williams & Wilkins, 1995, pp 845–868.

Zola-Morgan SM, Squire LR: Neuroanatomy of memory. *Ann Rev Neurosci* 16:547–563, 1993.

14

SLEEP, COMA, AND BRAIN DEATH

INTRODUCTION OF CLINICAL CASE

T. R., a 58-year-old man, was seen by his family physician because of constant sleepiness which interfered with his work and other activities. The patient stated that he rarely slept well and that his sleep was often punctuated by a series of awakenings. His wife confirmed this remark. She hastened to add that her husband snored quite loudly when he fell asleep and that each series of snores was followed by a silent period lasting 30 or 40 seconds. Examination revealed enlargement of the patient's adenoids and tonsils, but all other findings were normal. The patient was generally healthy, but he had gained 30 lbs since his last office visit, and his weight was now in the top quartile for someone of his age and height. The physician referred the man to a sleep clinic where he was scheduled for polysomnography.

SLEEP

The human nervous system cannot remain in a waking state for prolonged periods of time without suffering adverse effects. For reasons that are not entirely clear, we require regular periods of sleep, and nightly sleep time consumes approximately one-third of our life span. While sleeping, our normal sense of consciousness is suspended as we experience dreams and other sensations that revitalize the central nervous system (CNS). Despite the restful feeling acquired from a good night's sleep, the sleep state is not mediated by a simple decrease in neuronal activity throughout the brain. Rather, sleep is an active process that is mediated by dramatic changes in the pattern of neural activity in specific brain regions including the neocortex, thalamus, and certain brainstem nuclei.

Disruption of sleep is a common complaint heard by many physicians. It is estimated that 15% of the population has a chronic sleeping problem and that 20% may suffer from occasional bouts of insomnia. Insufficient sleep is an enormous public health problem underscored by the fact that 5%–10% of all adults habitually use hypnotic medications to fall asleep. Furthermore, industrialization has led to an increase in the number of night-workers whose sleep patterns may be severely disrupted. One consequence of this has been an increase in major accidents during the night, such as the nuclear incidents at Chernobyl and Three Mile Island, when the propensity for sleeping is strongest.

Neural Activity and Electroencephalography

In 1929, Hans Berger demonstrated the feasibility of displaying cortical activity in humans by amplifying the small electrical signals recorded by electrodes placed on the scalp. This procedure, called electroencephalography, is widely used to characterize the global features of cortical activity during wakefulness and different stages of sleep.

As discussed in Chapter 1, fluctuations in the membrane potential of a neuron are extremely small and must be recorded by a microelectrode placed inside the neuron. When a large group of neurons are excited or inhibited simultaneously, however, this produces a massive flow of ionic current that can be detected by electrodes located hundreds of microns away. Hence, synchronization of cortical activity results in a small electrical signal that can be recorded by an electrode on the overlying scalp. A record of these electrical signals, called an electroencephalogram (EEG), represents the time-course of changes in the summed electrical activity of large populations of cortical neurons. These changes in electrical activity are primarily the result of changes in postsynaptic potentials, not action potentials. Action potentials are too brief to make a significant contribution to the EEG unless large numbers of cortical neurons are discharging at precisely the same time.

The EEG is used in the diagnosis of sleep disorders and epilepsy.

Since scalp electrodes detect neural events only in the underlying cortex, electrodes must be placed at several sites over the frontal, parietal, temporal, and occipital lobes for a complete EEG (Figure 14-1). Electroencephalography is routinely performed to determine whether epileptic seizure activity originates from the hippocampus, the surrounding limbic structures, or from other cortical regions. For this reason, EEG electrodes are sometimes placed on the sphenoid bone or in the nasopharynx to detect paroxysmal events in the medial temporal lobe.

Sensory stimuli produce evoked potentials in the EEG.

Changes in EEG activity related to sensory stimuli are called evoked potentials or event-related potentials (ERPs). Depending on the modality of the stimulus, ERPs

FIGURE 14-1 ▶
Standard Electroencephalogram (EEG) Recording Sites. Top and side views of the human scalp showing the location of electrodes for electroencephalography. Abbreviations for recording sites: A = auricle; C = central; F = frontal; FP = frontal pole; O = occipital; P = parietal; T = temporal.

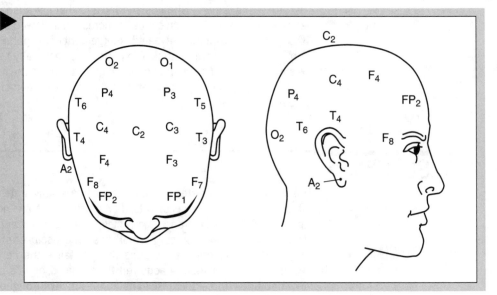

appear in one of the primary cortical regions that receive direct sensory projections from the thalamus. Cutaneous stimulation, for example, produces somatosensory-evoked potentials (SEPs) within the contralateral parietal cortex. Tones or flashes of light normally produce ERPs in the auditory or visual cortices, respectively. In patients who have sustained damage to a cranial nerve or to one of the ascending sensory pathways, the cortical ERPs for that particular modality are substantially reduced.

STATES OF CONSCIOUSNESS CORRELATED WITH EEG ACTIVITY

Changes in the amplitude and frequency of EEG activity provide a reliable indicator of changes in alertness and in the underlying activity of the cerebral cortex (Table 14-1). During the alert waking state, neuronal activity throughout the cerebral cortex tends to be desynchronized. Although certain groups of cortical neurons may display coordinated discharge patterns while processing information, most cortical neurons discharge at different times as they perform their perceptual, cognitive, or motor functions. Because cortical activity is desynchronized during waking periods, an EEG recorded from an alert individual with both eyes open contains low-amplitude, high-frequency waves. The waking EEG typically contains frequencies between 14 and 30 hertz (Hz), a bandwidth known as the beta range. During quiet resting with the eyes closed, the EEG shows prominent oscillations at 8–14 Hz, which are identified as alpha waves. During sleep, EEG activity slows, and larger amplitudes become prominent as more and more cortical neurons oscillate synchronously in the theta (4–8 Hz) or delta (0.5–4 Hz) frequency ranges.

◀ **TABLE 14-1**
Classification of EEG Activity

Classification	Frequency	Level of Arousal
Beta waves	14–30 Hz	Alert, eyes open
Alpha waves	8–14 Hz	Quiet waking, eyes closed
Theta waves	4–8 Hz	Drowsy, sleep stages 1 and 2
Delta waves	0.5–4 Hz	Deep sleep, stages 3 and 4

Clinical Evaluation of Sleep

To evaluate a patient's sleeping behavior, it is necessary to monitor several physiologic parameters in a laboratory that is equipped specifically for this purpose. In addition to recording EEG activity, a typical sleep laboratory also records an electro-oculogram (EOG) to detect rapid eye movements (REMs), and an electromyogram (EMG) to detect changes in muscle tone. This ensemble of records, known as a polysomnogram, provides the critical elements for characterizing sleep patterns in most individuals. Some sleep studies also measure changes in nasal airflow, respiratory movements, body temperature, or postural changes in body position.

SLEEP STAGES

A typical night's sleep is composed of a sequence of stages that are characterized by distinct shifts in the frequency and amplitude of the EEG (Figure 14-2). In a healthy adult, normal sleeping behavior follows a cyclic pattern in which the individual descends into deeper stages of non–rapid eye movement (NREM) sleep that are followed by progressively longer periods of REM sleep.

NREM Sleep. When an individual is resting quietly with eyes closed, the EEG contains low-voltage, fast-frequency alpha (8–14 Hz) rhythms. After becoming drowsy, sleep onset is marked by an abrupt shift to stage 1 sleep that is characterized by the presence of theta (4–8 Hz) waves and slow, rolling eye movements. Stage 1 represents a brief transitional period between wakefulness and true sleep and often does not reappear during the course of a night's sleep. As a person descends more deeply into stage 2 sleep, the EEG gradually becomes slower but is periodically interrupted by episodes of fast-frequency sleep spindles, and large-amplitude spikes that resemble the letter K (see Figure 14-2). Sleep spindles are 12–14 Hz waveforms that persist for 1–2 seconds and represent a specific type of interaction between the thalamus and cerebral cortex. Eventually, in stage 3 sleep, spindles occur less frequently, and slow EEG waves increase

*Large amplitude spikes in stage 2 sleep are called **K complexes**.*

Slow-wave sleep consists of delta waves (0.5–4 Hz).

in amplitude. Delta (0.5–4 Hz) waves appear irregularly in stage 3 sleep but are the main component of the EEG pattern during stage 4 of NREM sleep. In fact, stage 4 sleep is often called "slow-wave sleep" because this deep level of sleep is composed almost entirely of slow delta rhythms.

FIGURE 14-2 ▶

Polysomnography. *These electro-oculogram (EOG), electromyogram (EMG), and electroencephalogram (EEG) recordings illustrate the characteristic features of the different stages of sleep. The arrow in stage 2 indicates the presence of a K complex. (Source: Kales A: Sleep and dreams: recent research on clinical aspects. Ann Intern Med 68:1078–1104, 1968.)*

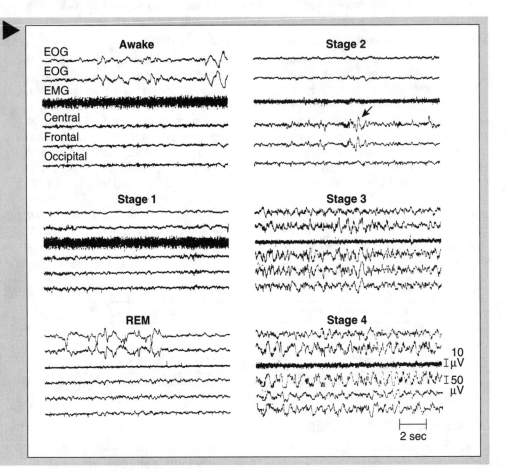

In experimental animals, total sleep deprivation disrupts homeostatic functions and eventually causes them to die. The chronic loss of NREM sleep is thought to be a major factor in their demise because selective deprivation of REM sleep alone does not produce serious consequences. Despite its obvious physiologic importance, the function of NREM sleep is not understood. Consistent with its restorative and revitalizing functions, slow-wave sleep reduces cerebral blood flow by 40% and produces a similar decline in oxygen consumption. This metabolic decrease is matched by a small, but significant, decrease in core body temperature. Indeed, a strong correlation exists between the circadian changes in body temperature and the propensity for sleep.

REM Sleep. At the end of each slow-wave sleep period, the EEG and other parameters show abrupt changes that signal the transition to REM sleep (Figure 14-3). During REM sleep, the EEG shows high-frequency, low-amplitude activity that resembles the desynchronized pattern of the waking state. Cerebral metabolism, as measured by cerebral blood flow and glucose consumption, increases 30%–40% over the resting wakeful state. For these reasons, REM sleep is often called paradoxical or active sleep.

As indicated by its name, REM sleep is characterized by rapid eye movements that are superimposed on a background of slower, rolling eye movements. The eye movements of REM sleep are driven by phasic bursts of neuronal activity that originate in the pontine tegmentum. Neuronal recordings from experimental animals during REM sleep indicate that REMs are correlated with bursts of neuronal discharges at numerous sites in the visual system including the oculomotor nuclei, the lateral geniculate nuclei, and the occipital cortex. Although recordings from the pons and lateral geniculate have been conducted only in experimental animals (Figure 14-4), the presence of pontine-

REMs are mediated by a burst of activity in the pons, lateral geniculate, and occipital cortex, which are called PGO spikes.

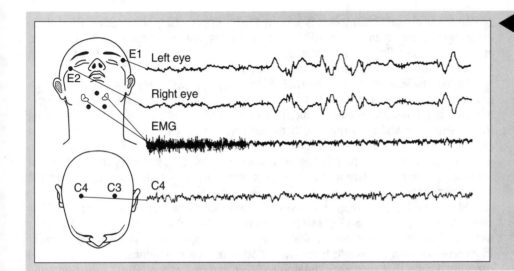

FIGURE 14-3
Transition to REM Sleep. The onset of a REM sleep period is marked by a sharp decrease in electromyogram (EMG) activity and the appearance of rapid eye movements as indicated by the electro-oculogram (EOG). Concomitantly, the electroencephalogram (EEG) waves shift to a lower amplitude and mixed frequency. C3 and C4 indicate central EEG recording sites. (Source: *Reprinted with permission from Kales A, Kales JD:* Evaluation and Treatment of Insomnia. *New York, NY: Oxford University Press, 1984, p. 6.*)

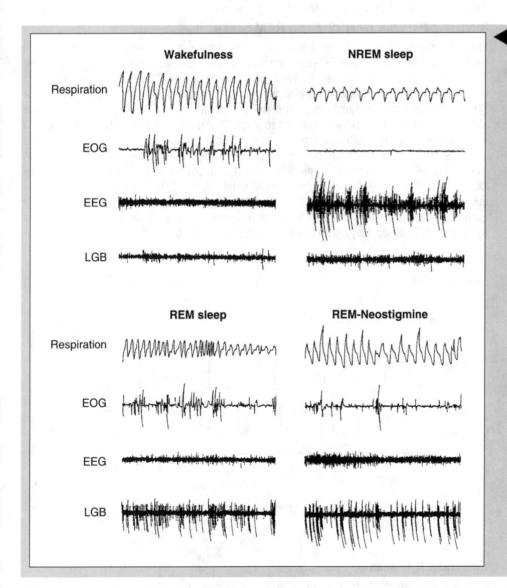

FIGURE 14-4
Wakefulness, NREM, and REM Sleep States. One-minute polygraphic recordings from a feline illustrate differences in the states of wakefulness, NREM sleep, and REM sleep. An injection of neostigmine (acetylcholinesterase inhibitor) into the medial pontine reticular formation induces a REM-like sleep state. EOG = electro-oculogram; EEG = electroencephalogram; LGB = lateral geniculate nucleus. (Source: *Reprinted with permission from Leonard TO, Lydic R:* Pontine nitric oxide modulates acetylcholine release, rapid eye movement sleep generation, and respiratory rate. *J Neurosci 17:774–785, 1997.*)

geniculate-occipital (PGO) spikes is assumed to be an essential component of REM sleep in humans. Other parameters of REM sleep, including changes in respiration, heart rate, and cerebral blood flow, are mediated by projections from the pontine tegmentum to sites located more caudally in the pons and medulla.

Unlike the waking state or the NREM sleep stages, REM sleep is associated with a profound loss of skeletal muscle tone. Only the extraocular muscles, the respiratory muscles, and the muscles controlling the ossicles of the middle ear remain active during REM sleep. The ability to regulate body temperature is lost, in part, because of the general paralysis of striated muscles. Furthermore, REM sleep is accompanied by a global suppression of sympathetic activity, one sign of which is pupillary constriction. All of these signs are consistent with a general reduction in homeostatic functions during the REM sleep stage.

Dreams occur during REM sleep.

Sleep studies on human volunteers indicate that most dreams occur during REM sleep. When awakened from REM sleep, more than 75% of the volunteers report that they were in the midst of a vivid dream. When they were awakened from NREM sleep, many of them reported having thought fragments or other mental experiences, but only a small percentage said that they were dreaming. Given the role of the lateral geniculate and striate cortex in mediating visual functions, PGO spikes are considered to be correlates of the visual images that are perceived during a dream.

RHYTHMIC PATTERN OF NREM AND REM SLEEP

The sequence of EEG activity during a night's sleep follows a predictable pattern (Figure 14-5). After sleep onset, the EEG shows a regular stepwise descent from stage 1 to stage 4, and this entire sequence usually takes about 60 minutes. The first abrupt shift from the slow-wave sleep of stage 4 to the desynchronized pattern of REM sleep occurs about 70–90 minutes after sleep onset. After the first REM sleep episode, which only lasts about 10 minutes, EEG activity returns to stage 2 and then descends through stages 3 and 4 of NREM sleep. Subsequently, a second REM episode appears about 90 minutes after the start of the first REM period. This alternating cycle between REM and NREM sleep is usually repeated four or five times during the course of a night's sleep. With the exception of the first REM period, most REM episodes last 20–30 minutes, and it takes about 90 minutes for a cycle of REM and NREM sleep to transpire. With each subsequent cycle, however, the proportion of NREM sleep devoted to stage 4 declines. By the end of the night, REM sleep may commence without passing through stage 4.

FIGURE 14-5 ▶
Periodic Pattern of Sleep. During a night of sleep, electroencephalogram (EEG) activity shifts between slow-wave sleep and REM sleep at regular intervals.

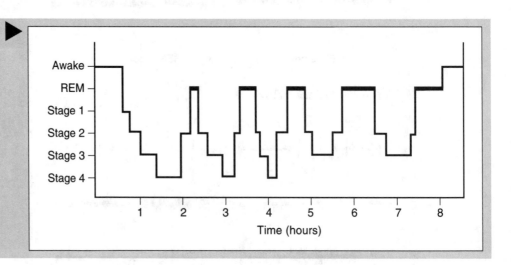

CIRCADIAN RHYTHMS

In humans and in most other vertebrates, sleep follows a circadian pattern. Although this pattern is strongly influenced by the alternating cycle of day and night, the brain has developed intrinsic mechanisms for controlling the circadian pattern of sleep and behavioral activity. Thus, when human subjects are placed in environments without clocks, windows, or other cues that might suggest the time of day, they continue to sleep at regular intervals and maintain a relatively normal circadian rhythm (Figure 14-6). In the absence of external temporal cues, however, the sleep-wake cycle usually lengthens to 25 or 26 hours. Based on this evidence, humans appear to have an internal clock that is reset each day and can be adjusted by seasonal changes in the onset and duration of daylight.

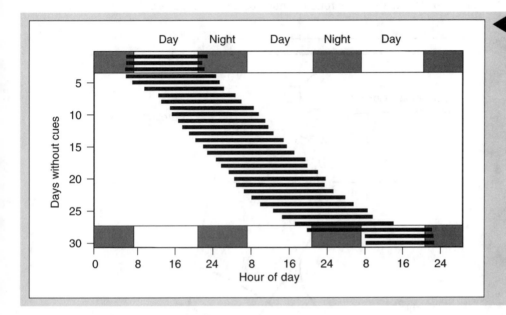

◀ **FIGURE 14-6**
Circadian Rhythms. *When cues about the time of day are removed, human subjects maintain a regular cycle of waking and sleeping but each cycle lengthens to 25 or 26 hours. The circadian pattern returns to a normal 24-hour cycle when time cues are reinstated.* Horizontal bars *represent waking hours.*

The brain region responsible for controlling circadian rhythms is the suprachiasmatic nucleus of the hypothalamus. Located above the optic chiasm, the suprachiasmatic nucleus receives fibers directly from the optic nerve to acquire information about the onset, intensity, and duration of daylight. In turn, the suprachiasmatic nucleus projects to the pontine tegmentum and other brainstem areas that control the different stages of sleep (see below). The role of the suprachiasmatic nucleus as a biologic clock is indicated by animal studies showing that damage to this structure severely disrupts the timing of the sleep-wake cycle. The total amount of REM and NREM sleep is unaffected following removal of the suprachiasmatic nucleus, but these sleep periods occur randomly and are no longer linked to nocturnal intervals. The exact mechanism by which the suprachiasmatic nucleus controls circadian rhythms is unclear but appears to involve cyclic changes in neural and hormonal activity. Evidence for a hormonal role is indicated by studies showing that following removal of the suprachiasmatic nucleus, an animal's circadian rhythm can be re-established by implanting a suprachiasmatic nucleus from a donor animal.

Neuroanatomy of Sleep

Changes in cortical activity during sleep are regulated by ascending projections from the thalamus and specific parts of the brainstem. High-voltage, slow-wave activity in the EEG during stages 3 and 4 is mediated by reverberating waves of synchronized activity flowing between the thalamus and cerebral cortex. Subsequent desynchronization of EEG activity during REM sleep occurs because thalamocortical synchronization is disrupted by depolarizing influences ascending from specific nuclei in the brainstem.

Slow EEG waves reflect synchronized oscillations in the discharges of thalamic and cortical neurons.

THALAMOCORTICAL INTERACTIONS AND CORTICAL SYNCHRONIZATION

The slow cortical oscillations of NREM sleep are a product of thalamic and cortical circuits working in concert with the intrinsic membrane properties of their constituent neurons. As indicated by Figure 14-7, the thalamocortical circuit that mediates EEG oscillations during slow-wave sleep is composed of three basic types of neurons. Thalamocortical neurons, which are located in almost all thalamic nuclei, send excitatory projections to widespread regions of the cerebral cortex, including sensory, motor, and association areas. These thalamocortical neurons also have collateral axons that terminate in the thalamic reticular nucleus, a slender nucleus that surrounds the lateral surface of the thalamus and is composed exclusively of GABAergic neurons which project to other parts of the thalamus (see Chapter 5). In essence, the reticular nucleus provides a recurrent inhibitory circuit for suppressing activity in thalamocortical neurons. Finally, excitatory corticothalamic projections, which originate from the deep layers of the cerebral cortex, terminate in the reticular nucleus and other parts of the thalamus.

FIGURE 14-7 ▶

Thalamocortical Circuits. Slow-wave sleep activity in the electroencephalogram (EEG) is mediated by interactions between neurons of the thalamus and cerebral cortex. The cerebral cortex and the relay nuclei of the thalamus have reciprocal excitatory connections and collateral projections to the reticular nucleus of the thalamus. The reticular nucleus contains GABAergic neurons that inhibit the thalamocortical relay neurons.

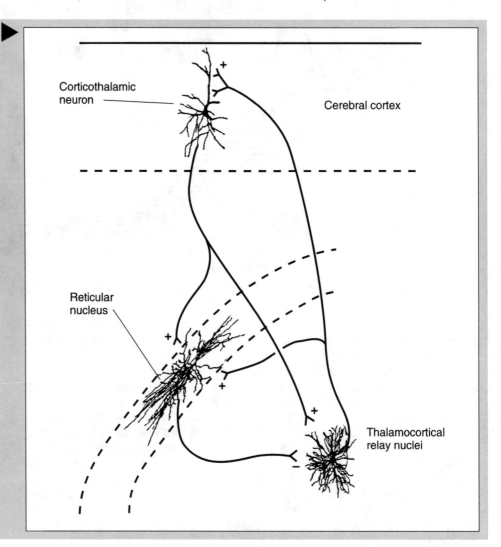

Corticothalamic neuron

Cerebral cortex

Reticular nucleus

Thalamocortical relay nuclei

Although the mechanisms by which cortical activity shifts from the high-frequency activity of wakefulness to the slow-wave activity of NREM sleep are not fully understood, it is known that delta-wave oscillations depend on neural mechanisms in the thalamus. Thalamocortical neurons have distinct voltage-gated conductances that enable them to oscillate between hyperpolarized and depolarized states (Figure 14-8). When a thalamocortical neuron is hyperpolarized, specific ion channels are activated that allow an inward, depolarizing flow of cations. This is called the hyperpolarization current (I_h) because it occurs when thalamocortical neurons are hyperpolarized. The depolarization produced by I_h activates a set of voltage-regulated calcium (Ca^{2+}) channels that permit a tremendous influx of Ca^{2+} ions into the neuron. This results in a prolonged Ca^{2+}-mediated low-threshold spike (LTS) that depolarizes the membrane potential sufficiently to produce a burst of sodium (Na^+)-driven action potentials. Subsequently, the Na^+ spikes inactivate the Ca^{2+} channels to prevent Ca^{2+} influx and allow the membrane potential to return to its original polarized state.

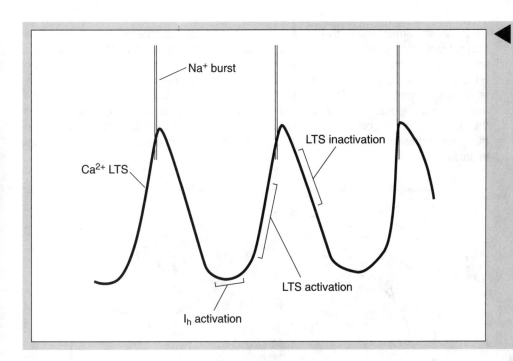

FIGURE 14-8
Delta Frequency Thalamocortical Rhythms. This trace shows rhythmic changes in the membrane potentials of a thalamocortical relay neuron. Following activation of the hyperpolarization current (I_h), the low-threshold spike (LTS) is mediated by a tremendous influx of calcium (Ca^{2+}). The Ca^{2+}-mediated LTS is of much longer duration than the sodium (Na^+)-mediated burst of action potentials. The LTS oscillates at a frequency of 1–4 Hz because of the interplay of voltage-regulated membrane currents (I_h and Ca^{2+}) and interactions with the inhibitory neurons of the reticular nucleus. See text for further details.

When thalamocortical neurons discharge, they also excite the inhibitory neurons of the reticular nucleus. Activation of this recurrent inhibitory circuit promotes oscillations by hyperpolarizing the membrane potential of the thalamocortical neurons at the same time that the Ca^{2+} spikes are inactivated. When the reticular neurons subsequently become inactive, as a result of loss of excitatory input from the thalamocortical neurons, the removal of inhibition allows the thalamocortical neurons to repeat their cycle of depolarization and LTS discharges. Hence, the intrinsic membrane properties of thalamocortical neurons, along with their reciprocal interactions with the reticular nucleus, produce oscillatory discharges in the delta frequency range (0.5–4 Hz). Benzodiazepines, which are widely prescribed to treat insomnia, induce sleep because they are GABAergic agonists that promote the oscillatory interactions between the reticular nucleus and the thalamocortical neurons. These oscillations are transmitted to the cerebral cortex via the thalamocortical pathways.

Pacemaker neurons in the reticular nucleus control thalamocortical oscillations.

Thalamocortical interconnections and the intrinsic membrane properties of these neurons also mediate oscillations in other frequency ranges during NREM sleep. Sleep spindles, for example, originate in the reticular nucleus and are transmitted to the cerebral cortex via the thalamocortical pathways. In addition, extremely slow oscillations (< 1 Hz) originating in the cerebral cortex become superimposed on the rhythmic activity originating in the thalamus to yield a variety of complex waveforms in both structures. Hence, the periodic nature of EEG activity during NREM sleep is a dynamic process that reflects the complex interplay between thalamus and cortex. The exact mechanisms by which these frequencies are initiated and modulated are the subject of current research.

ASCENDING BRAINSTEM PATHWAYS AND CORTICAL DESYNCHRONIZATION

Cortical desynchronization during REM sleep is mediated by increased activity in a set of ascending pathways that originate in the brainstem near the pons–midbrain junction. The first suggestion that such pathways might desynchronize cortical activity was provided by the work of Moruzzi and Magoun in 1949. They showed that electrical stimulation of the reticular formation in anesthetized cats causes the EEG to shift from slow-wave activity to a state of high-frequency desynchronized activity. Subsequently, they demonstrated that destruction of the ascending pathways from the rostral reticular formation produces behavioral stupor accompanied by low-frequency EEG waves in the delta range. These results led Moruzzi and Magoun to propose that an ascending reticular-activating system is responsible for stimulating the forebrain during periods of wakefulness.

Since the time of Moruzzi and Magoun, a large body of evidence indicates that cortical desynchronization during REM sleep is initiated and maintained by activity in a select group of pontine nuclei that project rostrally to the thalamus and other parts of the forebrain (Figure 14-9). Among these are the pedunculopontine tegmental (PPT) nucleus and the laterodorsal tegmental (LDT) nucleus, both of which are cholinergic and project to the thalamus and the nucleus basalis. The PPT and LDT also send cholinergic projections to the medial part of the pontine reticular formation (mPRF). The mPRF also projects to the thalamus and uses excitatory amino acid neurotransmitters to depolarize thalamocortical neurons.

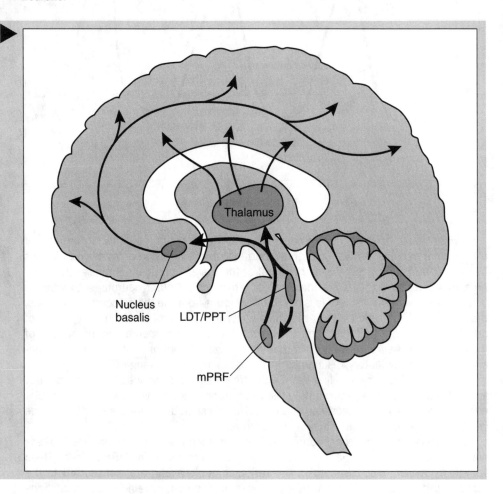

FIGURE 14-9 ▶
Brainstem Regulation of REM Sleep.
Sagittal view of the brain showing the location of the cholinergic laterodorsal tegmental (LDT) and pedunculopontine tegmental (PPT) nuclei, both of which project to the medial pontine reticular formation (mPRF). Together the LDT/PPT and mPRF activate the thalamus and the nucleus basalis in the forebrain. The thalamus and nucleus basalis send widespread excitatory projections to the cerebral cortex.

The LDT and PPT nuclei contain "REM-on" neurons; the mPRF contains "effector" neurons.

Involvement of the cholinergic LDT and PPT nuclei in REM sleep is supported by many experimental findings in animals. First, lesions of the LDT and PPT cause a marked reduction in REM sleep. Second, REM sleep is immediately preceded by an increase in neuronal activity in both of these brainstem nuclei. Third, direct application of cholinergic agonists into the mPRF produces cortical desynchronization and other signs of REM-like sleep (see Figure 14-4). These facts are consistent with evidence showing that mPRF neurons are excited by acetylcholine and discharge more frequently during REM sleep. Hence, the shift from EEG synchronization to desynchronization during REM sleep is mediated by prolonged thalamic depolarization triggered by the activation of ascending projections from the mPRF. Direct cholinergic projections from the LDT and PPT nuclei to the thalamus may also contribute to EEG desynchronization, but their primary role is to initiate REM sleep by activating the ascending projections from the mPRF. Consistent with this mechanism, neurons in the LDT/PPT nuclei serve as "REM-on" neurons, while those in the mPRF are considered "effector" neurons for REM sleep.

The periodic nature of REM sleep appears to be controlled by brainstem nuclei that inhibit the REM-on neurons of the PPT and LDT nuclei. Physiology experiments have shown that noradrenergic neurons in the locus ceruleus and serotonergic neurons in the

The locus ceruleus and the dorsal raphe nucleus contain "REM-off" neurons.

raphe nuclei are virtually silent during REM sleep but become increasingly active just before the end of each REM sleep episode. Furthermore, direct infusion of serotonin inhibits neuronal activity in the LDT/PPT nuclei. These findings suggest that serotonergic and noradrenergic neurons in the brainstem may act as "REM-off " neurons. According to many neurophysiologists, the pattern of periodic changes in the activity of REM-on and REM-off neurons suggests that reciprocal connections between these groups of neurons may control the duration of NREM and REM sleep periods (Figure 14-10).

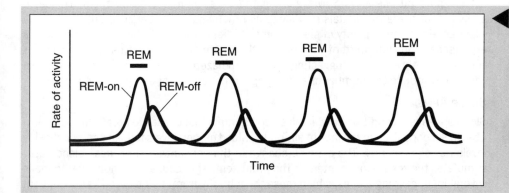

◀ **FIGURE 14-10**
Relative Activity of REM-on and REM-off Neurons. *The REM-on cholinergic neurons of the laterodorsal tegmental (LDT) and pedunculopontine tegmental (PPT) nuclei show periodic changes in activity that correspond to REM sleep. The end of the REM sleep period coincides with increasing activity of REM-off noradrenergic neurons in the locus ceruleus and REM-off serotonergic neurons in the dorsal raphe nucleus.*

Sleep Disorders

More than 50 specific types of sleep disorders have been identified, and each one can be classified into one of the following categories: (1) insomnias, (2) hypersomnias, (3) parasomnias, and (4) rhythm disruptions. The insomnias involve problems with initiating and maintaining sleep, whereas hypersomnias are characterized by excessive sleep or drowsiness. The parasomnias encompass a broad set of undesirable sleep-related behaviors such as sleepwalking and nocturnal enuresis (bed-wetting). Rhythm disruptions involve changes in circadian rhythm such as those caused by changing time zones (i.e., jet lag). Some of the more common sleep disorders are described in the following sections.

INSOMNIA

Insomnia, or an inability to obtain adequate sleep, is often a symptom of other problems. Transient insomnia lasts no more than a couple of weeks and is usually caused by the emotional upheaval associated with a specific event. Persistent insomnia may have many underlying causes including chronic pain, drug abuse, gastroesophageal reflux, respiratory difficulty, or psychiatric illness.

When a patient complains of insomnia, the physician must determine whether sleep disruption is symptomatic of an illness or problem that can be treated without prescribing sleeping pills. It has been estimated that emotional disturbances may account for almost two-third of the insomnias. Chronic anxiety and depression, for example, are commonly associated with insomnia and can exacerbate the inability to obtain sleep, which may potentiate the underlying psychopathology. Polysomnograms from depressed patients indicate that they obtain less slow-wave sleep and enter REM sleep much earlier than normal individuals. Since the primary complaint of many depressed patients is insomnia, many of these patients are not properly diagnosed and are prescribed sleeping pills instead of antidepressants.

Many insomniacs are awakened by events which they cannot identify. The most common of these are periodic limb movements that may occur during NREM sleep. Such leg movements usually consist of a triple flexion involving the ankle, knee, and hip. These movements last 2–3 seconds and may occur periodically at 20–40-second intervals for several minutes. In contrast to movement disorders, which are inhibited by sleep (e.g. extrapyramidal tremors, chorea), these periodic limb movements often begin while the person is awake and can occur during subsequent periods of sleep. Such leg movements are often associated with EEG arousal and cause the patient to be awakened. Since the patient is unaware of these movements while sleeping, their sleep behavior must be evaluated by polysomnography. Insomnia produced by periodic leg movements is usually treated with clonazepam, a benzodiazepine with sedative effects.

Unfortunately, many patients complaining of chronic insomnia show no irregularities in their polysomnograms. Compared to the amount of delta activity recorded in their EEG, most insomniacs underestimate the amount of sleep that they obtain. In fact, in studies in which insomniac patients were awakened from a deep sleep (as indicated by the presence of delta waves in the EEG), many of these patients claimed that they were not sleeping but were lying awake when the experimenter aroused them. Hence, it appears that these individuals may sleep as much as normal persons, but they do not experience the same quality of sleep. Some studies, however, indicate that insomniacs experience more intermittent awakenings than normal persons. This latter finding is consistent with evidence suggesting that benzodiazepines are effective hypnotics because they reduce the number of awakenings in the course of a night's sleep.

SLEEP APNEA

Sleep apnea is a condition in which a sleeping individual ceases to breath for periods of 15–30 seconds. Due to the lack of air intake, blood oxygen levels fall, and carbon dioxide levels rise significantly. The extreme change in the concentration of these blood gases stimulates the respiratory centers in the brainstem. This causes the individual to make several loud, gasping snores, which rouse them briefly from their sleep. The subsequent increase in air intake reinstates the blood gases to normal levels and allows the person to return to sleep until the cycle is repeated. Because of the constant shifting between periods of sleep and arousal, the individual is unrefreshed upon awakening and feels a pervasive sleepiness throughout the day.

Sleep apnea is usually associated with loud, periodic snoring. A series of 3–6 loud snores or gasps followed by a silent period of 20–50 seconds is repeated throughout the night. This pattern characterizes the obstructive sleep apnea (OSA) syndrome in which the airway collapses and airflow ceases despite persistent respiratory effort. Abnormalities in the upper airway such as narrow nasal passages, a deviated nasal septum, enlarged adenoids or tonsils, an enlarged tongue, or temporomandibular joint problems may cause OSA. This syndrome occurs more frequently among men than women, and occurs most commonly among obese adults between 40 and 60 years of age. Approximately two-thirds of the patients diagnosed with OSA are obese, and their symptoms are exacerbated by factors such as a gain in weight, alcohol consumption, or sleep deprivation.

Sleep apnea is associated with an increased risk of sudden death during sleep. Sleep apnea may occur in infants or young children and has been proposed as a factor in sudden infant death syndrome (SIDS). There is a high incidence of sleep apnea among the elderly, perhaps as high as 30% among persons greater than 65 years of age. Sleep apnea is also associated with adults who have chronic obstructive pulmonary disease, systemic hypertension, and a variety of cardiac arrhythmias while sleeping.

A polysomnogram is necessary to diagnose sleep apnea and to determine whether it is obstructive or central in origin. Obstructive apnea is characterized by respiratory effort in the absence of air flow because the airway is blocked. Central apnea is due to a lack of respiratory effort, presumably because the brainstem respiratory centers are inhibited; the airway remains open, but there is no air flow because the diaphragm does not contract. The distinction between central and obstructive apnea can be determined by monitoring respiratory movements. Some individuals have a mixed apnea involving a central component combined with obstruction of the airway.

NARCOLEPSY

Narcolepsy is a neurologic disorder characterized by increasing drowsiness and daytime sleep attacks that occur at inappropriate moments. These attacks last 5–30 minutes and may strike without warning while the patient is eating, speaking, or even driving. Thus, narcolepsy poses a serious health risk because these patients are prone to accidental injury while operating a car or other types of machinery.

Narcolepsy usually begins between 15 and 30 years of age, and excessive sleepiness is almost always the first sign of this disorder. Patients with narcolepsy need to sleep more frequently than normal individuals, and the narcoleptic sleep attack is essentially a minisleep that intrudes into the waking state. In addition to sleep attacks, narcoleptic patients also exhibit cataplexy, but this symptom may not appear for several months or years. Cataplexy is precipitated by strong emotional behaviors, such as laughing, and consists of an abrupt loss of muscle tone without any change in consciousness. During a typical cataplexic episode, the patient's head falls forward, their arms drop, and their knees buckle. In more severe cases, the patient collapses because all muscles except the muscles of respiration are completely paralyzed.

Many of the behavioral symptoms of narcolepsy are similar to those of REM sleep. Thus, narcoleptic patients may exhibit sleep paralysis, a global paralysis of voluntary muscles during the initial entry into sleep or on awakening from sleep. During these periods, narcoleptic patients also report hypnagogic hallucinations, which contain vivid auditory and visual sensations. Collectively, the presence of cataplexy, sleep paralysis, and sensory hallucinations appear to resemble the muscle atonia and dream state that normal individuals experience during REM sleep. The possibility that narcolepsy might represent the intrusion of REM sleep into the waking state is strongly suggested by polysomnographic recordings showing that narcoleptic patients enter the REM sleep state almost directly from the waking state. For diagnostic purposes, the presence of a sleep-onset REM period is considered a defining symptom of narcolepsy.

Narcolepsy represents the intrusion of REM sleep into the waking state.

The neural mechanisms underlying narcolepsy are unknown. Although damage to the upper brainstem or lower hypothalamus has sometimes produced narcoleptic symptoms, the neuropathologic findings in narcoleptic patients have been inconsistent. Narcolepsy has a genetic basis that is associated with inheritance of a class II antigen of the major histocompatibility complex on chromosome 6. The major histocompatibility complex is a cluster of genes that encode the molecules in the immune system responsible for recognizing antigens. Several pairs of monozygotic twins have been identified that are discordant for this disease, however, and this suggests that environmental factors should not be dismissed.

Despite a lack of knowledge concerning the neural basis of narcolepsy, it is well established that cataplexy can be controlled by medications that enhance synaptic transmission of the putative REM-off neurons. Tricyclic antidepressants, which block the reuptake of norepinephrine and serotonin, prevent cataplexy but are ineffective in the treatment of sleep attacks. Instead, excessive sleepiness is treated by psychomotor stimulants (e.g., methylphenidate, amphetamine) that elevate the level of alertness by increasing the synaptic release of catecholamines. Prolonged use of stimulants has serious side effects, however, and their intake can be minimized by scheduling daytime naps at appropriate times.

COMA AND BRAIN DEATH

The loss of consciousness that accompanies sleep is a normal and self-regulating process. In instances such as fainting, a loss of consciousness may represent a temporary reduction in cerebral blood flow, which is easily treated. In almost all other cases, however, loss of consciousness is a serious condition that can be produced by brain damage, drug overdose, hypothermia, or certain types of toxic-metabolic disorders. The comatose patient represents the ultimate challenge to the capabilities of the attending neurologist.

Neural Basis of Consciousness

Patients who are awake and aware of their surroundings are said to be conscious. The state of being conscious implies that a person has the capacity to perceive, learn, and engage in purposeful behavior. Because the conscious state is inherently introspective and is not easily accessible to scientific study, the biologic basis of consciousness is uncertain. Nonetheless, extensive study of patients with brain damage indicates that human consciousness depends on interactions between distinct systems in the brain (Figure 14-11). Cognitive functions, such as perception, memory, language, and the capacity to plan and execute motor behaviors, are mediated by a system that includes the cerebral cortex, basal ganglia, and the sensory specific nuclei of the thalamus. A second system, responsible for regulating attention, motivation, and emotional behavior, resides in limbic structures, such as the hypothalamus, the basal forebrain, the hippocampus, the amygdala, the cingulum, and the septal nuclei. Activation and arousal of the first two systems depend on a third neural system comprised of ascending projections from the reticular formation, the intralaminar nuclei of the thalamus, and the posterior hypothalamus.

FIGURE 14-11 ▶

Neural Basis of Consciousness. *Consciousness is an emergent property that depends on complex interactions between distinct systems within the brain. High-level cognitive functions (e.g., perception, awareness) are derived from processes in the telencephalon and the sensory-specific pathways of the thalamus. Affect, mood, attention, and motivation depend on structures in the limbic system. Rostral projections from the brainstem and the nonspecific nuclei of the thalamus activate the telencephalic and limbic structures.*

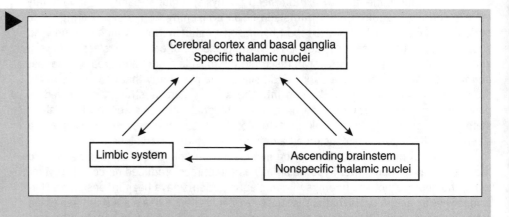

The functional division of consciousness into distinct systems suggests that consciousness has both qualitative and quantitative dimensions. Although certain structures within these systems may have specific neurologic functions, these systems are widely distributed throughout the neuraxis, and the functional boundaries between them are imprecise. Thus, relatively focal damage can affect more than one of these systems. Regardless of whether consciousness is affected by global or focal abnormalities, its character may change either partially or completely. The following sections focus on the changes that can be produced by abnormalities in the ascending projections from the brainstem, the nonspecific nuclei of the thalamus, and related structures.

Comatose States and Other Global Impairments in Consciousness

An isoelectric or flat EEG trace usually indicates brain death.

The term "comatose" is used to describe a state resembling deep sleep from which a patient cannot be aroused by internal or external stimuli. Comatose patients have no conscious awareness of themselves or their environment. The EEG shows abnormal patterns and, if coma deepens, the electrical activity of the EEG gradually decreases and may disappear. With the exception of patients who are deeply anesthetized or are suffering from severe hypothermia, the loss of EEG activity indicates brain death.

A vegetative state is a condition in which the patient has not regained conscious awareness following a severe brain injury, but the EEG contains rhythmic activity resembling sleep-wake cycles. Some signs of spontaneous arousal may appear, but the patient remains unconscious. Patients in a vegetative state present abnormal somatic signs and, if structural damage is present, may show defects in brain scans based on computerized tomography (CT) or magnetic resonance imaging (MRI). If the vegetative state persists over a long duration, the patient is said to have suffered "cognitive death" because only the neural mechanisms subserving certain autonomic functions remain intact.

The term "stupor" is used to describe a state in which a patient must receive constant noxious stimulation, such as shouting or shaking, to remain awake. Stupor caused by structural damage to the brain is associated with many abnormal clinical signs, whereas stupor caused by a chemical poisoning resembles a state of deep sleep. In either case, the EEG pattern is always abnormal in patients with stupor, and it can be distinguished from an EEG pattern representing normal sleep.

Diagnosis of the Comatose State

Many cases of coma are quickly diagnosed after obtaining an accurate history and performing a careful neurologic examination. In other instances, CT and MRI brain scans are necessary to determine the location of brain damage, and an EEG is indispensable for discerning coma from epilepsy or other conditions related to infectious or metabolic disorders. Coma can sometimes be difficult to distinguish from severe hysteria, depression, or drug overdose and may require the physician to exclude drug use or other diseases as possible causes. On rare occasions, coma might be considered erroneously in cases in which the patient is conscious but is unable to move or communicate because of severe paralysis. This "locked-in state" may result from severe postinfectious polyneuritis or bilateral damage to the descending motor pathways. Lesions that spare consciousness almost always spare the oculomotor pathways originating from the midbrain. Thus, locked-in patients can usually communicate by blinking or by making selected eye movements.

Coma can be distinguished from deep sleep on the basis of several criteria (Table 14-2). While a person in deep sleep can be aroused by vigorous and sustained external stimulation, this is not the case with a comatose individual. A comatose person does not exhibit REM activity, circadian rhythms, or any of the periodic changes that characterize normal sleep. Finally, normal sleep is an active process associated with wide fluctuations in the metabolic activity of the brain. In the comatose state, however, cerebral metabolism falls below the levels observed during deep slow-wave sleep.

> Patients who are conscious, but completely paralyzed, are in a "locked-in state."

◀ **TABLE 14-2**
Differences between Coma and Sleep

	Coma	*Sleep*
Behavior	Not arousable	Arousable to wakefulness
Movements	Motionless except for reflex responses	Spontaneous turnings, eye movements
EEG activity	REM activity absent	Periodic REM and NREM activity
Evoked potentials	Abnormal BAEPs after brainstem damage	Normal BAEPs and SEPs
Cortical metabolism	Declines 50%–60% below normal	Fluctuates with REM and NREM activity

Note. EEG = electroencephalogram; REM = rapid eye movement; BAEPs = brainstem auditory-evoked potentials; SEPs = somatosensory-evoked potentials.

The measurement of ERPs in the somatosensory and auditory systems has proven useful in evaluating comatose patients. Somatosensory-evoked potentials (SEPs) are induced by electrically stimulating the median or peroneal nerves. Recordings from electrodes placed over the spinal column, the brainstem, and the scalp have revealed the presence of distinct waves or potentials that correspond to the sequential activation of the spinal cord, the thalamus, and the cerebral cortex. Application of auditory stimuli produce a similar series of waves known as brainstem auditory-evoked potentials (BAEPs) which correspond to sequential transmission of activity from the auditory nerve (wave I) to the cochlear nuclei (wave II), the superior olives (wave III), the lateral lemnisci (wave IV), and finally to the inferior colliculi (wave V). The latency and size of the SEPs and BAEPs are often helpful for determining the brain regions that are functionally intact and those that are damaged. Because SEPs and BAEPs are resistent to anesthetics, they retain relatively normal waveforms even at drug doses that cause an isoelectric or flat EEG. Changes in the latency of SEPs, in particular, have value in predicting the outcome of coma. Comatose patients that lose cortical SEPs have never survived; bilateral disappearance of the SEPs usually precedes brain death by as much as 24 hours. By comparison, individuals who have normal bilateral SEPs shortly after injury or asphyxia have a 90% chance of regaining consciousness.

> SEPs and BAEPs are used to evaluate comatose patients.

Principal Causes of Coma

The causes of coma can be divided into two major categories: structural lesions and toxic-metabolic disorders (Table 14-3).

TABLE 14-3 ▶

Major Causes of Coma

Type of Coma	Neural Structures Affected	Causes and Mechanisms
Brain lesions, compression, or supratentorial damage	Bilateral cerebral hemispheres and bilateral posterior thalamus	Large infarcts, hemorrhages, tumors, neoplasms, and diencephalic herniation through tentorial notch
Infratentorial damage	Mesencephalic-pontine junction	Infarcts, hemorrhages, neoplasms, trauma, subdural hematoma, and uncal herniation
Toxic or metabolic disorders	Global and diffuse	Drugs, poisons, anoxia–ischemia, hypoglycemia, hepatic or renal failure, and encephalitis

STRUCTURAL LESIONS ASSOCIATED WITH COMA

Coma may result from destruction or compression of critical areas in the brainstem-diencephalic arousal system by trauma, hemorrhage, or neoplasms. In addition, the brainstem-diencephalic system can also be affected indirectly by the gradual enlargement of an intracranial mass located some distance away. Both types of structural lesions are classified with respect to the tentorium, the dural sheet located between the occipital lobe and the cerebellum.

Supratentorial Lesions. Coma is not frequently produced by cortical lesions unless large parts of the cortex are damaged bilaterally. In patients with large cortical wounds, the incidence of coma is nearly 30% when the damage involves only the left hemisphere, but is only 10% when the damage is restricted to the right hemisphere. These differential findings suggest that the integrity of the language processing areas is important for maintaining global consciousness. Coma is more likely to be induced by cortical hemorrhage because it is accompanied by massive cerebral swelling. By comparison, cortical lesions caused by embolic strokes may affect sensory, motor, or language functions but seldom result in coma.

Supratentorial lesions often affect consciousness by compressing the brain through the tentorial notch. Progressive enlargement of a tumor or other intracranial mass causes an increase in downward pressure on the brainstem, which results in herniation of the medial temporal lobe (uncal herniation) and protrusion of the medulla through the foramen magnum. Uncal herniation invariably affects the oculomotor nerve, and this loss of parasympathetic influence produces ipsilateral mydriasis (pupillary dilation). If the supratentorial lesion is unilateral, differential compression of the descending corticospinal tracts may cause asymmetrical limb movements and deep tendon reflexes. Compression of the caudal brainstem and its intrinsic nuclei causes abnormal respiratory patterns including Cheyne-Stokes breathing (rhythmic waxing and waning in the depth of respiration), hyperventilation, and apnea.

Infratentorial Lesions. Substantial data support the concept of a distributed nonspecific arousal system that originates from the central paramedian region of the lower thalamus, mesencephalon, and rostral pons. In most cases where coma is produced by an infratentorial lesion, noninvasive imaging techniques indicate widespread damage to the central tegmental area of the midbrain, and this damage usually extends into the thalamus or pons or, in some instances, into both regions. Damage restricted to only one segment of the neuraxis (i.e., the pons or the midbrain) rarely causes profound coma. Moreover,

Supratentorial lesions may produce coma by compressing the brainstem.

Infratentorial lesions resulting in coma usually cause extensive damage to the pontine and mesencephalic tegmentum.

infratentorial lesions that produce coma frequently spare the ascending sensory pathways and their relay nuclei in the brainstem. Thus, coma does not result from the loss of ascending sensory influences on the diencephalon.

Vascular lesions resulting in coma are more likely to involve both the thalamus and mesencephalon together. Such lesions are especially likely following occlusion of the perforating arteries arising from the basilar artery, the posterior cerebral arteries, or the posterior communicating arteries. Damage to the posterior thalamus alone may cause severe coma if the lesions are bilateral and involve the paramedian thalamus and related areas such as the posterior intralaminar complex, the central median nuclei, and the medial dorsal nuclei.

Patients who survive extensive damage to the rostral brainstem may persist in a comatose state for many months or years. Such patients eventually regain cyclic patterns of arousal and nonarousal in their EEG activity, but this pattern does not follow the normal sequence seen during sleep. Some patients who sustain severe damage to the pontine-mesencephalic junction may exhibit desynchronized EEG activity in the alpha range and are said to be in "alpha coma." In these patients, however, attempts to link particular EEG patterns to the integrity of specific neural structures have been disappointing. Although some patients may show EEG synchronization, which suggests the activation of neural structures involved in sleep, most neurologists regard coma as a pathologic process that disrupts the neural mechanisms controlling the sleep-wake cycle.

Virtually no individual has survived extensive damage to the caudal brainstem. The medulla and lower pons regulate respiration and cardiovascular functions, and damage to this region usually causes immediate death due to respiratory or circulatory failure. In rare cases where the patient did not die immediately because they were maintained on a ventilator, they are often paralyzed due to loss of the descending pyramidal tracts. Such patients do not descend into a comatose state; they remain conscious because of damage to areas in the caudal brainstem which must become active to induce sleep. Until death ensues, these patients are in a "locked-in state" and can communicate only by making a series of coded eye movements.

TOXIC-METABOLIC DISORDERS

Coma can be produced by many conditions that cause global neural depression. Metabolic coma usually has a gradual onset and can be caused by brain anoxia, ischemia, hypoglycemia, or exposure to a variety of drugs and poisons. The most common symptoms that precede metabolic coma include tremor, loss of postural control, and myoclonic limb movements (nonrhythmic jerks). Ocular movements are rarely affected unless the coma is severe.

RESOLUTION OF CLINICAL CASE

A polysomnogram revealed that T. R.'s excessive sleepiness was caused by OSA. Despite making respiratory movements, T. R. periodically ceased breathing during sleep because his airway became obstructed, possibly due to his enlarged adenoids and tonsils. Although surgical removal of the adenoids and tonsils might cure his problem, a more conservative approach would be to prescribe a weight-loss program in combination with nasal continuous positive airway pressure. Among obese patients who have moderate cases of OSA, weight loss alone is often successful. In more severe cases, an increase in nasal air pressure is the most effective treatment for managing OSA. The patient wears a tight-fitting mask that delivers pressurized air to keep the airway expanded between breaths.

REVIEW QUESTIONS

Directions: For each of the following questions, choose the **one best** answer.

1. Which of the following brain regions is responsible for initiating REM sleep?
    (A) Pedunculopontine and laterodorsal tegmental nuclei
    (B) Medial pontine reticular formation
    (C) Suprachiasmatic nucleus
    (D) Dorsal raphe nuclei
    (E) Locus ceruleus

2. Damage to which of the following brain regions is most likely to produce severe coma?
    (A) Medulla
    (B) Basal ganglia
    (C) Anterior thalamus
    (D) Right cerebral hemisphere
    (E) Pontine-mesencephalic junction

3. Which of the following conditions would most likely cause coma?
    (A) Cerebral infarction
    (B) Uncal herniation after a subdural hematoma
    (C) Occlusion of the medial striate artery
    (D) Contusion of the cerebellum
    (E) Transient ischemic attack

4. Which of the following symptoms is a general characteristic of normal sleep?
    (A) Apnea
    (B) Cataplexy
    (C) Abnormal latencies of somatic-evoked potentials (SEPs)
    (D) Fluctuations in cerebral metabolism
    (E) Diffuse slowing of electroencephalogram (EEG) activity below 8 Hz for several hours

5. A patient who periodically falls asleep during the day, often in response to emotional stimuli, is likely to have which of the following conditions?
    (A) Insomnia
    (B) Narcolepsy
    (C) Cognitive death
    (D) Obstructive sleep apnea (OSA)
    (E) Circadian rhythm disorder

ANSWERS AND EXPLANATIONS

1. The answer is A. The pedunculopontine and laterodorsal tegmental nuclei contain REM-on neurons that initiate REM sleep. These REM-on neurons activate effector neurons in the medial pontine reticular formation, which, in turn, depolarize the thalamus to produce cortical desynchronization during REM sleep. The locus ceruleus and dorsal raphe nuclei contain REM-off neurons that suppress the REM-on neurons toward the end of the REM sleep period. The suprachiasmatic nucleus is not involved in REM sleep.

2. The answer is E. One of the leading causes of coma is extensive damage to the brainstem tegmentum at the pontine-mesencephalic junction. Damage to the medulla usually causes immediate death because of cardiac or respiratory failure. Damage restricted to the cerebral cortex or to the posterior thalamus may result in coma if the damage occurs bilaterally. Extensive damage to the right cerebral hemisphere alone results in coma in less than 10% of the cases. The basal ganglia and the anterior thalamus have not been implicated in coma.

3. The answer is B. Uncal herniation compresses the rostral brainstem and, thus, damages the ascending pathways that regulate consciousness. Except in cases of extensive bilateral cortical damage, cerebral infarction may produce paralysis, aphasia, or a sensory deficit but not a loss of consciousness. The medial striate artery supplies the basal ganglia, a structure that has not been implicated in coma. A cerebellar contusion is unlikely to cause coma unless the cerebellum swells or hemorrhages, thereby compressing the underlying brainstem. Coma may result from prolonged ischemia or anoxia but is unlikely to develop from a transient episode of ischemia.

4. The answer is D. Cerebral blood flow and glucose consumption vary with the periodic changes in EEG activity that accompany REM and NREM sleep. Apnea is associated with abnormal sleep and can cause insomnia. Cataplexy is a defining symptom of narcolepsy. Abnormal latencies in the SEPs and diffuse slowing of EEG activity below 8 Hz are associated with coma.

5. The answer is B. The main symptom of narcolepsy is the prevalence of sleep attacks, many of which are prompted by emotional stimuli. Insomnia is characterized by an inability to sleep. Although OSA may increase sleepiness during the day, it does not provoke sudden sleep attacks. Cognitive death is a term used to describe the loss of cognitive functions that occurs when a patient is in a chronic vegetative state. Circadian rhythm disorders are characterized by changes in the onset and duration of sleep with respect to the time of day, not by periodic sleep attacks.

ADDITIONAL READING

Kales A, Kales JD: *Evaluation and Treatment of Insomnia.* New York, NY: Oxford University Press, 1984.

Lydic R, Biebuyck JF (eds): *Clinical Physiology of Sleep.* Bethesda, MD: American Physiological Society, 1988.

Plum F: Coma and related global disturbances of the human conscious state. In *Cerebral Cortex: Normal and Altered States of Function*, vol 9. Edited by Jones EG, Peters A. New York, NY: Plenum Press, 1991, pp 359–425.

Steriade M, McCarley RW: *Brainstem Control of Wakefulness and Sleep.* New York, NY: Plenum Press, 1990.

Steriade M, McCormick DA, Sejnowski TJ: Thalamocortical oscillations in the sleeping and aroused brain. *Science* 262:679–685, 1993.

INDEX

NOTE: An "f" after a page number denotes a figure; a "t" after a page number denotes a table.